I0510690

Gastroenterology: Clinical Perspectives

Gastroenterology: Clinical Perspectives

Edited by Cyrus Holt

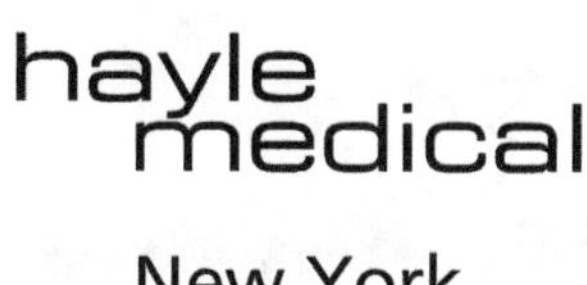

New York

Hayle Medical,
750 Third Avenue, 9th Floor,
New York, NY 10017, USA

Visit us on the World Wide Web at:
www.haylemedical.com

ISBN: 978-1-63241-890-6

Cataloging-in-Publication Data

Gastroenterology : clinical perspectives / edited by Cyrus Holt.
p. cm.
Includes bibliographical references and index.
ISBN 978-1-63241-890-6
1. Gastroenterology. 2. Digestive organs--Diseases. 3. Digestive organs--Diseases--Treatment. I. Holt, Cyrus.
RC801 .G37 2020
616.33--dc23

Table of Contents

Preface

Gastroenterology is a specialized field of medicine, which focuses on the diseases of the gastrointestinal (GI) tract or the digestive system. The GI tract is responsible for the digestion of food, absorption of nutrients and removal of wastes from the body. The diseases treated under the scope of gastroenterology are ulcers, acid reflux, hepatitis C, jaundice, pancreatitis, colon cancer, hemorrhoids, etc. The diagnosis of most of these conditions can be done non-surgically with the help of colonoscopies, endoscopic ultrasounds, sigmoidoscopies, liver biopsies, double balloon enteroscopies, endoscopic retrograde cholangiopancreatography, etc. Certain endoscopic procedures can also be used for the removal of polyps, esophageal and intestinal dilation, and for stemming blood loss, among others. The aim of this book is to present researches that have transformed the discipline of gastroenterology and aided its advancement. It traces the progress of this field and highlights some of its key aspects. It is an essential guide for both academicians and those who wish to pursue this discipline further.

Significant researches are present in this book. Intensive efforts have been employed by authors to make this book an outstanding discourse. This book contains the enlightening chapters which have been written on the basis of significant researches done by the experts.

Finally, I would also like to thank all the members involved in this book for being a team and meeting all the deadlines for the submission of their respective works. I would also like to thank my friends and family for being supportive in my efforts.

Editor

1

Antichronic Gastric Ulcer Effect of Zinc-Baicalin Complex on the Acetic Acid-Induced Chronic Gastric Ulcer Rat Model

Hui Yang,[1] **Yi Lu**,[2] **Xiao-Feng Zeng**,[3] **Ling Li**,[1] **Rong-Ping Zhang**,[1] **Zhong-Kun Ren**,[2] **and Xu Liu**[1]

[1]*Biomedical Engineering Center, Kunming Medical University, Kunming 650500, China*
[2]*Neurosurgery, The 1st Affiliated Hospital of Kunming Medical University, Kunming 650032, China*
[3]*School of Forensic Medicine, Kunming Medical University, Kunming 650500, China*

Correspondence should be addressed to Zhong-Kun Ren; renzhongkunbio@163.com and Xu Liu; liuxu1956@163.com

Academic Editor: Haruhiko Sugimura

Background. Baicalin (BA) has been shown to have anti-inflammatory and antioxidant activity. Zinc is a nutrient element. *Objective.* This study is aimed at investigating the antichronic gastric ulcer activity of Zn-Baicalin complex (BA-Zn) and its related mechanisms in an acetic acid-induced gastric ulcer rat model. *Results.* The severely ulcerated gastric mucosa of model rats had lower GSH-Px (52.21 ± 7.13) and SOD (7.03 ± 0.10) activity, and higher MDA (2.39 ± 0.03) content compared to sham rats. BA-Zn reduced the gastric ulcer index in a dose-dependent manner, significantly increased SOD activity and GSH-Px level, and reduced the MDA content and IL-8 and TNF-α levels in the gastric mucosa. BA-Zn (6.5 and 13 mg/kg) exerted a greater antiulcerogenic effect than both BA and zinc-gluconate, leading to a reduced ulcer index (18.43 ± 1.11, 15.00 ± 1.44), decreased MDA content (1.33 ± 0.07, 0.63 ± 0.01), and increased SOD activity (17.62 ± 0.11, 20.12 ± 0.32) and GSH-Px levels (102.12 ± 9.11, 120.25 ± 9.07). In addition, our results from Western blot suggested that BA-Zn (6.5 and 13 mg/kg) has a greater antiulcerogenic effect than both BA and zinc-gluconate. *Conclusion.* The BA-Zn complex possesses greater antichronic gastric ulcer properties compared to BA and zinc-gluconate due to its ability of oxidation resistance and anti-inflammatory effects.

1. Introduction

Peptic ulcers create a serious disease state in humans, are common worldwide, and have an increasing incidence rate. Gastric ulceration often increases the level of gastric acid secretion, can damage the gastric mucosal barrier, and penetrates the mucus layer [1, 2]. An ulcer model induced by acetic acid in rats resembles human chronic ulcers in both pathological features and healing process. Therefore, this model is more promising and useful for researchers to explore gastric ulcer. The pathogenesis of gastric ulcers is complex due to multifactorial and complex interaction between protective and destructive factors. Nonsteroidal anti-inflammatory drugs (NSAIDs) are the most commonly recommended medication and are comprehensively used to decrease clinical cases of pain and inflammation [3]. However, these drugs are known to induce intestinal ulcerations and hinder ulcer healing [4]. Traditional medicinal herbs and plants offer great promise in the treatment of many diseases and are an important source of new chemical substances with potential therapeutic effects to treat several diseases.

Chemical moieties isolated from plants have a long history of beneficial effects for treating ulcers. Baicalin (BA) is a flavonoid compound extracted and purified from the Chinese medicinal herb *Scutellaria baicalensis* Georgi, which has been demonstrated to have antiulcer, antipyretic, anti-inflammatory, analgesic, anticancer, antioxidant, and wound healing properties [5–10]. Zinc is essential for the maintenance of human cell functions. Moreover, it is reported that zinc can promote the healing of small intestinal mucosal damage. Zinc loss could significantly impair wound healing [11]. Zinc is also a free radical scavenger and anti-inflammatory agent, which can halt the progression of gastrointestinal disease and interrupt the associated inflammatory processes. Zinc complexes have always exerted potent antiulcer activity. Zinc-carnosine is a common antiulcer drug used in the treatment of gastric ulcers in Japan [12]. However, there is little research about the antichronic gastric ulcer ability of BA-Zn, and its related mechanism is still unclear.

It was reported that reactive oxygen species (ROS) played an important role in digestive disorders [13, 14]. In addition, oxygen free radical production and lipid peroxidation play an essential function in the development of gastric ulceration [15, 16]. Moreover, alterations to the antioxidant defense system in ulcerative disorders suggest a vital role for free radicals in ulcerations induced by acetic acid. Inflammatory cytokines such as IL-8 can also influence gastric ulcer healing [17, 18]. Thus, inflammatory cytokines are regarded as indicators of gastric ulcers.

In this study, we investigated whether the BA-Zn complex possesses antiulcer activity in a rat model of acetic acid-induced chronic gastric ulcer through free radical scavenging and anti-inflammatory activity.

2. Materials and Methods

2.1. Chemicals and Reagents. Baicalin (BA, Mw: 464.38) was purchased from Wanfang Chemical Company (Yunnan, China). The zinc complex of baicalin (BA-Zn, $Zn(C_{21}H_{17}O_{11})(CH_3COO)\cdot 3.5H_2O$, Mw: 632) was synthesized by the College of Pharmacy of Kunming Medical University. The LD50 of the zinc-baicalin (BA-Zn) complex is 4.76 g/kg·bw, and the ED50 is 1.042 mg/kg. IL-8, TNF-α, SOD, GSH-Px, and MDA kits were purchased from Nanjing Jiancheng Research Institute (Nanjing, China).

2.2. Preparation of BA-Zn. 500 ml of water was added to 50 g of BA in a beaker, stirring constantly, and making this into a suspension liquid, heating to 55°C at pH 6.5–7.0, then adding a zinc acetate-saturated solution, and mixing fully. This was then cooled to room temperature, and filtered for red precipitation. This was then washed with 75% ethanol and ddH_2O_2, respectively, and finally drying these precipitation at 60°C.

2.3. Animals. Healthy male Sprague-Dawley rats, 7 weeks old and weighing 180–200 g, were from the experimental animal center of Kunming Medical College (certificate number SCXK2005-0008). The Animal Ethics Committee agreement number is KMMU2015011. The animals were housed on a pathogen-free environment with a constant 12 h light/12 h dark cycle in a temperature-controlled central facility (18–22°C) with free access to normal chow and tap water for a week. All procedures were in accordance with the Animal Ethics Committee of Kunming Medical University and the Guide for the Care and Use of Laboratory Animals.

2.4. Experimental Protocol for Ulceration and Healing. Animals were divided randomly into eight experimental groups with 10 animals in each group: the sham group (water vehicle, p.o. (*per os*)), model group (chronic gastric ulcers), BA-Zn groups (3.25, 6.5, and 13 mg/kg BA-Zn, p.o.), BA group (4.6 mg/kg BA, p.o.), zinc-gluconate group (9.32 mg/kg, p.o.), and omeprazole group (4.0 mg/kg omeprazole, p.o.). Chronic gastric ulcers were induced with acetic acid according to the method of Okabe et al. [19]. Briefly, the rats were anesthetized with sodium pentobarbital (30 mg/kg, respectively, i.p. (intraperitoneal injection)), and then the abdomen was opened, and the stomach exposed. A solution of 80% acetic acid (v/v, 0.5 ml) was instilled into a cylinder (5 mm of diameter) that was applied to the serosal surface of the stomach and, after 1 min, was removed by aspiration; the area of contact was washed with sterile saline. Forty-eight hours after ulcer induction, the rats were orally treated with vehicle (sham: water, 1 mg/kg), BA (4.6 mg/kg), zinc-gluconate (9.32 mg/kg), omeprazole (4.0 mg/kg), and BA-Zn (3.25, 6.5, 13 mg/kg) once a day for 7days. On the day following the last treatment, all animals were alive. Then, the animals were euthanatized by an overdose of pentobarbital sodium (150 mg/kg, i.p.), and the stomachs were removed and opened for the measurement of the ulcer area (mm^2) as length (mm) × width (mm). The gastric ulcer tissue was used for the following tests.

2.5. Histological Preparation. A sample obtained from the middle of the gastric lesion was processed according to the conventional procedure and stained with hematoxylin-eosin. The stomachs were removed, filled with 5 ml of 10% formalin and allowed to stand for 5 min; then, these were cut open along the greater curvature. The longitudinal and abscissal lengths of the upper, opened part of the ulcer were measured with a micrometer that was attached to a stereoscopic microscope, and the product of both lengths (mm^2) is expressed in terms of the ulcer index (Table 1). After the ulcer size was measured, the stomach tissue was again immersed in 10% formalin for 24 h. The formalin-fixed tissues were then cut so that a small amount of the normal tissue surrounding the ulcer remained.

2.6. Hematoxylin and Eosin Staining. The stomach tissues were immediately fixed in 4% paraformaldehyde for 48 h at 4°C. Paraffin sections (5 μm) were prepared and then stained with hematoxylin and eosin (HE) according to standard procedures. Tissue were observed and microphotographed under a light microscope.

2.7. Detection of SOD Activity, GSH-Px, MDA, IL-8, and TNF-α Levels. Gastric tissue from the ulcerated portion of the stomach was excised, washed with distilled water, chopped, and homogenized at 3000 rpm in chilled Tris buffer (10 mM, pH 7.4) at a concentration of 10% w/v. Then, the homogenate was centrifuged at 9000 ×g at 4°C for 20 min and the supernatants were used for the determination of superoxide dismutase (SOD), methylenedioxyamphetamine (MDA), and GSH-Px (glutathione peroxidase) contents, as well as IL-8 and TNF-α expression levels by using the following detection kits purchased from Nanjing Jiancheng Biotechnology Co. Ltd.: a superoxide dismutase (SOD) assay kit (WST-1 method) (no. 20160914); glutathione peroxidase (GSH-Px) assay kit (colorimetric method) (no. 20160115); malondialdehyde (MDA) assay kit (TBA method) (no. 20161130); interleukin-8 assay kit (no. 20160815); and tumor necrosis factor-α assay kit (no. 20160703). The changes in

Table 1: Effect of BA-Zn on oxidant stress in rat mucosa induced by acetic acid.

Group	(mg/kg)	Ulcer index (mm^2)	SOD (U/mg)	MDA (μmol/l)	GSH-Px (U/l)
Sham	—	$0 \pm 0^{***}$	$22.09 \pm 0.09^{***}$	$0.91 \pm 0.06^{***}$	$136.09 \pm 9.09^{***}$
Model	—	28.35 ± 3.27	7.03 ± 0.10	2.39 ± 0.03	52.21 ± 7.13
BA	4.6	$24.38 \pm 2.30^{*}$	$12.09 \pm 0.13^{**}$	$3.54 \pm 0.04^{*}$	$85.07 \pm 7.11^{**}$
	3.25	$24.94 \pm 2.00^{*}$	6.75 ± 0.06	$1.75 \pm 0.07^{**}$	55.11 ± 6.06
BA-Zn	6.5	$18.43 \pm 1.11^{***}$	$17.62 \pm 0.11^{***}$	$1.33 \pm 0.07^{***}$	$102.12 \pm 9.11^{***}$
	13	$15.00 \pm 1.44^{***}$	$20.12 \pm 0.32^{***}$	$0.63 \pm 0.01^{***}$	$120.25 \pm 9.07^{***}$
Zinc-gluconate	9.32	$23.71 \pm 2.00^{*}$	$9.07 \pm 0.33^{*}$	2.00 ± 0.12	$80.35 \pm 6.77^{*}$
Omeprazole	4	$15.35 \pm 1.22^{***}$	$19.32 \pm 0.09^{***}$	$1.00 \pm 0.11^{***}$	$107.12 \pm 9.05^{***}$

$^{*}P < 0.05$, $^{**}P < 0.01$, and $^{***}P < 0.001$, vs. the model group.

absorbance were determined using a spectrophotometer; the results are expressed as U/l and μmol/l for GSH-Px and MDA, U/mg protein for SOD activity, and ng/ml for IL-8 and TNF-α levels.

2.8. Western Blot Analysis. Western blot analysis was used for the protein expression levels of SOD1, TNF-α, and IL-8. Total proteins of tissues were extracted with lysis buffer (Beyotime, China). The insoluble protein lysate was removed by centrifugation at 10,000 ×g for 10 min at 4°C. Total proteins were separated by 10% sodium dodecyl sulfate-polyacrylamide gel electrophoresis (SDS-PAGE), followed by blocking in 5% skim milk on a PVDF membrane. The membranes were hybridized with primary antibodies (Proteintech, USA) for 2 h at 4°C and then with secondary antibodies (Proteintech, USA) for 2 h at room temperature. The bands were developed using an enhanced chemiluminescence (ECL) detection system (EMD Millipore, USA) for horseradish peroxidase (HRP). The relative amounts of the various proteins were analyzed. β-Actin was used as a loading control. The results were quantified using ImageJ software.

2.9. Statistical Analysis. All the results were expressed as mean ± SD. Statistical comparisons were made between drug-treated groups and acetic acid groups. The data was statistically analyzed by one-way analysis of variance (ANOVA) (Tukey's post hoc test) using GraphPad Prism software version 5.0a (GraphPad Software Inc., California, USA). $P < 0.05$ was considered to be statistically significant.

3. Results

3.1. BA-Zn Protects against Acetic Acid-Induced Gastric Lesions. The molecular formula of BA-Zn is $Zn(C_{21}H_{17}O_{11})(CH_3COO)\cdot 3.5H_2O$, and it has a molecular weight of 632 g/mol (Figure 1). The macroscopic appearance of the gastric tissue is shown in Figure 2. Rats treated with only water (Figure 2(a)) showed a normal glandular stomach. Figure 2(b) shows the deep ulceration and severe edematous changes in the gastric mucosa of the model group that was induced with 80% acetic acid and treated with water daily. By contrast, rats treated with BA-Zn (3.25, 6.5, or 13 mg/kg) or BA, zinc-gluconate, or omeprazole showed less severe ulceration and less edema in the gastric mucosa induced by 80% acetic acid (Figures 2(c)–2(h)).

As shown in Figure 3(a), the microscopic histological appearance of the gastric tissue and the normal gastric epithelium was observed in the sham group. The application of acetic acid induced the disruption of the superficial region of the gastric gland with loss of epithelial cells, as well as pronounced edema of the submucosa and degradation of the mucosa in the model group (Figure 3(b)).

BA-Zn (3.25, 6.5, and 13 mg/kg) and omeprazole markedly reduced the severity of gastric ulcers (swelling, destruction, and extensive destruction on the surface of the epithelium) and promoted marginal regeneration of the epithelium compared to the model group (Figures 3(c)–3(e) and 3(h)). In the BA (4.6 mg/kg) and zinc-gluconate- (9.32 mg/kg) treated groups, the severity of the gastric ulcers was also inhibited (Figures 3(f) and 3(g)).

In all animals from all the groups that survived, the longitudinal and abscissal lengths of the upper, opened part of the ulcer were measured with a micrometer that was attached to a stereoscopic microscope, and the product of both lengths (mm^2) was expressed in terms of the ulcer index. As shown in Table 1, the sham group showed no ulcer index, and administration of BA-Zn at doses of 3.25, 6.5, and 13 mg/kg decreased the gastric ulcer index to 24.94 ± 2.00 ($P < 0.05$), 18.43 ± 1.11 ($P < 0.001$), and $15.00 \pm 1.44\ mm^2$ ($P < 0.001$) (12.0%, 35.0%, and 47.1% protection, respectively), compared to the ulcer index of the model group which was $28.35 \pm 3.27\ mm^2$. BA (4.6 mg/kg) reduced the gastric ulcer index to 24.38 ± 2.30 ($P < 0.05$) compared to that of the model group. Zinc-gluconate (9.32 mg/kg) also reduced the gastric ulcer index to 23.71 ± 2.00 ($P < 0.05$) compared to that of the model group. Moreover, zinc-gluconate had a higher gastric ulcer index than the BA-Zn group (6.5 and 13 mg/kg, $P < 0.001$, respectively). It indicated that BA-Zn (6.5 and 13 mg/kg) has a stronger healing effect than zinc-gluconate. Omeprazole (4.0 mg/kg), the positive control drug, demonstrated a potency for reducing the gastric ulcer index ($15.35 \pm 1.22\ mm^2$; $P < 0.001$ compared to the model group). BA-Zn (13 mg/kg) showed the best potency for reducing the gastric ulcer index, which was the same as omeprazole.

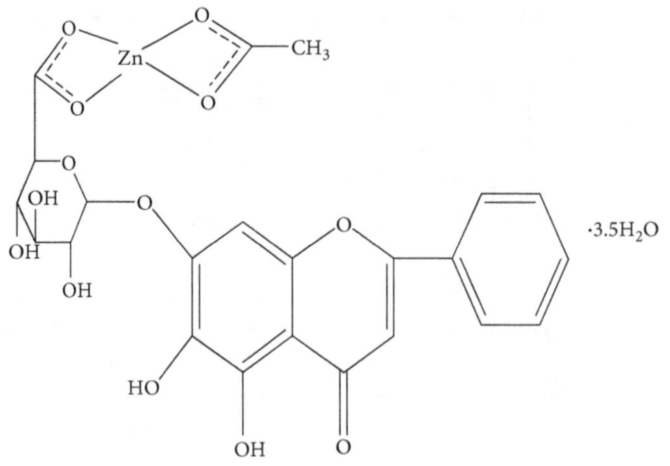

$$\cdot 3.5H_2O$$

FIGURE 1: Structural formula of BA-Zn.

3.2. BA-Zn Suppressed Oxidative Stress in Acetic Acid-Induced Gastric Tissue of Rats. Increased oxidative stress was shown in the ulcerated gastric mucosa of the model group, and this group also had significantly decreased SOD and GSH-Px activities and an increased level of lipid peroxidation (MDA) content compared to those of the sham group ($P < 0.001$).

As shown in Table 1, SOD activity in the mucosa of the model group was significantly lower (7.03 ± 0.10 U/mg protein) than in the sham group (22.09 ± 0.09 U/mg protein; $P < 0.001$). BA-Zn treatment at 6.5 and 13 mg/kg significantly increased the SOD activity to 17.62 ± 0.11 and 20.12 ± 0.32 U/mg protein ($P < 0.001$ and $P < 0.001$), respectively, compared to that of the model group (7.03 ± 0.10 U/mg protein). Moreover, the administration of 6.5 and 13 mg/kg BA-Zn led to higher SOD activity than did the administration of BA (17.62 ± 0.11 and 20.12 ± 0.32 vs. 12.09 ± 0.13 U/mg protein; $P < 0.05$ and $P < 0.01$), and these also markedly increased SOD activity than that of the zinc-gluconate group (9.07 ± 0.33 U/mg protein; $P < 0.001$). It indicated that BA-Zn has a stronger antioxidative effect than BA and zinc-gluconate. Zinc-gluconate (9.32 mg/kg) significantly increased SOD activity to 9.07 ± 0.33 U/mg protein ($P < 0.05$) compared to that of the model group (7.03 ± 0.10 U/mg protein). Omeprazole (4.0 mg/kg) demonstrated an increase in SOD activity (19.32 ± 0.09 U/mg protein; $P < 0.001$, compared to that of the model group).

GSH-Px levels in the gastric mucosa of the model group were significantly lower than in the sham group (52.21 ± 7.13 vs. 136.09 ± 9.09 U/l; $P < 0.001$). Administration of 6.5 and 13 mg/kg BA-Zn significantly increased the GSH-Px level in a dose-dependent manner ($P < 0.001$ and $P < 0.001$, respectively, compared to that of the model group). Moreover, the administration of 6.5 and 13 mg/kg BA-Zn led to increased GSH-Px activity compared to that of the BA group (102.12 ± 9.11 and 120.25 ± 9.07 vs. 85.07 ± 7.11 U/l; $P < 0.05$), and the administration of 6.5 and 13 mg/kg BA-Zn also markedly increased GSH-Px activity compared to that of the zinc-gluconate group (80.35 ± 6.77 U/l; $P < 0.001$). It indicated that BA-Zn has a stronger antioxidative effect than BA and zinc-gluconate. Zinc-gluconate (9.32 mg/kg) significantly increased GSH-Px activity to 80.35 ± 6.77 U/l ($P < 0.05$) compared to that of the model group (52.21 ± 7.13 U/l). Omeprazole (4.0 mg/kg) demonstrated an increase in GSH-Px activity (107.12 ± 9.05 U/l; $P < 0.001$ compared to that of the model group).

The inhibitory effects of BA-Zn on lipid peroxidation (MDA) are shown in Table 1. The MDA content in the gastric mucosa of the model group was higher than in the sham group (2.39 ± 0.03 vs. 0.91 ± 0.06 μmol/l; $P < 0.001$). Treatment with 3.25, 6.5, and 13 mg/kg BA-Zn significantly decreased the MDA content to 1.75 ± 0.07, 1.33 ± 0.07, and 0.63 ± 0.01 μmol/l ($P < 0.01$, $P < 0.001$, and $P < 0.001$, respectively, compared to that of the model group). Moreover, the administration of 3.25, 6.5, and 13 mg/kg BA-Zn led to lower MDA activity than BA (1.75 ± 0.07, 1.33 ± 0.07, and 0.63 ± 9.01 vs. 3.54 ± 0.04 μmol/l; $P < 0.05$) and the zinc-gluconate group (2.00 ± 0.12 μmol/l; $P < 0.001$), indicating that BA-Zn had a stronger antioxidative effect than BA and zinc-gluconate. Zinc-gluconate (9.32 mg/kg) showed a decrease in MDA content (2.00 ± 0.12 μmol/l; $P < 0.05$ compared to that the model group). Omeprazole (4.0 mg/kg) also demonstrated a decrease in MDA content (1.00 ± 0.11 μmol/l; $P < 0.001$ compared to that of the model group).

3.3. Effect of BA-Zn on the Concentration of TNF-α and IL-8. As shown in Table 2, the level of TNF-α in the model group was significantly higher than in the sham group (2.73 ± 0.10 vs. 0.72 ± 0.09 ng/ml; $P < 0.001$). The administration of 3.25, 6.5, and 13 mg/kg BA-Zn significantly decreased the TNF-α concentration in a dose-dependent manner (1.95 ± 0.06, 1.62 ± 0.11, and 1.12 ± 0.32; $P < 0.05$, $P < 0.001$, and $P < 0.001$, respectively, compared to that of the model group). Zinc-gluconate (9.32 mg/kg) demonstrated a decreased TNF-α level (2.00 ± 0.11 ng/ml; $P < 0.05$ compared to that of the model group). Administration of 6.5 and 13 mg/kg BA-Zn significantly decreased the TNF-α concentration compared to that of the zinc-gluconate group (2.00 ± 0.11 ng/ml; $P < 0.001$). Omeprazole (4.0 mg/kg) demonstrated a decreased TNF-α concentration (1.32 ± 0.09 ng/ml; $P < 0.001$ compared to that of the model group).

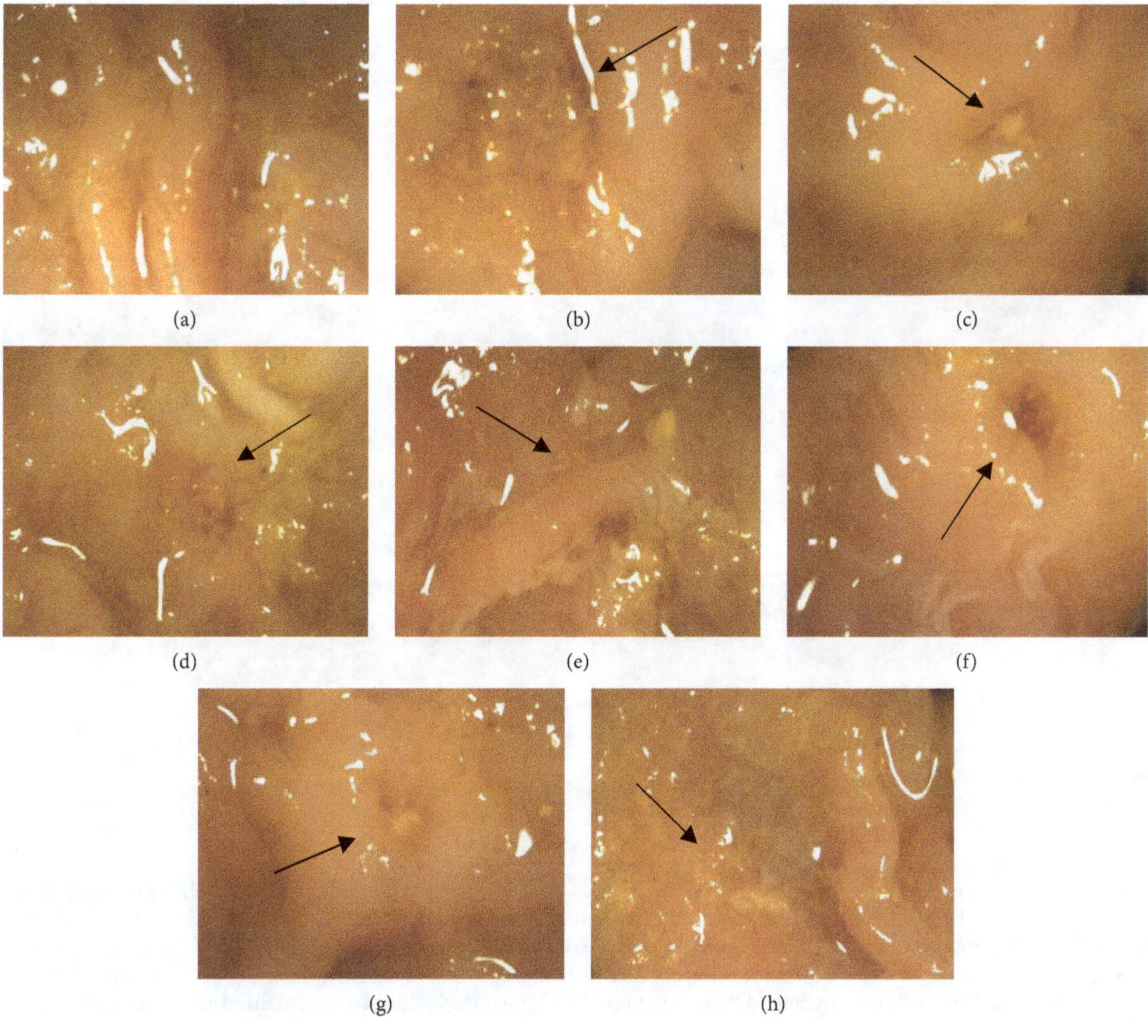

FIGURE 2: Appearances of acetic acid-induced gastric ulcers in different groups: (a) the sham group treated daily with water, (b) an ulceration from the model group induced by acetic acid, (c–e) an ulceration from the BA-Zn group induced by acetic acid and treated daily with BA-Zn (3.25, 6.5, and 13 mg/kg, p.o.), (f) an ulceration from the BA group induced by acetic acid and treated daily with BA (4.6 mg/kg, p.o.), (g) an ulceration from the zinc-gluconate group induced by acetic acid and treated daily with zinc-gluconate (9.32 mg/kg, p.o.), and (h) an ulceration from the omeprazole group induced by acetic acid and treated daily with omeprazole (4.0 mg/kg, p.o.). Black arrows indicate ulcer location.

The level of IL-8 in the model group was significantly higher than in the sham group (0.69 ± 0.03 vs. 0.21 ± 0.06 ng/ml; $P < 0.01$). Administration of 3.25, 6.5, and 13 mg/kg BA-Zn significantly decreased the IL-8 level in a dose-dependent manner (0.36 ± 0.07, 0.33 ± 0.07, and 0.29 ± 0.01; $P < 0.01$, $P < 0.01$, and $P < 0.001$, respectively, compared to that of the model group). Zinc-gluconate (9.32 mg/kg) demonstrated a decreased IL-8 level (0.60 ± 0.01 ng/ml; $P < 0.05$ compared to that of the model group). Administration of 3.25, 6.5, and 13 mg/kg BA-Zn significantly decreased the IL-8 concentration compared to that of the zinc-gluconate group (0.60 ± 0.01 ng/ml; $P < 0.001$). Omeprazole (4.0 mg/kg) also demonstrated a decreased IL-8 level (0.45 ± 0.01 ng/ml; $P < 0.05$ compared to the model group).

To further demonstrate the effect of BA-Zn on the concentration of SOD, TNF-α, and IL-8 in the above groups, Western blot assays were used to detect the expression levels of these proteins. In Figure 4(a) and 4(b), we reveal that BA-Zn treatment significantly increased SOD expression compared to that in the model and zinc-gluconate groups. BA-Zn also significantly decreased the expression of TNF-α and IL-8 compared to that in the model and zinc-gluconate groups. In summary, the above results indicate that BA-Zn had better antioxidative and anti-inflammatory effects than both BA and zinc-gluconate.

4. Discussion

Gastric ulcer is a common dysfunction of the digestive system, and an increasing number of people worldwide are suffering damage from ulcers. The acetic acid-induced ulcer model resembles human chronic ulcers in both pathological features and aspects of the healing process [20, 21]; thus, it is the most useful model for us to use when investigating gastric ulcers. Previous studies have demonstrated that experimental gastric ulcers have many histological and ultrastructural abnormalities, including a reduced height, marked dilation of gastric glands, and increased connective tissue, that may

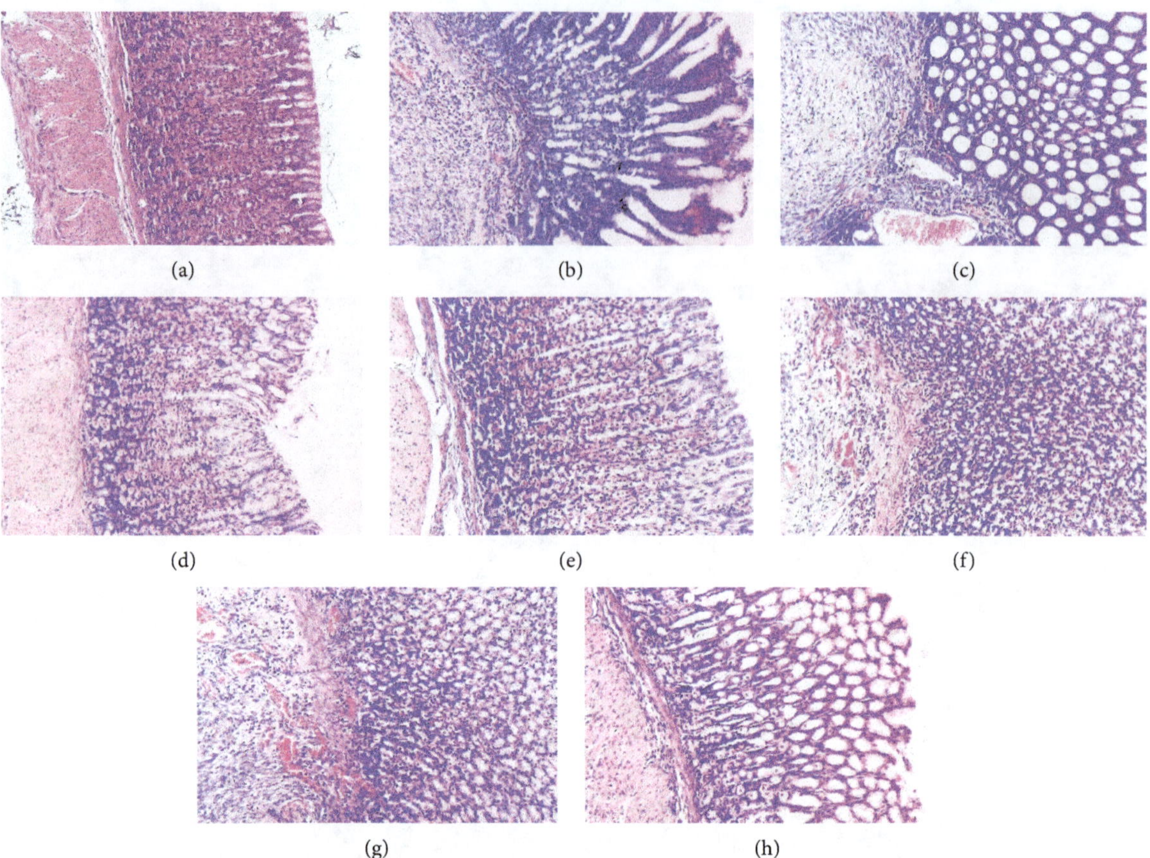

Figure 3: Photomicrographs of acetic acid-induced gastric ulcers from different groups: (a) sham group, (b) HE staining of the model group induced by acetic acid, (c–e) HE staining of the BA-Zn group induced by acetic acid and treated daily with BA-Zn (3.25, 6.5, and 13 mg/kg, p.o.), (f) HE staining of the BA group induced by acetic acid and treated daily with BA (4.6 mg/kg, p.o.), (g) HE staining of the zinc-gluconate group induced by acetic acid and treated daily with zinc-gluconate (9.32 mg/kg, p.o.), and (h) HE staining of the omeprazole group induced by acetic acid and treated daily with omeprazole (4.0 mg/kg, p.o.). The HE stained slides were visualized under a bright field microscope with 20x magnification.

Table 2: Concentration of TNF-α and IL-8 in rat mucosa induced by acetic acid.

Group	(mg/kg)	TNF-α (ng/ml)	IL-8 (ng/ml)
Sham	—	$0.72 \pm 0.09^{***}$	$0.21 \pm 0.06^{**}$
Model	—	2.73 ± 0.10	0.69 ± 0.03
BA	4.6	$1.91 \pm 0.13^{*}$	$0.54 \pm 0.04^{*}$
	3.25	$1.95 \pm 0.06^{*}$	$0.36 \pm 0.07^{**}$
BA-Zn	6.5	$1.62 \pm 0.11^{***}$	$0.33 \pm 0.07^{**}$
	13	$1.12 \pm 0.32^{***}$	$0.29 \pm 0.01^{***}$
Zinc-gluconate	9.32	$2.00 \pm 0.11^{*}$	$0.60 \pm 0.01^{*}$
Omeprazole	4	$1.32 \pm 0.09^{***}$	$0.45 \pm 0.01^{*}$

$^{*}P < 0.05$, $^{**}P < 0.01$, and $^{***}P < 0.001$, vs. the model group.

interfere with the mucosal defense system and cause ulcer recurrence with some ulcerogenic factors [22, 23].

In recent years, chemical drugs used for the treatment of gastric ulcers have induced many side effects. Recently, newly developed drugs with herbal origins may offer reduced side effects compared with chemical drugs [24]. In folk knowledge, medicinal plants have been used for the treatment of various disorders. More and more medicinal plants with various therapeutic properties, especially for the treatment of gastritis and gastric ulcers, have been identified [25–27]. However, few traditional Chinese medicinal plants for gastric ulcer treatment have been studied. Currently, because of the lack of effective and applicable pharmacological treatments for gastric ulcer, more and more people have focused on traditional medicines. The investigation of the therapeutic functions of traditional medicinal herbs in gastric ulcer offer promising potential.

Scutellaria baicalensis is a popular medicinal herb used in traditional Chinese medicine, and it is used for the treatment of high fevers, ulcers, inflammation, and even cancer. The main bioactive flavonoids in *Scutellaria baicalensis* include baicalein, baicalin (BA) (baicalein-7-glucuronide), wogonin, wogonoside (wogonin-7-glucuronide), oroxylin A, and oroxylin A-7-glucuronide. *Scutellaria baicalensis* and its flavones have been studied for their various pharmacological activities, including anti-inflammatory [28], antibacterial [29], neuroprotective [30], anticonvulsant [31], antiviral [32], antitumor [33], and antioxidant [34] activities. BA is the most popular bioactive flavonoid for treating ulcers. However, the

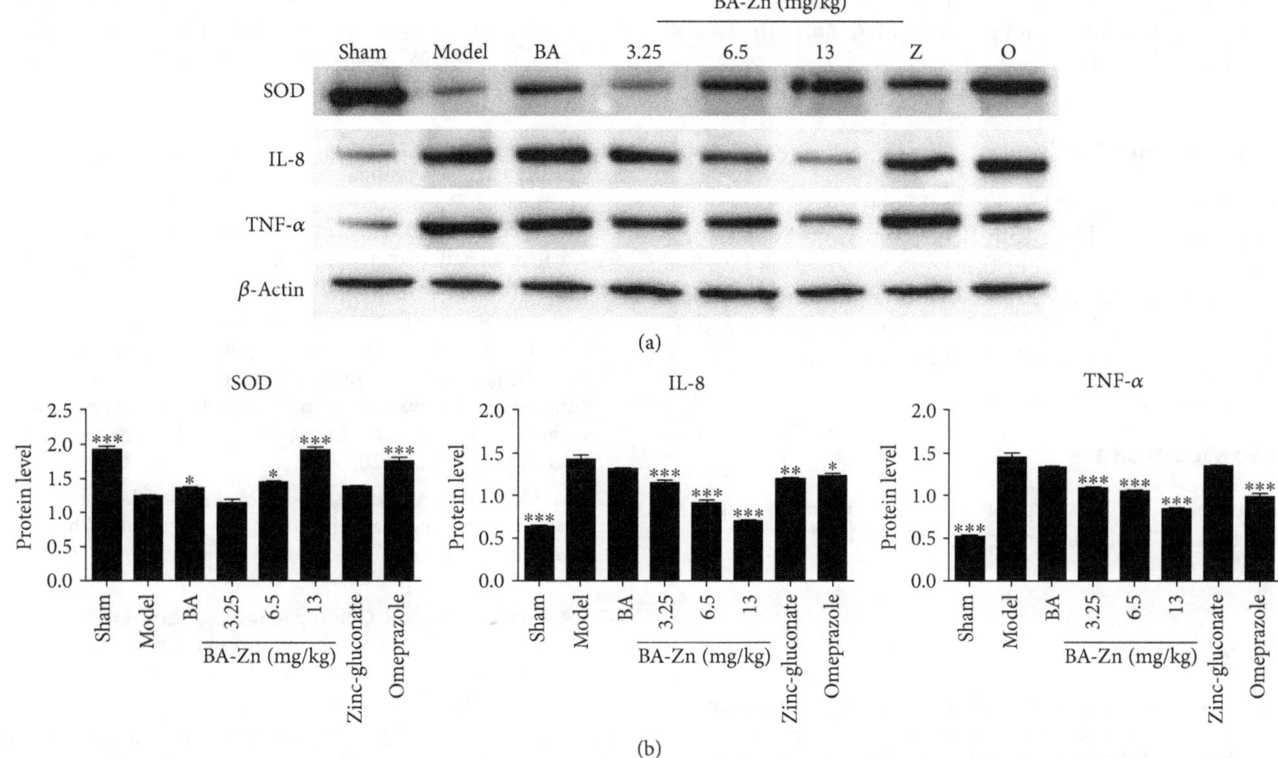

Figure 4: Western blot analysis of SOD, TNF-α, and IL-8 expression. (a) The protein expression levels of SOD, TNF-α, and IL-8 were analyzed by Western blot analysis. β-Actin was used as a loading control. (b) Quantification of SOD, TNF-α, and IL-8 protein expression levels using ImageJ software. Z: zinc-gluconate, O: omeprazole. $^{*}P < 0.05$, $^{**}P < 0.01$, and $^{***}P < 0.001$, vs. the model group.

antichronic gastric ulcer effects of BA alone or in complex have not yet been elucidated.

In this paper, we examined the effects of BA-Zn, BA, and zinc-gluconate and related mechanisms on gastric ulcer healing in an acetic acid-induced gastric ulcer rat model. It has been reported that zinc-gluconate has a protective effect on gastric ulcers [35]. Acetic acid induces a state of acute stress in the gastric mucosa, subsequently inducing gastric ulcers. Moreover, acetic acid-induced gastric ulceration leads to chronic oxidative stress with decreased SOD activity and GSH-Px expression levels and increased lipid peroxidation (MDA). It is well known that SOD, GSH-Px, and MDA play important roles in protecting the gastric mucosa against various damaging agents [36, 37]. GSH-Px also plays an important role in protecting against oxidative gastric mucosal injury [38]. MDA is currently regarded as a reliable index of ROS-induced mucosal injury [39]. Therefore, the detection of SOD, GSH-Px, and MDA contents can reflect and indicate the level of oxidative stress. In addition, increased concentrations of TNF-α and IL-8 were detected in the ulcerated gastric mucosa. BA-Zn (13 mg/kg) significantly accelerated the healing of gastric ulcers, through an increase in SOD and GSH-Px activity and a decrease in MDA, IL-8, and TNF-α contents. We also detected the levels of SOD, IL-8, and TNF-α by Western blot. We found that BA-Zn significantly accelerated ulcer healing by decreasing oxidative stress and attenuating inflammation. In our results, zinc-gluconate also has a protective effect on gastric ulcers, but BA-Zn has much stronger protective and healing abilities in gastric ulcers. On the basis of our data, BA-Zn (13 mg/kg) has greater antigastric ulcer abilities than either BA or zinc-gluconate.

Collectively, BA-Zn presents important ulcer-healing properties in the model of chronic ulcer induced by acetic acid in rats. Omeprazole is one of the most popular drugs used for the therapeutic control of gastroduodenal ulcers in humans. In our work, BA-Zn also exerted an antiulcerogenic effect similar to that of omeprazole against the development of acetic acid-induced gastric ulcers in rats using antioxidant and anti-inflammatory abilities. Therefore, the BA-Zn complex may become a potential and promising drug for the treatment of human gastroduodenal ulcers. In summary, our study indicates that BA-Zn promotes ulcer healing by decreasing oxidative stress and attenuating inflammation in an acetic acid-induced gastric ulcer rat model. However, additional studies are needed to explore the novel mechanisms of BA-Zn and determine whether other mechanisms are also involved in the antiulcer effects of this complex.

5. Conclusion

In conclusion, BA-Zn facilitates the healing of acetic-induced chronic ulcers in rats through its antioxidant and anti-inflammatory properties. The results of this study provide a foundation for the clinical application of BA-Zn in the treatment of gastroduodenal ulcers.

Authors' Contributions

This study was designed by Xu Liu. Experimental work was done by Hui Yang, Zhong-Kun Ren, Yi Lu, Xiao-Feng Zeng, and Ling Li. The first draft of this paper was written by Hui Yang and reviewed by Xu Liu and Rong-Ping Zhang. Zhong-Kun Ren and Yi Lu reviewed the methodology and results. All authors reviewed and approved the final version.

Acknowledgments

The present study was supported by the Yunnan Applied Basic Research Projects (Grant no. 2005C00092).

References

[1] J. L. Goldstein, J. Aisenberg, F. Lanza et al., "A multicenter, randomized, double-blind, active-comparator, placebo-controlled, parallel-group comparison of the incidence of endoscopic gastric and duodenal ulcer rates with valdecoxib or naproxen in healthy subjects aged 65 to 75 years," *Clinical Therapeutics*, vol. 28, no. 3, pp. 340–351, 2006.

[2] G. H. Heeba, M. K. A. Hassan, and R. S. Amin, "Gastroprotective effect of simvastatin against indomethacin-induced gastric ulcer in rats: role of nitric oxide and prostaglandins," *European Journal of Pharmacology*, vol. 607, no. 1–3, pp. 188–193, 2009.

[3] P. A. Gladding, M. W. I. Webster, H. B. Farrell, I. S. L. Zeng, R. Park, and N. Ruijne, "The antiplatelet effect of six non-steroidal anti-inflammatory drugs and their pharmacodynamic interaction with aspirin in healthy volunteers," *The American Journal of Cardiology*, vol. 101, no. 7, pp. 1060–1063, 2008.

[4] A. Lanas, M. A. Perez-Aisa, F. Feu et al., "A nationwide study of mortality associated with hospital admission due to severe gastrointestinal events and those associated with nonsteroidal antiinflammatory drug use," *The American Journal of Gastroenterology*, vol. 100, no. 8, pp. 1685–1693, 2005.

[5] B. Cryer and K. W. Mahaffey, "Gastrointestinal ulcers, role of aspirin, and clinical outcomes: pathobiology, diagnosis, and treatment," *Journal of Multidisciplinary Healthcare*, vol. 7, pp. 137–146, 2014.

[6] J. Lu, J. S. Wang, and L. Y. Kong, "Anti-inflammatory effects of Huang-Lian-Jie-Du decoction, its two fractions and four typical compounds," *Journal of Ethnopharmacology*, vol. 134, no. 3, pp. 911–918, 2011.

[7] J. M. Hwang, T. H. Tseng, Y. Y. Tsai et al., "Protective effects of baicalein on tert-butyl hydroperoxide-induced hepatic toxicity in rat hepatocytes," *Journal of Biomedical Science*, vol. 12, no. 2, pp. 389–397, 2005.

[8] J. Dou, L. Chen, G. Xu et al., "Effects of baicalein on Sendai virus in vivo are linked to serum baicalin and its inhibition of hemagglutinin-neuraminidase," *Archives of Virology*, vol. 156, no. 5, pp. 793–801, 2011.

[9] M. Y. Yun, J. H. Yang, D. K. Kim et al., "Therapeutic effects of baicalein on atopic dermatitis-like skin lesions of NC/Nga mice induced by *Dermatophagoides pteronyssinus*," *International Immunopharmacology*, vol. 10, no. 9, pp. 1142–1148, 2010.

[10] J. H. Liu, H. Wann, M. M. Chen et al., "Baicalein significantly protects human retinal pigment epithelium cells against H_2O_2-induced oxidative stress by scavenging reactive oxygen species and downregulating the expression of matrix metalloproteinase-9 and vascular endothelial growth factor," *Journal of Ocular Pharmacology and Therapeutics*, vol. 26, no. 5, pp. 421–429, 2010.

[11] P. D. Zalewski, A. Q. Truong-Tran, D. Grosser, L. Jayaram, C. Murgia, and R. E. Ruffin, "Zinc metabolism in airway epithelium and airway inflammation: basic mechanisms and clinical targets. A review," *Pharmacology & Therapeutics*, vol. 105, no. 2, pp. 127–149, 2005.

[12] M. Odashima, M. Otaka, M. Jin et al., "Zinc L-carnosine protects colonic mucosal injury through induction of heat shock protein 72 and suppression of NF-κB activation," *Life Sciences*, vol. 79, no. 24, pp. 2245–2250, 2006.

[13] A. Bhattacharyya, R. Chattopadhyay, S. Mitra, and S. E. Crowe, "Oxidative stress: an essential factor in the pathogenesis of gastrointestinal mucosal diseases," *Physiological Reviews*, vol. 94, no. 2, pp. 329–354, 2014.

[14] L. Chanudom and J. Tangpong, "Anti-inflammation property of *Syzygium cumini* (L.) Skeels on indomethacin-induced acute gastric ulceration," *Gastroenterology Research and Practice*, vol. 2015, Article ID 343642, 12 pages, 2015.

[15] L. M. da Silva, A. Allemand, D. A. G. B. Mendes et al., "Ethanolic extract of roots from *Arctium lappa* L. accelerates the healing of acetic acid-induced gastric ulcer in rats: involvement of the antioxidant system," *Food and Chemical Toxicology*, vol. 51, pp. 179–187, 2013.

[16] S. K. Jaiswal, C. V. Rao, B. Sharma, P. Mishra, S. Das, and M. K. Dubey, "Gastroprotective effect of standardized leaf extract from *Argyreia speciosa* on experimental gastric ulcers in rats," *Journal of Ethnopharmacology*, vol. 137, no. 1, pp. 341–344, 2011.

[17] A. A. El-Fakhry, M. A. El-Daker, R. I. Badr et al., "Association of the CagA gene positive *Helicobacter pylori* and tissue levels of interleukin-17 and interleukin-8 in gastric ulcer patients," *The Egyptian Journal of Immunology*, vol. 19, no. 1, pp. 51–62, 2012.

[18] Y. W. Yin, A. M. Hu, Q. Q. Sun et al., "Association between interleukin-8 gene −251 T/A polymorphism and the risk of peptic ulcer disease: a meta-analysis," *Human Immunology*, vol. 74, no. 1, pp. 125–130, 2013.

[19] S. Okabe, J. L. A. Roth, and C. J. Pfeiffer, "A method for experimental, penetrating gastric and duodenal ulcers in rats. Observations on normal healing," *The American Journal of Digestive Diseases*, vol. 16, no. 3, pp. 277–284, 1971.

[20] K. Takagi, S. Okabe, and R. Saziki, "A new method for the production of chronic gastric ulcer in rats and the effect of several drugs on its healing," *Japanese Journal of Pharmacology*, vol. 19, no. 3, pp. 418–426, 1969.

[21] S. Okabe and K. Amagase, "An overview of acetic acid ulcer models—the history and state of the art of peptic ulcer research," *Biological & Pharmaceutical Bulletin*, vol. 28, no. 8, pp. 1321–1341, 2005.

[22] A. Tarnawski, J. Stachura, W. J. Krause, T. G. Douglass, and H. Gergely, "Quality of gastric ulcer healing: a new, emerging concept," *Journal of Clinical Gastroenterology*, vol. 13, Supplement 1, pp. S42–S47, 1991.

[23] A. S. Tarnawski, "Cellular and molecular mechanisms of gastrointestinal ulcer healing," *Digestive Diseases and Sciences*, vol. 50, Supplement 1, pp. S24–S33, 2005.

[24] M. Arun and V. V. Asha, "Gastroprotective effect of *Dodonaea viscosa* on various experimental ulcer models," *Journal of Ethnopharmacology*, vol. 118, no. 3, pp. 460–465, 2008.

[25] A. Alkofahi and A. H. Atta, "Pharmacological screening of the anti-ulcerogenic effects of some Jordanian medicinal plants in rats," *Journal of Ethnopharmacology*, vol. 67, no. 3, pp. 341–345, 1999.

[26] S. Khennouf, H. Benabdallah, K. Gharzouli et al., "Effect of tannins from *Quercus suber* and *Quercus coccifera* leaves on ethanol-induced gastric lesions in mice," *Journal of Agricultural and Food Chemistry*, vol. 51, no. 5, pp. 1469–1473, 2003.

[27] S. Bhattacharya, S. R. Chaudhuri, S. Chattopadhyay, and S. K. Bandyopadhyay, "Healing properties of some Indian medicinal plants against indomethacin-induced gastric ulceration of rats," *Journal of Clinical Biochemistry and Nutrition*, vol. 41, no. 2, pp. 106–114, 2007.

[28] B. Q. Li, T. Fu, W. H. Gong et al., "The flavonoid baicalin exhibits anti-inflammatory activity by binding to chemokines," *Immunopharmacology*, vol. 49, no. 3, pp. 295–306, 2000.

[29] J. Wu, D. Hu, and K. X. Wang, "Study of *Scutellaria baicalensis* and Baicalin against antimicrobial susceptibility of *Helicobacter pylori* strains in vitro," *Zhong yao cai = Zhongyaocai = Journal of Chinese Medicinal Materials*, vol. 31, no. 5, pp. 707–710, 2008.

[30] A. M. Y. Lin, Y. H. Ping, G. F. Chang et al., "Neuroprotective effect of oral S/B remedy (*Scutellaria baicalensis* Georgi and *Bupleurum scorzonerifolfium* Willd) on iron-induced neurodegeneration in the nigrostriatal dopaminergic system of rat brain," *Journal of Ethnopharmacology*, vol. 134, no. 3, pp. 884–891, 2011.

[31] S. Y. Yoon, I. C. dela Pena, C. Y. Shin et al., "Convulsion-related activities of *Scutellaria* flavones are related to the 5,7-dihydroxyl structures," *European Journal of Pharmacology*, vol. 659, no. 2-3, pp. 155–160, 2011.

[32] L. Chen, J. Dou, Z. Su et al., "Synergistic activity of baicalein with ribavirin against influenza A (H1N1) virus infections in cell culture and in mice," *Antiviral Research*, vol. 91, no. 3, pp. 314–320, 2011.

[33] M. Li-Weber, "New therapeutic aspects of flavones: the anticancer properties of *Scutellaria* and its main active constituents wogonin, baicalein and baicalin," *Cancer Treatment Reviews*, vol. 35, no. 1, pp. 57–68, 2009.

[34] D. E. Shieh, L. T. Liu, and C. C. Lin, "Antioxidant and free radical scavenging effects of baicalein, baicalin and wogonin," *Anticancer Research*, vol. 20, no. 5A, pp. 2861–2865, 2000.

[35] B. Bandyopadhyay and S. K. Bandyopadhyay, "Protective effect of zinc gluconate on chemically induced gastric ulcer," *The Indian Journal of Medical Research*, vol. 106, pp. 27–32, 1997.

[36] S. S. Poulsen, "On the role of epidermal growth factor in the defence of the gastroduodenal mucosa," *Scandinavian Journal of Gastroenterology*, vol. 128, pp. 20–23, 1987.

[37] S. Kwiecień, T. Brzozowski, P. C. H. Konturek, and S. J. Konturek, "The role of reactive oxygen species in action of nitric oxide-donors on stress-induced gastric mucosal lesions," *Journal of Physiology and Pharmacology*, vol. 53, 4 Part 2, pp. 761–773, 2002.

[38] I. Chattopadhyay, U. Bandyopadhyay, K. Biswas, P. Maity, and R. K. Banerjee, "Indomethacin inactivates gastric peroxidase to induce reactive-oxygen-mediated gastric mucosal injury and curcumin protects it by preventing peroxidase inactivation and scavenging reactive oxygen," *Free Radical Biology & Medicine*, vol. 40, no. 8, pp. 1397–1408, 2006.

[39] M. Maes, P. Ruckoanich, Y. S. Chang, N. Mahanonda, and M. Berk, "Multiple aberrations in shared inflammatory and oxidative & nitrosative stress (IO&NS) pathways explain the co-association of depression and cardiovascular disorder (CVD), and the increased risk for CVD and due mortality in depressed patients," *Progress in Neuro-Psychopharmacology and Biological Psychiatry*, vol. 35, no. 3, pp. 769–783, 2011.

2

Superior Mesenteric Artery Syndrome: Clinical, Endoscopic, and Radiological Findings

Emanuele Sinagra,[1,2] Dario Raimondo,[1] Domenico Albano,[3] Valentina Guarnotta,[4] Melania Blasco,[5] Sergio Testai,[6] Marta Marasà,[6] Vincenzo Mastrella,[6] Valerio Alaimo,[6] Valentina Bova,[6] Giovanni Albano,[6] Dario Sorrentino,[6] Giovanni Tomasello,[2,7] Francesco Cappello,[2,7] Angelo Leone,[8] Francesca Rossi,[1] Massimo Galia,[3] Roberto Lagalla,[3] Federico Midiri,[3] Gaetano Cristian Morreale,[9] Georgios Amvrosiadis,[9] Guido Martorana,[10] Marcello Giuseppe Spampinato,[10] Vittorio Virgilio,[11,12] and Massimo Midiri[3]

[1]*Gastroenterology and Endoscopy Unit, Fondazione Istituto G. Giglio, Contrada Pietra Pollastra Pisciotto, 90015 Cefalù, Italy*
[2]*Euro-Mediterranean Institute of Science and Technology (IEMEST), 90100 Palermo, Italy*
[3]*Department of Radiology, DIBIMED, University of Palermo, Via del Vespro 127, 90127 Palermo, Italy*
[4]*Section of Cardio-Respiratory and Endocrine-Metabolic Diseases, Biomedical Department of Internal and Specialist Medicine (DIBIMIS), University of Palermo, Piazza delle Cliniche 2, 90127 Palermo, Italy*
[5]*Internal Medicine Unit, Fondazione Istituto G. Giglio, Contrada Pietra Pollastra Pisciotto, 90015 Cefalù, Italy*
[6]*Radiology Unit, Fondazione Istituto G. Giglio, Contrada Pietra Pollastra Pisciotto, 90015 Cefalù, Italy*
[7]*Department of Experimental Biomedicine and Clinical Neuroscience, Section of Human Anatomy, University of Palermo, 90100 Palermo, Italy*
[8]*BioNec, Section of Histology, Department of Experimental and Clinical Neurosciences, University of Palermo, Palermo, Italy*
[9]*Gastroenterology Unit, PO. V. Cervello, via Trabucco, 90146 Palermo, Italy*
[10]*Surgery Unit, Fondazione Istituto G. Giglio, Contrada Pietra Pollastra Pisciotto, 90015 Cefalù, Italy*
[11]*Strategic Direction, Fondazione Istituto Giuseppe Giglio, Cefalù, Italy*
[12]*Division of Vascular Surgery, Garibaldi Hospital, Catania, Italy*

Correspondence should be addressed to Emanuele Sinagra; emanuelesinagra83@googlemail.com

Academic Editor: Riccardo Casadei

Background. The superior mesenteric artery (SMA) syndrome is a rare entity presenting with upper gastrointestinal tract obstruction and weight loss. Studies to determine the optimal methods of diagnosis and treatment are required. *Aims and Methods.* This study aims at analyzing the clinical presentation, diagnosis, and management of SMA syndrome. Ten cases of SMA syndrome out of 2074 esophagogastroduodenoscopies were suspected. A contrast-enhanced computed tomography (CECT) scan was performed to confirm the diagnosis. After, a gastroenterologist and a nutritionist personalized the therapy. Furthermore, we compared the demographical, clinical, endoscopic, and radiological parameters of these cases with a control group consisting of 10 cases out of 2380 EGDS of initially suspected (but not radiologically confirmed) SMA over a follow-up 2-year period (2015-2016). *Results.* The prevalence of SMA syndrome was 0.005%. Median age and body mass index were 23.5 years and 21.5 kg/m^2, respectively. Symptoms developed between 6 and 24 months. Median aortomesenteric angle and aorta-SMA distance were 22 and 6 mm, respectively. All patients improved on conservative treatment. In our series, a marked (>5 kg) weight loss ($p = 0.006$) and a long-standing presentation (more than six months in 80% of patients) ($p = 0.002$) are significantly related to a diagnosis of confirmed SMA syndrome at CECT after an endoscopic suspicion. A "resembling postprandial distress syndrome dyspepsia" presentation may be helpful to the endoscopist in suspecting a latent SMA syndrome ($p = 0.02$). The narrowing of both the aortomesenteric angle ($p = 0.001$) and the aortomesenteric distance ($p < 0.001$) was significantly associated with the diagnosis of SMA after an endoscopic suspicion; however, the narrowing of the aortomesenteric distance seemed to be more accurate, rather than the narrowing of the aortomesenteric angle. *Conclusion.* SMA syndrome represents a diagnostic and therapeutic challenge. Our results show the following findings: the importance of the endoscopic suspicion of SMA syndrome; the preponderance of a long-standing and chronic onset; a female preponderance; the importance of the nutritional counseling for the treatment; no need of surgical intervention; and better diagnostic accuracy of the narrowing of the aorta-SMA distance. Larger prospective studies are needed to clarify the best diagnosis and management of the SMA syndrome.

1. Introduction

The superior mesenteric artery (SMA) syndrome is a rare entity, usually presenting with acute or chronic upper gastrointestinal tract obstruction and weight loss, due to the compression of the third part of the duodenum between the abdominal aorta and the SMA itself [1]. It represents an atypical cause of proximal intestinal obstruction, which occurs most frequently in young patients presenting with an important weight loss [2]. An abnormal low insertion of the SMA or a high insertion of the angle of Treitz that dislocates the duodenum to a cranial position may support this condition. Among the most frequent causes of SMA syndrome, the best recognized are an acquired anatomic abnormality occurring after scoliosis surgery, spinal trauma, abdominal surgery (e.g., total proctocolectomy and ileal J-pouch anal anastomosis), burns (since causing a hypercatabolic state), anorexia nervosa, and finally neoplastic diseases and malabsorptive states, which may be related to prolonged wasting conditions [2–6]. Patients with SMA syndrome may present both acutely and insidiously, thus making the diagnosis of the SMA syndrome as challenging and often delayed. Furthermore, the optimal treatment of SMA syndrome also remains a challenge. Indeed, after the diagnosis, conservative treatment with nutritional support and positioning should be tried first, and surgery may represent a lasting therapeutic option in case of failure. To date, few and small-number studies analyzed all these features of this syndrome, also due to the rarity of SMA syndrome. For this reason, studies to determine the optimal methods of diagnosis and treatment are essential. This study aims at analyzing the clinical presentation, diagnosis, and management of SMA syndrome.

2. Materials and Methods

Over a 2-year period (2013-2014), 10 cases of SMA syndrome out of 2074 esophagogastroduodenoscopies (EGDS) were initially suspected (see Table 1). In this setting, a pulsatile extrinsic compression in the third portion of the duodenum represented, to date, the most reliable finding which could guide the endoscopist to suspect SMA syndrome.

Once EGDS was performed, and once SMA syndrome was suspected after upper endoscopy, contrast-enhanced computed tomography (CECT) scan was performed on these patients to confirm the diagnosis.

CECT scan was done on a multidetector scanner with routine protocol comprising of no enhanced phase followed by arterial and portal phases performed after the administration of a bolus of 80–100 ml of nonionic iodinated contrast agent (Iohexol, Omnipaque 300, GE Healthcare, Princeton, NJ). The values for the study were obtained in the arterial phase using reformatted images: maximum intensity projection and multiplanar reconstruction with selected axial and sagittal images. In this setting, the CECT axial section should show the compression of the third part of the duodenum between the SMA and abdominal aorta, with proximal duodenal (and gastric) dilation. Furthermore, at the sagittal multiplanar reconstruction CECT, the angle between the SMA and aorta was measured at the origin. In adults, SMA usually forms an angle of 45° with the aorta, with the normal angle ranging from 25° to 60° [7], while clinical SMA syndrome manifestations appear if the angle drops below 25°. It is believed that values of this angle may be lower for pediatric patients [2].

On the other hand, the perpendicular distance between the SMA and aorta was measured at the site where the duodenum crosses between the lower border of the duodenum (D3) and the midpoint of the duodenal loop which is crossing at that site (D2). Further criteria for the diagnosis of SMA syndrome included an aortomesenteric distance of less than 8–10 mm [8], measured at the site where the duodenum crosses between D3 and D2.

Furthermore, we compared the demographical, clinical, endoscopic, and radiological parameters of these cases with a control group consisting of 10 cases out 2380 EGDS of initially suspected (but not radiologically confirmed) SMA over a follow-up 2-year period (2015-2016).

The Statistical Packages for Social Science SPSS version 17 (SPSS, Inc.) was used for data analysis. The analysis was performed at the group level. The normality of quantitative variables was tested with the Shapiro-Wilk test. Data were presented as the median and interquartile ranges for continuous variables. The Mann–Whitney test was used to compare the numerical variables in the two groups of patients (patients with SMA and controls). A p value < 0.05 was considered statistically significant.

Once the diagnosis of SMA syndrome was confirmed, the patients were referred to a gastroenterologist and to a nutritionist to discuss a personalized approach of therapy; furthermore, for each patient, a surgical consultation was proposed.

3. Results

In our series, we prospectively evaluated 10 cases of SMA (2 males, 8 females), with a prevalence of 0.005% (see Table 2). Median age was 40 years (range 14–40), and the median body mass index was 21.5 kg/m^2. Symptoms developed between 6 and 24 months (median 18 months).

In the control group, we prospectively evaluated 10 cases of endoscopically suspected (but not confirmed through CECT) SMA (1 male, 9 females), with a prevalence of 0.003% (see Table 2).

Table 1: Demographical, clinical, endoscopic, and radiological findings of patients with superior mesenteric artery syndrome.

	Patient 1	Patient 2	Patient 3	Patient 4	Patient 5	Patient 6	Patient 7	Patient 8	Patient 9	Patient 10
Hospital admission	Not	Not	Not	Yes (14 days)	Not	Yes (12 days)	Not	Not	Not	Not
Age	34	17	14	40	23	38	23	24	25	23
Sex	Female	Female	Female	Male	Female	Female	Male	Female	Female	Female
Weight (kg)	45	84	50	45	60	40	65	43	47	43
Body mass index (kg/m^2)	20	28	22	19	23	18	22	15	21.5	21.5
Weight loss before the diagnosis (kg)	10	5	6	10	6	20	16	5	6	5
Comorbidities	Anorexia nervosa	GP6DH deficiency	None	Crohn's disease	None	Spina bifida	None	Anorexia nervosa	None	None
Further endoscopic findings	None	*Helicobacter pylori*-related gastritis	Grade A esophagitis	Cardial incontinence	Cardial incontinence	None	Hiatal ernia; *Helicobacter pylori*-related gastritis	Cardial incontinence	Cardial incontinence	None
Onset (months)	12	12	12	6	24	18	18	6	18	18
Clinical presentation	Dismotility-like dyspepsia	Dismotility-like dyspepsia	Dismotility-like dyspepsia	Otherwise unexplained weight loss	Reflux-like dyspepsia	Otherwise unexplained weight loss	Dismotility-like dyspepsia	Dismotility-like dyspepsia	Reflux-like dyspepsia	Dismotility-like dyspepsia
Diagnosis	Upper endoscopy, abdominal computed tomography	Upper endoscopy, abdominal computed tomography	Upper endoscopy, abdominal computed tomography	Upper endoscopy, abdominal computed tomography	Upper endoscopy, abdominal computed tomography	Upper endoscopy, abdominal computed tomography	Upper endoscopy, abdominal computed tomography	Upper endoscopy, abdominal computed tomography	Upper endoscopy, abdominal computed tomography	Upper endoscopy, abdominal computed tomography
Aortomesenteric angle	23	38	15	15	46	24	20	21	22	22
Aorta-superior mesenteric artery distance	6	5	5	4	6	6	6	5	6	6
Treatment	Conservative	Conservative	Conservative	Conservative	Conservative	Conservative	Conservative	Conservative	Conservative	Conservative

Table 2: Characteristics of patients with SMA and control group.

Parameters	Patients with SMA ($N = 10$) Median (IR)	Control group ($N = 10$) Median (IR)	p
Age (years)	40 (14–65)	34.5 (17–53)	0.912
Body mass index (kg/m^2)	22 (15–28)	23 (17–26)	0.315
Weight decrease (kg)	6 (5–20)	0.5 (0–13)	0.006
Onset of symptoms	14 (6–24)	2.5 (0–15)	0.002
Aortomesenteric angle (mm)	22 (15–46)	74.5 (25–87)	0.001
Aorta-SMA distance (mm)	6 (4–6)	11 (10–12)	<0.001
	Subjects (%)	*Subjects* (%)	
Gender			
Male	2 (20%)	1 (10%)	
Female	8 (80%)	9 (90%)	0.540
Hospitalization	2 (20%)	1 (10%)	0.531
Comorbidities	5 (50%)	8 (80%)	0.160
Clinical symptoms at onset			
Postprandial distress syndrome	7 (70%)	2 (20%)	0.025
Otherwise unexplained weight loss	2 (20%)	2 (20%)	1
Gastroesophageal reflux disease	1 (10%)	1 (10%)	1
Epigastric pain syndrome	0 (0)	5 (50%)	0.010
Further endoscopic findings			
Helicobacter pylori presence	2 (20%)	3 (30%)	0.606
Erosive gastroesophageal reflux disease	1 (10%)	2 (20%)	0.531
Cardial incontinence	4 (40%)	4 (40%)	1
Hiatal hernia	1 (10%)	4 (40%)	0.121
D-G reflux	0 (0)	2 (20%)	0.136
Celiac disease	0 (0)	1 (10%)	0.305
Gastric polyps	0 (0)	1 (10%)	0.305

Furthermore, in the follow-up period, we detected further 2 cases (both females) of SMA syndrome that were suspected at the EGDS and successively confirmed at CECT.

In this last group, 2 out of 10 patients refused to undergo CECT to confirm the initially suspected SMA, because they improved conservatively after, respectively, gluten avoidance (since celiac disease was concurrently suspected at the EGDS and successively confirmed at the histological analysis) and after *Helicobacter pylori* eradication. In this group, median age was 34.5 years (range 17–53), and the median body mass index was 23 kg/m^2. Symptoms developed between 0 and 15 months (median 2.5 months).

The most common presentation in the SMA group was "postprandial distress syndrome (epigastric pain and discomfort, nausea, and vomiting) dyspepsia" ($p = 0.02$), according to Rome IV criteria, and weight loss (median weight loss before diagnosis was 6 kg), while in the control group, the most common presentation was "epigastric pain syndrome" dyspepsia ($p = 0.01$), according to Rome IV criteria, with a less marked weight loss (median weight loss before diagnosis was 0.5 kg).

Premorbid conditions were present in 5 patients (anorexia nervosa in 2 patients and G6PDH deficiency, spina bifida, and Crohn's disease in 3 patients), whereas other metabolic and haematological comorbidities were observed in the control group (Figure 1). Only 2 of 10 patients of the SMA group and 1 in the control group were hospitalized, due to severe malnutrition. Median aortomesenteric angle was 22° ($p = 0.001$), and median aorta-SMA distance was 6 mm ($p < 0.001$).

With regard to the control group, both the radiological parameters were significantly associated with the diagnosis of SMA after an endoscopic suspicion.

Interestingly, all the patients improved on conservative treatment in spite of the surgical consultation proposed to each patient. Treatment strategies involved a conservative measure such as nasogastric decompression (in the two hospitalized patients) and hyperalimentation followed by oral feeding and frequent small meals, through a close clinical follow-up under the supervision of a gastroenterologist and a nutritionist.

Figures 2–4 show some representative cases of our study population.

4. Discussion

SMA syndrome represents still a diagnostic and therapeutic challenge. Its prevalence is 0.1–0.3% [9], according to the literature arising from imaging-based studies. To our knowledge, the present study is the first that shows a prevalence of

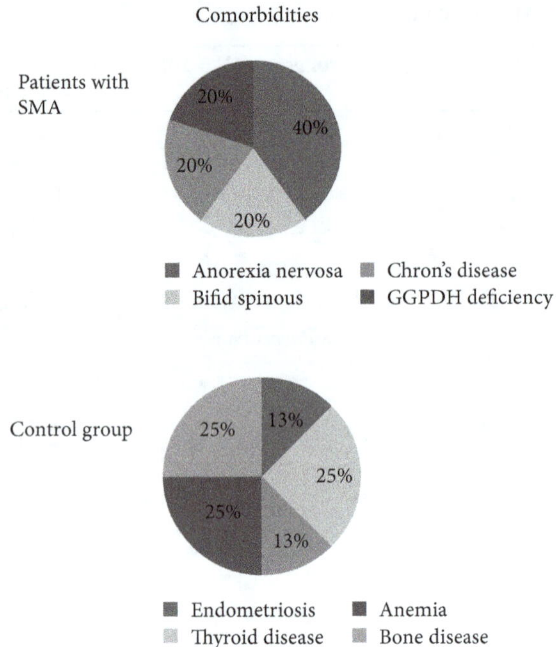

Figure 1: Percentage of patients with comorbidities in both groups (SMA and controls).

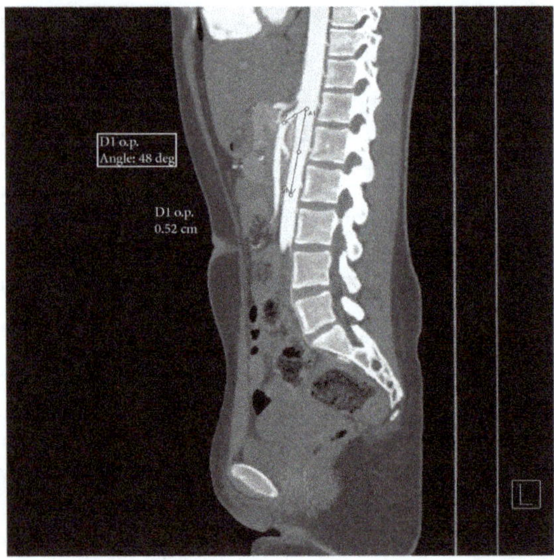

Figure 2: Sagittal reconstruction of a CECT scan showing the narrowing of the aortomesenteric angle and the reduction of the aorta-SMA distance (patient 1).

SMA syndrome based only on endoscopic findings, which could justify the relatively lower prevalence of this disease with regard to imaging studies. Interestingly, Merrett et al. published in 2009 a series of eight cases of SMA syndrome in which only one upper endoscopy suspected a possible obstruction of the third part of the duodenum [10].

Usually, SMA syndrome can present with an acute occurrence, such as a duodenal obstruction, or more insidiously, such as our patients who presented with long-standing vague abdominal pain, early satiety, anorexia, and recurrent episodes of abdominal pain associated with vomiting [11]. However, the diagnosis of the SMA syndrome is difficult and often delayed and complicated, due to its insidious presentation [1].

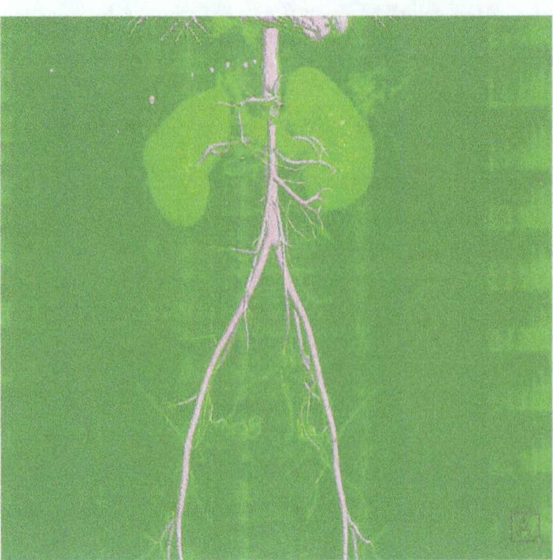

Figure 3: 3-D angiographic reconstruction of a CECT scan showing the narrowing of the aortomesenteric angle and the reduction of the aorta-SMA distance, in the same patient (patient 1).

In our series (see Table 2), a marked (>5 kg) weight loss ($p = 0.006$) and a long-standing presentation (more than six months in the 80% of patients) ($p = 0.002$) are significantly related to a diagnosis of confirmed SMA syndrome at CECT after an endoscopic suspicion. A "resembling postprandial distress syndrome dyspepsia" presentation may be helpful to the endoscopist in suspecting a latent SMA syndrome, similar to what emerged in our study.

However, this condition affects female patients, older children, adolescents, and even underweight individuals with a history of rapid weight loss [12, 13]. In our series, we confirmed a female preponderance and a higher prevalence of the syndrome in the young-adult age group, even if there was no statistical difference with regard to age and sex ratio between the SMA group and the control group.

Upper endoscopic examination may show a pulsatile extrinsic compression indicative of this syndrome, even if only an "experienced" endoscopist may recognize this particular finding. Advances in imaging, such as in CT and magnetic resonance imaging (MRI), have dramatically helped with clear visualization of the aortomesenteric angle and of the aortomesenteric distance, thus improving the diagnostic rate [14].

CECT criteria for the diagnosis of SMA syndrome include an aortomesenteric angle of less than 22° and an aortomesenteric distance of less than 8–10 mm [8]. Usually, the aortomesenteric angle and distance significantly correlate with BMI in a normal population [15]. In our cohort, both the parameters were significantly associated with the diagnosis of SMA after an endoscopic suspicion; however, the narrowing of the aortomesenteric distance seemed to be more

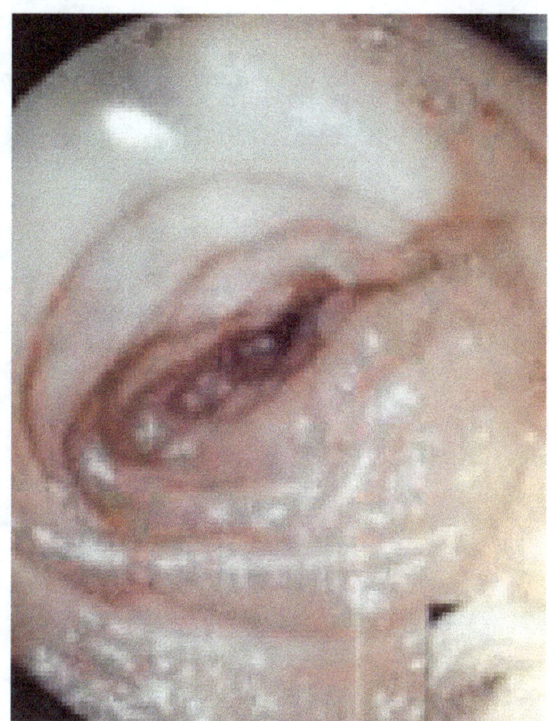

FIGURE 4: Endoscopic view showing the narrowing of the third part of the duodenum due to a pulsating extrinsic compression.

accurate, rather than the narrowing of the aortomesenteric angle, as diagnostic criterion for SMA syndrome, as previously suggested [16].

Furthermore, both CECT and MRI are helpful to assess intra-abdominal and retroperitoneal fat [8] and to identify other problems that may require intervention, like compression of the left renal vein that results in renal vein thrombosis.

Therefore, in the appropriate clinical context, detailed history as well as endoscopic and imaging findings could raise the diagnostic yield in the case of suspicion for the diagnosis of SMA syndrome. In fact, a delay in the diagnosis can potentially lead to many complications [1].

With regard to the treatment of SMA syndrome, although many patients require surgery, in our series, all the patients were taken under close clinical follow-up by both the gastroenterologist and the nutritionist. Treatment strategies involved conservative measures such as nasogastric decompression (in the two hospitalized patients) and hyperalimentation followed by oral feeding and frequent small meals, with parallel initiation of nutritional support, prokinetics, and proton pump inhibitors. Posturing techniques at the times of meals and motility agents may be helpful in these patients [17]. The role of nutritional counseling seemed to be particularly useful in the management of our patients during the follow-up.

All the patients, despite that a surgical consultation was proposed, did not require any surgical intervention, in contrast with previous studies [18], with the exception of isolated reports [11].

All the patients underwent a close clinical follow-up under the supervision of both the nutritionist and the gastroenterologist. A further endoscopical or radiological follow-up was not proposed, since guidelines about the follow-up of SMA syndrome do not exist, due to the invasiveness of upper endoscopy (in fact, once that the diagnosis was established, we did not consider a second look by endoscopy as useful) and due to the concern inherent to the exposure to ionizing radiation (since the patients experienced a positive clinical response).

In conclusion, with regard to a previously published series, our results show the following significant aspects: the importance of the endoscopic suspicion of SMA syndrome, when confirmed by CECT scan; the preponderance of a long-standing and chronic onset; a female preponderance; the importance of nutritional counseling in the therapeutic approach; the absence of a need for surgical intervention; and the better diagnostic accuracy of the narrowing of the aorta-SMA distance, rather than the narrowing of the aortomesenteric angle. However, further prospective studies, with a larger number of patients, are needed to clarify the best way to diagnose and manage the SMA syndrome.

Disclosure

The authors disclose that an earlier version of this work was presented as an abstract as shown at the following link: https://www.ueg.eu/education/document/superior-mesenteric-artery-syndrome-clinical-endoscopic-and-radiological-findings /122777/.

Authors' Contributions

Emanuele Sinagra designed the study. Emanuele Sinagra, Gaetano Cristian Morreale, Georgios Amvrosiadis, Domenico Albano, Valentina Guarnotta, and Melania Blasco wrote the paper. Sergio Testai, Federico Midiri, Giovanni Albano, Dario Sorrentino, Valerio Alaimo, Valentina Bova, Marta Marasà, and Vincenzo Mastrella collected and acquired radiological data. Guido Martorana, Francesco Cappello, Giovanni Tomasello, Marcello Giuseppe Spampinato, Massimo Midiri, and Dario Raimondo analyzed the data. Vittorio Virgilio supervised the work. All the authors critically revised the article and approved the final version to be published.

References

[1] E. Sinagra, L. M. Montalbano, C. Linea et al., "Delayed-onset superior mesenteric artery syndrome presenting as oesophageal peptic stricture," *Case Reports in Gastroenterology*, vol. 6, no. 1, pp. 94–102, 2012.

[2] V. Zaraket and L. Deeb, "Wilkie's syndrome or superior mesenteric artery syndrome: fact or fantasy?," *Case Reports in Gastroenterology*, vol. 9, no. 2, pp. 194–199, 2015.

[3] A. I. Tsirikos, R. E. Anakwe, and A. D. L. Baker, "Late presentation of superior mesenteric artery syndrome following scoliosis surgery: a case report," *Journal of Medical Case Reports*, vol. 2, no. 1, p. 9, 2008.

[4] G. H. Ballantyne, S. M. Graham, L. Hammers, and I. M. Modlin, "Superior mesenteric artery syndrome following ileal J-pouch anal anastomosis. An iatrogenic cause of early postoperative obstruction," *Diseases of the Colon and Rectum*, vol. 30, no. 6, pp. 472–474, 1987.

[5] J. M. Reckler, R. Majo, H. M. BRUCK et al., "Superior mesenteric artery syndrome as a consequence of burn injury," *The Journal of Trauma*, vol. 12, no. 11, pp. 979–985, 1972.

[6] P. A. Verhoef and A. Rampal, "Unique challenges for appropriate management of a 16-year-old girl with superior mesenteric artery syndrome as a result of anorexia nervosa: a case report," *Journal of Medical Case Reports*, vol. 3, no. 1, p. 127, 2009.

[7] L. S. Pasumarthy, D. E. Ahlbrandt, and J. W. Srour, "Abdominal pain in a 20-year-old woman," *Cleveland Clinic Journal of Medicine*, vol. 77, no. 1, pp. 45–50, 2010.

[8] M. E. Rabie, O. Ogunbiyi, A. S. Al Qahtani, S. B. M. Taha, A. El Hadad, and I. El Hakeem, "Superior mesenteric artery syndrome: clinical and radiological considerations," *Surgery Research and Practice*, vol. 2015, Article ID 628705, 5 pages, 2015.

[9] T. Welsch, M. W. Büchler, and P. Kienle, "Recalling superior mesenteric artery syndrome," *Digestive Surgery*, vol. 24, no. 3, pp. 149–156, 2007.

[10] N. D. Merrett, R. B. Wilson, P. Cosman, and A. V. Biankin, "Superior mesenteric artery syndrome: diagnosis and treatment strategies," *Journal of Gastrointestinal Surgery*, vol. 13, no. 2, pp. 287–292, 2009.

[11] C. Foster and A. Choudhary, "Severe malnutrition causing superior mesenteric artery syndrome in an adolescent with Triple A syndrome," *Journal of Pediatric Endocrinology and Metabolism*, vol. 29, no. 10, pp. 1221–1224, 2016.

[12] P. Vulliamy, V. Hariharan, J. Gutmann, and D. Mukherjee, "Superior mesenteric artery syndrome and the "nutcracker phenomenon"," *BMJ Case Reports*, vol. 2013, 2013.

[13] A. Bhagirath Desai, D. Sandeep Shah, C. Jagat Bhatt, K. Umesh Vaishnav, and B. Salvi, "Measurement of the distance and angle between the aorta and superior mesenteric artery on CT scan: values in Indian population in different BMI categories," *The Indian Journal of Surgery*, vol. 77, no. S2, pp. 614–617, 2015.

[14] B. Unal, A. Aktaş, G. Kemal et al., "Superior mesenteric artery syndrome: CT and ultrasonography findings," *Diagnostic and Interventional Radiology*, vol. 11, no. 2, pp. 90–95, 2005.

[15] H. Ozkurt, M. M. Cenker, N. Bas, S. M. Erturk, and M. Basak, "Measurement of the distance and angle between the aorta and superior mesenteric artery: normal values in different BMI categories," *Surgical and Radiologic Anatomy*, vol. 29, no. 7, pp. 595–599, 2007.

[16] O. J. Arthurs, U. Mehta, and P. A. K. Set, "Nutcracker and SMA syndromes: what is the normal SMA angle in children?," *European Journal of Radiology*, vol. 81, no. 8, pp. e854–e861, 2012.

[17] Z. Naseem, G. Premaratne, and R. Hendahewa, ""Less is more": non operative management of short term superior mesenteric artery syndrome," *Annals of Medicine and Surgery*, vol. 4, no. 4, pp. 428–430, 2015.

[18] S. Y. Yao, R. Mikami, and S. Mikami, "Minimally invasive surgery for superior mesenteric artery syndrome: a case report," *World Journal of Gastroenterology*, vol. 21, no. 45, pp. 12970–12975, 2015.

3

Noninvasive Biomarkers of Colorectal Cancer: Role in Diagnosis and Personalised Treatment Perspectives

Gianluca Pellino,[1,2] Gaetano Gallo,[3,4] Pierlorenzo Pallante,[5] Raffaella Capasso,[6] Alfonso De Stefano,[7] Isacco Maretto,[8] Umberto Malapelle,[9] Shengyang Qiu,[10] Stella Nikolaou,[10] Andrea Barina,[8] Giuseppe Clerico,[4] Alfonso Reginelli,[11] Antonio Giuliani,[12] Guido Sciaudone,[1] Christos Kontovounisios,[10,13] Luca Brunese,[6] Mario Trompetto,[4] and Francesco Selvaggi[1]

[1]*Unit of General Surgery, Department of Medical, Surgical, Neurological, Metabolic and Ageing Sciences, Università degli Studi della Campania "Luigi Vanvitelli", Piazza Miraglia 2, 80138 Naples, Italy*
[2]*Colorectal Surgery Unit, Hospital Universitario y Politécnico La Fe, Valencia, Spain*
[3]*Department of Medical and Surgical Sciences, OU of General Surgery, University of Catanzaro, Catanzaro, Italy*
[4]*Department of Colorectal Surgery, Clinic S. Rita, Vercelli, Italy*
[5]*Institute of Experimental Endocrinology and Oncology (IEOS), National Research Council (CNR), Via S. Pansini 5, Naples, Italy*
[6]*Department of Medicine and Health Sciences, University of Molise, Via Francesco de Sanctis 1, 86100 Campobasso, Italy*
[7]*Department of Abdominal Oncology, Division of Abdominal Medical Oncology, Istituto Nazionale per lo Studio e la Cura dei Tumori, "Fondazione G. Pascale, " IRCCS, Naples, Italy*
[8]*1st Surgical Clinic, Department of Surgical, Oncological, and Gastroenterological Sciences, University of Padua, Padua, Italy*
[9]*Dipartimento di Sanità Pubblica, Università degli Studi di Napoli Federico II, Naples, Italy*
[10]*Department of Colorectal Surgery, Royal Marsden Hospital, London, UK*
[11]*Department of Internal and Experimental Medicine, Magrassi-Lanzara, Institute of Radiology, Università degli Studi della Campania "Luigi Vanvitelli", Piazza Miraglia 2, 80138 Naples, Italy*
[12]*Department of Medicine and Health Sciences "V. Tiberio", University of Molise, Campobasso, Italy*
[13]*Department of Surgery and Cancer, Chelsea and Westminster Hospital Campus, Imperial College London, London, UK*

Correspondence should be addressed to Francesco Selvaggi; fselvaggi@hotmail.com

Academic Editor: Alessandro Passardi

Colorectal cancer (CRC) is the third leading cause of cancer-related deaths worldwide. It has been estimated that more than one-third of patients are diagnosed when CRC has already spread to the lymph nodes. One out of five patients is diagnosed with metastatic CRC. The stage of diagnosis influences treatment outcome and survival. Notwithstanding the recent advances in multidisciplinary management and treatment of CRC, patients are still reluctant to undergo screening tests because of the associated invasiveness and discomfort (e.g., colonoscopy with biopsies). Moreover, the serological markers currently used for diagnosis are not reliable and, even if they were useful to detect disease recurrence after treatment, they are not always detected in patients with CRC (e.g., CEA). Recently, translational research in CRC has produced a wide spectrum of potential biomarkers that could be useful for diagnosis, treatment, and follow-up of these patients. The aim of this review is to provide an overview of the newer noninvasive or minimally invasive biomarkers of CRC. Here, we discuss imaging and biomolecular diagnostics ranging from their potential usefulness to obtain early and less-invasive diagnosis to their potential implementation in the development of a bespoke treatment of CRC.

1. Introduction

Colorectal cancer (CRC) is the third most common cancer among men and women and the third leading cause of cancer-related deaths in the world, with an incidence of 1.2 million new cases and 608,700 deaths annually [1].

Metastasis accounts for approximately 90% of CRC-related deaths; this is mainly due to the absence of an ideal method of screening [2]. Detection of CRC at an early stage may confer a 90% 5-year survival rate, compared to 12% if distant metastasis occurs [3, 4].

One of the primary targets of screening is the identification of advanced colorectal adenomas.

The currently available screening modalities, such as the guaiac-based faecal occult blood test (gFOBT) and carcinoembryonic antigen (CEA) test, are effective but limited by low specificity and sensitivity. Sigmoidoscopy and colonoscopy are invasive, have certain morbidity risks, and require cumbersome preparatory procedures that lead to a low participation rate.

The gFOBT has been associated with a reduction of 15–33% in CRC-related mortality, particularly if the test is performed every 1 or 2 years [5, 6]. Despite being noninvasive, inexpensive, and easily applicable, it has low accuracy, particularly regarding the detection of preneoplastic lesions; it also has a low specificity rate leading to a high number of unnecessary colonoscopies [7, 8]. The new, more sensitive version of an antibody-based globin test, known as immunochemical FOBT or faecal immunochemical test (FIT), is inconvenient because the specimen needs to be sent to a laboratory for testing [9]. Nowadays, colonoscopy is the gold standard for the early diagnosis of CRC [10], but it has several risks such as bleeding, perforation, missed adenoma/cancer, and related death.

The ideal CRC biomarker should be easily and quantitatively measured, highly specific, and sensitive, as well as reliable and reproducible [11]. It should be able to stratify between different risk-based populations, selecting patients who really need a second-line test (endoscopic and radiologic investigations). Ideally, this aim can be achieved with a noninvasive and inexpensive method, using easily available biological samples such as urine, breath, serum, and faeces.

Despite the advances made over the last years, no single test is currently able to diagnose and monitor the posttreatment course of CRC patients. Herein, we review the current status of noninvasive biomarkers in CRC and provide insights for their implementation in the clinical management of patients.

2. Circulating Biomarkers and Eliminated Metabolites

2.1. Genetic and Epigenetic Alterations and CRC. Genetic and epigenetic changes characterizing the carcinogenesis of CRC are essential for the identification and development of an ideal biomarker [12]. Genetic markers are based on the identification of mutations in a subset of genes, including p53, APC, KRAS, NRAS, and DNA repair genes such as hMSH1 (human mutS homolog 1) or hMLSH2 [13, 14]. Unfortunately, this approach has a modest diagnostic sensitivity for invasive cancers and advanced benign tumors [15]. Epigenetic alterations include DNA methylation, microRNA (miRNA) expression, histone modification, and chromatin remodelling. They represent inheritable changes in gene expression without modifications to the DNA sequence.

DNA methylation consists in the enzymatic addition of a methyl group to cytosine in 5-position. The process is catalyzed by DNA methyltransferases and usually entails a covalent linkage within a CG dinucleotide sequence, termed CpG transcription [16].

Owing to their high tissue specificity and critical role in oncogenesis, miRNAs have the potential to be reliable biomarkers for the diagnosis and classification of CRC as well as for predicting treatment outcomes in the near future [17–19]. Several studies have recently demonstrated the role of miRNAs obtained from different body fluids (such as plasma, serum, urine, saliva, and tissues) in the pathogenesis of CRC (including metastasis spread [20]) with subsequent implications on treatment and prognosis [21].

The improvement of validated protocols and the discovery of new technologies such as next-generation sequencing (NGS) [22] allow a very careful evaluation of the whole miRNAome in different samples.

miRNAs are small single-stranded, noncoding RNAs, discovered in 1993 as developmental regulators in *Caenorhabditis elegans* [23, 24], with a length of 18–25 nucleotides [25]. Their aberrant expression patterns have been detected in various types of malignancies including breast cancer, lung cancer, pancreatic cancer, ovarian cancer, and CRC [26–28], playing an essential role as posttranscriptional regulators of carcinogenesis, progression, invasion, angiogenesis, and metastasis [25, 29–34].

They suppress translation or induce mRNA degradation by binding to the 3′ untranslated region (UTR) of their target genes [35]. More than 50% of the discovered human miRNA genes are localized in fragile chromosomal regions that are susceptible to amplification, deletion, or translocation during the natural history of CRC [36, 37]. This makes them the most promising future predictive markers for the diagnosis and prognosis of CRC; additionally, they could aid to determine the therapeutic response to chemotherapeutic drugs.

After several enzymatic reactions, the mature miRNA is integrated into the RNA-induced silencing complex (RISC) to then negatively regulate the expression of hundreds of target mRNAs by translation inhibition or mRNA degradation. This is achieved by the recognition of complementary sites on the target mRNA [38]. Consequently, miRNAs are able to give us more prognostic and diagnostic information than mRNAs. miRNAs also modulate T and B lymphocyte activation (both the innate and adaptive immune responses [39]), thus helping cancer cells avoid recognition by the immune system in the blood/lymph vessels.

Lastly, they target inflammatory signalling molecules, thereby inducing or inhibiting chronic inflammation and inflammation-related cancers. This is confirmed by studies on the expression of KRAS, which is inversely correlated with miR 143 [40] and c-Myc, which can promote tumoral growth via miR 17-92 [41]. Both miR 324-5p and miR 122 are involved in the regulation of TNF-alfa [42], CUEDC2 [43], and NOD2 [44].

2.1.1. Plasmatic miRNAs. Several miRNAs are dysregulated in the plasma of patients with CRC [45, 46]. They can either circulate freely or be in exosomes. Thanks to their small size, miRNAs are well protected from endogenous degradation [47–49] and can remain stable for a long period of time, in contrast to the fast degradation of mRNAs and proteins. Furthermore, cancer cells secrete some miRNAs into systemic circulation [48], confirming their central role in CRC screening.

The number of aberrantly expressed miRNAs in CRC tissues has rapidly grown due to the increasing number of studies on the topic [28, 50]. As an example, miR 17-92a has an oncogenic function because it is upregulated during the well-known adenoma-to-carcinoma sequence [51, 52].

miR 21, one of the most extensively investigated oncogenic miRNAs, is highly correlated with CRC cell proliferation, invasion, lymph node metastasis, and advanced clinical stage [53–55]. It is overexpressed in colorectal adenomas when compared with normal colonic mucosa [54]. It participates in the multistep process of CRC carcinogenesis, regulates several pathways such as MAPK and WNT/Beta-catenin [56–58], and its level decreases after surgical removal of CRC [59].

Other evaluated miRNAs are linked with hepatic metastasis. These can also be useful for early detection of CRC, as predictors of recurrence of CRC (stages II and III), and to determine the probability of resistance to preoperative chemoradiotherapy (CRT) in a CRC cell line [46, 60–67]. miR 92a is overexpressed in serum, plasma, and stool of patients with advanced adenoma, when compared to controls [66–68].

2.1.2. Faecal miRNAs. Exfoliated faecal colonocytes or tumor-secreted miRNAs are directly and continuously released from tumors into the intestinal lumen, providing a rationale for a stool-based miRNA test for the diagnosis of CRC [11, 69]. Furthermore, miRNAs in faeces correlate with the grading of the tumor [70]. Faecal miR 135b is elevated in CRC and adenomatous tissue samples in contrast to adjacent healthy tissue [71], whereas miR 106a can decrease the number of false negatives when using a gFOBT [72]. Unfortunately, the stool environment is much more complex (compared to plasma) and its testing requires a certain volume and density of the sample for each assay.

2.1.3. miRNAs, Diet, and Lifestyle. In CRC, there is a clear link between lifestyle, diet, and epigenetic factors expressed in an aberrant way. However, it is still debated whether changes in lifestyle can modify epigenetic mechanisms and reduce the risk of CRC progression.

Tarallo et al. [73] demonstrated the modulatory effect of different dietary habits on a panel of miRNAs; the highest differences in the expression (in stool and plasma samples) of miR 17-92 cluster among people with vegan, vegetarian, or omnivorous diet habits.

Several recent studies show that fish; oil-fed animals; vitamins A, D, and E; and minerals such as selenium and resveratrol (trans-3,4′,5′-trihydroxystilbene) can modify the levels of expressed miRNAs [73–79].

Various recent studies demonstrate a clear relationship between miRNA expression and CRC [80]. These new diagnostic possibilities are highly influencing the current research in the CRC field.

Endogenous miRNAs, packed and protected from the action of RNase (in contrast with rapid degradation of mRNA and proteins), allow us to discriminate normal colonic mucosa, colon adenomas, and carcinomas. The possibility of miRNA-based therapies, inhibiting oncogenic miRNAs or restoring tumor suppressor miRNAs, could open a new scenario in the treatment of CRC, despite the bias on the different methods for evaluating the population, methodology of collection of the used samples, and quantification methods.

2.1.4. Methylated DNA. Increased concentrations of circulating methylated DNA have been reported in the blood of cancer patients [81–83]. *SEPT9* is one of the most widely studied genes with an important role in the early diagnosis of CRC as well as in metastatic CRC.

In the PRESEPT study, Church and coworkers [84] found 666 (9.7%) advanced and 2359 (34.3%) nonadvanced adenomas in the 6874 patients who underwent colonoscopy. Among them, circulating methylated *SEPT9* has been identified in 9.6% of the advanced adenomas and 7.7% of the nonadvanced adenomas.

Barault et al. [85] identified candidate biomarkers of CRC analysing the methylation profile of CRC cell lines. Methylated ctDNA enables, in association with CT scan, the tracking of tumor response in metastatic CRC patients treated with chemotherapy (FOLFOX, FOLFIRI, ± bevacizumab) and targeted agents (panitumumab). They validated its use in monitoring metastatic CRC response to therapy, including chemotherapy, targeted therapy, and temozolomide in a longitudinal study. Furthermore, several authors evaluated the diagnostic performance of SEPT9 assay along with other blood-based methylated genes. The association of SEPT9 with TAC1 methylation assay yielded a sensitivity of 73.1% and a specificity of 92.3% [86] while its association with *TMEFF2* and *ALX4* further increased both sensitivity (80.7%) and specificity (90.0%) [87].

2.2. Neurotensins and CRC. There is increasing recognition that cancers of the gastrointestinal tract (pancreas as well as other organs) express receptors for various endogenous host hormones. This raises the possibility that hormones can play a role in the proliferation of these cancers and therefore highlights the potential of these hormonal signalling pathways as targets for novel cancer diagnostic and therapeutic strategies. One of these promising candidates in CRC is the tridecapeptide neurotensin (NT) [88, 89]. NT was first isolated in 1973 from the bovine hypothalamus and digestive tract [90]. Its physiological functions are those of a neurotransmitter in the central nervous system and of a hormone in the periphery. There is increasing evidence of the role it plays in CRC.

Some colonic tumors synthesise and release NT, resulting in autocrine control and cellular proliferation [91]. Physiological levels of NT appear to stimulate the growth of many human CRC cell lines (SW480, SW620, HT29, HCT116, and Cl.19A) expressing the NT receptor 1 (NTR1) [92]. NT accelerates colonic cancer carcinogenesis in animal models. For example, rats injected with both a CRC carcinogen and NT demonstrate a significant increase in the number, size, and invasiveness of colon tumors [93]. Administration of NT by itself significantly stimulated growth in murine colon tumors as well as human colon cancers xenografted into mice; it also resulted in a significant decrease in survival [94].

In humans, NT mRNA, peptide, and receptor were found in resected CRC specimens as well as four well-known human cancer cell lines *in vitro*. In surgical specimens where NT was identified in cancer cells, it was absent in adjacent normal bowel mucosa [91].

Gui et al. examined NTR1 expression in human CRC by measuring NTR1 mRNA in normal colonic mucosa, adenomas, and colonic adenocarcinomas. NTR1 mRNA expression was undetectable in epithelial cells of normal colonic epithelium, but it was expressed in adenomas and adenocarcinomas. Higher expression levels were seen in adenocarcinomas when compared to adenomas. Tissue from lymphovascular invasion showed even higher expression levels of NTR1 than that from the rest of the tumor. These results suggest that increased NTR1 expression may be an early event during colonic tumorigenesis that can also contribute to tumor progression and aggressive behaviour in colonic adenocarcinomas [95].

Evaluation of blood NT levels in colorectal cancer was recently conducted using 56 colorectal cancer patients and 15 controls; early evidence suggests that NT levels could differentiate between cancer and noncancer patient groups.

2.3. Liquid Biopsy. Biopsies have a central role in disease management, particularly in cancer patients. They allow clinicians to diagnose, determine a treatment course, and evaluate prognosis. In addition to specifying the histological nature of the disease, tissue biopsies are used to determine the genetic features of the tumor. This information can be used to treat patients with drugs tailored to the genetic makeup of their tumor and to give predictive and prognostic information.

However, although tissue biopsies are critical in the decision-making process, they have limitations. A single biopsy represents a snapshot of the complexity of molecular tumor alterations and tends to underestimate the real intratumoral heterogeneity [96]. Moreover, molecular targeted therapies may require multiple biopsies to accurately evaluate both the intratumoral heterogeneity and the genome modifications occurring during treatment because cancer genomes are also unstable and tend to change over time. Obtaining multiple biopsies at baseline and during the treatments is challenging owing to patient discomfort, procedural complications, costs, tumor accessibility, and the potential risk of tumor seeding.

In the field of precision medicine, the term liquid biopsy (LB) refers to those genetic tests performed on a biological component extracted from body fluids, in particular, from whole blood. This sample can be used to obtain circulating tumor cells (CTC), circulating tumor DNA (ctDNA), and exosomes [97, 98]; these components represent a small fraction of the total biological elements actively or passively released into the blood through metastisation processes, necrosis, or apoptosis. Today, many clinical trials have aimed to investigate the role of LBs in the management of metastatic CRC (mCRC) patients, specifically by analysing the role of CTC, ctDNA, and exosomes as alternative biological sources to monitor tumor evolution and response in a dynamic manner, considering that cancer is not a "molecularly stable" disease [99–101]. In addition, an LB represents a key approach to analyse, through a noninvasive and simple blood test, the molecular heterogeneity among different tumor sites in the same patient (primary tumor versus distant metastasis) to define the best target for a therapeutic approach or to monitor patients with no clinically detectable disease after surgery and standard therapy [99–106].

Plasma DNA that is analysed on CTC or on ctDNA has been suggested as an alternative way to evaluate tumor genomes [106–112]. CTCs are cancer cells derived from tumors that are released into the bloodstream through a process known as the epithelial-mesenchymal transition (EMT), from either a primary or metastatic site. In the past years, the simple presence of CTCs was an indicator of a poorer prognosis in CRC and other cancer types, such as breast, prostate, and lung cancer. CTC molecular characterization represents an attractive real-time option to monitor metastatic diffusion before instrumental detection [98–100].

Plasma cell-free DNA (cfDNA) is the result of DNA fragments that are released into circulation from both normal and tumor cells. Since CTC and ctDNA are valid sources to evaluate tumor genomes and can be considered as "surrogates" of tissue biopsies, they can be defined as LB. Initially, both CTC and ctDNA were used as simple quantitative markers. The analysis of clinical relevant mutations can also be feasible in a simple way by using ctDNA, even if it represents a small fraction of the total cfDNA released into the blood by healthy cells or primary cancer cells or directly by CTCs. Additionally, the quantity of cfDNA has a prognostic role in mCRC patients, and, overall, cfDNA levels have been demonstrated to be higher in cancer patients, when compared to healthy controls [101, 103, 105, 106].

In another recent study, Strickler et al. [113] reported results from clinical cfDNA testing of 1397 patients with advanced CRC. They compared these results with three large CRC tumor tissue sequencing cohorts. Evidence of ctDNA in the blood was similar to recent studies in colon cancer. Furthermore, authors identified a previously unreported cluster of EGFR extracellular domain (ECD) mutations involving V441 and S442 that accounted for 25% of all ECD mutations, representing an important and novel mechanism of resistance to EGFR blockade.

Analysis of plasma samples may offer several advantages in determining KRAS mutation status in patients who have progressed on EFGR target therapy. Siena et al. [114] studied the mechanism of secondary resistance in EGFR inhibitor-treated patients finding new *KRAS* mutations in 7.1% and 57.1% of patients whose tumor genotype was determined

Table 1

Potential applications of LB in CRC
Early diagnosis
Assessment of molecular heterogeneity of overall disease
Identification of genetic alterations for targeted therapy
Evaluation of tumor response after preoperative treatments
Monitoring of minimal residual disease
Assessment of evolution of resistance in real time

using tissuebased and plasmabased analyses, respectively, during treatment with the combination of irinotecan and panitumumab.

Exosomes are very interesting, small endocytic membrane vesicles that are initially isolated from the peripheral circulation of cancer patients and play a central role in the communication processes among cells by activation of surface ligands or by transferring of molecules among the cells. Exosomes can either manipulate the local and systemic environment, allowing cancer growth and dissemination, or modulate the immune system to elicit or suppress an antitumor response. In addition, exosomes represent a good source of DNA fragments, proteins, mRNA, miRNA, and other biological molecules and are protected by a lipid bilayer membrane, which confers a high degree of stability. Recently, many studies on exosomes demonstrate either a prognostic or predictive value, emphasizing their potentiality in clinical practice. A genome-wide expression profile of miRNAs has been shown to be significantly different among primary lung cancers and corresponding noncancerous lung tissues and thus has shown to have a potential role as a diagnostic marker [98, 105].

Therefore, in the near future, an integrated analysis of ctDNA, CTC, and exosomes could be used in a clinical setting for mCRC to refine patient therapy selection and management.

Currently, there is an increasing interest in the evaluation of genomic features available from LB.

The concept behind LB and its possible clinical applications in CRC is summarized in Table 1.

2.3.1. LB as a Diagnostic Biomarker. The first effort towards the clinical use of cfDNA from LB was the simple quantitative evaluation of plasma DNA. A significant difference in cfDNA levels was found in healthy subjects compared to cancer patients. Heitzer et al. [115] found that, compared to healthy subjects, stage IV CRC patients ($n = 32$) showed higher cfDNA levels with substantial variability. Moreover, a third of patients had a biphasic size distribution of plasma DNA fragments, and this finding was associated with increased CTC numbers and an elevated concentration of KRAS-mutated plasma DNA fragments. Therefore, CRC patients show not only higher levels of cfDNA but also a specific pattern of tumor DNA fragmentation.

Frattini et al. [116] performed a quantitative analysis of plasma DNA in 70 CRC patients and 20 healthy subjects at baseline and during follow-up. In a subset of CRC patients, they also compared the KRAS mutation and the p16INK4a promoter hypermethylation in tissue samples and in cfDNA. They found that plasma DNA levels are useful for diagnosing cancer as well as determining disease-free status and the presence of recurrence.

Unfortunately, the fraction of ctDNA originating from tumor cells is between 0.01% and more than 90%, and it can vary greatly [117].

2.3.2. LB as a Prognostic Biomarker. Clinical, radiological, histopathological, and molecular factors are widely used as prognostic factors of rectal cancer. Tumor alterations in LB could have the potential to be associated with prognosis. Lecomte et al. [118] evaluated KRAS mutations and epigenetic alterations such as hypermethylation of a cyclin-dependent kinase inhibitor in cfDNA of 8 stage I, 21 stage II, 16 stage III, and 13 stage IV CRC patients. KRAS mutations and epigenetic alterations were found in 20 to 50% of these patients, and all of the patients without evidence of KRAS mutations or epigenetic alterations showed a 2-year survival rate. They also found an association between plasma ctDNA levels and the prognosis of CRC patients. These findings were confirmed by Diehl et al. [117], who demonstrated that CRC patients who relapsed within 1 year after surgery had higher ctDNA levels at the time of recurrence.

Bertorelle et al. [119] evaluated the association between RNA-hTERT (telomere-specific reverse transcriptase) plasma levels and the overall survival of stage II CRC patients, for whom the value of adjuvant chemotherapy is still debated. Compared to patients with low hTERT levels, those with high hTERT levels showed a significantly poorer survival rate (hazard ratio = 3.30, 95% CI 1.98–5.52), suggesting that hTERT levels could support the decision of performing adjuvant chemotherapy in stage II CRC patients.

In the CAPRI-GOIM trial, conducted by Normanno et al. [120], 340 KRAS exon-2 wild-type metastatic CRC patients received first-line cetuximab plus FOLFIRI. Tumor samples were analysed using NGS while BEAMing (digital PCR technology combines emulsion PCR with magnetic beads and flow cytometry for the highly sensitive detection and quantification of mutant tumor DNA molecules) has been used to search for KRAS and NRAS mutations in plasma samples. They concluded that ctDNA may replace tumor tissue analysis.

2.3.3. LB as a Predictive Biomarker. The prediction of tumor responses to a neoadjuvant therapy is clinically relevant because it can allow for treatment modifications before or during the treatment and, ultimately, to a tailored therapy that avoids inefficient, toxic, and costly approaches. Moreover, a treatment fails when resistance develops against chemotherapeutic agents, as observed for KRAS in CRC patients [121]. In this setting, LB could be preferable to tissue biopsies to monitor molecular changes throughout therapy (e.g., biological drugs), thus avoiding repeated tumor tissue sampling; it could also be useful to detect drug resistance before it becomes clinically evident. Kuo et al. [122] compared KRAS mutations in cfDNA and primary tumor tissues and demonstrated that the detection rate of KRAS mutations

Table 2: Imaging Biomarkers.

Modality	Parameters	Application
CT	Anatomical and functional imaging (DCET-CT)	Staging and treatment response
MRI	Anatomical and functional imaging (DWI, DCE-MRI, TA)	Diagnosis, local staging, prognostic evaluation, treatment response
PET-CI	Metabolic and anatomical imaging	Diagnosis, staging and treatment response
PET-MRI	Metabolic and anatomical imaging	Diagnosis, staging, prognostic evaluation, treatment response

was 50% in plasma and 28.8% in resected primary tumor tissue with an agreement of 78.8%. Diaz et al. [123] showed that, in CRC patients without KRAS mutations, treatment with panitumumab induced mutations in 38% of cases within 5 and 6 months following treatment. In a blind prospective study, Thierry et al. [109] compared KRAS and BRAF mutation statuses in tumor tissue and cfDNA of mCRC patients. They showed a 100% diagnostic specificity and sensitivity for the BRAF V600E mutation and a 98% specificity and 92% sensitivity for the KRAS mutation by cfDNA analysis. In 98 clinically stage II-III rectal patients who underwent neoadjuvant CRT, RNA-hTERT plasma levels were found to be a promising biomarker of tumor response [124]. The posttherapy levels of hTERT statistically decreased, and the difference of cfRNA levels between post- and preneoadjuvant therapy independently predicted tumor response. Agostini el al. [125] evaluated the role of cfDNA as a predictor of tumor response in rectal cancer patients who underwent neoadjuvant CRT. Based on the findings that cfDNA arising from tumor cells can be recognized on the basis of fragment lengths (compared to physiological cfDNA), they found that the longer fragments of cfDNA (derived from tumor cells) and, in particular, the ratio between long and short fragments (derived from apoptosis), were associated with tumor response to neoadjuvant therapy.

2.3.4. LB as a Biomarker of Tumor Relapse. Another promising clinical application of an LB is the detection of tumor relapse after a curative treatment. Currently, local or distant recurrence is detected by clinical data and radiological imaging. These methods are costly with a questionable cost-effective value. An LB has the potential to overcome this limitation. Diehl et al. [117] demonstrated that it was possible to detect disease recurrence by monitoring tumor-specific alterations in the plasma of CRC patients after surgery with almost 100% sensitivity and specificity. The persistence of tumor alterations in cfDNA after a radical surgery was associated with an incomplete resection, thus allowing clinicians a very early identification of residual disease in patients. Frattini et al. [116] reported the role of cfDNA as a promising biomarker of recurrence; however, CEA determination is currently, even with its limitations, the only widely accepted biomarker used in clinical practice.

Resection radicality is one of the most important predictors for local recurrence and overall survival. In the largest prospective trial of minimal residual disease (MRD) to date, Tie et al. [126] performed next-generation-sequencing of 1046 plasma samples from 230 patients with resected stage II colorectal cancer. Thanks to the early decreases in ctDNA amounts in patients with metastatic disease, they demonstrated that plasma tumor DNA is a better marker for recurrence than carcinoembryonic antigen (CEA), which is currently used in the clinical setting.

The biological principles behind an LB are widely accepted, and the future applications are appealing. Although many studies support the role of LB as a new noninvasive tool in cancer detection and cancer-treatment settings, few studies have focused on the impact of using LB in the diagnosis and treatment of rectal cancer. Moreover, because this research topic is still relatively new, it is quite difficult to translate early findings into clinical applications. In addition, there are many technical aspects that differ between studies with a lack of standardization, which makes clinical application even more difficult. These considerations led to the conclusion that, although there is a solid theoretical basis and increasing evidence for its potential clinical use, the inclusion of LB into the clinical decision-making process for CRC diagnosis and treatment will require more time.

3. Imaging

The use of imaging in CRC has significantly evolved over the last decade, playing a key role in providing answers concerning diagnosis, staging, treatment optimization, and follow-up [126–131]. The imaging modalities currently available for CRC assessment (Table 2) can be divided into two main types: anatomical and functional. Anatomical imaging modalities still remain the mainstay, with computed tomography (CT) imaging suited for colon tumor evaluation and magnetic resonance imaging (MRI) optimal for rectal tumor assessment. However, with the development of new tracer and contrast agents, the evolution of fusion technologies between fludeoxyglucose positron emission tomography (FDG-PET) and MRI and the development of functional MRI techniques may offer new perspectives into cancer perfusion, metabolic, and molecular phenotypes [132]. During recent years, MRI has gained wide acceptance in the assessment of CRC and is considered the first-choice imaging modality for the primary staging and restaging after CRT [133–135]. In particular, despite CT, MRI is an imaging technique that provides functional data in addition to structural and anatomic details. Diffusion-weighted MRI (DW-MRI) and dynamic contrast-enhanced MRI (DCE-MRI) tools can allow to evaluate biological and functional modifications induced by treatment, also aiming to predict clinical outcomes in the setting of adjuvant therapies [136].

DW-MRI investigates and highlights the random movement ("diffusion") of water protons in the extracellular space of biological tissues and derives its imaging contrast from these differences. The diffusion of water molecules in biological tissues depends on many factors and is mainly influenced by cellular density [134, 137]. In tissues with low cellularity, water molecules can freely diffuse resulting in a low DW-MRI signal. On the contrary, this mobility is impeded or "restricted" in tissues with high cellularity (e.g., a tumor) due to reduced extracellular space, resulting in a high DWI-MRI signal. Water proton diffusion can be quantified by the means of the apparent diffusion coefficient (ADC), which reflects the degree of restriction of water molecules (diffusion), indirectly reflecting tissue cellularity [134, 136].

Recognizing these properties, DW-MRI can be a useful tool to detect CRC in cases where the identification of cancer with conventional MRI sequences and CT may be difficult. This technique is useful in cases including malignant transformation within nonspecific mural thickening, desmoplastic reaction, fibrotic or inflammatory changes due to inflammatory bowel disease (IBD), pelvic extraintestinal malignancy, or radiotherapy [138–141]. The addition of DWI-MRI to the conventional T2-weighted sequences improves lesion conspicuity of rectal cancer with 96% sensitivity and a positive predictive value of up to 100% [142, 143]. In this regard, Barral et al. reported that DW-MRI is able to reveal malignant foci in rectal involvement by IBD [140]. Similarly, several studies suggested that DWI-MRI also increases the sensitivity for the diagnosis of colon cancer, with the ability to discriminate between colon cancer and acute diverticulitis in patients with uncertain CT findings (due to a pseudotumoral diverticulitis pattern [142–145]). The use of DWI-MRI could also aid to exceed the limitation of conventional MRI sequences in discriminating between T2 and T3 cancer because the former may present with a desmoplastic reaction resembling cancer invasion.

By quantitative analysis, the ADC value of rectal cancer is reported to be significantly lower than that of a normal rectal wall, with a threshold ADC value of $1.240 \times 10{-}3\ mm^2/s$ having a sensitivity of 94% and a specificity of 100% for the diagnosis of rectal cancer [146]. The ADC value has been proposed as a potential biomarker for rectal cancer because it seems to correlate with tumor aggressiveness [147, 148]. ADC values correlate with mesorectal fascia invasion, lymph node involvement, histological differentiation, CA 19-9 and Ki-67 levels, and AgNOR counts [148, 149]. It also helps to differentiate between mucinous carcinoma and tubular adenocarcinoma [150].

DW-MRI is now more commonly used to assess early tumor changes and response after treatment [151, 152]. Treatment-induced cellular death and vascular changes can precede tumor size variation; thus, ADC variations may be a useful biomarker of treatment outcome for drugs that induce apoptosis and neoadjuvant CRT in locally advanced cancer [151]. In the literature, although controversial, it has been found that rectal cancer with low ADC values ($<1.0 \times 10{-}3$ mm2/s) has a better response to CRT [153, 154]. Similarly, it has been demonstrated that liver metastasis with a high ADC baseline value shows a poor response to chemotherapy because it is commonly characterized by necrosis and cellular membrane disruption, suggesting an aggressive phenotype [155]. Another approach by Cai et al. showed that the signal intensity and signal intensity ratio of the tumor on DWI-MRI was more accurate than ADC measurements to assess complete tumor response [156].

Treatment-induced change is often preceded by perfusion alterations as changes of permeability, blood volume, and blood flow [157]. Because capillary perfusion influences the delivery of drugs to cancer cells, measurement of capillary perfusion by DCE-MRI is described as a surrogate marker for evaluating the efficacy of chemotherapy with bevacizumab [158]. Thanks to the fast imaging acquisition after intravenous contrast medium administration, DCE-MRI is an attractive modality for assessing antiangiogenic cancer treatments because it reveals changes in cancer vascularization and even predicts cancer shrinkage, otherwise reflecting a prognostic tumor phenotype [133, 158]. The improvement of postprocessing and the implementation of more complex algorithms of extraction of the signal decrease in DWI-MRI allow to separate tissue diffusivity and microcapillary perfusion. In detail, the biexponential model is based on the intravoxel incoherent motion (IVIM) theory introduced by Le Bihan et al., as a method useful to assess both perfusion and diffusion [159, 160]. This method could allow an early diagnosis of tumor response to CRT or new therapeutic agents like antiangiogenics [161, 162].

Heterogeneity is a well-recognized feature of malignancy associated with increased tumor aggression and treatment resistance. Texture analysis (TA) is an emerging image processing algorithm that can quantify heterogeneity of cancers. Recently, it has been reported that textural features of rectal cancer, assessed by textural analysis (TexRAD) using a filtration-histogram technique of T2-weighted pre- and post-CRT, can predict the outcome before undergoing surgery and could potentially select patients for individual therapy [163].

Malignant cells have high glucose metabolism, and the differential uptake of 18FDG by cancer cells can be used to detect both the short- and the long-term tumor responses, which either are not evident on CT or foresee a decrease in tumor size [164]. Integrated FDG-PET-CT provides complementary metabolic information that allows the detection of malignant disease in morphologically normal organs or at unexpected sites that can be easily overlooked on cross-sectional imaging [165]. The combination of metabolic and anatomical imaging increases sensitivity and specificity of cancer detection and is useful to evaluate treatment response [136, 166]. When assessed by FDG-PET-CT, metabolic response to therapy correlates with clinical response, tumor biology, and disease-free survival in CRC patients [166]. However, unlike CT scans, a validated scheme for assessing cancer response to therapy with FDG-PET-CT is not available [128]. In addition to FDG, other PET radiotracers can be employed to image intracellular processes targeted for therapy. Indicators of cellular proliferation include 18F-FLT, 11C-choline, and 18F-choline, whereas 15O-water and 18-F-FMISO indicate perfusion and hypoxia, respectively [136]. Hypoxia is known to contribute to CRT resistance, leading to angiogenesis and potential development of metastasis [165]. An imaging biomarker for radioresistance, such as 18-F-FMISO, could be employed to determine any differentials within the cancer and used to modulate radiotherapy in order to appropriately vary the radiation field and also to identify resistant areas that can be selectively dose escalated [137].

A novel approach of molecular imaging using PET-CT is the employment of radiolabelled antibodies or antibody fragments, such as 89Zr-rituximab, which allows to assess the distribution and availability among cancer cells of the epidermal growth factor receptor [167, 168]. This may support decision making for the selection of patients likely to benefit from therapy, identification of dose-limiting tissue, and optimization therapeutic planning [168].

Recently, thanks to new fusion technologies, a hybrid PET-MRI machine became available allowing functional imaging with simultaneously acquired PET and MRI data, changing the management of cancer patients [169–172]. This hybrid tool exceeds some limitations of FDG-PET-CT by allowing better soft tissue evaluation, more accurate T-staging, and improved characterization of small liver lesions and by providing better anatomical details for surgical planning while minimizing radiation exposure [169]. By adding functional MRI to PET, PET/MRI may further improve diagnostic accuracy in the differentiation of scar tissue for recurrence of CRC [172].

4. Nanotechnology and CRC Diagnosis

In recent years, nanotechnologies have made striking improvements in the diagnosis and treatment of human cancers. Specifically, they have enabled the development of nanomedicine, a new branch of medicine based on the use of nanomaterials in different activities, research, and clinical settings to improve the diagnosis and treatment of diseases [173]. Their applications in medicine are possible because nanoparticles (NPs) are resistant to oxidation, are easy to generate, and are full of interesting optical properties [174]. Additionally, other important characteristics such as biocompatibility, adaptable toxicity, dimension and surface chemical features, and a good stability in biological fluids and tissues [169] permit us to use them as active nanosystems in biomedicine [175–178].

In addition, because they are very small (nanometric scale), they are able to directly interact with cell and subcellular structures, although in a nonselective manner [175–177]. In principle, this could limit the utilization of NPs for specific applications; however, the organic groups and molecules linked to the NP surface (functionalization) allow to overcome this problem [174], thus improving the quality of the NP (based on the chemical groups linked on its surface, it can be used in different applications [174]). Further improvements to NPs include linking polyethylene glycol (PEG) molecules to its surface (to avoid passive extravasation and to increase their half-life in the circulation [168–180]) and the optimization of functionalization protocols that otherwise tend to generate agglomeration and agglutination of NPs [181, 182]. Finally, the addition of specific fragments capable of recognizing particular cell surfaces allows the NPs to transfer, accumulate, and promote the internalization of NP in a specific manner by tumor cells [183, 184].

4.1. Nanotechnologies in Noninvasive Diagnosis. Nanobioconjugates produced as previously described have been successfully used in the diagnosis of colorectal cancer [185]; in particular, various types of applications lead to an effective improvement of diagnostic techniques.

First of all, we know that, although MRI represents an indispensable noninvasive tool for diagnosis (it does not use ionizing radiation like computer tomography), it is still not sufficiently adequate to achieve 3D resolutions in real time [174]. However, this method is undergoing several improvements thanks to the use of magnetic nanobioconjugates as a contrast medium (magnetic particle imaging (MPI)), which help to increase the specificity and sensitivity of detection [174]. Among the NPs used effectively in these imaging techniques, we include iron oxide and nanobioconjugates constituted by liposomes, micelles, and dendrimers carrying paramagnetic ions [183, 186]. In addition, NPs have been used in a new noninvasive imaging technique (not employing ionizing radiation) defined as photoacoustic tomography, which combines ultrasound with the optical contrast provided by nanocages, carbon nanotubes, and gold speckled silica particles [187, 188]. Magnetic nanocrystals have also been used for multimodal diagnosis employing MPI and fluorescence [175]. As far as CRC is concerned, successful applications have been made with quantum dots (QD) [185]. These NPs are constituted by nanocrystals of a semiconductor and are capable of emitting fluorescence following excitation. Their particular optical characteristics provide them a series of advantages in several applications for cancer, including CRC [189, 190]. In particular, one study [191] reported an improvement of the immunohistochemical evaluation using QD in the procedure (QD-IHC). This methodology could be also applied to the immunocytochemical evaluation of antigens on the surface of living cells in a noninvasive manner, opening new perspectives in the evaluation of CTC in clinical practice [191]. Other studies demonstrated their eminent role in *in vivo* MRI diagnosis [192] and in CRC targeting of QD linked to bevacizumab [193]. In the latter case, noninvasive nanoprobes were able to detect CRC expressing high levels of VEGF. Additional methodologies, which take advantage of the useful characteristics of QD, are currently being evaluated and applied in the field of CRC diagnosis.

Another class of NPs employed in the analysis of CRC is constituted by dendrimers [185]. These are macromolecular structures that, starting from a centre, are formed by the addition of several repeated and branching elements. Similar to other NPs, these features conferred them the opportunity to be used in several applications of cancer nanomedicine [194, 195].

5. Bespoke Treatment: Role of Biomarkers in Clinical Setting

For many years, chemotherapy for mCRC was based simply on the combination of 5-fluorouracil (5-FU) plus levamisole

(LV), a treatment that could improve median survival up to 11 months [196]. During the last 20 years, the association of oxaliplatin or irinotecan with 5-FU/LV led to an improvement in the outcome of patients affected by mCRC [197, 198]. Independently from the first-line therapy choice, patients receiving all available anti-CRC drugs may report a prolonged overall survival (OS) exceeding even 2 years [199]. The introduction of target therapies (bevacizumab, cetuximab, panitumumab, aflibercept, and regorafenib) has further ameliorated overall survival in the metastatic setting. As these agents are active on processes controlling cell growth, survival, angiogenesis, and spread following selective pathways, the efficacy of these drugs depends on a strict selection linked to particular molecular profiles.

The combination of mAbs binding to the vascular endothelial growth factor and EGFR with chemotherapy in mCRC has been shown to improve the efficacy, thus increasing treatment options [200, 201].

With the aim to optimize treatments, it is now well recognized that the variable responses among mCRC patients are influenced by the molecular profile of the tumor, which is specific and different among all individuals. Therefore, it is essential to individualize these different molecular aspects.

In the management of mCRC, several prognostic and predictive biomarkers have been identified over the past years and they can be used to define a personalised treatment for patients. Prognostic biomarkers identify patients regardless of treatment and may provide details about the disease prognosis. Predictive biomarkers help categorize patients potentially benefiting from a specific treatment or that show resistance [202] towards it. Thus, many analyses were conducted to identify tumor-related predictive factors aimed to suggest treatment responses [203].

The Erb family of cell membrane receptors includes HER1/erbB1 (EGFR), HER2/c-neu (ErbB-2), HER3 (ErbB-3), and HER4 (ErbB-4) [204]. As the EGFR gene was initially identified as an oncogene, it has become progressively the main target of biologic agents, prompting the development of anti-EGFR mAbs and tyrosine kinase inhibitors (TKIs). mAbs cetuximab (an anti-IgG1) and panitumumab (an anti-IgG2) act by binding to the extracellular domain site of the receptor, whereas erlotinib and gefitinib, two EGFR TKIs, compete with the binding site of ATP to the TK portion of the receptor, resulting in the inhibition of EGFR autophosphorylation. Both strategies (mAb and TKI) suspend the intracellular downstream signalling transmission.

The first clinical trials exploring the efficacy of anti-EGFR mAbs enrolled patients whose tumors expressed high levels of EGFR; however, overall response rates (ORRs) were low [205], which suggested the need of identifying additional factors potentially affecting the response to these agents [206]. Lièvre et al. were the first to identify a relation between mutant KRAS and poor responsiveness to EGFR-targeted treatments [207]. Thirty patients treated with cetuximab combined with irinotecan as second/third-line treatment were considered. KRAS mutations were detected in 13 of the 30 (43%) patients. None of the responders (0/11) had KRAS mutations, whereas 68.4% (13/19) of nonresponders presented them ($p = 0.0003$). The OS was significantly higher in wild-type KRAS (KRAS-WT) patients than in patients carrying a KRAS mutation (median OS: 16.3 versus 6.9 months, respectively, $p = 0.016$).

The next challenge was to understand why KRAS-mutated tumors did not respond to anti-EGFR mAbs. In this context, studies focused on key signalling molecule downstream of EGFR, including mutations in the KRAS, NRAS, BRAF, and PIK3CA genes and PTEN protein expression.

In the EGFR/RAS/RAF/MEK/ERK kinase downstream path, the KRAS protein is a GTPase that normally binds to the interior fragment of the cell wall. It conveys external signals from the receptor to the nucleus, regulating cell cycle (growth, proliferation, and apoptosis). The KRAS gene is located on the short arm of chromosome 12. Patients harboring point mutations in the KRAS gene generally have mutations within codon 12 at exon 2 (82%–87%), codon 13 (13%–18%), codon 61 (exon 3), and codon 146 (exon 4) [208]. In wild-type subjects, the activity of anti-EGFR mAbs on the external part of the receptor causes conformational changes blocking the RAS/RAF/MEK/ERK transmission. KRAS mutations impede EGFR activity for the constitutive activation of the intracellular fragment of the KRAS protein. In mCRC patients, the incidence of KRAS mutations is about 30%–45% [209].

Two randomized clinical trials comparing panitumumab or cetuximab with no active care in pretreated and chemorefractory mCRC patients [121, 208] demonstrated that KRAS mutant patients do not benefit from anti-EGFR mAbs. In the CO.17 [121] and AMGEN [208] studies, only KRAS-WT patients treated with cetuximab (median OS: 9.5 months versus 4.8 months) or panitumumab (median PFS: 12.3 weeks versus 7.3 weeks) had a survival benefit over best supportive care. In the cohort of patients with KRAS mutations, mAbs did not prolong PFS or OS.

The Cetuximab Combined With Irinotecan in First-Line Therapy for Metastatic Colorectal Cancer (CRYSTAL) phase III trial enrolled 599 patients to receive FOLFIRI plus cetuximab and 599 patients in the arm with FOLFIRI alone [210]. Sixty-four percent of the cases were exon 2-KRAS-WT; in these patients, both the risk of disease progression (HR of PFS: 0.68 [95% CI 0.50–0.94]) and that of death (HR of OS: 0.84 [95% CI 0.64 to 1.11] were lower in cetuximab-treated patients. No difference in PFS or OS was reported in the experimental arm in mutated patients.

The role of KRAS as a prognostic biomarker in CRC is quite controversial. The CO.17 study [121] analysed the prognostic involvement of KRAS status by assessing the interaction between KRAS status and survival in patients receiving best supportive care alone. There were no significant differences in median OS in either KRAS-WT or KRAS-MUT patients (4.8 months versus 4.6 months, resp.).

Similarly, Kim et al. [211] found that clinical outcomes did not differ between KRAS-WT and KRAS-MUT mCRC patients treated with chemotherapy alone. The RASCAL Collaborative Group evaluated the prognostic role of KRAS among thousands of patients with any-stage CRC [212, 213]. They found that KRAS-MUT patients presented shorter PFS and OS compared to wild-type patients. The RASCAL-2 study concluded that the G12 V mutation in the KRAS gene at codon 12 increases the risk of relapse or death only in Dukes' C CRC [213].

The retrospective analysis performed on mCRC patients in the MRC FOCUS trial [214] showed that KRAS mutations have a modest negative prognostic impact on OS (HR = 1.24; 95% CI 1.06–1.46; $p = 0.008$), but not on PFS (HR = 1.14; 95% CI 0.98–1.36; $p = 0.09$).

Neuroblastoma-ras (NRAS) is a member of the RAS oncogene family and is located on chromosome 1. The product of this gene is a GTPase enzyme membrane protein that shuttles between the Golgi apparatus and the cellular membrane. KRAS, BRAF, and NRAS mutations are mutually exclusive [215]. In CRC, the NRAS mutation rate is 3%–5% [216]. NRAS mutations are associated with the lack of response to cetuximab treatment. In the study by De Roock et al., NRAS-MUT patients treated with either cetuximab or panitumumab (2.6% of 644 KRAS-WT subjects) had a significantly lower ORR than NRAS-WT patients (7.7% versus 38.1%). PFS and OS did not differ statistically between mutated and wild-type patients.

A retrospective evaluation of biomarkers from patients enrolled in the PRIME trial indicated that NRAS plays an important role in predicting the efficacy of panitumumab treatment. Among the 656 patients with KRAS-WT exon 2, 108 (17%) had other mutations in KRAS exon 3 or 4, in NRAS exons 2, 3, or 4, or in BRAF exon 15 [217]. Patients with KRAS-WT exon 2 tumors bearing any RAS mutation did not achieve any benefit from panitumumab (median OS 17.1 months versus 17.1 months; $p = 0.12$). "All RAS" wild-type tumors (namely, wild type for KRAS exons 2/3/4 and for NRAS exons 2/3/4) significantly benefited from the combination treatment (median OS 25.8 months versus 20.2 months HR = 0.77; 95% CI 0.64–0.94; $p = 0.009$).

To elucidate the mechanisms of resistance to anti-EGFR antibodies, Bertotti et al. [218] performed a whole-exome analysis of 129 tumors in patient-derived xenografts detecting mutations in ERBB2, EGFR, FGFR1, PDGFRA, and MAP2K1 that could be potential mechanisms of primary resistance to anti-EGFR antibody therapy in CRC. Furthermore, investigation showed that amplifications and mutations in the tyrosine kinase receptor adaptor gene (IRS2) may contribute to the increased sensitivity to anti-EGFR therapy, representing a potential biomarker to predict full response to anti-EGFR-related CRC therapy.

Following these results, retrospective subanalyses were done on all the surviving wild-type patients enrolled in the CRYSTAL and OPUS trials. The results confirmed the important role of RAS mutational status in the optimal management of mCRC. Mutated patients do not benefit from anti-EGFR treatment, to the extent that this treatment could even be detrimental compared with chemotherapy alone. Therefore, in a real-life setting, the RAS mutational analysis has become essential and mandatory before beginning an anti-EGFR-based treatment.

5.1. BRAF. The BRAF protein is a cytoplasmic serine-threonine kinase bearing mutations in approximately 8%–10% of sporadic CRC [219]. The BRAF protein is one of the main effectors of KRAS; it is located immediately after KRAS effectors and it must be phosphorylated by KRAS to be activated. The point mutation V600E causes a CTG to CAG substitution at codon 600, which leads to a constitutive activation of the RAS/RAF/MEK/ERK cascade, similar to KRAS mutations.

In the retrospective analysis performed by Di Nicolantonio and colleagues, 113 tumor samples treated with cetuximab or panitumumab (with or without chemotherapy) were analysed and 79 KRAS-WT patients were identified. In this cohort, 11 (13.9%) patients were BRAF mutants and none of them responded to treatment.

In the CRYSTAL study [210], 9% (59 of 625) of patients carried BRAF mutations and they reported limited benefits from treatment with a shorter median OS in both arms, compared with the KRAS-WT and BRAF-WT population whose survival was 21.6 and 25.1 months, respectively. BRAF-MUT status was unrelated to cetuximab efficacy; thus, the authors concluded that BRAF mutation is a negative prognostic biomarker and not a predictive factor. Moreover, in the combined analysis of the CRYSTAL and OPUS results [220], a BRAF mutation was considered a negative prognostic marker in conclusion. In fact, survival times were lower in the BRAF-MUT population irrespective of therapy administered.

A BRAF mutation was also considered a negative prognostic biomarker in the PRIME trial [217]. In fact, patients with RAS-WT but BRAF-MUT tumors had a worse PFS and OS compared to subjects with wild-type RAS and BRAF tumors. In the RAS-WT/BRAF-MUT subgroup, the addition of panitumumab to chemotherapy produced a small benefit (difference was not statistically significant) in term of DFS and OS ($p = 0.12$ and 0.76, resp.).

The negative prognostic role of BRAF was also explored in clinical trials that enrolled patients to receive an intensive chemotherapy regimen plus an anti-VEGF treatment. The TRIBE trial compared the effect of bevacizumab plus the standard chemotherapy FOLFIRI with the association of 5-fluorouracil, irinotecan, levamisole, and oxaliplatin (FOLFOXIRI schedule). Final results of this trial showed a better outcome with the experimental arm; results showed an improvement of median PFS, OS, and ORR. A subset analysis was also performed in BRAF-MUT patients. Among the assessed patients, 28 (7%) BRAF-MUT patients reported a median OS of 13.7 months, significantly short if compared with the 37.1 months calculated for all wild-type patients [221].

It has been recently debated if a BRAF mutation could be considered a negative predictive factor too. Two meta-analyses were published in 2015 highlighting BRAF function. Pietrantonio et al. [222] assessed the negative predictive role covered by this mutation, which was mainly exerted towards anti-EGFR treatment. Rowland et al. [223] concluded that a BRAF mutation could only be considered as a negative prognostic biomarker (based on a not-significant interaction test and on the absence of a sufficient amount of data).

In conclusion, a BRAF mutation should be considered a negative prognostic biomarker rather than a negative predictive factor influencing anti-EGFR mAbs. BRAF-MUT patients have a poorer prognosis than BRAF-WT patients, irrespective of schedule of chemotherapy. These patients may benefit from anti-EGFR mAb treatment, but to a significantly lesser extent than BRAF-WT patients.

5.2. HER-2. The HER family of tyrosine kinase receptors consists of EGFR, HER2 (ErbB2), HER3, and HER4. They are responsible for cell survival and proliferation via signalling through the RAS-RAF-ERK and PI3K-PTEN-AKT pathways [224].

HER2 is a potential therapeutic target in patients with CRCs, and it is overexpressed in 25–35% of human breast cancers [225]. The level and incidence of HER2 overexpression in primary CRCs appear to be different.

In 2012, The Cancer Genome Atlas (TCGA) Network published the most comprehensive systematic molecular characterization of CRC to date, revealing genomic amplifications or mutations of the tyrosine kinase-encoding gene *ERBB2* in 7% of colorectal tumors, suggesting a novel potential therapeutic target for this cancer [226].

Several studies have assessed HER2 overexpression in CRC, with some reporting membranous expression, varying in the range 2.1–11% in [227–233], and others reporting cytoplasmic overexpression in the range 47.4–68.5% [230, 234, 235].

Kavuri and colleagues [236] studied the effect of ERBB2-targeted therapy in *ERBB2*-mutated CRC demonstrating that engineered intestinal cell lines that host *ERBB2* mutations are highly sensitive to irreversible EGFR/ERBB2 tyrosine kinase inhibitors, neratinib and afatinib, with these inhibitors inducing effective inhibition of ERBB2 and its downstream pathways.

Furthermore, xenografts from these cells lines were also sensitive to both neratinib and the combination of neratinib and trastuzumab. Interestingly, single-agent neratinib in a patient-derived xenograft (PDX) harboring *ERBB2* L866M mutation and amplification resulted in tumor stabilization and not in tumor regression as in the case of the combination of trastuzumab and neratinib. This result has been confirmed in another PDX harboring *ERBB2* S310Y mutation. Both PDX models were resistant to trastuzumab alone.

Anti-EGFR therapies, including cetuximab and panitumumab, have improved the prognosis of patients with CRC, particularly in the case of wild-type *KRAS* genes, in which these agents exhibit greater effectiveness [210, 237–239]. KRAS activities downstream the EGFR pathway and its spontaneous activation because mutation promotes cell proliferation despite the presence of anti-EGFR antibody [240].

In the previously described trial, sequencing CRC tumors with *ERBB2* mutation, Kavuri et al. [236] found that 50% (6/12) had a coccurring *KRAS* mutation.

Similarly, Kloth et al. [241] reported that three of 14 of *ERBB2*-mutated MSI CRC harbored *KRAS* mutation. Even though this cooccurrence could be justified in hypermutated MSI tumors, it is a surprising finding in the nonhypermutated tumors. Above all, several studies have exclusively evaluated mutant or amplified *ERBB2* as a target in tumors or models lacking such *KRAS* alterations. Further studies will be needed to better define both the etiology of this cooccurrence as well as the therapeutic consequences.

Based on promising preclinical studies in *ERBB2*-amplified CRC [242, 243], Siena et al. [244] conducted a phase II clinical trial of dual ERBB2 blockade. Patients with *ERBB2*-amplified, *KRAS* exon 2 wild-type, metastatic CRC who progressed after multiple lines of therapy, were treated with trastuzumab and lapatinib. Of 913 patients screened, 44 (4.8%) were found to be *ERBB2* amplified. Among 23 patients treated with dual anti-ERBB2 therapy, 8 (35%) patients had an objective response.

Similarly, trastuzumab and pertuzumab demonstrated response rates of 23% and disease control rates of 69% in the colorectal arm of a basket study [245]. These results were consistent with those of Valtorta et al [246].

Recent studies do suggest that HER2 overexpression by gene amplification may indeed be related to poor outcome in *KRAS* wt metastatic CRC patients treated with cetuximab or panitumumab [247].

In a study of 137 patient-derived xenograft (PDX) tumors, conducted by Hurwitz and colleagues, HER2 amplification was found in 13.6% of cases in patients with cetuximab-resistant, *KRAS* wild-type tumors [243].

Although patients with *HER2* amplification were resistant to anti-EGFR antibody therapy, other treatment strategies, including lapatinib or trastuzumab, can overcome cetuximab resistance in CRCs [242]. Finally, in addition to the previously reported trial conducted by Siena et al. [244], Deeken et al. [248] concluded that the combination of cetuximab and lapatinib provided a partial response in some patients with CRC who were resistant to anti-EGFR antibody therapy.

5.3. MSI-H. There are two molecular pathways in colorectal carcinogenesis. One is chromosomal instability (CIN) and the other is microsatellite instability (MSI) [249, 250].

High-level microsatellite instability (MSI-H) CRCs constitute approximately 15% of all CRCs in Western countries [251–253], more frequent in the early than the late stage of disease. The cause of MSI-H colorectal cancers is a deficiency of the DNA mismatch repair (MMR) system characterized by unstable microsatellites, a type of simple DNA sequence repeat. Its role consists in the postreplicative control of newly synthesised DNA strands and the correction of polymerase misincorporation events [254, 255].

MSI-H colorectal cancers can occur as sporadic tumors, because of methylation of promoter regions of the hMLH1 during tumorigenesis [256], or in the context of hereditary nonpolyposis colorectal cancer (HNPCC) or Lynch syndrome (LS) [257] with mutations of DNA MMR genes, primarily hMLH1, hMSH2, hMSH6, and hPMS2.

A defect in MMR is not manifested until both alleles of an MMR gene are inactivated (even if LS is dominantly inherited, a second hit on the other allele is required). MSI status can be determined by DNA testing. In particular, five microsatellite markers recommended by the National Cancer Institute (NCI) workshop have been used for MSI analysis: BAT25, BAT26, D2S123, D5S346, and D17S250 [256].

Two or more of the five markers are required to confirm the presence of MSI-H. Conversely, a low level of MSI (MSI-L) is assigned when only one unstable markers is detected. MSI-H CRC is known to have well-defined clinicopathological and molecular features. In fact, MSI-H CRC are preferentially located in the proximal colon and frequently associated with a less advanced cancer stage, extracellular mucin production, medullary carcinoma and poorly differentiated carcinoma, tumor-infiltrating lymphocytes, a Crohn's-like lymphoid reaction, and a *BRAF* V600E mutation [258–260]. Furthermore, it is associated with favorable survival in comparison with MSS/MSI-L. Interestingly, it is associated with chemotherapy resistance (i.e., adjuvant 5-FU-based chemotherapy) [261–265] but patients with metastatic disease are good candidates for immune-targeted therapy such nivolumab or pembrolizumab [266–268]. Conversely, several studies supporting MSI-H as a predictive factor for improved response to irinotecan- or irinotecan-based chemotherapy in CRC patients have been reported [269, 270].

6. Conclusive Remarks

CRC is a complex biological process involving multiple steps and genes, including genetic and epigenetic [271] factors, germline and somatic mutations, and chromosomal aberrations [272].

The three most important pathways of CRC carcinogenesis are the EGFR signalling pathway, with the involvement of KRAS and BRAF, the DNA mismatch repair (MMR), and the fields of epigenetics such aberrant hypermethylation and microRNAs (miRNAs) expression.

Over the recent years, several biomarkers of CRC have been proposed and encouraging progress has been made in our understanding the behaviour of CRC at a molecular level. Even if further validation studies are needed, assessing the role of biomarkers in experimental models and in patients could open new perspectives concerning a patient-tailored approach. Moreover, they could increase CRC screening uptake, given their limited invasiveness.

Acknowledgments

The authors would like to express their gratitude to Anna Ari Colace, Alessia di Gilio, and Rosaria di Martino, Staff of Centro di Servizio (SBA)—Università degli Studi della Campania "Luigi Vanvitelli"—for their support in retrieving the full text of some of the included articles.

References

[1] A. Jemal, F. Bray, M. M. Center, J. Ferlay, E. Ward, and D. Forman, "Global cancer statistics," *CA: a Cancer Journal for Clinicians*, vol. 61, no. 2, pp. 69–90, 2011.

[2] I. J. Fidler, "The pathogenesis of cancer metastasis: the 'seed and soil' hypothesis revisited," *Nature Reviews. Cancer*, vol. 3, no. 6, pp. 453–458, 2003.

[3] American Cancer Society, *Colorectal Cancer Facts & Figures 2011–2013*, American Cancer Society, Atlanta, 2011, http://www.cancer.org/research/cancerfactsfigures/colorectalcancerfactsfigures/colorectal-cancer-facts-figures-2011-2013-page.

[4] American Cancer Society, *Cancer Facts & Figures 2012*, American Cancer Society, Atlanta, 2012, http://www.cancer.org/research/cancerfactsstatistics/cancerfactsfigures2012/.

[5] J. S. Mandel, J. H. Bond, T. R. Church et al., "Reducing mortality from colorectal cancer by screening for fecal occult blood. Minnesota Colon Cancer Control Study," *The New England Journal of Medicine*, vol. 328, no. 19, pp. 1365–1371, 1993.

[6] D. Lieberman, "Colon cancer screening and surveillance controversies," *Current Opinion in Gastroenterology*, vol. 25, no. 5, pp. 422–427, 2009.

[7] J. E. Allison, I. S. Tekawa, L. J. Ransom, and A. L. Adrain, "A comparison of fecal occult-blood tests for colorectal-cancer screening," *The New England Journal of Medicine*, vol. 334, no. 3, pp. 155–160, 1996.

[8] L. G. van Rossum, A. F. van Rijn, R. J. Laheij et al., "Random comparison of guaiac and immunochemical fecal occult blood tests for colorectal cancer in a screening population," *Gastroenterology*, vol. 135, no. 1, pp. 82–90, 2008.

[9] C. G. Fraser, C. M. Matthew, N. A. G. Mowat, J. A. Wilson, F. A. Carey, and R. J. C. Steele, "Immunochemical testing of individuals positive for guaiac faecal occult blood test in a screening programme for colorectal cancer: an observational study," *The Lancet Oncology*, vol. 7, no. 2, pp. 127–131, 2006.

[10] H. I. Meissner, N. Breen, C. N. Klabunde, and S. W. Vernon, "Patterns of colorectal cancer screening uptake among men and women in the United States," *Cancer Epidemiology, Biomarkers & Prevention*, vol. 15, no. 2, pp. 389–394, 2006.

[11] A. Link, F. Balaguer, Y. Shen et al., "Fecal MicroRNAs as novel biomarkers for colon cancer screening," *Cancer Epidemiology, Biomarkers & Prevention*, vol. 19, no. 7, pp. 1766–1774, 2010.

[12] L. J. W. Bosch, B. Carvalho, R. J. A. Fijneman et al., "Molecular tests for colorectal cancer screening," *Clinical Colorectal Cancer*, vol. 10, no. 1, pp. 8–23, 2011.

[13] T. F. Imperiale, D. F. Ransohoff, S. H. Itzkowitz, B. A. Turnbull, M. E. Ross, and Colorectal Cancer Study Group, "Fecal DNA versus fecal occult blood for colorectal-cancer screening in an average-risk population," *The New England Journal of Medicine*, vol. 351, no. 26, pp. 2704–2714, 2004.

[14] S. Gout and J. Huot, "Role of cancer microenvironment in metastasis: focus on colon cancer," *Cancer Microenvironment*, vol. 1, no. 1, pp. 69–83, 2008.

[15] D. A. Lieberman, "Clinical practice. Screening for colorectal cancer," *The New England Journal of Medicine*, vol. 361, no. 12, pp. 1179–1187, 2009.

[16] M. Kulis and M. Esteller, "2-DNA Methylation and Cancer," *Advances in Genetics*, vol. 70, pp. 27–56, 2010.

[17] M. van Engeland, S. Derks, K. M. Smits, G. A. Meijer, and J. G. Herman, "Colorectal cancer epigenetics: complex simplicity," *Journal of Clinical Oncology*, vol. 29, no. 10, pp. 1382–1391, 2011.

[18] G. A. Calin and C. M. Croce, "MicroRNA signatures in human cancers," *Nature Reviews Cancer*, vol. 6, no. 11, pp. 857–866, 2006.

[19] S. Muhammad, K. Kaur, R. Huang et al., "MicroRNAs in colorectal cancer: role in metastasis and clinical perspectives,"

World Journal of Gastroenterology, vol. 20, no. 45, pp. 17011–17019, 2014.

[20] Y. B. Zheng, K. Xiao, G. C. Xiao et al., "MicroRNA-103 promotes tumor growth and metastasis in colorectal cancer by directly targeting LATS2," *Oncology Letters*, vol. 12, no. 3, pp. 2194–2200, 2016.

[21] O. Slaby, M. Svoboda, J. Michalek, and R. Vyzula, "MicroRNAs in colorectal cancer: translation of molecular biology into clinical application," *Molecular Cancer*, vol. 8, no. 1, p. 102, 2009.

[22] J. Hamfjord, A. M. Stangeland, T. Hughes et al., "Differential expression of miRNAs in colorectal cancer: comparison of paired tumor tissue and adjacent normal mucosa using high-throughput sequencing," *PLoS One*, vol. 7, no. 4, article e34150, 2012.

[23] R. C. Lee, R. L. Feinbaum, and V. Ambros, "The C. elegans heterochronic gene *lin-4* encodes small RNAs with antisense complementarity to *lin-14*," *Cell*, vol. 75, no. 5, pp. 843–854, 1993.

[24] B. Wightman, I. Ha, and G. Ruvkun, "Posttranscriptional regulation of the heterochronic gene *lin-14* by *lin-4* mediates temporal pattern formation in C. elegans," *Cell*, vol. 75, no. 5, pp. 855–862, 1993.

[25] D. Sayed and M. Abdellatif, "MicroRNAs in development and disease," *Physiological Reviews*, vol. 91, no. 3, pp. 827–887, 2011.

[26] Y. Okugawa, Y. Toiyama, and A. Goel, "An update on microRNAs as colorectal cancer biomarkers: where are we and what's next?," *Expert Review of Molecular Diagnostics*, vol. 14, no. 8, pp. 999–1021, 2014.

[27] Y. Hayashita, H. Osada, Y. Tatematsu et al., "A polycistronic microRNA cluster, *miR-17-92*, is overexpressed in human lung cancers and enhances cell proliferation," *Cancer Research*, vol. 65, no. 21, pp. 9628–9632, 2005.

[28] M. Z. Michael, S. M. O' Connor, N. van Holst Pellekaan, G. P. Young, and R. J. James, "Reduced accumulation of specific microRNAs in colorectal neoplasia," *Molecular Cancer Research*, vol. 1, no. 12, pp. 882–891, 2003.

[29] B. Zhang, X. Pan, G. P. Cobb, and T. A. Anderson, "microRNAs as oncogenes and tumor suppressors," *Developmental Biology*, vol. 302, no. 1, pp. 1–12, 2007.

[30] D. P. Bartel, "MicroRNAs: genomics, biogenesis, mechanism, and function," *Cell*, vol. 116, no. 2, pp. 281–297, 2004.

[31] E. R. Fearon and B. Vogelstein, "A genetic model for colorectal tumorigenesis," *Cell*, vol. 61, no. 5, pp. 759–767, 1990.

[32] L. Ma, J. Teruya-Feldstein, and R. A. Weinberg, "Tumour invasion and metastasis initiated by microRNA-10b in breast cancer," *Nature*, vol. 449, no. 7163, pp. 682–688, 2007.

[33] W. K. K. Wu, P. T. Y. Law, C. W. Lee et al., "MicroRNA in colorectal cancer: from benchtop to bedside," *Carcinogenesis*, vol. 32, no. 3, pp. 247–253, 2011.

[34] J. Folkman and M. Klagsbrun, "Angiogenic factors," *Science*, vol. 235, no. 4787, pp. 442–447, 1987.

[35] D. Hanahan and R. A. Weinberg, "Hallmarks of cancer: the next generation," *Cell*, vol. 144, no. 5, pp. 646–674, 2011.

[36] B. Bierie and H. L. Moses, "Tumour microenvironment: TGFβ: the molecular Jekyll and Hyde of cancer," *Nature Reviews. Cancer*, vol. 6, no. 7, pp. 506–520, 2006.

[37] M. Bockhorn, R. K. Jain, and L. L. Munn, "Active versus passive mechanisms in metastasis: do cancer cells crawl into vessels, or are they pushed?," *The Lancet Oncology*, vol. 8, no. 5, pp. 444–448, 2007.

[38] G. M. Arndt, L. Dossey, L. M. Cullen et al., "Characterization of global microRNA expression reveals oncogenic potential of miR-145 in metastatic colorectal cancer," *BMC Cancer*, vol. 9, no. 1, p. 374, 2009.

[39] J. E. Fish, M. M. Santoro, S. U. Morton et al., "miR-126 regulates angiogenic signaling and vascular integrity," *Developmental Cell*, vol. 15, no. 2, pp. 272–284, 2008.

[40] S. Paget, "The distribution of secondary growths in cancer of the breast. 1889," *Cancer Metastasis Reviews*, vol. 8, no. 2, pp. 98–101, 1989.

[41] M. Dews, A. Homayouni, D. Yu et al., "Augmentation of tumor angiogenesis by a Myc-activated microRNA cluster," *Nature Genetics*, vol. 38, no. 9, pp. 1060–1065, 2006.

[42] D. Ye, S. Guo, R. al-Sadi, and T. Y. Ma, "MicroRNA regulation of intestinal epithelial tight junction permeability," *Gastroenterology*, vol. 141, no. 4, pp. 1323–1333, 2011.

[43] Y. Chen, S. X. Wang, R. Mu et al., "Dysregulation of the MiR-324-5p-CUEDC2 axis leads to macrophage dysfunction and is associated with colon cancer," *Cell Reports*, vol. 7, no. 6, pp. 1982–1993, 2014.

[44] Y. Chen, C. Wang, Y. Liu et al., "miR-122 targets NOD2 to decrease intestinal epithelial cell injury in Crohn's disease," *Biochemical and Biophysical Research Communications*, vol. 438, no. 1, pp. 133–139, 2013.

[45] E. K. O. Ng, W. W. S. Chong, H. Jin et al., "Differential expression of microRNAs in plasma of patients with colorectal cancer: a potential marker for colorectal cancer screening," *Gut*, vol. 58, no. 10, pp. 1375–1381, 2009.

[46] Z. Huang, D. Huang, S. Ni, Z. Peng, W. Sheng, and X. Du, "Plasma microRNAs are promising novel biomarkers for early detection of colorectal cancer," *International Journal of Cancer*, vol. 127, no. 1, pp. 118–126, 2010.

[47] A. B. Hui, W. Shi, P. C. Boutros et al., "Robust global microRNA profiling with formalin-fixed paraffin- embedded breast cancer tissues," *Laboratory Investigation*, vol. 89, no. 5, pp. 597–606, 2009.

[48] P. S. Mitchell, R. K. Parkin, E. M. Kroh et al., "Circulating microRNAs as stable blood-based markers for cancer detection," *Proceedings of the National Academy of Sciences of the United States of America*, vol. 105, no. 30, pp. 10513–10518, 2008.

[49] X. Chen, Y. Ba, L. Ma et al., "Characterization of microRNAs in serum: a novel class of biomarkers for diagnosis of cancer and other diseases," *Cell Research*, vol. 18, no. 10, pp. 997–1006, 2008.

[50] G. A. Calin, C. D. Dumitru, M. Shimizu et al., "Frequent deletions and down-regulation of micro- RNA genes *miR15* and *miR16* at 13q14 in chronic lymphocytic leukemia," *Proceedings of the National Academy of Sciences of the United States of America*, vol. 99, no. 24, pp. 15524–15529, 2002.

[51] Y. Ma, P. Zhang, F. Wang et al., "Elevated oncofoetal miR-17-5p expression regulates colorectal cancer progression by repressing its target gene *P130*," *Nature Communications*, vol. 3, no. 1, p. 1291, 2012.

[52] A. Tsuchida, S. Ohno, W. Wu et al., "miR-92 is a key oncogenic component of the miR-17-92 cluster in colon cancer," *Cancer Science*, vol. 102, no. 12, pp. 2264–2271, 2011.

[53] N. Oue, K. Anami, A. J. Schetter et al., "High miR-21 expression from FFPE tissues is associated with poor survival and

response to adjuvant chemotherapy in colon cancer," *International Journal of Cancer*, vol. 134, no. 8, pp. 1926–1934, 2014.

[54] A. J. Schetter, S. Y. Leung, J. J. Sohn et al., "MicroRNA expression profiles associated with prognosis and therapeutic outcome in colon adenocarcinoma," *JAMA*, vol. 299, no. 4, pp. 425–436, 2008.

[55] Y. Toiyama, M. Takahashi, K. Hur et al., "Serum miR-21 as a diagnostic and prognostic biomarker in colorectal cancer," *Journal of the National Cancer Institute*, vol. 105, no. 12, pp. 849–859, 2013.

[56] F. Meng, R. Henson, H. Wehbe-Janek, K. Ghoshal, S. T. Jacob, and T. Patel, "MicroRNA-21 regulates expression of the PTEN tumor suppressor gene in human hepatocellular cancer," *Gastroenterology*, vol. 133, no. 2, pp. 647–658, 2007.

[57] F. Talotta, A. Cimmino, M. R. Matarazzo et al., "An autoregulatory loop mediated by miR-21 and PDCD4 controls the AP-1 activity in RAS transformation," *Oncogene*, vol. 28, no. 1, pp. 73–84, 2009.

[58] A. Kawakita, S. Yanamoto, S. Yamada et al., "MicroRNA-21 promotes oral cancer invasion via the Wnt/β-catenin pathway by targeting DKK2," *Pathology Oncology Research*, vol. 20, no. 2, pp. 253–261, 2014.

[59] K. Lee and L. R. Ferguson, "MicroRNA biomarkers predicting risk, initiation and progression of colorectal cancer," *World Journal of Gastroenterology*, vol. 22, no. 33, pp. 7389–7401, 2016.

[60] W. Tang, Y. Zhu, J. Gao et al., "MicroRNA-29a promotes colorectal cancer metastasis by regulating matrix metalloproteinase 2 and E-cadherin via KLF4," *British Journal of Cancer*, vol. 110, no. 2, pp. 450–458, 2014.

[61] L. G. Wang and J. Gu, "Serum microRNA-29a is a promising novel marker for early detection of colorectal liver metastasis," *Cancer Epidemiology*, vol. 36, no. 1, pp. e61–e67, 2012.

[62] T.-Y. Kuo, E. Hsi, I.-P. Yang, P.-C. Tsai, J.-Y. Wang, and S.-H. H. Juo, "Computational analysis of mRNA expression profiles identifies microRNA-29a/c as predictor of colorectal cancer early recurrence," *PLoS One*, vol. 7, no. 2, article e31587, 2012.

[63] R. Aharonov, "Tumor microRNA-29a expression and the risk of recurrence in stage II colon cancer," *International Journal of Oncology*, vol. 40, no. 6, pp. 2097–2103, 2012.

[64] J. Gao, N. Li, Y. Dong et al., "miR-34a-5p suppresses colorectal cancer metastasis and predicts recurrence in patients with stage II/III colorectal cancer," *Oncogene*, vol. 34, no. 31, pp. 4142–4152, 2015.

[65] J. Salendo, M. Spitzner, F. Kramer et al., "Identification of a microRNA expression signature for chemoradiosensitivity of colorectal cancer cells, involving miRNAs-320a, -224, -132 and let7g," *Radiotherapy & Oncology*, vol. 108, no. 3, pp. 451–457, 2013.

[66] G. H. Liu, Z. G. Zhou, R. Chen et al., "Serum miR-21 and miR-92a as biomarkers in the diagnosis and prognosis of colorectal cancer," *Tumor Biology*, vol. 34, no. 4, pp. 2175–2181, 2013.

[67] C. W. Wu, S. S. M. Ng, Y. J. Dong et al., "Detection of miR-92a and miR-21 in stool samples as potential screening biomarkers for colorectal cancer and polyps," *Gut*, vol. 61, no. 5, pp. 739–745, 2012.

[68] H. B. Le, W. Y. Zhu, D. D. Chen et al., "Evaluation of dynamic change of serum miR-21 and miR-24 in pre- and post-operative lung carcinoma patients," *Medical Oncology*, vol. 29, no. 5, pp. 3190–3197, 2012.

[69] Y. Koga, M. Yasunaga, A. Takahashi et al., "MicroRNA expression profiling of exfoliated colonocytes isolated from feces for colorectal cancer screening," *Cancer Prevention Research*, vol. 3, no. 11, pp. 1435–1442, 2010.

[70] F. E. Ahmed, C. D. Jeffries, P. W. Vos et al., "Diagnostic microRNA markers for screening sporadic human colon cancer and active ulcerative colitis in stool and tissue," *Cancer Genomics & Proteomics*, vol. 6, no. 5, pp. 281–295, 2009.

[71] C. W. Wu, S. C. Ng, Y. Dong et al., "Identification of microRNA- 135b in stool as a potential noninvasive biomarker for colorectal cancer and adenoma," *Clinical Cancer Research*, vol. 20, no. 11, pp. 2994–3002, 2014.

[72] Y. Koga, N. Yamazaki, Y. Yamamoto et al., "Fecal miR-106a Is a useful marker for colorectal cancer patients with false-negative results in immunochemical fecal occult blood test," *Cancer Epidemiology, Biomarkers & Prevention*, vol. 22, no. 10, pp. 1844–1852, 2013.

[73] S. Tarallo, B. Pardini, G. Mancuso et al., "MicroRNA expression in relation to different dietary habits: a comparison in stool and plasma samples," *Mutagenesis*, vol. 29, no. 5, pp. 385–391, 2014.

[74] P. A. Northcott, A. Fernandez-L, J. P. Hagan et al., "The miR-17/92 polycistron is up-regulated in sonic hedgehog-driven medulloblastomas and induced by N-myc in sonic hedgehog-treated cerebellar neural precursors," *Cancer Research*, vol. 69, no. 8, pp. 3249–3255, 2009.

[75] A. Bonauer, G. Carmona, M. Iwasaki et al., "MicroRNA-92a controls angiogenesis and functional recovery of ischemic tissues in mice," *Science*, vol. 324, no. 5935, pp. 1710–1713, 2009.

[76] O. Hänninen, A. L. Rauma, K. Kaartinen, and M. Nenonen, "Vegan diet in physiological health promotion," *Acta Physiologica Hungarica*, vol. 86, no. 3-4, pp. 171–180, 1999.

[77] K. W. Witwer, "XenomiRs and miRNA homeostasis in health and disease: evidence that diet and dietary miRNAs directly and indirectly influence circulating miRNA profiles," *RNA Biology*, vol. 9, no. 9, pp. 1147–1154, 2012.

[78] K. W. Witwer, M. A. McAlexander, S. E. Queen, and R. J. Adams, "Real-time quantitative PCR and droplet digital PCR for plant miRNAs in mammalian blood provide little evidence for general uptake of dietary miRNAs: limited evidence for general uptake of dietary plant xenomiRs," *RNA Biology*, vol. 10, no. 7, pp. 1080–1086, 2013.

[79] A. Bye, H. Røsjø, S. T. Aspenes, G. Condorelli, T. Omland, and U. Wisløff, "Circulating microRNAs and aerobic fitness–the HUNT-study," *PLoS One*, vol. 8, no. 2, article e57496, 2013.

[80] "miRBase," [updated 2013 June; cited 2014 June 6]. http://www.miRbase.org/index.shtml.

[81] B. M. Evers, *Molecular Mechanisms in Gastrointestinal Cancer*, R.G. Landes, 1999.

[82] L. J. Herrera, S. Raja, W. E. Gooding et al., "Quantitative analysis of circulating plasma DNA as a tumor marker in thoracic malignancies," *Clinical Chemistry*, vol. 51, no. 1, pp. 113–118, 2005.

[83] S. Sabbioni, E. Miotto, A. Veronese et al., "Multigene methylation analysis of gastrointestinal tumors: TPEF emerges as a frequent tumor-specific aberrantly methylated marker that can be detected in peripheral blood," *Molecular Diagnosis*, vol. 7, no. 3-4, pp. 201–207, 2003.

[84] T. R. Church, M. Wandell, C. Lofton-Day et al., "Prospective evaluation of methylated *SEPT9* in plasma for detection of asymptomatic colorectal cancer," *Gut*, vol. 63, no. 2, pp. 317–325, 2014.

[85] L. Barault, A. Amatu, G. Siravegna et al., "Discovery of methylated circulating DNA biomarkers for comprehensive non-invasive monitoring of treatment response in metastatic colorectal cancer," *Gut*, vol. 0, pp. 1–11, 2017.

[86] Y. Liu, C. K. Tham, S. Y. K. Ong et al., "Serum methylation levels of *TAC1 SEPT9* and *EYA4* as diagnostic markers for early colorectal cancers: a pilot study," *Biomarkers*, vol. 18, no. 5, pp. 399–405, 2013.

[87] Q. He, H. Y. Chen, E. Q. Bai et al., "Development of a multiplex MethyLight assay for the detection of multigene methylation in human colorectal cancer," *Cancer Genetics and Cytogenetics*, vol. 202, no. 1, pp. 1–10, 2010.

[88] L. E. Heasley, "Autocrine and paracrine signaling through neuropeptide receptors in human cancer," *Oncogene*, vol. 20, no. 13, pp. 1563–1569, 2001.

[89] R. P. Thomas, M. R. Hellmich, C. M. Townsend Jr, and B. M. Evers, "Role of gastrointestinal hormones in the proliferation of normal and neoplastic tissues," *Endocrine Reviews*, vol. 24, no. 5, pp. 571–599, 2003.

[90] R. Carraway and S. E. Leeman, "The isolation of a new hypotensive peptide, neurotensin, from bovine hypothalami," *The Journal of Biological Chemistry*, vol. 248, no. 19, pp. 6854–6861, 1973.

[91] B. M. A. R. K. Evers, J. Ishizuka, D. H. Chung, C. M. Townsend JR., and J. C. Thompson, "Neurotensin expression and release in human colon cancers," *Annals of Surgery*, vol. 216, no. 4, pp. 423–431, 1992.

[92] J. J. Maoret, Y. Anini, C. Rouyer-Fessard, D. Gully, and M. Laburthe, "Neurotensin and a non-peptide neurotensin receptor antagonist control human colon cancer cell growth in cell culture and in cells xenografted into nude mice," *International Journal of Cancer*, vol. 80, no. 3, pp. 448–454, 1999.

[93] M. Tasuta, H. Iishi, M. Baba, and H. Taniguchi, "Enhancement by neurotensin of experimental carcinogenesis induced in rat colon by azoxymethane," *British Journal of Cancer*, vol. 62, no. 3, pp. 368–371, 1990.

[94] K. Yoshinaga, B. M. Evers, M. Izukura et al., "Neurotensin stimulates growth of colon cancer," *Surgical Oncology*, vol. 1, no. 2, pp. 127–134, 1992.

[95] X. Gui, G. Guzman, P. R. Dobner, and S. H. S. Kadkol, "Increased neurotensin receptor-1 expression during progression of colonic adenocarcinoma," *Peptides*, vol. 29, no. 9, pp. 1609–1615, 2008.

[96] M. Gerlinger, A. J. Rowan, S. Horswell et al., "Intratumor heterogeneity and branched evolution revealed by multiregion sequencing," *The New England Journal of Medicine*, vol. 366, no. 10, pp. 883–892, 2012.

[97] C. Bedin, M. V. Enzo, P. Del Bianco, S. Pucciarelli, D. Nitti, and M. Agostini, "Diagnostic and prognostic role of cell-free DNA testing for colorectal cancer patients," *International Journal of Cancer*, vol. 140, no. 8, pp. 1888–1898, 2017.

[98] C. Rolfo, M. Castiglia, D. Hong et al., "Liquid biopsies in lung cancer: the new ambrosia of researchers," *Biochimica et Biophysica Acta (BBA) - Reviews on Cancer*, vol. 1846, no. 2, pp. 539–546, 2014.

[99] E. Kidess-Sigal, H. E. Liu, M. M. Triboulet et al., "Enumeration and targeted analysis of *KRAS*, *BRAF* and *PIK3CA* mutations in CTCs captured by a label-free platform: comparison to ctDNA and tissue in metastatic colorectal cancer," *Oncotarget*, vol. 7, no. 51, pp. 85349–85364, 2016.

[100] C. R. C. Tan, L. Zhou, and W. S. El-Deiry, "Circulating tumor cells versus circulating tumor DNA in colorectal cancer: pros and cons," *Current Colorectal Cancer Reports*, vol. 12, no. 3, pp. 151–161, 2016.

[101] J. Zhou, L. Chang, Y. Guan et al., "Application of circulating tumor DNA as a non-invasive tool for monitoring the progression of colorectal cancer," *PLoS One*, vol. 11, no. 7, article e0159708, 2016.

[102] U. Malapelle, A. De Stefano, C. Carlomagno, C. Bellevicine, and G. Troncone, "Next-generation sequencing in the genomic profiling of synchronous colonic carcinomas: comment on Li *et al*(2015)," *Journal of Clinical Pathology*, vol. 68, no. 11, pp. 946-947, 2015.

[103] U. Malapelle, P. Pisapia, D. Rocco et al., "Next generation sequencing techniques in liquid biopsy: focus on non-small cell lung cancer patients," *Translational Lung Cancer Research*, vol. 5, no. 5, pp. 505–510, 2016.

[104] J. A. Denis, A. Patroni, E. Guillerm et al., "Droplet digital PCR of circulating tumor cells from colorectal cancer patients can predict *KRAS* mutations before surgery," *Molecular Oncology*, vol. 10, no. 8, pp. 1221–1231, 2016.

[105] J. J. Jones, B. E. Wilcox, R. W. Benz et al., "A plasma-based protein marker panel for colorectal cancer detection identified by multiplex targeted mass spectrometry," *Clinical Colorectal Cancer*, vol. 15, no. 2, pp. 186–194.e13, 2016.

[106] A. Willms, C. Müller, H. Julich et al., "Tumour- associated circulating microparticles: a novel liquid biopsy tool for screening and therapy monitoring of colorectal carcinoma and other epithelial neoplasia," *Oncotarget*, vol. 7, no. 21, pp. 30867–30875, 2016.

[107] E. Crowley, F. Di Nicolantonio, F. Loupakis, and A. Bardelli, "Liquid biopsy: monitoring cancer- genetics in the blood," *Nature Reviews Clinical Oncology*, vol. 10, no. 8, pp. 472–484, 2013.

[108] C. Bettegowda, M. Sausen, R. J. Leary et al., "Detection of circulating tumor DNA in early- and late-stage human malignancies," *Science Translational Medicine*, vol. 6, no. 224, p. 224ra24, 2014.

[109] A. R. Thierry, F. Mouliere, S. el Messaoudi et al., "Clinical validation of the detection of *KRAS* and *BRAF* mutations from circulating tumor DNA," *Nature Medicine*, vol. 20, no. 4, pp. 430–435, 2014.

[110] E. Heitzer, M. Auer, P. Ulz, J. B. Geigl, and M. R. Speicher, "Circulating tumor cells and DNA as liquid biopsies," *Genome Medicine*, vol. 5, no. 8, p. 73, 2013.

[111] K. C. A. Chan, P. Jiang, C. W. M. Chan et al., "Noninvasive detection of cancer-associated genome-wide hypomethylation and copy number aberrations by plasma DNA bisulfite sequencing," *Proceedings of the National Academy of Sciences of the United States of America*, vol. 110, no. 47, pp. 18761–18768, 2013.

[112] K. C. A. Chan, P. Jiang, Y. W. L. Zheng et al., "Cancer genome scanning in plasma: detection of tumor-associated copy number aberrations, single- nucleotide variants, and tumoral heterogeneity by massively parallel sequencing," *Clinical Chemistry*, vol. 59, no. 1, pp. 211–224, 2013.

[113] J. H. Strickler, J. M. Loree, L. G. Ahronian et al., "Genomic landscape of cell-free DNA in patients with colorectal cancer," *Cancer Discovery*, vol. 8, no. 2, pp. 164–173, 2018.

[114] S. Siena, A. Sartore-Bianchi, R. Garcia-Carbonero et al., "Dynamic molecular analysis and clinical correlates of tumor evolution within a phase II trial of panitumumab-based therapy in metastatic colorectal cancer," *Annals of Oncology*, vol. 29, no. 1, pp. 119–126, 2018.

[115] E. Heitzer, M. Auer, E. M. Hoffmann et al., "Establishment of tumor-specific copy number alterations from plasma DNA of patients with cancer," *International Journal of Cancer*, vol. 133, no. 2, pp. 346–356, 2013.

[116] M. Frattini, et al.G. Gallino, S. Signoroni et al., "Quantitative and qualitative characterization of plasma DNA identifies primary and recurrent colorectal cancer," *Cancer Letters*, vol. 263, no. 2, pp. 170–181, 2008.

[117] F. Diehl, K. Schmidt, M. A. Choti et al., "Circulating mutant DNA to assess tumor dynamics," *Nature Medicine*, vol. 14, no. 9, pp. 985–990, 2008.

[118] T. Lecomte, A. Berger, F. Zinzindohoué et al., "Detection of free-circulating tumor-associated DNA in plasma of colorectal cancer patients and its association with prognosis," *International Journal of Cancer*, vol. 100, no. 5, pp. 542–548, 2002.

[119] R. Bertorelle, M. Briarava, E. Rampazzo et al., "Telomerase is an independent prognostic marker of overall survival in patients with colorectal cancer," *British Journal of Cancer*, vol. 108, no. 2, pp. 278–284, 2013.

[120] N. Normanno, R. Esposito Abate, M. Lambiase et al., "*RAS* testing of liquid biopsy correlates with the outcome of metastatic colorectal cancer patients treated with first-line FOLFIRI plus cetuximab in the CAPRI-GOIM trial," *Annals of Oncology*, vol. 29, no. 1, pp. 112–118, 2018.

[121] C. S. Karapetis, S. Khambata-Ford, D. J. Jonker et al., "*K-ras* mutations and benefit from cetuximab in advanced colorectal cancer," *The New England Journal of Medicine*, vol. 359, no. 17, pp. 1757–1765, 2008.

[122] Y.-B. Kuo, J.-S. Chen, C.-W. Fan, Y.-S. Li, and E.-C. Chan, "Comparison of *KRAS* mutation analysis of primary tumors and matched circulating cell-free DNA in plasmas of patients with colorectal cancer," *Clinica Chimica Acta*, vol. 433, pp. 284–289, 2014.

[123] L. A. Diaz Jr, R. T. Williams, J. Wu et al., "The molecular evolution of acquired resistance to targeted EGFR blockade in colorectal cancers," *Nature*, vol. 486, no. 7404, pp. 537–540, 2012.

[124] S. Pucciarelli, E. Rampazzo, M. Briarava et al., "Telomere-specific reverse transcriptase (hTERT) and cell-free RNA in plasma as predictors of pathologic tumor response in rectal cancer patients receiving neoadjuvant chemoradiotherapy," *Annals of Surgical Oncology*, vol. 19, no. 9, pp. 3089–3096, 2012.

[125] M. Agostini, S. Pucciarelli, M. V. Enzo et al., "Circulating cell-free DNA: a promising marker of pathologic tumor response in rectal cancer patients receiving preoperative chemoradiotherapy," *Annals of Surgical Oncology*, vol. 18, no. 9, pp. 2461–2468, 2011.

[126] J. Tie, Y. Wang, C. Tomasetti et al., "Circulating tumor DNA analysis detects minimal residual disease and predicts recurrence in patients with stage II colon cancer," *Science Translational Medicine*, vol. 8, no. 346, article 346ra92, 2016.

[127] R. B. Iyer, P. M. Silverman, R. A. DuBrow, and C. Charnsangavej, "Imaging in the diagnosis, staging, and follow-up of colorectal cancer," *American Journal of Roentgenology*, vol. 179, no. 1, pp. 3–13, 2002.

[128] E. McKeown, D. W. Nelson, E. K. Johnson et al., "Current approaches and challenges for monitoring treatment response in colon and rectal cancer," *Journal of Cancer*, vol. 5, no. 1, pp. 31–43, 2014.

[129] L.-F. de Geus-Oei, D. Vriens, H. W. M. van Laarhoven, W. T. A. van der Graaf, and W. J. G. Oyen, "Monitoring and predicting response to therapy with ^{18}F-FDG PET in colorectal cancer: a systematic review," *Journal of Nuclear Medicine*, vol. 50, Supplement 1, pp. 43S–54S, 2009.

[130] N. Maggialetti, R. Capasso, D. Pinto et al., "Diagnostic value of computed tomography colonography (CTC) after incomplete optical colonoscopy," *International Journal of Surgery*, vol. 33, Suppl 1, pp. S36–S44, 2016.

[131] V. Cuccurullo, F. Cioce, A. Sica et al., "Gastroenteric diseases in the third millennium: a rational approach to optimal imaging technique and patient selection," *Recenti Progressi in Medicina*, vol. 103, no. 11, pp. 426–430, 2012.

[132] H. C. Thoeny and B. D. Ross, "Predicting and monitoring cancer treatment response with diffusion- weighted MRI," *Journal of Magnetic Resonance Imaging*, vol. 32, no. 1, pp. 2–16, 2010.

[133] J. P. B. O'Connor, C. J. Rose, A. Jackson et al., "DCE-MRI biomarkers of tumour heterogeneity predict CRC liver metastasis shrinkage following bevacizumab and FOLFOX-6," *British Journal of Cancer*, vol. 105, no. 1, pp. 139–145, 2011.

[134] M. Barral, C. Eveno, C. Hoeffel et al., "Diffusion-weighted magnetic resonance imaging in colorectal cancer," *Journal of Visceral Surgery*, vol. 153, no. 5, pp. 361–369, 2016.

[135] R. G. H. Beets-Tan and G. L. Beets, "Local staging of rectal cancer: a review of imaging," *Journal of Magnetic Resonance Imaging*, vol. 33, no. 5, pp. 1012–1019, 2011.

[136] A. Zaniboni, G. Savelli, C. Pizzocaro, P. Basile, and V. Massetti, "Positron emission tomography for the response evaluation following treatment with chemotherapy in patients affected by colorectal liver metastases: a selected review," *Gastroenterology Research and Practice*, vol. 2015, Article ID 706808, 7 pages, 2015.

[137] E. Van Cutsem, H. M. Verheul, P. Flamen et al., "Imaging in colorectal cancer: progress and challenges for the clinicians," *Cancers*, vol. 8, no. 9, 2016.

[138] T. L. F. Nguyen, P. Soyer, P. Fornès, P. Rousset, R. Kianmanesh, and C. Hoeffel, "Diffusion-weighted MR imaging of the rectum: clinical applications," *Critical Reviews in Oncology/Hematology*, vol. 92, no. 3, pp. 279–295, 2014.

[139] M. Barral, A. Dohan, M. Allez et al., "Gastrointestinal cancers in inflammatory bowel disease: an update with emphasis on imaging findings," *Critical Reviews in Oncology/Hematology*, vol. 97, pp. 30–46, 2016.

[140] M. Barral, C. Hoeffel, M. Boudiaf et al., "Rectal cancer in inflammatory bowel diseases: MR imaging findings," *Abdominal Imaging*, vol. 39, no. 3, pp. 443–451, 2014.

[141] G. Pellino, R. Marcellinaro, G. Sciaudone et al., "Large bowel cancer in the setting of inflammatory bowel disease: features and management with a focus on rectal cancer," *European Surgery*, vol. 48, no. 4, pp. 191–202, 2016.

[142] S. X. Rao, M. S. Zeng, C. Z. Chen et al., "The value of diffusion- weighted imaging in combination with T_2-weighted

imaging for rectal cancer detection," *European Journal of Radiology*, vol. 65, no. 2, pp. 299–303, 2008.

[143] T. Ichikawa, S. M. Erturk, U. Motosugi et al., "High-b value diffusion- weighted MRI for detecting pancreatic adenocarcinoma: preliminary results," *American Journal of Roentgenology*, vol. 188, no. 2, pp. 409–414, 2007.

[144] E. Öistämö, F. Hjern, L. Blomqvist, A. Von Heijne, and M. Abraham-Nordling, "Cancer and diverticulitis of the sigmoid colon. Differentiation with computed tomography versus magnetic resonance imaging: preliminary experiences," *Acta Radiologica*, vol. 54, no. 3, pp. 237–241, 2013.

[145] A. Reginelli, M. G. Pezzullo, M. Scaglione, M. Scialpi, L. Brunese, and R. Grassi, "Gastrointestinal disorders in elderly patients," *Radiologic Clinics of North America*, vol. 46, no. 4, pp. 755–771, 2008.

[146] P. Soyer, M. Lagadec, M. Sirol et al., "Free-breathing diffusion-weighted single-shot echo-planar MR imaging using parallel imaging (GRAPPA 2) and high *b* value for the detection of primary rectal adenocarcinoma," *Cancer Imaging*, vol. 10, no. 1, pp. 32–39, 2010.

[147] Y. Sun, T. Tong, S. Cai, R. Bi, C. Xin, and Y. Gu, "Apparent diffusion coefficient (ADC) value: a potential imaging biomarker that reflects the biological features of rectal cancer," *PLoS One*, vol. 9, no. 10, article e109371, 2014.

[148] L. Curvo-Semedo, D. M. J. Lambregts, M. Maas, G. L. Beets, F. Caseiro-Alves, and R. G. H. Beets-Tan, "Diffusion-weighted MRI in rectal cancer: apparent diffusion coefficient as a potential noninvasive marker of tumor aggressiveness," *Journal of Magnetic Resonance Imaging*, vol. 35, no. 6, pp. 1365–1371, 2012.

[149] M. Akashi, Y. Nakahusa, T. Yakabe et al., "Assessment of aggressiveness of rectal cancer using 3-T MRI: correlation between the apparent diffusion coefficient as a potential imaging biomarker and histologic prognostic factors," *Acta Radiologica*, vol. 55, no. 5, pp. 524–531, 2014.

[150] K. Nasu, Y. Kuroki, and M. Minami, "Diffusion-weighted imaging findings of mucinous carcinoma arising in the anorectal region: comparison of apparent diffusion coefficient with that of tubular adenocarcinoma," *Japanese Journal of Radiology*, vol. 30, no. 2, pp. 120–127, 2012.

[151] A. R. Padhani, G. Liu, D. Mu-Koh et al., "Diffusion-weighted magnetic resonance imaging as a cancer biomarker: consensus and recommendations," *Neoplasia*, vol. 11, no. 2, pp. 102–125, 2009.

[152] D. M. Koh, M. Blackledge, A. R. Padhani et al., "Whole-body diffusion-weighted MRI: tips, tricks, and pitfalls," *American Journal of Roentgenology*, vol. 199, no. 2, pp. 252–262, 2012.

[153] O. Schaefer and M. Langer, "Detection of recurrent rectal cancer with CT, MRI and PET/CT," *European Radiology*, vol. 17, no. 8, pp. 2044–2054, 2007.

[154] E. Arriola, M. Navarro, D. Parés et al., "Imaging techniques contribute to increased surgical rescue of relapse in the follow-up of colorectal cancer," *Diseases of the Colon & Rectum*, vol. 49, no. 4, pp. 478–484, 2006.

[155] D. M. Koh, E. Scurr, D. Collins et al., "Predicting response of colorectal hepatic metastasis: value of pretreatment apparent diffusion coefficients," *American Journal of Roentgenology*, vol. 188, no. 4, pp. 1001–1008, 2007.

[156] P. Q. Cai, Y. P. Wu, X. An et al., "Simple measurements on diffusion-weighted MR imaging for assessment of complete response to neoadjuvant chemoradiotherapy in locally advanced rectal cancer," *European Radiology*, vol. 24, no. 11, pp. 2962–2970, 2014.

[157] S. H. Tirumani, K. W. Kim, M. Nishino et al., "Update on the role of imaging in management of metastatic colorectal cancer," *Radiographics*, vol. 34, no. 7, pp. 1908–1928, 2014.

[158] S. De Bruyne, N. Van Damme, P. Smeets et al., "Value of DCE-MRI and FDG-PET/CT in the prediction of response to preoperative chemotherapy with bevacizumab for colorectal liver metastases," *British Journal of Cancer*, vol. 106, no. 12, pp. 1926–1933, 2012.

[159] D. M. Koh, D. J. Collins, and M. R. Orton, "Intravoxel incoherent motion in body diffusion-weighted MRI: reality and challenges," *American Journal of Roentgenology*, vol. 196, no. 6, pp. 1351–1361, 2011.

[160] D. Le Bihan, E. Breton, D. Lallemand, M. L. Aubin, J. Vignaud, and M. Laval-Jeantet, "Separation of diffusion and perfusion in intravoxel incoherent motion MR imaging," *Radiology*, vol. 168, no. 2, pp. 497–505, 1988.

[161] M.-K. Ganten, M. Schuessler, T. Bauerle et al., "The role of perfusion effects in monitoring of chemoradiotherapy of rectal carcinoma using diffusion-weighted imaging," *Cancer Imaging*, vol. 13, no. 4, pp. 548–556, 2013.

[162] Y. Xiao, J. Pan, Y. Chen, Y. Chen, Z. He, and X. Zheng, "Intravoxel incoherent motion-magnetic resonance imaging as an early predictor of treatment response to neoadjuvant chemotherapy in locoregionally advanced nasopharyngeal carcinoma," *Medicine*, vol. 94, no. 24, article e973, 2015.

[163] O. Jalil, A. Afaq, B. Ganeshan et al., "Magnetic resonance based texture parameters as potential imaging biomarkers for predicting long-term survival in locally advanced rectal cancer treated by chemoradiotherapy," *Colorectal Disease*, vol. 19, no. 4, pp. 349–362, 2017.

[164] A. D. Van den Abbeele, "The lessons of GIST—PET and PET/CT: a new paradigm for imaging," *The Oncologist*, vol. 13, Supplement 2, pp. 8–13, 2008.

[165] R. A. Herbertson, A. F. Scarsbrook, S. T. Lee, N. Tebbutt, and A. M. Scott, "Established, emerging and future roles of PET/CT in the management of colorectal cancer," *Clinical Radiology*, vol. 64, no. 3, pp. 225–237, 2009.

[166] M. Gauthé, M. Richard-Molard, W. Cacheux et al., "Role of fluorine 18 fluorodeoxyglucose positron emission tomography/computed tomography in gastrointestinal cancers," *Digestive and Liver Disease*, vol. 47, no. 6, pp. 443–454, 2015.

[167] N. E. Makris, R. Boellaard, A. van Lingen et al., "PET/CT-derived whole-body and bone marrow dosimetry of ^{89}Zr-Cetuximab," *Journal of Nuclear Medicine*, vol. 56, no. 2, pp. 249–254, 2015.

[168] V. Sforza, E. Martinelli, F. Ciardiello et al., "Mechanisms of resistance to anti-epidermal growth factor receptor inhibitors in metastatic colorectal cancer," *World Journal of Gastroenterology*, vol. 22, no. 28, pp. 6345–6361, 2016.

[169] A. D. Culverwell, F. U. Chowdhury, and A. F. Scarsbrook, "Optimizing the role of FDG PET-CT for potentially operable metastatic colorectal cancer," *Abdominal Imaging*, vol. 37, no. 6, pp. 1021–1031, 2012.

[170] G. Pellino, E. Nicolai, O. A. Catalano et al., "PET/MR versus PET/CT imaging: impact on the clinical management of small-bowel Crohn's disease," *Journal of Crohn's and Colitis*, vol. 10, no. 3, pp. 277–285, 2016.

[171] O. A. Catalano, M. S. Gee, E. Nicolai et al., "Evaluation of quantitative PET/MR enterography biomarkers for discrimination of inflammatory strictures from fibrotic strictures in Crohn disease," *Radiology*, vol. 278, no. 3, pp. 792–800, 2016.

[172] C. Buchbender, T. A. Heusner, T. C. Lauenstein, A. Bockisch, and G. Antoch, "Oncologic PET/MRI, part 1: tumors of the brain, head and neck, chest, abdomen, and pelvis," *Journal of Nuclear Medicine*, vol. 53, no. 6, pp. 928–938, 2012.

[173] A. Bartoş, D. Bartoş, B. Szabo et al., "Recent achievements in colorectal cancer diagnostic and therapy by the use of nanoparticles," *Drug Metabolism Reviews*, vol. 48, no. 1, pp. 27–46, 2016.

[174] R. Subbiah, M. Veerapandian, and K. S. Yun, "Nanoparticles: functionalization and multifunctional applications in biomedical sciences," *Current Medicinal Chemistry*, vol. 17, no. 36, pp. 4559–4577, 2010.

[175] S. R. Grobmyer, N. Iwakuma, P. Sharma, and B. M. Moudgil, "What is cancer nanotechnology?," *Methods in Molecular Biology*, vol. 624, pp. 1–9, 2010.

[176] F. Alexis, J. W. Rhee, J. P. Richie, A. F. Radovic-Moreno, R. Langer, and O. C. Farokhzad, "New frontiers in nanotechnology for cancer treatment," *Urologic Oncology*, vol. 26, no. 1, pp. 74–85, 2008.

[177] K. B. Hartman, L. J. Wilson, and M. G. Rosenblum, "Detecting and treating cancer with nanotechnology," *Molecular Diagnosis & Therapy*, vol. 12, no. 1, pp. 1–14, 2008.

[178] K. Cho, X. Wang, S. Nie, Z. G. Chen, and D. M. Shin, "Therapeutic nanoparticles for drug delivery in cancer," *Clinical Cancer Research*, vol. 14, no. 5, pp. 1310–1316, 2008.

[179] T. Lammers, W. E. Hennink, and G. Storm, "Tumour-targeted nanomedicines: principles and practice," *British Journal of Cancer*, vol. 99, no. 3, pp. 392–397, 2008.

[180] A. Llevot and D. Astruc, "Applications of vectorized gold nanoparticles to the diagnosis and therapy of cancer," *Chemical Society Reviews*, vol. 41, no. 1, pp. 242–257, 2012.

[181] S. G. Grancharov, H. Zeng, S. Sun et al., "Bio-functionalization of monodisperse magnetic nanoparticles and their use as biomolecular labels in a magnetic tunnel junction based sensor," *The Journal of Physical Chemistry B*, vol. 109, no. 26, pp. 13030–13035, 2005.

[182] G. Kickelbick and U. S. Schubert, "Advances in nanophase materials and nanotechnology," in *Functionalization and Surface Treatment of Nanoparticles*, M. I. Baraton, Ed., pp. 91–102, American Scientific Publishers, Valencia, CA, USA, 2003.

[183] G. Bajaj and Y. Yeo, "Tumor targeted nanoparticles: state of the art and remaining challenges," in *Nanoparticulate Drug Delivery Systems Strategies, Technologies and Applications*, Y. Yeo, Ed., pp. 12–21, Wiley, New Jersey, 2013.

[184] D. Peer, J. M. Karp, S. Hong, O. C. Farokhzad, R. Margalit, and R. Langer, "Nanocarriers as an emerging platform for cancer therapy," *Nature Nanotechnology*, vol. 2, no. 12, pp. 751–760, 2007.

[185] V. Buddolla, S. Kim, and K. Lee, "Recent insights into nanotechnology development for detection and treatment of colorectal cancer," *International Journal of Nanomedicine*, vol. 11, pp. 2491–2504, 2016.

[186] K. H. Bae, K. Lee, C. Kim, and T. G. Park, "Surface functionalized hollow manganese oxide nanoparticles for cancer targeted siRNA delivery and magnetic resonance imaging," *Biomaterials*, vol. 32, no. 1, pp. 176–184, 2011.

[187] A. De La Zerda, C. Zavaleta, S. Keren et al., "Carbon nanotubes as photoacoustic molecular imaging agents in living mice," *Nature Nanotechnology*, vol. 3, no. 9, pp. 557–562, 2008.

[188] X. Yang, S. E. Skrabalak, Z. Y. Li, Y. Xia, and L. V. Wang, "Photoacoustic tomography of a rat cerebral cortex in vivo with au nanocages as an optical contrast agent," *Nano Letters*, vol. 7, no. 12, pp. 3798–3802, 2007.

[189] M. Fang, C. W. Peng, D. W. Pang, and Y. Li, "Quantum dots for cancer research: current status, remaining issues, and future perspectives," *Cancer Biology & Medicine*, vol. 9, no. 3, pp. 151–163, 2012.

[190] W.-J. Zeng, C.-W. Peng, J.-P. Yuan, R. Cui, and Y. Li, "Quantum dot-based multiplexed imaging in malignant ascites: a new model for malignant ascites classification," *International Journal of Nanomedicine*, vol. 10, no. 1, pp. 1759–1768, 2015.

[191] S. Wang, W. Li, D. Yuan, J. Song, and J. Fang, "Quantitative detection of the tumor-associated antigen large external antigen in colorectal cancer tissues and cells using quantum dot probe," *International Journal of Nanomedicine*, vol. 11, pp. 235–247, 2016.

[192] X. Xing, B. Zhang, X. Wang, F. Liu, D. Shi, and Y. Cheng, "An "imaging-biopsy" strategy for colorectal tumor reconfirmation by multipurpose paramagnetic quantum dots," *Biomaterials*, vol. 48, pp. 16–25, 2015.

[193] M. Gazouli, P. Bouziotis, A. Lyberopoulou et al., "Quantum dots-bevacizumab complexes for *in vivo* imaging of tumors," *In Vivo*, vol. 28, no. 6, pp. 1091–1095, 2014.

[194] L. P. Wu, M. Ficker, J. B. Christensen, P. N. Trohopoulos, and S. M. Moghimi, "Dendrimers in medicine: therapeutic concepts and pharmaceutical challenges," *Bioconjugate Chemistry*, vol. 26, no. 7, pp. 1198–1211, 2015.

[195] E. Abbasi, S. F. Aval, A. Akbarzadeh et al., "Dendrimers: synthesis, applications, and properties," *Nanoscale Research Letters*, vol. 9, no. 1, p. 247, 2014.

[196] Meta-Analysis Group in Cancer, "Modulation of fluorouracil by leucovorin in patients with advanced colorectal cancer: evidence in terms of response rate. Advanced colorectal cancer meta-analysis project," *Journal of Clinical Oncology*, vol. 10, no. 6, pp. 896–903, 1992.

[197] A. de Gramont, A. Figer, M. Seymour et al., "Leucovorin and fluorouracil with or without oxaliplatin as first-line treatment in advanced colorectal cancer," *Journal of Clinical Oncology*, vol. 18, no. 16, pp. 2938–2947, 2000.

[198] J. Y. Douillard, D. Cunningham, A. D. Roth et al., "Irinotecan combined with fluorouracil compared with fluorouracil alone as first-line treatment for metastatic colorectal cancer: a multicentre randomised trial," *The Lancet*, vol. 355, no. 9209, pp. 1041–1047, 2000.

[199] A. Grothey and D. Sargent, "Overall survival of patients with advanced colorectal cancer correlates with availability of fluorouracil, irinotecan, and oxaliplatin regardless of whether doublet or single- agent therapy is used first line," *Journal of Clinical Oncology*, vol. 23, no. 36, pp. 9441-9442, 2005.

[200] H. Hurwitz, L. Fehrenbacher, W. Novotny et al., "Bevacizumab plus irinotecan, fluorouracil, and leucovorin for metastatic colorectal cancer," *The New England Journal of Medicine*, vol. 350, no. 23, pp. 2335–2342, 2004.

[201] D. Cunningham, Y. Humblet, S. Siena et al., "Cetuximab monotherapy and cetuximab plus irinotecan in irinotecan-

refractory metastatic colorectal cancer," *The New England Journal of Medicine*, vol. 351, no. 4, pp. 337–345, 2004.

[202] R. Dienstmann, E. Vilar, and J. Tabernero, "Molecular predictors of response to chemotherapy in colorectal cancer," *The Cancer Journal*, vol. 17, no. 2, pp. 114–126, 2011.

[203] B. Markman, F. Javier Ramos, J. Capdevila, and J. Tabernero, "EGFR and KRAS in colorectal cancer," *Advances in Clinical Chemistry*, vol. 51, pp. 71–119, 2010.

[204] V. Heinemann, S. Stintzing, T. Kirchner, S. Boeck, and A. Jung, "Clinical relevance of EGFR- and KRAS-status in colorectal cancer patients treated with monoclonal antibodies directed against the EGFR," *Cancer Treatment Reviews*, vol. 35, no. 3, pp. 262–271, 2009.

[205] E. Van Cutsem, M. Peeters, S. Siena et al., "Open-label phase III trial of panitumumab plus best supportive care compared with best supportive care alone in patients with chemotherapy- refractory metastatic colorectal cancer," *Journal of Clinical Oncology*, vol. 25, no. 13, pp. 1658–1664, 2007.

[206] S. Siena, A. Sartore-Bianchi, F. Di Nicolantonio, J. Balfour, and A. Bardelli, "Biomarkers predicting clinical outcome of epidermal growth factor receptor-targeted therapy in metastatic colorectal cancer," *JNCI: Journal of the National Cancer Institute*, vol. 101, no. 19, pp. 1308–1324, 2009.

[207] A. Lièvre, J.-B. Bachet, D. le Corre et al., "*KRAS* mutation status is predictive of response to cetuximab therapy in colorectal cancer," *Cancer Research*, vol. 66, no. 8, pp. 3992–3995, 2006.

[208] R. G. Amado, M. Wolf, M. Peeters et al., "Wild-type *KRAS* is required for panitumumab efficacy in patients with metastatic colorectal cancer," *Journal of Clinical Oncology*, vol. 26, no. 10, pp. 1626–1634, 2008.

[209] R. Wong and D. Cunningham, "Using predictive biomarkers to select patients with advanced colorectal cancer for treatment with epidermal growth factor receptor antibodies," *Journal of Clinical Oncology*, vol. 26, no. 35, pp. 5668–5670, 2008.

[210] E. van Cutsem, C.-H. Köhne, E. Hitre et al., "Cetuximab and chemotherapy as initial treatment for metastatic colorectal cancer," *The New England Journal of Medicine*, vol. 360, no. 14, pp. 1408–1417, 2009.

[211] S. T. Kim, K. H. Park, J. S. Kim, S. W. Shin, and Y. H. Kim, "Impact of *KRAS* mutation status on outcomes in metastatic colon cancer patients without anti-epidermal growth factor receptor therapy," *Cancer Research and Treatment*, vol. 45, no. 1, pp. 55–62, 2013.

[212] H. J. N. Andreyev, A. R. Norman, P. A. Clarke, D. Cunningham, and J. R. Oates, "Kirsten ras mutations in patients with colorectal cancer: the multicenter "RASCAL" study," *JNCI: Journal of the National Cancer Institute*, vol. 90, no. 9, pp. 675–684, 1998.

[213] H. J. N. Andreyev, A. R. Norman, D. Cunningham et al., "Kirsten ras mutations in patients with colorectal cancer: the 'RASCAL II' study," *British Journal of Cancer*, vol. 85, no. 5, pp. 692–696, 2001.

[214] S. D. Richman, M. T. Seymour, P. Chambers et al., "*KRAS* and *BRAF* mutations in advanced colorectal cancer are associated with poor prognosis but do not preclude benefit from oxaliplatin or irinotecan: results from the MRC FOCUS trial," *Journal of Clinical Oncology*, vol. 27, no. 35, pp. 5931–5937, 2009.

[215] E. Hawkes and D. Cunningham, "Relationship between colorectal cancer biomarkers and response to epidermal growth factor receptor monoclonal antibodies," *Journal of Clinical Oncology*, vol. 28, no. 28, pp. e529–e531, 2010.

[216] W. de Roock, B. Claes, D. Bernasconi et al., "Effects of *KRAS*, *BRAF*, *NRAS*, and *PIK3CA* mutations on the efficacy of cetuximab plus chemotherapy in chemotherapy-refractory metastatic colorectal cancer: a retrospective consortium analysis," *The Lancet Oncology*, vol. 11, no. 8, pp. 753–762, 2010.

[217] J. Y. Douillard, K. S. Oliner, S. Siena et al., "Panitumumab-FOLFOX4 treatment and RAS mutations in colorectal cancer," *The New England Journal of Medicine*, vol. 369, no. 11, pp. 1023–1034, 2013.

[218] A. Bertotti, E. Papp, S. Jones et al., "The genomic landscape of response to EGFR blockade in colorectal cancer," *Nature*, vol. 526, no. 7572, pp. 263–267, 2015.

[219] F. Di Nicolantonio, M. Martini, F. Molinari et al., "Wild-type *BRAF* is required for response to panitumumab or cetuximab in metastatic colorectal cancer," *Journal of Clinical Oncology*, vol. 26, no. 35, pp. 5705–5712, 2008.

[220] C. Bokemeyer, E. V. Cutsem, P. Rougier et al., "Addition of cetuximab to chemotherapy as first-line treatment for *KRAS* wild-type metastatic colorectal cancer: pooled analysis of the CRYSTAL and OPUS randomised clinical trials," *European Journal of Cancer*, vol. 48, no. 10, pp. 1466–1475, 2012.

[221] C. Cremolini, F. Loupakis, C. Antoniotti et al., "FOLFOXIRI plus bevacizumab versus FOLFIRI plus bevacizumab as first-line treatment of patients with metastatic colorectal cancer: updated overall survival and molecular subgroup analyses of the open-label, phase 3 TRIBE study," *The Lancet Oncology*, vol. 16, no. 13, pp. 1306–1315, 2015.

[222] F. Pietrantonio, F. Petrelli, A. Coinu et al., "Predictive role of BRAF mutations in patients with advanced colorectal cancer receiving cetuximab and panitumumab: a meta-analysis," *European Journal of Cancer*, vol. 51, no. 5, pp. 587–594, 2015.

[223] A. Rowland, M. M. Dias, M. D. Wiese et al., "Meta-analysis of BRAF mutation as a predictive biomarker of benefit from anti-EGFR monoclonal antibody therapy for RAS wild-type metastatic colorectal cancer," *British Journal of Cancer*, vol. 112, no. 12, pp. 1888–1894, 2015.

[224] A. Wells, "EGF receptor," *The International Journal of Biochemistry & Cell Biology*, vol. 31, no. 6, pp. 637–643, 1999.

[225] S. Paik, R. Hazan, E. R. Fisher et al., "Pathologic findings from the National Surgical Adjuvant Breast and Bowel Project: prognostic significance of erbB-2 protein overexpression in primary breast cancer," *Journal of Clinical Oncology*, vol. 8, no. 1, pp. 103–112, 1990.

[226] The Cancer Genome Atlas Network, "Comprehensive molecular characterization of human colon and rectal cancer," *Nature*, vol. 487, no. 7407, pp. 330–337, 2012.

[227] D. O. Kavanagh, G. Chambers, L. O' Grady et al., "Is overexpression of HER-2 a predictor of prognosis in colorectal cancer?," *BMC Cancer*, vol. 9, no. 1, p. 1, 2009.

[228] A. H. Marx, E. C. Burandt, M. Choschzick et al., "Heterogenous high-level HER-2 amplification in a small subset of colorectal cancers," *Human Pathology*, vol. 41, no. 11, pp. 1577–1585, 2010.

[229] A. Ooi, T. Takehana, X. Li et al., "Protein overexpression and gene amplification of *HER-2* and *EGFR* in colorectal cancers: an immunohistochemical and fluorescent *in situ*

hybridization study," *Modern Pathology*, vol. 17, no. 8, pp. 895–904, 2004.

[230] T. Osako, M. Miyahara, S. Uchino, M. Inomata, S. Kitano, and M. Kobayashi, "Immunohistochemical study of c-erbB-2 protein in colorectal cancer and the correlation with patient survival," *Oncology*, vol. 55, no. 6, pp. 548–555, 1998.

[231] F. Sclafani, A. Roy, D. Cunningham et al., "HER2 in high-risk rectal cancer patients treated in EXPERT-C, a randomized phase II trial of neoadjuvant capecitabine and oxaliplatin (CAPOX) and chemoradiotherapy (CRT) with or without cetuximab," *Annals of Oncology*, vol. 24, no. 12, pp. 3123–3128, 2013.

[232] W. S. Lee, Y. H. Park, J. N. Lee, J. H. Baek, T. H. Lee, and S. Y. Ha, "Comparison of HER2 expression between primary colorectal cancer and their corresponding metastases," *Cancer Medicine*, vol. 3, no. 3, pp. 674–680, 2014.

[233] D. R. Nathanson, A. T. Culliford, J. Shia et al., "HER 2/*neu* expression and gene amplification in colon cancer," *International Journal of Cancer*, vol. 105, no. 6, pp. 796–802, 2003.

[234] M. L. Caruso and A. M. Valentini, "Immunohistochemical p53 overexpression correlated to c-erbB-2 and cathepsin D proteins in colorectal cancer," *Anticancer Research*, vol. 16, no. 6B, pp. 3813–3818, 1996.

[235] S. S. Park and S. W. Kim, "Activated Akt signaling pathway in invasive ductal carcinoma of the breast: correlation with HER2 overexpression," *Oncology Reports*, vol. 18, no. 1, pp. 139–143, 2007.

[236] S. M. Kavuri, N. Jain, F. Galimi et al., "HER2 activating mutations are targets for colorectal cancer treatment," *Cancer Discovery*, vol. 5, no. 8, pp. 832–841, 2015.

[237] A. F. Sobrero, J. Maurel, L. Fehrenbacher et al., "EPIC: phase III trial of cetuximab plus irinotecan after fluoropyrimidine and oxaliplatin failure in patients with metastatic colorectal cancer," *Journal of Clinical Oncology*, vol. 26, no. 14, pp. 2311–2319, 2008.

[238] C. Bokemeyer, I. Bondarenko, J. T. Hartmann et al., "Efficacy according to biomarker status of cetuximab plus FOLFOX-4 as first-line treatment for metastatic colorectal cancer: the OPUS study," *Annals of Oncology*, vol. 22, no. 7, pp. 1535–1546, 2011.

[239] J. Y. Douillard, S. Siena, J. Cassidy et al., "Randomized, phase III trial of panitumumab with infusional fluorouracil, leucovorin, and oxaliplatin (FOLFOX4) versus FOLFOX4 alone as first-line treatment in patients with previously untreated metastatic colorectal cancer: the PRIME study," *Journal of Clinical Oncology*, vol. 28, no. 31, pp. 4697–4705, 2010.

[240] S. M. Leto and L. Trusolino, "Primary and acquired resistance to EGFR-targeted therapies in colorectal cancer: impact on future treatment strategies," *Journal of Molecular Medicine*, vol. 92, no. 7, pp. 709–722, 2014.

[241] M. Kloth, V. Ruesseler, C. Engel et al., "Activating ERBB2/HER2 mutations indicate susceptibility to pan-HER inhibitors in Lynch and Lynch-like colorectal cancer," *Gut*, vol. 65, no. 8, pp. 1296–1305, 2016.

[242] K. Yonesaka, K. Zejnullahu, I. Okamoto et al., "Activation of ERBB2 signaling causes resistance to the EGFR-directed therapeutic antibody cetuximab," *Science Translational Medicine*, vol. 3, no. 99, pp. 99ra86–99ra86, 2011.

[243] A. Bertotti, G. Migliardi, F. Galimi et al., "A molecularly annotated platform of patient-derived xenografts ("xenopatients") identifies HER2 as an effective therapeutic target in cetuximab-resistant colorectal cancer," *Cancer Discovery*, vol. 1, no. 6, article 22586653, pp. 508–523, 2011.

[244] S. Siena, A. Sartore-Bianchi, L. Trusolino et al., "Trastuzumab and lapatinib in HER2-amplified metastatic colorectal cancer patients (mCRC): the HERACLES trial," *Journal of Clinical Oncology*, vol. 33, Supplement 15, p. 3508, 2015.

[245] H. Hurwitz, J. D. Hainsworth, C. Swanton et al., "Targeted therapy for gastrointestinal (GI) tumors based on molecular profiles: early results from MyPathway, an open-label phase IIa basket study in patients with advanced solid tumors," *Journal of Clinical Oncology*, vol. 34, Supplement 4, p. 653, 2016.

[246] E. Valtorta, C. Martino, A. Sartore-Bianchi et al., "Assessment of a HER2 scoring system for colorectal cancer: results from a validation study," *Modern Pathology*, vol. 28, no. 11, pp. 1481–1491, 2015.

[247] V. Martin, L. Landi, F. Molinari et al., "HER2 gene copy number status may influence clinical efficacy to anti-EGFR monoclonal antibodies in metastatic colorectal cancer patients," *British Journal of Cancer*, vol. 108, no. 3, pp. 668–675, 2013.

[248] J. F. Deeken, H. Wang, D. Subramaniam et al., "A phase 1 study of cetuximab and lapatinib in patients with advanced solid tumor malignancies," *Cancer*, vol. 121, no. 10, pp. 1645–1653, 2015.

[249] C. Lengauer, K. W. Kinzler, and B. Vogelstein, "Genetic instability in colorectal cancers," *Nature*, vol. 386, no. 6625, pp. 623–627, 1997.

[250] B. Vogelstein, E. R. Fearon, S. R. Hamilton et al., "Genetic alterations during colorectal-tumor development," *The New England Journal of Medicine*, vol. 319, no. 9, pp. 525–532, 1988.

[251] M. S. Pino and D. C. Chung, "Microsatellite instability in the management of colorectal cancer," *Expert Review of Gastroenterology & Hepatology*, vol. 5, no. 3, pp. 385–399, 2014.

[252] A. de la Chapelle and H. Hampel, "Clinical relevance of microsatellite instability in colorectal cancer," *Journal of Clinical Oncology*, vol. 28, no. 20, pp. 3380–3387, 2010.

[253] C. R. Boland and A. Goel, "Microsatellite instability in colorectal cancer," *Gastroenterology*, vol. 138, no. 6, pp. 2073–2087.e3, 2010.

[254] J. Jiricny, "The multifaceted mismatch-repair system," *Nature Reviews Molecular Cell Biology*, vol. 7, no. 5, pp. 335–346, 2006.

[255] R. R. Iyer, A. Pluciennik, V. Burdett, and P. L. Modrich, "DNA mismatch repair: functions and mechanisms," *Chemical Reviews*, vol. 106, no. 2, pp. 302–323, 2006.

[256] C. R. Boland, S. N. Thibodeau, S. R. Hamilton et al., "A National Cancer Institute Workshop on Microsatellite instability for cancer detection and familial pre-disposition: development of international criteria for the determination of microsatellite instability in colorectal cancer," *Cancer Research*, vol. 58, no. 22, pp. 5248–5257, 1998.

[257] H. T. Lynch, M. W. Shaw, C. W. Magnuson, A. L. Larsen, and A. J. Krush, "Hereditary factors in cancer: study of two large midwestern kindreds," *Archives of Internal Medicine*, vol. 117, no. 2, pp. 206–212, 1966.

[258] S. Ogino, K. Nosho, G. J. Kirkner et al., "CpG island methylator phenotype, microsatellite instability, *BRAF* mutation and clinical outcome in colon cancer," *Gut*, vol. 58, no. 1, pp. 90–96, 2009.

[259] M. A. Jenkins, S. Hayashi, A. M. O'Shea et al., "Pathology features in Bethesda guidelines predict colorectal cancer microsatellite instability: a population-based study," *Gastroenterology*, vol. 133, no. 1, pp. 48–56, 2007.

[260] G. Deng, I. Bell, S. Crawley et al., "*BRAF* mutation is frequently present in sporadic colorectal cancer with methylated hMLH1, but not in hereditary nonpolyposis colorectal cancer," *Clinical Cancer Research*, vol. 10, no. 1, pp. 191–195, 2004.

[261] S. Popat, R. Hubner, and R. S. Houlston, "Systematic review of microsatellite instability and colorectal cancer prognosis," *Journal of Clinical Oncology*, vol. 23, no. 3, pp. 609–618, 2005.

[262] C. Guastadisegni, M. Colafranceschi, L. Ottini, and E. Dogliotti, "Microsatellite instability as a marker of prognosis and response to therapy: a meta-analysis of colorectal cancer survival data," *European Journal of Cancer*, vol. 46, no. 15, pp. 2788–2798, 2010.

[263] P. Benatti, R. Gafà, D. Barana et al., "Microsatellite instability and colorectal cancer prognosis," *Clinical Cancer Research*, vol. 11, no. 23, pp. 8332–8340, 2005.

[264] R. Jover, P. Zapater, A. Castells et al., "The efficacy of adjuvant chemotherapy with 5-fluorouracil in colorectal cancer depends on the mismatch repair status," *European Journal of Cancer*, vol. 45, no. 3, pp. 365–373, 2009.

[265] G. Des Guetz, O. Schischmanoff, P. Nicolas, G. Y. Perret, J. F. Morere, and B. Uzzan, "Does microsatellite instability predict the efficacy of adjuvant chemotherapy in colorectal cancer? A systematic review with meta-analysis," *European Journal of Cancer*, vol. 45, no. 10, pp. 1890–1896, 2009.

[266] https://clinicaltrials.gov/ct2/show/NCT02060188?term=CHECKMATE+142&rank=1.

[267] https://clinicaltrials.gov/ct2/show/NCT02460198?term=KEYNOTE+164&rank=1.

[268] https://clinicaltrials.gov/ct2/show/NCT02563002?term=KEYNOTE+177&rank=1.

[269] M. M. Bertagnolli, D. Niedzwiecki, C. C. Compton et al., "Microsatellite instability predicts improved response to adjuvant therapy with irinotecan, fluorouracil, and leucovorin in stage III colon cancer: cancer and leukemia group B protocol 89803," *Journal of Clinical Oncology*, vol. 27, no. 11, pp. 1814–1821, 2009.

[270] D. Fallik, F. Borrini, V. Boige et al., "Microsatellite instability is a predictive factor of the tumor response to irinotecan in patients with advanced colorectal cancer," *Cancer Research*, vol. 63, no. 18, pp. 5738–5744, 2003.

[271] W. M. Grady and J. M. Carethers, "Genomic and epigenetic instability in colorectal cancer pathogenesis," *Gastroenterology*, vol. 135, no. 4, pp. 1079–1099, 2008.

[272] A. V. Kudryavtseva, A. V. Lipatova, A. R. Zaretsky et al., "Important molecular genetic markers of colorectal cancer," *Oncotarget*, vol. 7, no. 33, pp. 53959–53983, 2016.

4

Feasibility, Safety, and Efficacy of Pressurized Intraperitoneal Aerosol Chemotherapy (PIPAC) for Peritoneal Metastasis

Florian Kurtz,[1] Florian Struller,[1] Philipp Horvath,[1] Wiebke Solass,[2] Hans Bösmüller,[2] Alfred Königsrainer,[1] and Marc A. Reymond[1,3]

[1]*Dept. of General Surgery, Karls-Eberhard University Tübingen, Germany*
[2]*Institute of Pathology, Karls-Eberhard University Tübingen, Germany*
[3]*National Center for Pleura and Peritoneum, Comprehensive Cancer Center South-Western Germany, Tübingen, Stuttgart, Germany*

Correspondence should be addressed to Marc A. Reymond; marc.reymond@yahoo.de

Academic Editor: Charles Honore

Introduction. Pressurized intraperitoneal aerosol chemotherapy (PIPAC) is a novel drug delivery system with superior pharmacological properties for treating peritoneal metastasis (PM). Safety and efficacy results of PIPAC with cisplatin/doxorubicin or oxaliplatin from a registry cohort are presented. *Methods.* IRB-approved registry study. Retrospective analysis. No predefined inclusion criteria, individual therapeutic recommendation by the interdisciplinary tumor board. Safety assessment with CTCAE 4.0. Histological assessment of tumor response by an independent pathologist using the 4-tied peritoneal regression grading system (PRGS). Mean PRGS and ascites volume were assessed at each PIPAC. *Results.* A total of 142 PIPAC procedures were scheduled in 71 consecutive patients with PM from gastric ($n = 26$), colorectal ($n = 17$), hepatobiliary/pancreatic ($n = 9$), ovarian ($n = 6$), appendiceal ($n = 5$) origin, pseudomyxoma peritonei ($n = 4$), and other tumors ($n = 3$). Mean age was 58 ± 13 years. Patients were heavily pretreated. Mean PCI was 19 ± 13. Laparoscopic nonaccess rate was 11/142 procedures (7.7%). Mean number of PIPAC/patient was 2. All patients were eligible for safety analysis. There was no procedure-related mortality. There were 2.8% intraoperative and 4.9% postoperative complications. 39 patients underwent more than one PIPAC and were eligible for efficacy analysis, and PRGS could be assessed in 36 of them. In 24 patients (67%), PRGS improved or remained unchanged at PIPAC#2, reflecting tumor regression or stable disease. Ascites was present in 24 patients and diminished significantly under therapy. Median survival was 11.8 months (95% CI: 7.45–16.2 months) from PIPAC#1. *Conclusion.* PIPAC is feasible, safe, and well-tolerated and can induce histological regression in a significant proportion of pretreated PM patients. This trial is registered with NCT03210298.

1. Introduction

In spite of recent progress in systemic palliative chemotherapy, prognosis of peritoneal metastasis remains dismal [1]. The cytotoxic effect of chemotherapy might be improved by the use of intraperitoneal drug delivery, when malignant disease is confined to the peritoneal cavity. Improved cytotoxicity is based on the theoretical potential for increased exposure of the tumor to antineoplastic agents [2].

However, two pharmacokinetic problems appear to limit the effectiveness of intraperitoneal chemotherapy: poor tumor penetration by the drug and incomplete irrigation of serosal surfaces by the drug-containing solution [3, 4] Moreover, intraperitoneal chemotherapy is hampered by dose-limiting local toxicity, so that its clinical use remains fairly limited [5]. Thus, there is a considerable research effort for developing next-generation drug delivery systems for intraperitoneal chemotherapy that maximizes local efficacy while limiting systemic side effects [6].

One of these new intraperitoneal cytotoxic drug delivery systems is pressurized intraperitoneal aerosol chemotherapy (PIPAC), which is gaining rapid clinical acceptance in the palliative therapy of peritoneal metastasis worldwide. The rationale of PIPAC is based on the use of a pressurized therapeutic aerosol [7] with superior pharmacological properties, in particular, a deeper drug tissue penetration [8, 9], a higher drug tissue concentration [10], and a more homogeneous distribution than with liquid chemotherapy [11, 12]. Increased drug penetration under pressure had been previously demonstrated in other animal models [13, 14]. Moreover, hyperpressure obtained by gas administration during laparoscopy decreases the venous blood outflow from the abdomen, which might result in an increased time of drug tissue contact [15]. PIPAC allows a significant dose reduction and therefore largely prevents systemic organ toxicity [16, 17]. Promising results have been published in peritoneal metastasis of gastric [18, 19], ovarian [20, 21], colorectal [22], pancreatic [23, 24], and hepatobiliary [25] origins. A recent systemic review of the literature concluded that PIPAC is feasible, safe, and well-tolerated and that preliminary good response rates call for a prospective analysis of oncological efficacy [26].

Meanwhile, at least 15 prospective clinical trials are ongoing evaluating oncological efficacy of PIPAC in multiple indications with various drugs, including cisplatin, oxaliplatin, doxorubicin, and nab-paclitaxel [27]. However, these studies only cover selected groups of patients so that registry data are needed for highlighting PIPAC results in the other patients and in rare indications. In the present paper, we report about our experience gained with PIPAC since July 2016 at a tertiary cancer center offering all other therapeutic options for peritoneal metastasis, including in particular palliative systemic chemotherapy, intraperitoneal chemotherapy, intraperitoneal virotherapy [28], cytoreductive surgery, and hyperthermic intraperitoneal chemotherapy (HIPEC).

Here, we demonstrate that PIPAC is feasible in a large number of patients with peritoneal metastasis in the salvage situation, that PIPAC is safe, and that encouraging survival figures and significant ascites reduction has been observed.

2. Patients and Methods

2.1. Study Design. This is a registry study on a cohort of consecutive patients, starting with the first patient treated with PIPAC in our institution. No patient was excluded. Data were entered prospectively into a patient registry, and analysis was retrospective. No primary/secondary endpoint was predefined.

2.2. Ethical and Regulatory Framework. The international PIPAC patient registry was approved by the Ethics Committee, Ruhr-University Bochum, on Jan 11, 2016 (reference 15-5280), and by the data protection officer of the State of North Rhine-Westphalia, Germany. Each patient gave his/her written informed consent both for the PIPAC procedure and for data storage management and analysis. The registry is hosted by an independent quality control organization (AnInstitut für Qualitätssicherung in der Operativen Medizin gGmbH, Otto-von-Guericke Universität Magdeburg) [29]. Although cisplatin, doxorubicin, and/or oxaliplatin is routinely used in clinical practice worldwide for locoregional therapy in peritoneal disease and has been the object of multiple randomized controlled trials [30–37], none of these drugs is currently approved for intraperitoneal delivery. Therefore, PIPAC was applied "off-label."

2.3. Patient Selection. Each patient was presented in the interdisciplinary tumor board (ZGO) of the Comprehensive Cancer Center, University Hospital Tübingen, Germany. PIPAC therapy was recommended on an individual basis; no inclusion or exclusion criteria were predefined. Patients with extraperitoneal metastases (with the exception of isolated pleural effusion) were not treated. Complete or partial bowel obstruction, presence of gastric discharge tube, or very poor general condition (Karnofsky < 50%) was considered a palliative situation, and the patients were referred to a palliative care unit. If the tumor board recommended cytoreductive surgery and HIPEC, then the patient was not considered for a PIPAC therapy.

2.4. Technique of PIPAC. After the creation of a standard CO_2 pneumoperitoneum, two access trocars (Kii®, Applied Medical, Düsseldorf, Germany) were inserted through the abdominal wall. A staging laparoscopy with the determination of the peritoneal cancer index (PCI) was followed by multiple peritoneal biopsies in all abdominal quadrants. Tightness of the abdomen was verified. A disposable nebulizer (Capnopen®, Capnomed GmbH, Villingendorf, Germany) was introduced under videoscopic control into the abdomen through one of the trocars and connected with a high-pressure injector through a dedicated high-pressure line. Patients with peritoneal metastasis of colorectal or, by analogy, of appendicular origin were treated with oxaliplatin 92 mg/m^2 BSA diluted into 150 ml Glc 5%. All other patients were treated sequentially by doxorubicin 1.5 mg/m^2 BSA diluted into 50 ml 0.9% saline, then with cisplatin 15 mg/m^2 BSA diluted into 150 ml 0.9% saline. The cytotoxic solutions were nebulized into the expanded peritoneal cavity under an upstream pressure of 20 bar. Then, the therapeutic capnoperitoneum was maintained in a steady state at a pressure of 12 mmHg at a temperature of 37°C for 30 min. Thereafter, the capnoperitoneum was deflated through a closed aerosol waste system (CAWS) and the procedure was terminated.

2.5. Occupational Health Safety. The following safety measures were taken to exclude any exposure of the personnel [38]: first, the tightness of the abdomen was documented via zero-flow CO_2. Second, the procedure was performed in an operating room equipped with a laminar airflow. Third, the chemotherapy injections were remote-controlled, and no personnel remained in the operating room during the application.

2.6. PIPAC Cycles. PIPAC was repeated at 6-week intervals; in the case of major or complete histological regression, this interval was extended to 3 months. In the cases of combined treatment (systemic and intraperitoneal chemotherapy), a minimum delay of two weeks (bevacizumab: 4 weeks) between the last application of systemic chemotherapy and PIPAC was observed. Systemic chemotherapy could be started immediately (in practice 1 week) after PIPAC application.

2.7. Efficacy Assessment. Histological regression was assessed by an independent pathologist (Department of Pathology, University of Tübingen, Germany) by grading tumor biopsies taken during each PIPAC. Patients eligible for histological tumor response assessment had at least 2 PIPAC cycles. Histopathological tumor regression was graded according to the 4-tied peritoneal regression grading system (PRGS) [39]. Ascites was removed at the beginning of each PIPAC procedure, and the volume was measured. Analysis has been performed on 25 patients who presented with ≥300 ml ascites at PIPAC 1. All 25 patients were included in the analysis, independently of the number of PIPAC cycles received. PCI was not used as response criteria, due to the large subjectivity in the macroscopic judgement of lesions (tumor vs. scar).

2.8. Safety Assessment. Adverse events were graded according to the Common Terminology Criteria for Adverse Events (CTCAE) version 4.0 [40]. Surgical complications were graded according to the Dindo-Clavien classification [41].

2.9. Follow-Up. The mean follow-up was 10.4 ± 4.2 months. The closing date was October 17, 2017. A staging CT-scan was recommended every 3 months. Patients and/or general practitioners were contacted by phone and/or email.

2.10. Statistical Analysis. All p values are two-tailed, and a p value of less than 0.05 was considered statistically significant. Values are given as means or medians, where appropriate. We performed a multivariable logistic regression model (Cox) with survival as the dependent variable and PCI, Karnofsky index, PRGS, time point of peritoneal metastasis (synchronous vs. metachronous), number of previous chemotherapy lines, and presence of ascites (yes/no) as independent variables. Survival was modelled in a Kaplan-Meier survival curve. We used SPSS 24 for Windows (SPSS Inc., Chicago, IL, USA) for statistical analysis and SigmaPlot 13 (Systat Software Inc., San José, CA, USA) for creating graphs.

3. Results

3.1. Patients and Procedures. A total of 142 PIPAC procedures were scheduled in 71 patients with peritoneal metastasis and gastric cancer ($n = 26$), colorectal cancer ($n = 17$), hepatobiliary/pancreatic cancer ($n = 9$), ovarian cancer ($n = 6$), appendiceal cancer ($n = 5$), pseudomyxoma peritonei ($n = 4$), and other tumors ($n = 3$). The mean age of this cohort was 58 ± 13 years. The Karnofsky index was 80.3 ± 14.7. Ascites (300 ml and more) and pleural effusion were present in 24 and three patients, respectively. 42/71 patients received combined systemic chemotherapy and PIPAC. Patients' characteristics including the number of previous chemotherapy lines are shown in Table 1.

3.2. Feasibility. The patient flowchart is detailed in Figure 1. The laparoscopic nonaccess rate was 11/142 procedures (7.7%; eight primary, three secondary nonaccess). Thus, 24, 19, 13, six, and one patients underwent successfully one, two, three, four, and six PIPAC, respectively, totalizing 131 successful procedures. The mean number of PIPACs administered was two (minimum one, maximum six).

Table 1: Patient characteristics.

Variable	Value
Number of patients	71
Sex (M : F)	28 : 43
Age, years (±SD)	58 ± 13
Organ of origin	
(i) Gastric	26 (36.6%)
(ii) Colorectal	17 (23.9%)
(iii) Hepatobiliary-pancreatic	9 (12.7%)
(iv) Ovarian	6 (8.5%)
(v) Appendiceal	5 (7.0%)
(vi) PMP	4 (5.6%)
(vii) CUP, mesothelioma, yolk sac, prostate	3 (4.2%)
Extraperitoneal metastasis	
(i) Malignant pleural effusion	3 (4.2%)
(ii) Others	0
Peritoneal Cancer Index (PCI), mean ± SD	19.3 ± 12.5
Karnofsky Index before first PIPAC, mean ± SD	80.3 ± 14.7
Previous surgery	
(i) CRS and HIPEC	10 (14.1%)
(ii) Gastrectomy	11 (15.5%)
(iii) Colectomy	11 (15.5%)
(iv) Hysterectomy and adnexectomy	5 (7.0%)
(v) Laparotomy	9 (12.7%)
(vi) Laparoscopy	4 (5.6%)
(vii) Other surgeries	14 (19.7%)
(viii) None	7 (9.9%)
Previous systemic chemotherapy	
(i) None	11 (15.5%)
(ii) 1 line	18 (25.4%)
(iii) 2 lines	17 (23.9%)
(iv) 3 lines	10 (14.1%)
(v) >3 lines	15 (21.1%)
Simultaneous chemotherapy	42 (59.1%)

The mean operating time was 103 ± 30.7 min. The procedures were performed by six different surgeons, including two residents.

3.3. Safety. All 71 patients were eligible for safety analysis. Complications and side effects are detailed in Table 2.

(i) Intraoperative complications: there were four (2.8% procedures) intraoperative complications: one lung aspiration ad induction of narcosis, one bowel laceration in a patient with tumoral adherence to the abdominal wall, one bowel puncture with the Veres needle, and one bleeding requiring laparotomy. All surgical complications were repaired intraoperatively, and the patients recovered uneventfully. In all four patients, application of PIPAC was postponed to a later point of time

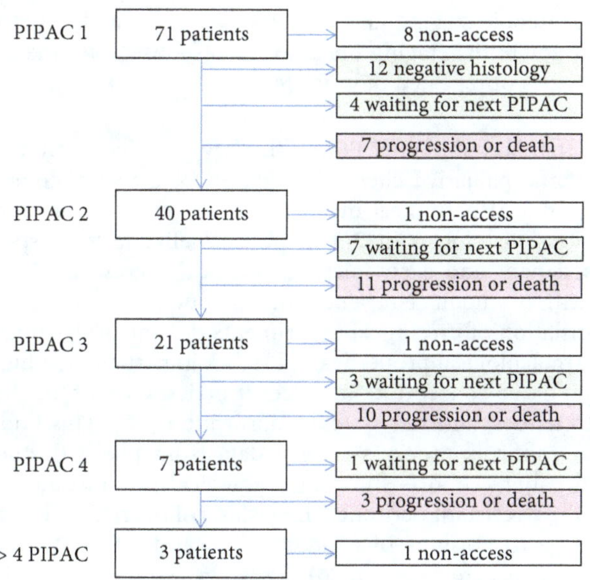

Figure 1: Patient flowchart.

Table 2: Adverse events.

Intraoperative			
Type of complication			
(i) Bowel injury		2#	
(ii) Lung aspiration		1	
(iii) Bleeding		1	
Total		4 (5.6%)	
Postoperative		Dindo-Clavien	CTCAE
Type of complication			
(i) Abdominal wall infiltration	2	1	N/A
(ii) Leucopenia	1	N/A	3
(iii) Ascites leakage	1	1	N/A
(iv) Nausea/vomiting	1	2	2
(v) Hematoma, transfusion	1	2	N/A
(vi) Hospital mortality	1*	5	5
Total		7 (9.9%)	

#detected and repaired intraoperatively; *ASA IV patient, 4500 ml ascites, unrelated to procedure.

(ii) Postoperative complications: there were seven postoperative complications (4.9% procedures): two patients developed abdominal wall infiltration because of localized leakage of the toxic aerosol, one patient under systemic chemotherapy (cisplatin/gemcitabine) developed moderate leucopenia (2970/μl) on postoperative day 3, and one patient under chronic anticoagulation developed an important intramural hematoma in the abdominal wall that was treated conservatively but required postoperative blood transfusion. In one patient, ascites leaked postoperatively through a trocar incision and necessitated a bedside skin suture. There were no procedure-related mortality and one hospital death (patient classified ASA IV, with 4500 ml ascites developed cardiopulmonary decompensation with fatal outcome on postoperative day 12)

3.4. Efficacy. 39 patients underwent more than one PIPAC and were eligible for efficacy analysis. No radiological evaluation according to RECIST criteria was performed. Histological analysis was performed by an independent pathologist who could compare the current with previous biopsies. Peritoneal grading regression score (PRGS) could be calculated in 36 of these 39 patients. In 24 patients (67%), PRGS improved or remained unchanged at PIPAC#2, reflecting tumor regression or stable disease. In the remaining 12 patients, PRGS deteriorated under therapy. At PIPAC#2, 10/39 patients (26%) had a complete histological regression (PRGS = 1) in multiple peritoneal biopsies as well as in a local peritoneal peritonectomy sample. Ascites volume diminished between PIPAC#1 and PIPAC#3 (Figure 2); in patients with an initial ascites volume equal or superior to 300 ml, this difference was significant (ANOVA, $p = 0.03$).

3.5. Survival. The mean follow-up for all patients was 10.7 ± 4.4 months from PIPAC#1. At the end of the follow-up, 36/71 patients were alive, 19 were dead, and 6 were lost to follow-up. For all organs of origin together, the median survival from the first PIPAC was 11.8 months (95% CI: 7.45–16.2 months). Figure 3 shows the overall survival from the first PIPAC depending on histology. The median survival from the first PIPAC was 6.8 months in ovarian cancer (median: 3–4th line situation), 6.8 months also in gastric cancer (2nd line situation), and 11.8 months in hepatobiliary-pancreatic tumors (3rd line situation) and was not reached after 11.8 months for colorectal cancer (3-4th line situation), pseudomyxoma peritonei (2-3rd line situation), and mesothelioma (2nd line situation).

4. Discussion

In the last few years, encouraging feasibility data regarding the application of PIPAC with low-dose cisplatin and doxorubicin or oxaliplatin in previously heavily pretreated patients with peritoneal metastasis have been published by several independent groups [17, 42]. Promising safety and efficacy results have been published in peritoneal metastasis of gastric [18, 19], ovarian [20, 21], colorectal [22], pancreatic [23, 24], and hepatobiliary [25] origins. Survey data on a total of 832 PIPAC procedures in 349 patients obtained from 9 centers have recently shown that the technique is well standardized with regard to indications, technical aspects, safety protocol, and treatment regimen so that results can be easily compared and even pooled between centers [43].

The results of this registry study on consecutive patients with advanced, pretreated peritoneal metastasis confirm that PIPAC is feasible, safe, and well-tolerated, which is in accordance with the above studies and with two systematic reviews [26, 44].

In the present cohort, the primary nonaccess rate was 8/71 patients = 11.2%. This figure is in line with the literature and confirms that nonaccess to the abdomen is a

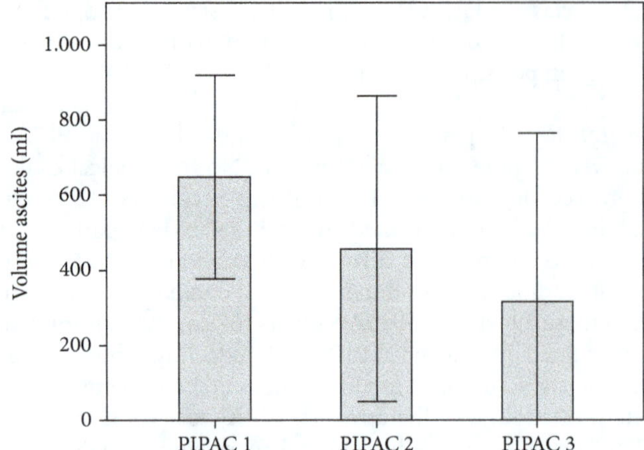

FIGURE 2: Ascites volume at PIPAC#1, PIPAC#2, and PIPAC#3. There is a significant decrease of ascites volume under therapy (ANOVA, $p = 0.03$).

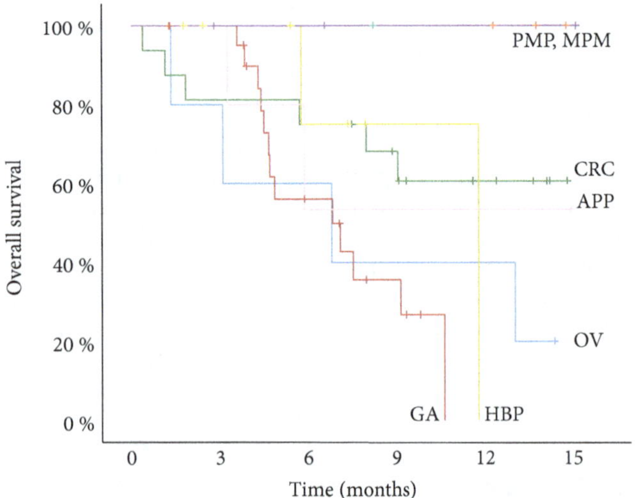

FIGURE 3: Overall survival probability (Kaplan-Meyer) of pretreated patients with pseudomyxoma peritonei (PMP), malignant peritoneal mesothelioma (MESO), and peritoneal metastasis of colorectal (CRC), appendiceal (APP), ovarian (OV), hepatobiliary-pancreatic (HBP), and gastric (GC) origins. Survival calculated from the date of first PIPAC.

limitation of PIPAC, as it is the case in any staging laparoscopy after a previous abdominal surgery. However, the nonaccess rate appears to be influenced by patient selection, with a maximal risk of access failure in patients having received previous CRS and HIPEC. It is important to note that nonaccess is not harmful (as a rule). Thus, since there is no good alternative therapeutic option in the case of relapse, previous CRS and HIPEC are not an absolute contraindication for PIPAC.

A particular methodological problem of the available cohort studies on PIPAC is their heterogeneity and the difficulty of assessing objectively tumor response in peritoneal metastasis [45]. Contrast-enhanced CT-scan has a low sensitivity for small-volumetric peritoneal lesions [46], so that laparoscopic staging and biopsies are increasingly used not only for initial staging but also for response assessment on the basis of repeated biopsies [47].

In this cohort, after PIPAC therapy combined or not with systemic palliative chemotherapy, an objective histological response of peritoneal metastasis has been observed across various histologies in 2/3 of patients eligible for response assessment and a complete histological regression in one-fourth of them. This encouraging finding is the clinical translation of preclinical experiments documenting superior pharmacological properties of PIPAC, in particular, a higher drug tissue concentration, a deeper penetration of the drugs into tissues, and less systemic absorption [12]. This finding also confirms previous clinical data from phase II studies and patient cohorts showing histological response rates for therapy-resistant peritoneal metastasis of ovarian, colorectal, and gastric origins of 62–88, 71–86, and 70–100 percent, respectively (reviewed in 26). Thus, the results of this cohort fit well into the research map in this field and contribute to the body of evidence supporting the clinical efficacy of PIPAC as a palliative therapy of peritoneal metastasis.

Another promising finding in this study is significant ascites control already after the first cycle of intraperitoneal chemotherapy as PIPAC. The positive effect of PIPAC on ascites has already been reported in other studies [21, 48] and appears independent from the type of primary tumor and might contribute to the stabilization of the quality of life reported after PIPAC in several clinical studies [21, 45, 49] and patient cohorts [48, 50, 51].

Although the number of cases is limited, survival figures are encouraging. For example, the median survival of (heavily pretreated) patients with peritoneal metastasis of hepatobiliary-pancreatic origin was 11.8 months since first PIPAC. This survival time is unexpectedly long but confirms indeed a previous report with a median survival of 14 months (range 10–20) since the diagnosis of peritoneal metastasis [23]. The median survival of pretreated patients with peritoneal metastasis of gastric origin was 6.8 months, which is similar to our results (6.4 months) obtained within the framework of a phase II clinical trial in peritoneal metastasis of gastric origin in the salvage situation [49].

The registry data presented here are of exploratory nature, and caution is warranted in their interpretation. Extrapolation of these data to other patient cohorts or their use for individual therapeutic decisions is not permissible. However, the experimental finding remains that, in our patient cohort, PIPAC was safe and able to reverse platin resistance in the majority of patients, most of them having been heavily pretreated beforehand. Notably, objective tumor regression in the peritoneal tumor nodes was achieved with local administration of a dose of chemotherapy reduced by an order of magnitude (ten times) as compared to a systemic dose. This significant dose reduction contributes probably to the good tolerability of the procedure in the patients treated. In parallel to the high histological response rate, survival appears encouraging in this cohort and this is also in line with the superior survival statistics of four phase II trials examining the efficacy of PIPAC in advanced peritoneal metastasis [19, 21, 45, 49]. Several prospective randomized trials will now be required to confirm these encouraging results in each tumor entity with various potential treatment regimens.

Disclosure

MAR is a holder of several patents on PIPAC technology and receives royalties from Capnomed GmbH, Villingendorf, Germany.

Funding

This study was funded by institutional funds.

References

[1] L. A. Lambert, "Looking up: recent advances in understanding and treating peritoneal carcinomatosis," *CA: A Cancer Journal for Clinicians*, vol. 65, no. 4, pp. 284–298, 2015.

[2] M. Markman, "Intraperitoneal antineoplastic drug delivery: rationale and results," *The Lancet Oncology*, vol. 4, no. 5, pp. 277–283, 2003.

[3] R. L. Dedrick and M. F. Flessner, "Pharmacokinetic problems in peritoneal drug administration: tissue penetration and surface exposure," *Journal of the National Cancer Institute*, vol. 89, no. 7, pp. 480–487, 1997.

[4] M. F. Flessner, "Pharmacokinetic problems in peritoneal drug administration: an update after 20 years," *Pleura and Peritoneum*, vol. 1, no. 4, pp. 183–191, 2016.

[5] M. Markman, "Chemotherapy: limited use of the intraperitoneal route for ovarian cancer-why?," *Nature Reviews. Clinical Oncology*, vol. 12, no. 11, pp. 628–630, 2015.

[6] G. R. Dakwar, M. Shariati, W. Willaert, W. Ceelen, S. C. De Smedt, and K. Remaut, "Nanomedicine-based intraperitoneal therapy for the treatment of peritoneal carcinomatosis - mission possible?," *Advanced Drug Delivery Reviews*, vol. 108, pp. 13–24, 2017.

[7] M. A. Reymond, B. Hu, A. Garcia et al., "Feasibility of therapeutic pneumoperitoneum in a large animal model using a microvaporisator," *Surgical Endoscopy*, vol. 14, no. 1, pp. 51–55, 2000.

[8] W. Solass, R. Kerb, T. Mürdter et al., "Intraperitoneal chemotherapy of peritoneal carcinomatosis using pressurized aerosol as an alternative to liquid solution: first evidence for efficacy," *Annals of Surgical Oncology*, vol. 21, no. 2, pp. 553–559, 2014.

[9] W. Solass, A. Herbette, T. Schwarz et al., "Therapeutic approach of human peritoneal carcinomatosis with Dbait in combination with capnoperitoneum: proof of concept," *Surgical Endoscopy*, vol. 26, no. 3, pp. 847–852, 2012.

[10] V. Khosrawipour, T. Khosrawipour, A. J. P. Kern et al., "Distribution pattern and penetration depth of doxorubicin after pressurized intraperitoneal aerosol chemotherapy (PIPAC) in a post-mortem swine model," *Journal of Cancer Research and Clinical Oncology*, vol. 142, no. 11, pp. 2275–2280, 2016.

[11] W. Solaß, A. Hetzel, G. Nadiradze, E. Sagynaliev, and M. A. Reymond, "Description of a novel approach for intraperitoneal drug delivery and the related device," *Surgical Endoscopy*, vol. 26, no. 7, pp. 1849–1855, 2012.

[12] C. Eveno, A. Haidara, I. Ali, C. Pimpie, M. Mirshahi, and M. Pocard, "Experimental pharmacokinetics evaluation of chemotherapy delivery by PIPAC for colon cancer: first evidence for efficacy," *Pleura and Peritoneum*, vol. 2, no. 2, pp. 103–110, 2017.

[13] P. Jacquet, O. A. Stuart, D. Chang, and P. H. Sugarbaker, "Effects of intra-abdominal pressure on pharmacokinetics and tissue distribution of doxorubicin after intraperitoneal administration," *Anti-Cancer Drugs*, vol. 7, no. 5, pp. 596–603, 1996.

[14] P. Esquis, D. Consolo, G. Magnin et al., "High intra-abdominal pressure enhances the penetration and antitumor effect of intraperitoneal cisplatin on experimental peritoneal carcinomatosis," *Annals of Surgery*, vol. 244, no. 1, pp. 106–112, 2006.

[15] C. B. Tempfer, "Pressurized intraperitoneal aerosol chemotherapy as an innovative approach to treat peritoneal carcinomatosis," *Medical Hypotheses*, vol. 85, no. 4, pp. 480–484, 2015.

[16] A. Blanco, U. Giger-Pabst, W. Solass, J. Zieren, and M. A. Reymond, "Renal and hepatic toxicities after pressurized intraperitoneal aerosol chemotherapy (PIPAC)," *Annals of Surgical Oncology*, vol. 20, no. 7, pp. 2311–2316, 2013.

[17] M. Robella, M. Vaira, and M. De Simone, "Safety and feasibility of pressurized intraperitoneal aerosol chemotherapy (PIPAC) associated with systemic chemotherapy: an innovative approach to treat peritoneal carcinomatosis," *World Journal of Surgical Oncology*, vol. 14, no. 1, p. 128, 2016.

[18] G. Nadiradze, U. Giger-Pabst, J. Zieren, D. Strumberg, W. Solass, and M. A. Reymond, "Pressurized intraperitoneal aerosol chemotherapy (PIPAC) with low-dose cisplatin and doxorubicin in gastric peritoneal metastasis," *Journal of Gastrointestinal Surgery*, vol. 20, no. 2, pp. 367–373, 2016.

[19] V. Khomyakov, A. Ryabov, A. Ivanov et al., "Bidirectional chemotherapy in gastric cancer with peritoneal metastasis combining intravenous XELOX with intraperitoneal chemotherapy with low-dose cisplatin and doxorubicin administered as a pressurized aerosol: an open-label, Phase-2 study (PIPAC-GA2)," *Pleura and Peritoneum*, vol. 1, no. 3, pp. 159–166, 2016.

[20] C. B. Tempfer, I. Celik, W. Solass et al., "Activity of pressurized intraperitoneal aerosol chemotherapy (PIPAC) with cisplatin and doxorubicin in women with recurrent, platinum-resistant ovarian cancer: preliminary clinical experience," *Gynecologic Oncology*, vol. 132, no. 2, pp. 307–311, 2014.

[21] C. B. Tempfer, G. Winnekendonk, W. Solass et al., "Pressurized intraperitoneal aerosol chemotherapy in women with recurrent ovarian cancer: a phase 2 study," *Gynecologic Oncology*, vol. 137, no. 2, pp. 223–228, 2015.

[22] C. Demtröder, W. Solass, J. Zieren, D. Strumberg, U. Giger-Pabst, and M. A. Reymond, "Pressurized intraperitoneal aerosol chemotherapy with oxaliplatin in colorectal peritoneal

metastasis," *Colorectal Disease*, vol. 18, no. 4, pp. 364–371, 2016.

[23] M. Graversen, S. Detlefsen, J. K. Bjerregaard, P. Pfeiffer, and M. B. Mortensen, "Peritoneal metastasis from pancreatic cancer treated with pressurized intraperitoneal aerosol chemotherapy (PIPAC)," *Clinical & Experimental Metastasis*, vol. 34, no. 5, pp. 309–314, 2017.

[24] T. Khosrawipour, V. Khosrawipour, and U. Giger-Pabst, "Pressurized intra peritoneal aerosol chemotherapy in patients suffering from peritoneal carcinomatosis of pancreatic adenocarcinoma," *PLoS One*, vol. 12, no. 10, article e0186709, 2017.

[25] T. A. Falkenstein, T. O. Götze, M. Ouaissi, C. B. Tempfer, U. Giger-Pabst, and C. Demtröder, "First clinical data of pressurized intraperitoneal aerosol chemotherapy (PIPAC) as salvage therapy for peritoneal metastatic biliary tract cancer," *Anticancer Research*, vol. 38, no. 1, pp. 373–378, 2018.

[26] F. Grass, A. Vuagniaux, H. Teixeira-Farinha, K. Lehmann, N. Demartines, and M. Hübner, "Systematic review of pressurized intraperitoneal aerosol chemotherapy for the treatment of advanced peritoneal carcinomatosis," *The British Journal of Surgery*, vol. 104, no. 6, pp. 669–678, 2017.

[27] http://www.clinicaltrials.gov, consulted on January 03, 2018.

[28] U. M. Lauer, M. Schell, J. Beil et al., "Phase I study of oncolytic vaccinia virus GL-ONC1 in patients with peritoneal carcinomatosis," *Clinical Cancer Research*, vol. 24, no. 18, pp. 4388–4398, 2018.

[29] http://www.an-institut.de, consulted on January 03, 2018.

[30] Z. He, T. T. Zhao, H. M. Xu et al., "Efficacy and safety of intraperitoneal chemotherapy in patients with advanced gastric cancer: a cumulative meta-analysis of randomized controlled trials," *Oncotarget*, vol. 8, no. 46, pp. 81125–81136, 2017.

[31] L. Elit, T. K. Oliver, A. Covens et al., "Intraperitoneal chemotherapy in the first-line treatment of women with stage III epithelial ovarian cancer: a systematic review with metaanalyses," *Cancer*, vol. 109, no. 4, pp. 692–702, 2007.

[32] E. A. Levine, K. I. Votanopoulos, P. Shen et al., "A multicenter randomized trial to evaluate hematologic toxicities after hyperthermic intraperitoneal chemotherapy with oxaliplatin or mitomycin in patients with appendiceal tumors," *Journal of the American College of Surgeons*, vol. 226, no. 4, pp. 434–443, 2018.

[33] W. J. van Driel, S. N. Koole, K. Sikorska et al., "Hyperthermic intraperitoneal chemotherapy in ovarian cancer," *New England Journal of Medicine*, vol. 378, no. 3, pp. 230–240, 2018.

[34] D. M. Provencher, C. J. Gallagher, W. R. Parulekar et al., "OV21/PETROC: a randomized gynecologic cancer intergroup phase II study of intraperitoneal versus intravenous chemotherapy following neoadjuvant chemotherapy and optimal debulking surgery in epithelial ovarian cancer," *Annals of Oncology*, vol. 29, no. 2, pp. 431–438, 2018.

[35] D. K. Armstrong, B. Bundy, L. Wenzel et al., "Intraperitoneal cisplatin and paclitaxel in ovarian cancer," *The New England Journal of Medicine*, vol. 354, no. 1, pp. 34–43, 2006.

[36] J. L. Walker, D. K. Armstrong, H. Q. Huang et al., "Intraperitoneal catheter outcomes in a phase III trial of intravenous versus intraperitoneal chemotherapy in optimal stage III ovarian and primary peritoneal cancer: a gynecologic oncology group study," *Gynecologic Oncology*, vol. 100, no. 1, pp. 27–32, 2006.

[37] S. Bonvalot, A. Cavalcanti, C. le Péchoux et al., "Randomized trial of cytoreduction followed by intraperitoneal chemotherapy versus cytoreduction alone in patients with peritoneal sarcomatosis," *European Journal of Surgical Oncology*, vol. 31, no. 8, pp. 917–923, 2005.

[38] W. Solass, U. Giger-Pabst, J. Zieren, and M. A. Reymond, "Pressurized intraperitoneal aerosol chemotherapy (PIPAC): occupational health and safety aspects," *Annals of Surgical Oncology*, vol. 20, no. 11, pp. 3504–3511, 2013.

[39] W. Solass, C. Sempoux, S. Detlefsen, N. J. Carr, and F. Bibeau, "Peritoneal sampling and histological assessment of therapeutic response in peritoneal metastasis: proposal of the peritoneal regression grading score (PRGS)," *Pleura and Peritoneum*, vol. 1, no. 2, pp. 99–107, 2016.

[40] *Common Terminology Criteria for Adverse Events (CTCAE) version 4.0 (v4.03: June 14, 2010)*, U.S. Department of Health and Human Services, National Institutes of Health, National Cancer Institute, Bethesda, MD, USA, 2009.

[41] D. Dindo, N. Demartines, and P. A. Clavien, "Classification of surgical complications: a new proposal with evaluation in a cohort of 6336 patients and results of a survey," *Annals of Surgery*, vol. 240, no. 2, pp. 205–213, 2004.

[42] M. Hübner, H. Teixeira Farinha, F. Grass et al., "Feasibility and safety of pressurized intraperitoneal aerosol chemotherapy for peritoneal carcinomatosis: a retrospective cohort study," *Gastroenterology Research and Practice*, vol. 2017, Article ID 6852749, 7 pages, 2017.

[43] M. Nowacki, M. Alyami, L. Villeneuve et al., "Multicenter comprehensive methodological and technical analysis of 832 pressurized intraperitoneal aerosol chemotherapy (PIPAC) interventions performed in 349 patients for peritoneal carcinomatosis treatment: an international survey study," *European Journal of Surgical Oncology*, vol. 44, no. 7, pp. 991–996, 2018.

[44] C. Tempfer, U. Giger-Pabst, Z. Hilal, A. Dogan, and G. A. Rezniczek, "Pressurized intraperitoneal aerosol chemotherapy (PIPAC) for peritoneal carcinomatosis: systematic review of clinical and experimental evidence with special emphasis on ovarian cancer," *Archives of Gynecology and Obstetrics*, vol. 298, no. 2, pp. 243–257, 2018.

[45] M. Graversen, S. Detlefsen, J. K. Bjerregaard, C. W. Fristrup, P. Pfeiffer, and M. B. Mortensen, "Prospective, single-center implementation and response evaluation of pressurized intraperitoneal aerosol chemotherapy (PIPAC) for peritoneal metastasis," *Therapeutic Advances in Medical Oncology*, vol. 10, 2018.

[46] Y. Satoh, T. Ichikawa, U. Motosugi et al., "Diagnosis of peritoneal dissemination: comparison of ^{18}F-FDG PET/CT, diffusion-weighted MRI, and contrast-enhanced MDCT," *AJR. American Journal of Roentgenology*, vol. 196, no. 2, pp. 447–453, 2011.

[47] W. P. Ceelen, "Scoring histological regression in peritoneal carcinomatosis: does it count?," *Pleura and Peritoneum*, vol. 1, no. 2, pp. 65-66, 2016.

[48] C. B. Tempfer, G. A. Rezniczek, P. Ende, W. Solass, and M. A. Reymond, "Pressurized intraperitoneal aerosol chemotherapy with cisplatin and doxorubicin in women with peritoneal carcinomatosis: a cohort study," *Anticancer Research*, vol. 35, no. 12, pp. 6723–6729, 2015.

[49] F. Struller, P. Horvath, W. Solass, F. J. Weinreich, A. Konigsrainer, and M. A. Reymond, "Pressurized intraperitoneal aerosol chemotherapy with low-dose cisplatin and

doxorubicin (PIPAC C/D) in patients with gastric cancer and peritoneal metastasis (PIPAC-GA1)," *Journal of Clinical Oncology*, vol. 35, Supplement 4, p. 99, 2017.

[50] H. Teixeira Farinha, F. Grass, A. Kefleyesus et al., "Impact of pressurized intraperitoneal aerosol chemotherapy on quality of life and symptoms in patients with peritoneal carcinomatosis: a retrospective cohort study," *Gastroenterology Research and Practice*, vol. 2017, Article ID 4596176, 10 pages, 2017.

[51] K. Odendahl, W. Solass, C. Demtröder et al., "Quality of life of patients with end-stage peritoneal metastasis treated with pressurized intraperitoneal aerosol chemotherapy (PIPAC)," *European Journal of Surgical Oncology*, vol. 41, no. 10, pp. 1379–1385, 2015.

5

The Association of Nil Per Os (NPO) Days with Necrotizing Enterocolitis

Yongming Wang,[1,2] Xiaoyu Li,[1,2] and Chunbao Guo[1,3]

[1] *Ministry of Education Key Laboratory of Child Development and Disorders, Children's Hospital, Chongqing Medical University, Chongqing, China*
[2] *Department of Neonatology, Children's Hospital, Chongqing Medical University, Chongqing, China*
[3] *Department of Pediatric General Surgery and Liver Transplantation, Children's Hospital, Chongqing Medical University, Chongqing, China*

Correspondence should be addressed to Xiaoyu Li; lxy0061@163.com and Chunbao Guo; guochunbao@foxmail.com

Academic Editor: Per Hellström

Background. Enteral feeds are an essential part of care for infants and may be a potential risk factor in NEC development. The present study objective was to evaluate the relationship between nil per os (NPO) and clinical outcomes in infants with NEC. *Methods.* This was a retrospective review of 196 premature, low-birth-weight infants with NEC from January 1, 2011, to October 31, 2016, at four academic tertiary care hospitals. The patients were evaluated based on the median nil per os (NPO) days (5.6 days) in longer NPO (6.3 ± 1.1 days) versus shorter NPO groups (4.2 ± 0.9 days). *Results.* Patients who experienced longer than 5.6 NPO days were more likely associated with perforated NEC (odds ratio (OR), 2.01; 95% confidence interval (CI), 1.07–3.76; $p = 0.021$), stage III NEC (OR, 1.81; 95% CI, 0.97–3.38; $p = 0.042$), and longer duration of mechanical ventilation (OR, 0.17; 95% CI, 0.08–0.98; $p = 0.005$) than the shorter duration group of 5.6 NPO days. For the secondary outcomes, there was a trend towards earlier birth ($p = 0.083$), longer NICU length of stay ($p = 0.093$), and higher mortality ($p = 0.10$) in the longer NPO cohort ($p = 0.057$). The incidence of bacterial sepsis and short bowel syndrome also increased as the length of NPO increased. There was no statistically significant difference in nutritional variables between the two groups within the in-hospital period. *Conclusion.* Longer NPO time was associated with the severity of NEC and more injurious clinical outcomes, as demonstrated by rates of surgical intervention and duration of mechanical ventilation.

1. Introduction

Necrotizing enterocolitis (NEC) is a major gastrointestinal emergency in neonates that affects approximately 6 to 7% of very-low-birth-weight (VLBW) infants born weighing less than 1500 g [1–3]. Numerous factors are thought to be associated with the pathogenesis of NEC, including prematurity, infection, red blood cell transfusion, enteral feeding, and bacterial colonization, which often lead to an inflammatory state and the clinical manifestation of NEC [4–6]. Enteral feeding of the premature gut, which has served as a therapeutic and preventive strategy in the management of NEC, has been implicated in both the pathogenesis and development of NEC [7, 8]. The current clinical practice includes a widely varied, cautious, delayed approaches to feeding very-low-birth-weight (VLBW) infants for fear of NEC, which may cause postnatal growth restriction.

It is thought that the proteins and carbohydrates derived from enteral nutrition provide substrates for bacterial growth and fermentation, which are possible risk factors for NEC. Conversely, enteral nutrition can prevent microbial overgrowth and prevent inflammation in the preterm gut [9]. The common thought is that early human milk enteral feeding appears to be a prevention strategy to reduce the occurrence of NEC. In contrast, withholding feedings and enforcing nil per os (NPO) in infants may have their own unintended consequences, including duodenal mucosal atrophy, impaired intestinal function, abnormal gut permeability, and subsequent feeding intolerance [10]. Furthermore, only parenteral feeding has been associated with various complications, including central line infections, liver disease, and alteration of the intestinal flora in the premature gut [11]. Several studies have shown that enteral nutrition has trophic effects that can minimize some of the intestinal problems caused by total parenteral nutrition [12, 13]. The potential for increasing the risk for NEC by delaying or interrupting enteral nutrition lies in the aforementioned benefits of enteral nutrition as it impacts gastrointestinal immune function, maturation, and integrity.

Currently, there are few published studies addressing whether or not there is any relationship between delayed or interrupted enteral nutrition and the development of NEC in extremely preterm neonates. We hypothesized that a longer duration of NPO (NPO days) would increase NEC severity in premature, low-birth-weight infants. We therefore conducted the present study to address the association between the number and percentage of nil per os (NPO) days and NEC in extremely preterm neonates, especially in the context of developing countries.

2. Materials and Methods

2.1. Patient Cohort. A retrospective review of the hospital-based cohort for NEC from January 1, 2011, to October 31, 2016, was performed in 4 newborn intensive care units (NICUs) at Yongchuan Hospital, Children's Hospital of Chongqing Medical University, Sanxia Hospital, and Jinan Maternity and Child Care Hospital with the approval of the institutional review board at each site. Infants eligible for inclusion had a diagnosis of NEC and Bell's stage ≥ stage 2 during the study period if they were premature (<37-week gestational age) at birth and had a very low birth weight (≤1500 g). Exclusion criteria included infants conceived from in vitro fertilization (IVF), acute pulmonary bacterial infection, major congenital anomalies (congenital heart disease), and gastrointestinal abnormalities (imperforate anus, intestinal atresia, or Hirschsprung disease), or infants without the information needed for outcome measures. All infants with NEC were followed up in the hospital's outpatient clinic until at least 3 months of corrected age. The diagnosis of NEC was defined using Bell's criteria and modified by Walsh and Kliegman [13], including clinical findings of abdominal distension, feeding intolerance, and radiographic findings (the presence of pneumatosis intestinalis, pneumoperitoneum, and/or portal gas). The SNAP-II (Score for Neonatal Acute Physiology, version II) was calculated from the data from the 1st day of life. The data pertaining to NEC that had been recorded by physicians or nurses during patient hospitalization were collected from the electronic medical records of patients, including demographic information, diagnosis, clinical management, laboratory data, mortality, length of stay (LOS), and discharge summaries.

2.2. Clinical Management and Follow-Up. All the patients were subjected to the same medical program, including feeding regimen, fluid resuscitation, parenteral nutrition support, and perioperative broad-spectrum antibiotics, if necessary. Here, the feeding regimen was directed by the discretion of the clinicians. Breast milk and human milk fortifier was primarily administered for enteral nutrition and initiated on the first day with 20 mL/kg/day and advanced by 30 mL/kg/day until maximum enteral feedings of 170 mL/kg/day were attained. If mother's milk was unavailable, a 20 cal/oz premature formula could be substituted for breast milk. All feeds were given as bolus by nasogastric tube at 2-hour intervals. Data on the type of milk or volume of milk were not collected. The feeds were discontinued for feeding intolerance and mechanical ventilation. NPO days were defined as days when an infant received no enteral nutrition over a 24-hour period. The number of NPO days from the day of life to the development of NEC was calculated. The primary outcome measure was the proportion of patients with perforated NEC and Bell's staging III. Surgical NEC was defined as NEC requiring either drainage or exploratory laparotomy. The secondary outcomes included in-hospital mortality within 90 days, total parenteral nutrition for 90 days, and the length of hospital stay for patients surviving 90 days.

2.3. Statistical Analysis. Statistical analyses were performed using the SPSS statistical package version 22 (SPSS Inc., Chicago, IL). Student's t-test and Mann-Whitney U test were used for comparison of parametric variables, which are described as the means ± standard deviation (the mean ± SD of the variable), and nonparametric continuous variables, which are described as medians and interquartile ranges (IQRs), respectively. Chi-square or Fisher's exact tests were used to compare categorical variables. The relative risks for postoperative variables were assessed using cross-tabulation (odds ratio (OR)) or multivariate logistic regression analysis (risk ratio (RR)). The conditional logistic regression model was used to investigate the association of the NPO day with the clinical outcome of NEC. We adjusted for the presence of a PDA, inotrope use (yes/no), antibiotic use (yes/no), and SNAP-II scores in the model (based on $p < 0.1$ in univariate analyses). The statistical significance was evaluated using a two-tailed 95% confidence interval (CI), and a P value less than 0.05 was considered statistically significant.

3. Results

3.1. Demographic Data. There were a total of 243 preterm infants followed for NEC diagnosis managed at our institution eligible for analysis during the study period, and 47 cases were excluded due to incomplete information ($n = 29$) and intestinal malformation ($n = 18$). The demographic characteristics of the infants are shown in Table 1. Sixty-five percent of the infants ($n = 128$) were male, and the average gestational age (GA) and birth weight of the patients were 26 ± 3.8 weeks and 1013 ± 306 g, respectively. Twenty-five percent of the infants (48, 24.5%) were assessed with over stage 3 disease by Bell's staging (Table 1), 58 (29.6%) of the included infants underwent surgical intervention after a median time period of 9 days (range: 2–19), and the remaining 138 infants were managed medically. Enteral feeding prior to NEC onset was identified in more than 77.6% ($n = 152$) of the included infants. Forty-six infants (23.5%) needed assisted ventilation,

TABLE 1: Baseline demographics and clinical characteristics for the eligible cohort ($n = 196$).

Variables	
Male : female	128 : 68
Gestational age (wk)	26.7 ± 3.8
Birth weight (g)	1013 ± 306
NPO (days)	5.6 ± 1.6
Bell's stage ≥ stage 3	48 (24.5)
History of enteral feeding, n (%)	152 (77.6)
Respiratory support, n (%)	46 (23.5)
Probiotics, n (%)	36 (12.8)
Age at diagnosis of NEC (days)	21 (5–35)
APGAR scores at 5 minutes	8.1 ± 1.3
SNAP-II scores	18.8 ± 12.6
Vasopressor use at enrollment, n (%)	59 (30.1)

and 45 infants (23.0%) needed hemodynamic support by fluid expansion with the administration of vasoactive amines. The median age at diagnosis was 13 days, and there were 69 cases (35.2%) with probiotic administration.

To explore clinical outcomes associated with NPO days, the corrected NPO days were dichotomized as "longer" or "shorter" based on the median amount of NPO days (5.6 days, Table 1). In the longer NPO group, an average of 6.3 ± 1.2 NPO days occurred before developing NEC compared with 4.2 ± 0.9 days to development of NEC in the shorter NPO group (Table 2). The baseline characteristics and clinical status of the two groups are reported in Table 2. No differences were observed for some of the baseline characteristics, including sex ($p = 0.52$), APGAR scores (at 5 minutes) ($p = 0.36$), probiotic usage ($p = 0.29$), or other disease severity in perforated necrotizing enterocolitis. Patients in the longer NPO group were more likely to be younger at birth ($p = 0.083$) and had a lower birth weight ($p = 0.101$) than were those with low NPO days, although no statistical significance was observed. With respect to some maternal features, such as maternal age ($p = 0.24$) or delivery mode (cesarean or vaginal) ($p = 0.44$), there was no difference among the two groups, which suggested that the study population reasonably represented the spectrum of neonates with necrotizing enterocolitis in our institutions. No differences in other clinical status, such as basic laboratory measures or vasopressor use at onset of NEC ($p = 0.38$), were found between the two groups.

3.2. Outcomes of Patients according to NPO Days. According to the established criteria, a comparison of the outcomes between the two groups is summarized in Table 3. Patients who experienced longer than 5.6 NPO days were more likely associated with perforated NEC (odds ratio (OR), 2.01; 95% confidence interval (CI), 1.07–3.76; $p = 0.021$) and stage III NEC (OR, 1.81; 95% CI, 0.97–3.38; $p = 0.042$). Furthermore, neonates in the longer NPO group required a significantly longer duration of mechanical ventilation (OR, 0.17; 95% CI, 0.08–0.98. $p = 0.005$) and had a higher rate of death prior to discharge than did those with fewer NPO days, although no significant differences were found ($p = 0.10$) (Table 3). The cause of death was primarily attributed to pan-intestinal NEC in 29 infants. The remaining deaths resulted from sepsis ($n = 11$) and severe short bowel ($n = 8$). There was no death that occurred after stoma closure. There were no significant differences in the rates of dependence on parenteral nutrition 90 days after surgery for the 76 patients surviving at least 90 days postoperatively ($p = 0.30$).

No significant differences were found in nutritional variables between the two groups within the in-hospital period (albumin and prealbumin). A higher proportion of neonates with more NPO days were diagnosed with culture-proven sepsis ($p = 0.16$) and short bowel syndrome ($p = 0.17$) than the proportions of those patients with fewer NPO days, but there were no statistically significant differences (Table 3). The majority of sepsis (65%) in the case population occurred within 72 hours or concurrent with the diagnosis of NEC. The mean hospitalization time in the NICU ($p = 0.093$) was longer in the group with longer NPO days, but this difference was not significant.

4. Discussion

In this study, we identified a statistically significant association between the length of NPO days and the severity and mortality of NEC in premature infants. In this study, the length of NPO time before the development of NEC was dichotomized to facilitate comparison between NEC patients in premature, low-birth-weight infants. In our research, patients who experienced more NPO days developed NEC at an earlier age and had higher rates of perforation. Due to the higher incidence of perforated NEC in those experiencing more NPO days, there was also a higher need for surgery or longer hospital stay.

To the best of our knowledge, few studies have directly investigated the impact of delayed or interrupted enteral intake on NEC onset or severity [14]. In our study, we tried to address this question and found that patients who were on a longer NPO restriction developed NEC at an earlier age and had a higher rate of perforation than those who had fewer NPO days. Although no studies have looked directly at the impact of NPO on NEC severity, a few have examined the effects of delayed enteral feeding on NEC onset. A recent study found that more NPO days were associated with a higher rate of NEC [15]. Our study was specifically aimed at exploring the potential negative consequences of keeping infants NPO, suggesting that the length of time spent with NPO can be a risk factor for NEC severity. Of course, this finding should be taken in the context of the other known risk factors for NEC in preterm infants. Feeds were discontinued due to feeding intolerance and mechanical ventilation. Since feeding intolerance and mechanical ventilation may be signs of NEC, NEC in itself may lead to longer fasting times, which may confound the results. We cannot comment on the indication for NPO status or whether the NPO days were primarily during the first few days of life and due to a delayed initiation of feeds. Enteral nutrition might promote gastrointestinal colonization with symbiotic organisms that form the intestinal microbiome, decrease

TABLE 2: Baseline demographics of eligible patients based on NPO days (chi-square test and Student's t-test).

Characteristics	Longer NPO ($n = 98$)	Shorter NPO ($n = 98$)	p values
Male : female	65 : 34	63 : 34	0.52
Gestational age (wk)	25.8 ± 2.9	27.4 ± 3.1	0.083
Birth weight (g)	964 ± 296	1125 ± 314	0.101
Probiotics, n (%)	16 (16.3)	20 (20.4)	0.29
APGAR scores at 5 minutes	8.1 ± 1.2	8.2 ± 1.1	0.36
SNAP-II scores	17.9 ± 12.3	19.6 ± 11.9	0.15
Cesarean delivery, n (%)	65 (66.3)	67 (68.4)	0.44
Maternal age (years)	29.6 ± 5.8	30.3 ± 4.7	0.24
SGA infant, n (%)	11 (11.2)	12 (12.2)	0.35
Transfusion preoperation, n (%)	17 (17.3)	13 (13.3)	0.28
Vasopressor use at enrollment, n (%)	28 (28.6)	31 (31.6)	0.38
Respiratory support, n (%)	24 (24.5)	22 (22.4)	0.43
First platelet count (onset of symptoms) (10^9/L)	288.2 ± 95.2	297.6 ± 88.6	0.16
Hemoglobin (g/L)	136.2 ± 41.3	129.8 ± 39.5	0.32
First WBC (onset of symptoms) (10^9/L)	17.8 ± 3.7	17.2 ± 4.8	0.42
First procalcitonin (onset of symptoms) (ng/mL, normal value: 0–0.5)	5.9 ± 3.4	6.3 ± 3.2	0.14
First CRP (onset of symptoms) (mg/L, normal value: 0–10)	25.3 ± 9.7	24.8 ± 8.9	0.18
Albumin (g/L, normal range, 35–50)	29.2 ± 6.2	28.9 ± 5.8	0.12

TABLE 3: Patient outcomes based on the NPO days.

	Longer NPO ($n = 98$)	Shorter NPO ($n = 98$)	p values	Odds ratio (95% CI)
Perforated NEC	36 (36.7)	22 (22.4)	0.021	2.01 (1.07–3.76)
NEC stage				
Stage II	63 (64.3)	75 (76.5)		
Stage III	35 (35.7)	23 (3.5)	0.042	1.81 (0.97–3.38)
Mechanical ventilation (days)	13.7 ± 6.4	10.8 ± 5.3	0.005	0.17 (0.08–0.98)
Days to enteral feeds (median)	22.9 ± 12.3	23.2 ± 11.6	0.23	0.42 (0.28–1.62)
90-day parenteral nutrition dependence, n (%)	7 (7.1)	6 (6.1)	0.30	
NICU length of stay (days), mean ± SD	26.5 ± 13.2	23.2 ± 12.5	0.093	0.32 (0.18–1.09)
Bacterial sepsis, n (%)	18 (18.4)	12 (12.2)	0.16	
Albumin minimum (g/L, normal range, 35–50)	32.4 ± 6.2	33.7 ± 5.8	0.125	
Mortality, n (%)	28 (28.6)	20 (20.4)	0.10	1.56 (0.81–3.01)
Short bowel syndrome	7 (7.1)	3 (3.1)	0.17	

bacterial translocation, improve intestinal motility, and prevent microbial overgrowth, which are the preventative pathophysiologic mechanisms for NEC [16–18]. Inhibition of inflammatory pathways that promote the development of NEC is emerging as one example of microbiome-mediated protection of the gastrointestinal tract.

Other factors, such as infection, hypoxia, ischemia, formula milk [19], and prematurity, per se, have been considered important in the pathogenesis of NEC. Compared with the group with shorter NPO days, infants who experienced longer NPO time had higher incidences of PDA, inotrope use, and antibiotic use and higher SNAP-II scores. All these measures are indicative of confounding as these may be related to delayed introduction or interruption of feeds and are themselves associated with development of NEC. Therefore, certain authors argue that the risk of NEC should not be considered in isolation of other potential clinical outcomes while formulating feeding policies and practices for preterm infants [20]. Clinical studies have evaluated the effects of different feeding regimens on the incidence of NEC and outcomes in premature neonates [21]. The use of breast milk initially may be protective against NEC. We did use maternal breast milk or donor breast milk exclusively until the infant reached 1500 g and was on full feeding volume, then we introduced formula. This was due to the high cost of donor breast milk to our hospital. The reduction in the use of TPN was significant, and any reduction in exposure to TPN further reduces the risk for infections, as well as TPN-associated liver disease [22]. The fluids from supplemental TPN during NPO days likely aid in meeting the fluid requirements at the onset of NEC, ensuring that infants are still being sustained with parenteral fluids prior to the clinical onset of symptoms. The recent Cochrane reviews did not reveal a statistically significant effect of early enteral feeding practices on the risk of NEC or all-cause mortality in very preterm or VLBW infants. Moreover, approximately 80% of the infants in those reviews were growth restricted and had evidence of fetal circulatory distribution abnormalities [23]. However, we did observe a detrimental effect of TPN on the risk of NEC.

Inherent limitations of our study include its retrospective nature, where data regarding the NPO days was unavailable for certain patients, creating an inherent risk of selection bias. Second, there were a number of infants for whom life support was withdrawn, making it difficult to interpret the survival data. A majority of the babies were on mixed human milk and formula feeds. At discharge, however, a majority had made a successful transition to exclusive human milk feedings. Third, although the study shows benefits from feeding for preterm infants in the current cohort, the results should be interpreted with care, given the lack of long-term data to assess the impact of NPO days for overall physiological advancement. Finally, the median difference in the time to regain birth weight must be interpreted with caution, given the nonblinded design and absence of data regarding feeding practice postdischarge. The strength of our study is that it evaluates a fairly uniform patient population that was managed similarly at our institution. A larger, multi-institutional study may help better define the impact of NPO days on outcomes.

5. Conclusion

In the current study, we identified that neonates who spent more time NPO had an increased severity of disease, as evidenced by higher rates of perforated NEC. We speculate that delayed or interrupted provision of enteral intake to preterm neonates affects gut maturation and defenses and predisposes infants to the development of NEC in this already at-risk population. It will be necessary to conduct further prospective cohort studies to provide information about this association and the potential reasons for the development of NEC.

Authors' Contributions

Yongming Wang designed the manuscript, analyzed the data, and evaluated the manuscript. Xiaoyu Li performed the statistical measurements and analyzed the data. Chunbao Guo analyzed the data and wrote the paper.

Acknowledgments

We thank Prof. Xianqing Jin for providing technical assistance and for insightful discussions during the preparation of the manuscript. We thank Dr. Xiaoyong Zhang at the Wistar Institute, USA, for the help with the linguistic revision of the manuscript. The research was supported by the National Natural Science Foundation of China (nos. 30973440 and 30770950) and the key project of the Chongqing Natural Science Foundation (CSTC, 2008BA0021 and cstc2012jjA0155).

References

[1] J. Neu and W. A. Walker, "Necrotizing enterocolitis," *The New England Journal of Medicine*, vol. 364, no. 3, pp. 255–264, 2011.

[2] B. J. Stoll, N. I. Hansen, E. F. Bell et al., "Trends in care practices, morbidity, and mortality of extremely preterm neonates, 1993-2012," *JAMA*, vol. 314, no. 10, pp. 1039–1051, 2015.

[3] R. M. Patel, S. Kandefer, M. C. Walsh et al., "Causes and timing of death in extremely premature infants from 2000 through 2011," *The New England Journal of Medicine*, vol. 372, no. 4, pp. 331–340, 2015.

[4] D. B. McElhinney, H. L. Hedrick, D. M. Bush et al., "Necrotizing enterocolitis in neonates with congenital heart disease: risk factors and outcomes," *Pediatrics*, vol. 106, no. 5, pp. 1080–1087, 2000.

[5] M. C. W. Henry and R. L. Moss, "Neonatal necrotizing enterocolitis," *Seminars in Pediatric Surgery*, vol. 17, no. 2, pp. 98–109, 2008.

[6] Z. J. Kastenberg and K. G. Sylvester, "The surgical management of necrotizing enterocolitis," *Clinics in Perinatology*, vol. 40, no. 1, pp. 135–148, 2013.

[7] E. J. Kim, N. M. Lee, and S. H. Chung, "A retrospective study on the effects of exclusive donor human milk feeding in a short period after birth on morbidity and growth of preterm infants during hospitalization," *Medicine*, vol. 96, no. 35, article e7970, 2017.

[8] S. Amin, "Rapid feed advancement appears protective in very low birth weight infants," *The Journal of Pediatrics*, vol. 170, pp. 341–344, 2016.

[9] R. H. Siggers, J. Siggers, T. Thymann, M. Boye, and P. T. Sangild, "Nutritional modulation of the gut microbiota and immune system in preterm neonates susceptible to necrotizing enterocolitis," *The Journal of Nutritional Biochemistry*, vol. 22, no. 6, pp. 511–521, 2011.

[10] P. T. Sangild, R. H. Siggers, M. Schmidt et al., "Diet- and colonization-dependent intestinal dysfunction predisposes to necrotizing enterocolitis in preterm pigs," *Gastroenterology*, vol. 130, no. 6, pp. 1776–1792, 2006.

[11] J. Siggers, M. V. Østergaard, R. H. Siggers et al., "Postnatal amniotic fluid intake reduces gut inflammatory responses and necrotizing enterocolitis in preterm neonates," *American Journal of Physiology. Gastrointestinal and Liver Physiology*, vol. 304, no. 10, pp. G864–G875, 2013.

[12] R. H. Siggers, T. Thymann, B. B. Jensen et al., "Elective cesarean delivery affects gut maturation and delays microbial colonization but does not increase necrotizing enterocolitis in preterm pigs," *American Journal of Physiology. Regulatory, Integrative and Comparative Physiology*, vol. 294, no. 3, pp. R929–R938, 2008.

[13] M. C. Walsh and R. M. Kliegman, "Necrotizing enterocolitis: treatment based on staging criteria," *Pediatric Clinics of North America*, vol. 33, no. 1, pp. 179–201, 1986.

[14] R. Clyman, A. Wickremasinghe, N. Jhaveri et al., "Enteral feeding during indomethacin and ibuprofen treatment of a patent ductus arteriosus," *The Journal of Pediatrics*, vol. 163, no. 2, pp. 406–411.e4, 2013.

[15] M. Kirtsman, E. W. Yoon, C. Ojah, Z. Cieslak, S. K. Lee, and P. S. Shah, "Nil-per-os days and necrotizing enterocolitis in extremely preterm infants," *American Journal of Perinatology*, vol. 32, no. 8, pp. 785–794, 2015.

[16] B. Rusconi, M. Good, and B. B. Warner, "The microbiome and biomarkers for necrotizing enterocolitis: are we any closer to prediction?," *The Journal of Pediatrics*, vol. 189, pp. 40–47.e2, 2017.

[17] L. K. Barron, B. B. Warner, P. I. Tarr, W. D. Shannon, E. Deych, and B. W. Warner, "Independence of gut bacterial content and neonatal necrotizing enterocolitis severity," *Journal of Pediatric Surgery*, vol. 52, no. 6, pp. 993–998, 2017.

[18] M. Pammi, J. Cope, P. I. Tarr et al., "Intestinal dysbiosis in preterm infants preceding necrotizing enterocolitis: a systematic review and meta-analysis," *Microbiome*, vol. 5, no. 1, p. 31, 2017.

[19] N. J. Hall, S. Eaton, and A. Pierro, "Royal Australasia of surgeons guest lecture. Necrotizing enterocolitis: prevention, treatment, and outcome," *Journal of Pediatric Surgery*, vol. 48, no. 12, pp. 2359–2367, 2013.

[20] V. T. Le, M. A. Klebanoff, M. M. Talavera, and J. L. Slaughter, "Transient effects of transfusion and feeding advances (volumetric and caloric) on necrotizing enterocolitis development: a case-crossover study," *PLoS One*, vol. 12, no. 6, article e0179724, 2017.

[21] R. D. Christensen and J. L. Street, "Randomized, controlled trial of slow versus rapid feeding volume advancement in preterm infants," *The Journal of Pediatrics*, vol. 146, no. 5, pp. 710-711, 2005.

[22] T. J. Butler, L. J. Szekely, and J. L. Grow, "A standardized nutrition approach for very low birth weight neonates improves outcomes, reduces cost and is not associated with increased rates of necrotizing enterocolitis, sepsis or mortality," *Journal of Perinatology*, vol. 33, no. 11, pp. 851–857, 2013.

[23] J. Morgan, L. Young, and W. McGuire, "Slow advancement of enteral feed volumes to prevent necrotising enterocolitis in very low birth weight infants," *Cochrane Database of Systematic Reviews*, vol. 28, no. 3, p. CD001241, 2017.

6

Fucosterol Protects against Concanavalin A-Induced Acute Liver Injury: Focus on P38 MAPK/NF-κB Pathway Activity

Wenhui Mo,[1] Chengfen Wang,[2] Jingjing Li,[1] Kan Chen,[1] Yujing Xia,[1] Sainan Li,[1] Ling Xu,[3] Xiya Lu,[1] Wenwen Wang,[1] and Chuanyong Guo[1]

[1]*Department of Gastroenterology, Shanghai Tenth People's Hospital, Tongji University School of Medicine, Shanghai 200072, China*
[2]*Putuo District People's Hospital, Tongji University School of Medicine, Shanghai 200060, China*
[3]*Department of Gastroenterology, Shanghai Tongren Hospital, Shanghai Jiaotong University School of Medicine, Shanghai 200336, China*

Correspondence should be addressed to Ling Xu; xiaoling05@126.com and Chuanyong Guo; guochuanyong@hotmail.com

Academic Editor: Kazuhiko Uchiyama

Objective. Fucosterol is derived from the brown alga *Eisenia bicyclis* and has various biological activities, including antioxidant, anticancer, and antidiabetic properties. The aim of this study was to investigate the protective effects of fucosterol pretreatment on Concanavalin A- (ConA-) induced acute liver injury in mice, and to understand its molecular mechanisms. *Materials and Methods.* Acute liver injury was induced in BALB/c mice by ConA (25 mg/kg), and fucosterol (dissolved in 2% DMSO) was orally administered daily at doses of 25, 50, and 100 mg/kg. The levels of hepatic necrosis, apoptosis, and autophagy associated with inflammatory cytokines were measured at 2, 8, and 24 h. *Results.* Fucosterol attenuated serum liver enzyme levels and hepatic necrosis and apoptosis induced by TNF-α, IL-6, and IL-1β. Fucosterol also inhibited apoptosis and autophagy by upregulating Bcl-2, which decreased levels of functional Bax and Beclin-1. Furthermore, reduced P38 MAPK and NF-κB signaling were accompanied by PPARγ activation. *Conclusion.* This study showed that fucosterol could alleviate acute liver injury induced by ConA by inhibiting P38 MAPK/PPARγ/NF-κB signaling. These findings highlight that fucosterol is a promising potential therapeutic agent for acute liver injury.

1. Introduction

The liver is the largest organ within the abdominal cavity and undertakes important physiological processes. Liver injury is the basis of acute liver failure and is primarily caused by viral infections, drugs, food additives, alcohol, and radioactive damage [1]. Currently, the etiology of acute liver injury is unclear and treatment with glucocorticoids or azathioprine often results in severe side effects [2]. Therefore, it is important to establish an animal model to screen effective drugs.

Immune responses are mediated by different cells and cytokines in different injury models. Concanavalin A (ConA) is a plant agglutinin extracted from Brazilian rubber beans that was firstly used to study liver injury by Tiegs et al. [3]. ConA can modify the major histocompatibility complex (MHC) structure to produce inflammatory reactions, by activating macrophages and $CD4^+$ T cells, which release TNF-α, IL-1β, IL-6, and other inflammatory factors that damage hepatic cells [4]. Thus, ConA treatment is a good simulation of the clinical onset of AIH and viral hepatitis. The model also has the advantages of utilizing a simple extraction and causing liver-specific damage (injury to other organs is not obvious), thus providing a reliable animal model for clinical research in basic immunology [5]. The ConA-induced inflammatory process is mediated by a series of endogenous inflammatory factors. Peroxisome proliferator-activated receptors (PPARs) are ligand-activated transcription factors that regulate lipid metabolism, blood pressure, cell growth, and differentiation [6–8]. In recent years, PPARs have been found to play important roles in the pathogenesis of inflammation [9–12]. PPARs are divided into three subtypes, PPARα, PPARβ, and PPARγ, which all regulate inflammatory responses [11]. PPARγ is especially well characterized because of its close relation with inflammatory signaling pathways such as NF-κB, activator protein 1 (AP-1), and JAK/STAT [13].

Fucosterol is separated and purified by silica gel column chromatography from the ethanol extract of brown algae [14] and has many pharmacological effects on various human ailments, such as diabetes, cancer, inflammation, and oxidation. Jung et al. showed that fucosterol could inhibit LPS-induced nitric oxide and *tert*-butylhydroperoxide-induced reactive oxygen species along with suppressing inducible nitric oxide synthase and cyclooxygenase-2 [15]. Yoo et al. showed that fucosterol inhibited the expression of inducible nitric oxide synthase, TNF-α, and IL-6, as well as suppressed the NF-κB and P38 MAPK pathways in LPS-induced RAW264.7 macrophages [16]. However, the *in vivo* effects of fucosterol are still unclear for acute liver injury. We hypothesized that fucosterol may have a protective effect on ConA-induced inflammation, and that its anti-inflammatory mechanism could be associated with NF-κB and PPARγ in mice.

2. Materials and Methods

2.1. Animals. Male BALB/c mice weighing 20–25 g (6–8 weeks old) were purchased from Shanghai SLAC Laboratory Animal Co. Ltd. (Shanghai, China) and housed in a clean room at 23 ± 2°C, 50% humidity, with a 12 h light/dark cycle. Animals were permitted free access to food and water, and all experiments were performed according to the National Institutes of Health Guidelines for the Care and Use of Laboratory Animals. The experiments were also approved by the Animal Care and Use Committee of Tongji University, Shanghai, China.

2.2. Reagents. Fucosterol and anisomycin were purchased from Sigma-Aldrich (St. Louis, MO, USA) and dissolved in 2% DMSO. Antibodies purchased from Cell Signaling Technology (Danvers, MA, USA) included TNF-α, PPARγ, RXRα, IL-6, IL-1β, LC3, NF-κB p65, P38 MAPK, p-P38 MAPK, JNK, p-JNK, ERK, and p-ERK. Antibodies purchased from Proteintech (Chicago, IL, USA) included Beclin-1, Bax, Bcl-2, P62, and β-actin. Liver enzymes were detected and analyzed using microplate test kits (Nanjing Jiancheng Biotech, Nanjing, China) and the RNA PCR kit was purchased from Takara Biotechnology (Dalian, China). Enzyme-linked immunosorbent assay (ELISA) kits for TNF-α, IL-6, and IL-1β were acquired from eBioscience (San Diego, CA, USA). A terminal deoxynucleotidyl transferase dUTP nick-end labeling (TUNEL) apoptosis assay kit was purchased from Roche (Basel, Switzerland).

2.3. Experimental Design. Mice were housed in a warm humid environment and treated with or without fucosterol by gavage for 3 d. Then, ConA was dissolved in normal saline solution and injected via tail vein to induce acute liver injury as previously demonstrated [17]. All mice were randomly distributed to different groups as follows: group I, normal (saline) group ($n = 6$); group II, control (2% DMSO) group ($n = 18$); group III, fucosterol (100 mg/kg) group ($n = 18$); group IV, ConA (25 mg/kg) group ($n = 18$); group V, treatment group ($n = 54$): ConA (25 mg/kg) + fucosterol (25, 50, or 100 mg/kg).

All mice in groups I, II, and III were sacrificed after 3 d, while six mice were randomly selected from groups IV to V (6 from each dose) and sacrificed 2, 8, and 24 h after ConA injection. Blood and liver tissues were collected for further analysis. The results of preliminary experiments showed no significant differences in biochemical or pathological indicators of liver disease between groups I and II, so group II was selected as the experimental control group.

2.4. Serum Enzymes and Cytokines. Serum was separated by centrifugation at 4500 rpm at 4°C for 10 min. The supernatant was used to detect alanine aminotransferase (ALT), aspartate aminotransferase (AST), and cytokines including TNF-α, IL-6, and IL-1β according to the manufacturer's protocols.

2.5. Pathological Assessments. Fresh liver tissue was washed with saline, embedded in 4% paraffin, and then cut into 5 μm sections. After drying for 2 h in an incubator, nuclei and cytoplasm were stained with hematoxylin and eosin (HE). Specific pathological changes were observed under a light microscope.

2.6. Western Blot Analysis. Frozen liver tissue (100 mg) was homogenized in 600 μL of radioimmunoprecipitation assay (RIPA) lysis buffer containing protease inhibitors and phenylmethane-sulfonyl fluoride (PMSF) by incubating on ice for 40 min. Supernatant was collected for bicinchoninic acid (BCA) assay after centrifugation at 12,000 rpm for 15 min. Equal amounts of protein were separated by SDS-PAGE using standard techniques, and separated proteins were transferred to activated polyvinylidene fluoride membranes. Membranes were blocked using 5% nonfat dried milk, and primary antibodies (CST, 1 : 1000; Proteintech, 1 : 500) diluted in blocking buffer were incubated at 4°C overnight. The next day, membranes were washed with phosphate-buffered saline containing 0.1% Tween 20 and incubated with anti-rabbit or anti-mouse IgG secondary antibodies (1 : 2000) for 1 h at 37°C. The Odyssey two-color infrared laser imaging system (LI-COR Biosciences, Lincoln, NE, USA) was used to analyze band densities with β-actin as the internal loading control.

2.7. Quantitative Real-Time PCR (qRT-PCR). Total RNA was extracted from approximately 50 mg of liver tissue using TRIzol, chloroform, and isopropyl alcohol. After determining RNA concentration, a reverse transcription kit was used to transcribe RNA into cDNA. SYBR Green qRT-PCR was performed to determine gene expression levels using a 7900HT fast real-time PCR system (Applied Biosystems, Foster City, CA, USA) according to the provided protocol. Levels of target gene and β-actin were compared on the basis of the solubility curve. Primers used in qRT-PCR experiments are shown in Table 1.

Table 1: Nucleotide sequences of primers used for qRT-PCR.

Gene		Primer sequence (5′-3′)
TNF-α	Forward	CAGGCGGTGCCTATGTCTC
	Reverse	CGATCACCCCGAAGTTCAGTAG
IL-1β	Forward	GCCACGGCACAGTCATTGA
	Reverse	TGCTGATGGCCTGATTGTCTT
IL-6	Forward	CTGCAAGAGACTTCCATCCAG
	Reverse	AGTGGTATAGACAGGTCTGTTGG
Beclin-1	Forward	ATGGAGGGGTCTAAGGCGTC
	Reverse	TGGGCTGTGGTAAGTAATGGA
P62	Forward	GAGGCACCCCGAAACATGG
	Reverse	ACTTATAGCGAGTTCCCACCA
LC3-II	Forward	GACCGCTGTAAGGAGGTGC
	Reverse	AGAAGCCGAAGGTTTCTTGGG
PPARγ	Forward	GGAAGACCACTGCATTCCTT
	Reverse	GTAATCAGCAACCATTGGGTCA
Bax	Forward	AGACAGGGGCCTTTTTGCTAC
	Reverse	AATTCGCCGGAGACACTCG
Bcl-2	Forward	GCTACCGTCGTCGTGACTTCGC
	Reverse	CCCCACCGAACTCAAAGAAGG
β-Actin	Forward	GGCTGTATTCCCCTCCATCG
	Reverse	CCAGTTGGTAACAATGCCATGT

2.8. Immunohistochemistry. After the paraffin sections were dewaxed in dimethylbenzene and rehydrated through a graded series of alcohol, antigen retrieval was performed with citric acid-hydrogen phosphate two sodium buffers. Then, 3% hydrogen peroxide solution was added for 5 min to block endogenous peroxidase activity. After blocking with 5% bovine serum albumin at 37°C for 20 min and at room temperature for 10 min, antibodies (CST, 1 : 100; Proteintech, 1 : 50) were incubated with the sections overnight in a wet box at 4°C. The next day, the slices were washed with PBS and incubated with goat anti-rabbit secondary antibody for 30 min at room temperature. A diaminobenzidine kit was used to colorize the staining for imaging under a light microscope.

2.9. Transmission Electron Microscopy. Liver tissue was perfused with 2% glutaraldehyde buffered with 0.2 mmol/L cacodylate for 4 h. Sections were observed by transmission electron microscopy (JEM-1230; JEOL, Tokyo, Japan) to show autophagosomes after postfixation in 1% osmium tetroxide for 1 h.

2.10. Cell Culture and CCK8 Assay. The normal LO2 cells were cultured in RPMI-1640 culture medium (Thermo Fisher Scientific (China) Co. Ltd.) supplemented with 10% fetal bovine serum (Hyclone™ Fetal Bovine Serum, South American Origin), 100 U/mL of penicillin, and 100 g/mL of streptomycin (Gibco, Canada) in a humidified incubator at 37°C under 5% CO_2. The cells were plated at a density 2×10^4 cells/well in 96-well plates (100 μL of medium per well). The concentration of fucosterol was 20 μM and the anisomycin concentration was 0.1 μM. Cell viability was measured with the CCK8 assay at a wavelength of 450 nm. The LO2 were divided into four groups:

(1) Control group: no treatment

(2) Anisomycin group: treated with anisomycin diluted in DMSO at a concentration of 0.1 μM

(3) Fucosterol group: treated with fucosterol diluted in DMSO at concentration of 20 μM

(4) F + A group: treated with fucosterol (20 μM) and anisomycin (0.1 μM)

2.11. Statistical Analysis. All statistical analyses were calculated using SPSS V22.0 (IBM, Armonk, NY, USA). Experimental data are presented as the mean ± standard deviation and were compared by one-way analysis of variance using the Student-Newman-Keuls method. Differences were considered significant at $p < 0.05$. Histograms were created using GraphPad Prism v6.0 (GraphPad, San Diego, CA, USA).

3. Results

3.1. Fucosterol Pretreatment Ameliorated ConA-Induced Acute Liver Necrosis. Transaminases are primarily stored in hepatocytes and are the most sensitive indicators of hepatocyte necrosis. Figure 1(a) shows serum ALT and AST levels of mice from different groups, and these results indicated that fucosterol did not cause changes in liver enzymes at 2, 8, or 24 h. However, ALT and AST levels increased rapidly after ConA injection, peaking at 8 h. Fucosterol pretreatment decreased this trend in a dose-dependent manner at different time points. Then we examined nuclei and cytoplasm through HE staining, which visually indicated the extent of liver cell damage (Figure 1(b)). These results showed that liver cells in the ConA group demonstrated nuclear condensation and fragmentation, and the cell outline disappeared and was replaced by an amorphous, red-colored granular coagulation or liquefied substance. After fucosterol pretreatment, the area of necrosis decreased significantly with increasing drug concentration, and the most severe phenotypes were only present at 24 h. This indicated that the drug significantly reduced ConA-induced acute liver injury at 2, 8, and 24 h. As liver injury peaked at 8 h, we selected this time point for subsequent studies.

3.2. Fucosterol Inhibited Apoptosis in the ConA-Induced Acute Liver Injury Model. In addition to necrosis, apoptosis and autophagy are also important mechanisms of cell death. Therefore, we chose 8 h ConA treatment to further explore the effects fucosterol on apoptosis. Transcription of the antiapoptotic gene Bcl-2 was significantly decreased in the model group, whereas the proapoptotic Bax was increased. Fucosterol treatment significantly increased Bcl-2 transcription in a dose-dependent manner compared with the ConA group. In contrast, Bax was decreased in the fucosterol treatment groups (Figure 2(a)). Next, we detected Bcl-2 and Bax protein levels and localization in tissues using Western blot and immunohistochemistry, respectively (Figures 2(b) and

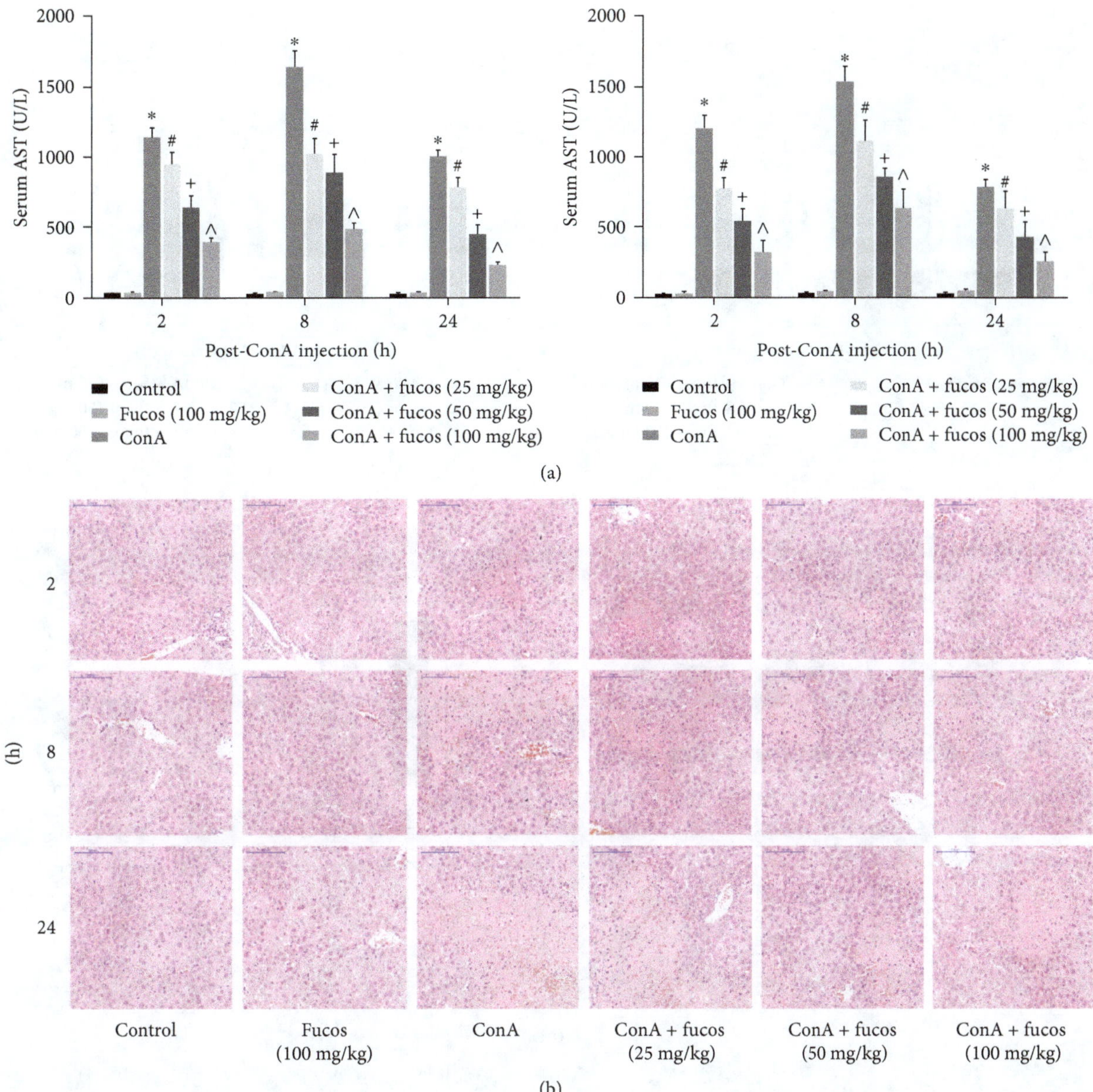

Figure 1: Effects of fucosterol on serum liver enzymes and acute liver injury pathology. (a) Serum ALT and AST levels 2, 8, and 24 h after ConA injection. Data are expressed as mean ± SD ($n = 6$, $^{*}P < 0.05$ for ConA versus control, $^{\#}P < 0.05$ for ConA + fucosterol (25 mg/kg) versus ConA, $^{+}P < 0.05$ for ConA + fucosterol (50 mg/kg) versus ConA + fucosterol (25 mg/kg), and $^{\wedge}P < 0.05$ for ConA + fucosterol (100 mg/kg) versus ConA + fucosterol (50 mg/kg)). (b) Hematoxylin and eosin staining of liver sections. Necrotic areas were imaged by digital microscopy; original magnification: 200x.

2(c)). Expression of Bcl-2 and Bax proteins were consistent with the mRNA results.

3.3. Fucosterol Reduced Autophagy Levels in the ConA-Induced Acute Liver Injury Model. Autophagy is a recently acknowledged cellular phenomenon that is related to programmed cell death. Thus, we also assessed autophagy levels, using Beclin-1, LC3, and P62 as autophagy markers. At the mRNA and protein level, Beclin-1 and LC-3 II were activated and showed increased expression in the ConA group, while autophagy levels were decreased after fucosterol treatment, which was most apparent at the maximum concentration (Figures 3(a) and 3(b)). Fucosterol had no obvious influence on autophagy in untreated normal animals. Inhibiting autophagy caused an accumulation of P62, so contrary to Beclin-1 and LC-3 II, P62 showed increased expression after fucosterol treatment. Furthermore, we performed immunohistochemical staining to directly observe autophagy levels *in vivo*, and the results were consistent with the expression data (Figure 3(c)). Autophagosomes with a bilayer membrane and autolysosomes after cytoplasmic degradation are important indicators of autophagy. We used transmission electron microscopy to show that the number of autophagosomes and autolysosomes increased after ConA injection,

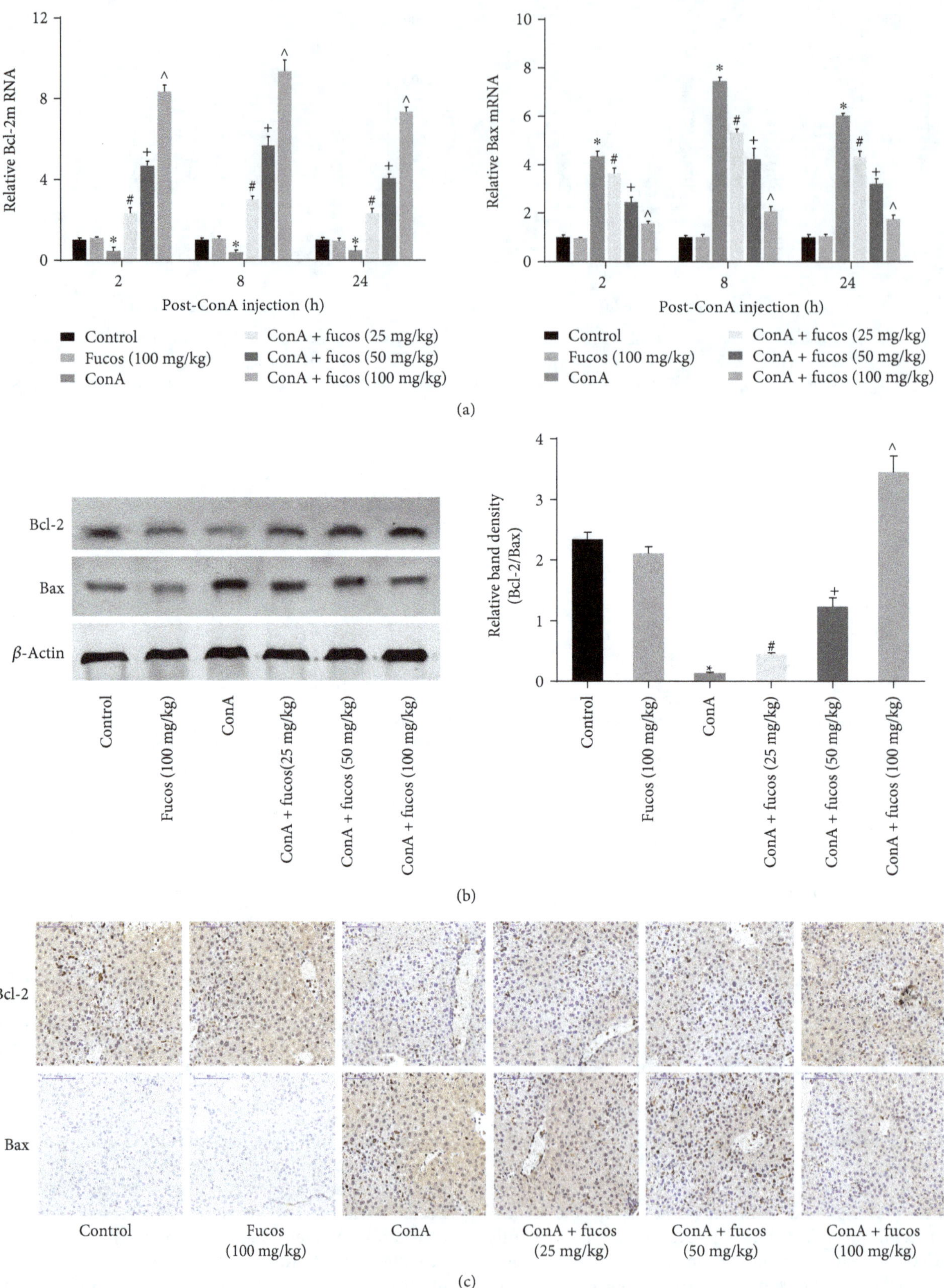

FIGURE 2: Effects of fucosterol on apoptosis in the acute liver injury model. (a) The expression of Bcl-2 and Bax mRNA were evaluated by quantitative real-time PCR. (b) Western blot and analysis of Bcl-2 and Bax protein levels. (c) Immunohistochemistry was used to detect Bcl-2 and Bax expression at 8 h ConA treatment. Original magnification: 200x. Data are expressed as mean ± SD ($n = 6$, $^{*}P < 0.05$ for ConA versus control, $^{\#}P < 0.05$ for ConA + fucosterol (25 mg/kg) versus ConA, $^{+}P < 0.05$ for ConA + fucosterol (50 mg/kg) versus ConA + fucosterol (25 mg/kg), and $^{\wedge}P < 0.05$ for ConA + fucosterol (100 mg/kg) versus ConA + fucosterol (50 mg/kg)).

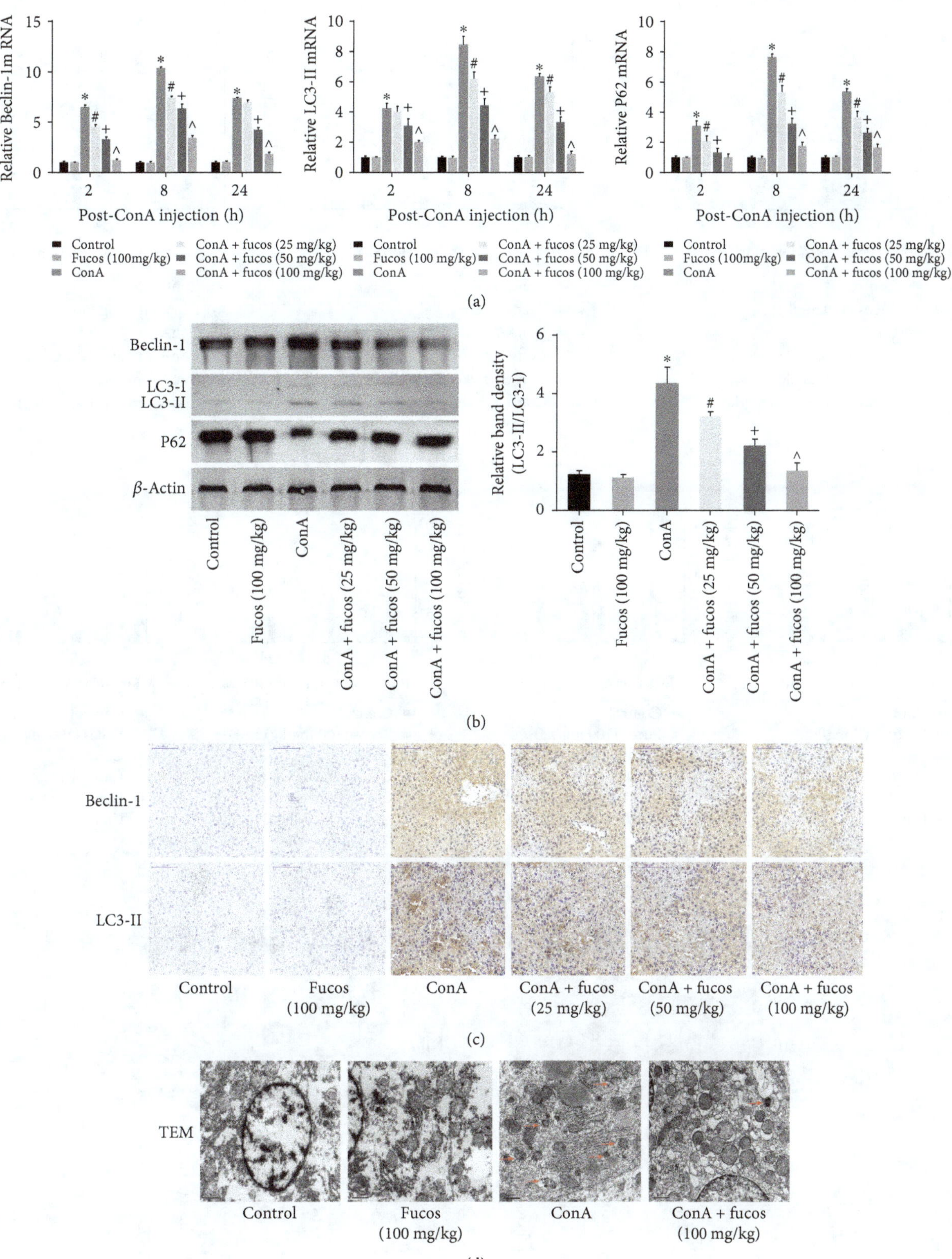

FIGURE 3: Effects of fucosterol on autophagy during acute liver injury. (a) The expression of Beclin-1, LC3-II, and P62 mRNA were evaluated by real-time PCR. (b) Western blot and analysis of Beclin-1, LC3-II, and P62 proteins. (c) Immunohistochemistry was used to detect the level of Beclin-1, LC3-II, and P62 expression at 8 h. Original magnification: 200x. (d) Autophagosome formation was detected in liver tissues with transmission electron microscopy at 8 h (magnification, ×10,000). Arrows indicate autophagosomes. Data are expressed as mean ± SD ($n = 6$, $^{*}P < 0.05$ for ConA versus control, $^{\#}P < 0.05$ for ConA + fucosterol (25 mg/kg) versus ConA, $^{+}P < 0.05$ for ConA + fucosterol (50 mg/kg) versus ConA + fucosterol (25 mg/kg), and $^{\wedge}P < 0.05$ for ConA + fucosterol (100 mg/kg) versus ConA + fucosterol (50 mg/kg)).

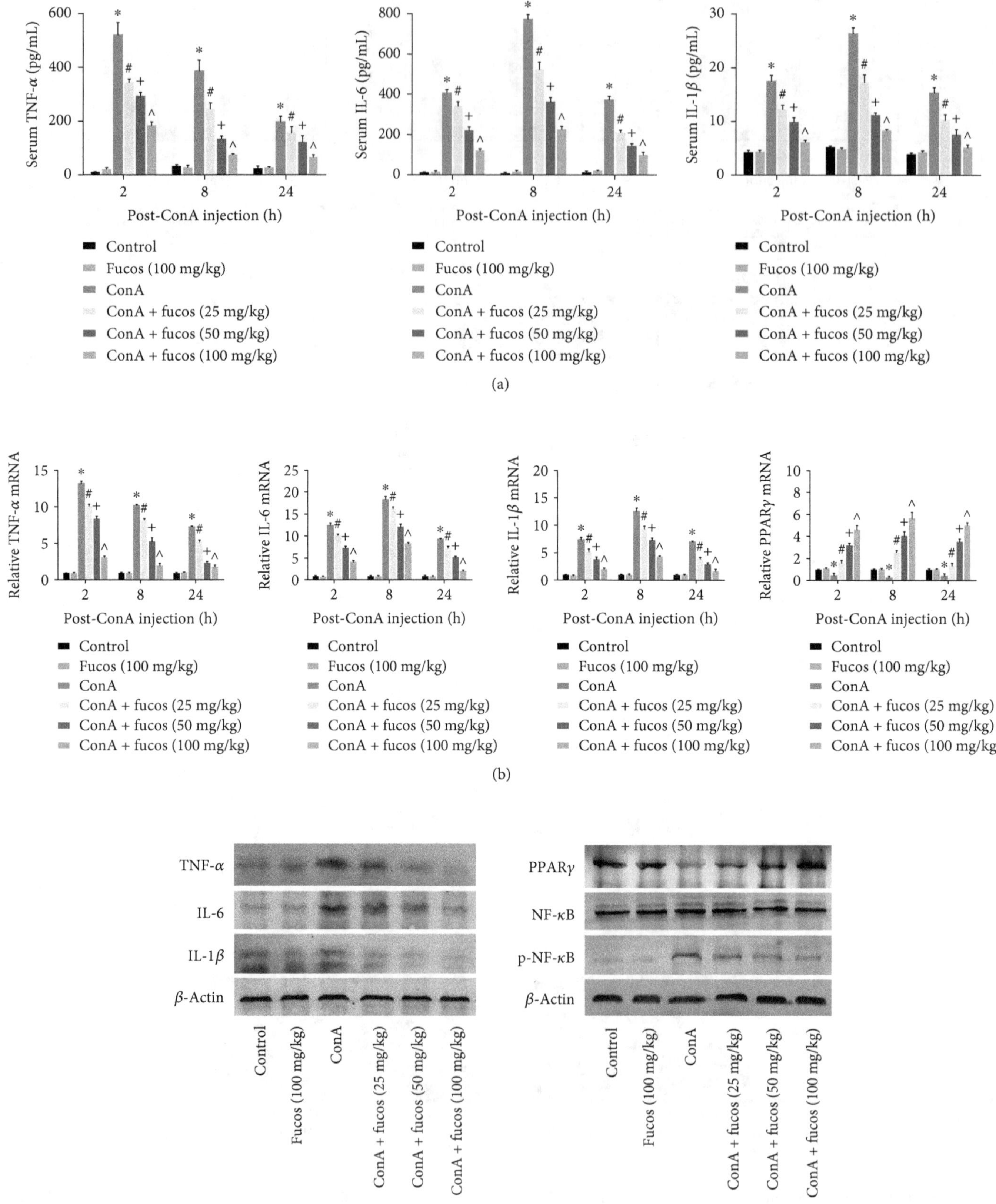

Figure 4: Continued.

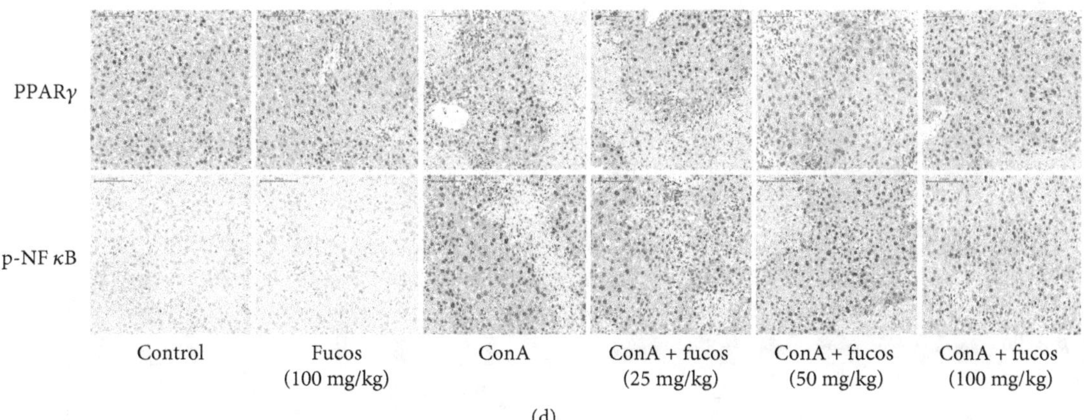

(d)

FIGURE 4: Effects of fucosterol on inflammatory factors in the acute liver injury model. (a) Serum levels of TNF-α, IL-6, and IL-1β 2, 8, and 24 h after ConA injection. (b) TNF-α, IL-6, IL-1β, and PPARγ mRNA levels were evaluated by quantitative real-time PCR. (c) Western blot and analysis of TNF-α, IL-6, IL-1β, PPARγ, NF-κB p65, and p-NF-κB p65 protein expression. (d) Immunohistochemistry was used to detect PPARγ and p-NF-κB p65 expression at 8 h. Original magnification: 200x. Data are expressed as mean ± SD ($n = 6$, $^*P < 0.05$ for ConA versus control, $^\#P < 0.05$ for ConA + fucosterol (25 mg/kg) versus ConA, $^+P < 0.05$ for ConA + fucosterol (50 mg/kg) versus ConA + fucosterol (25 mg/kg), and $^\wedge P < 0.05$ for ConA + fucosterol (100 mg/kg) versus ConA + fucosterol (50 mg/kg)).

and that fucosterol inhibited this trend (Figure 3(d)). These results suggest that fucosterol inhibited autophagy and reduced hepatocyte death *in vivo*.

3.4. Fucosterol Inhibited the Release of Inflammatory Factors and NF-κB p65 but Activated PPARγ in the ConA-Induced Acute Liver Injury Model. Inflammatory factors can activate neutrophils and lymphocytes causing necrosis or activate other signaling pathways that lead to apoptosis and autophagy. Therefore, inflammatory factors are also an important parameter in assessing cell damage. We evaluated TNF-α, IL-6, and IL-1β, the major mediators in ConA-induced liver injury, and found that their expression was consistent with the extent of necrosis, apoptosis, and autophagy. Serum TNF-α, IL-6, and IL-1β increased markedly after ConA treatment, while fucosterol pretreatment inhibited their release, and showed the greatest effect at the maximum concentration (Figure 4(a)). mRNA and protein levels of these inflammatory factors were also significantly decreased in liver tissue from the fucosterol treatment group compared with the ConA group, and the changes were statistically significant and in a concentration-dependent manner (Figure 4(b)). We further explored NF-κB p65 and its upstream pathway PPARγ, which play a major role in the release of inflammatory cytokines. These results showed that increased TNF-α, IL-6, and IL-1β release was associated with increased NF-κB p65 phosphorylation and decreased PPARγ expression. Immunohistochemistry showed a consistent trend with the Western blot data (Figure 4(c)). These data suggested that fucosterol may activate PPARγ, thereby inhibiting the NF-κB p65 pathway, which reduces the expression of inflammatory factors and subsequent necrosis and apoptosis.

3.5. Fucosterol Inhibited P38 MAPK Phosphorylation but Not JNK or ERK. We next sought to determine how fucosterol activated PPARγ, testing the hypothesis that the target may be a MAPK family member, based on these being upstream of PPARγ and on the pharmacological properties of fucosterol. Therefore, we examined the levels of P38 MAPK, JNK, and ERK phosphorylation. Western blot results showed that although ConA elevated phosphorylation levels of all MAPK family members, fucosterol only reduced the activated form of P38 MAPK, and had no effect on phosphorylated JNK or ERK (Figure 5(a)). Next, we examined p-P38 MAPK levels in liver tissue using immunohistochemistry, which confirmed the above results (Figure 5(b)). Furthermore, we investigated MKK3/6 activity, which is upstream of P38 MAPK, and these results were consistent with our hypothesis. In the ConA group, levels of phosphorylated MKK3/6 increased significantly, but with increasing fucosterol dosage, the trend of p-MKK3/6 and p-P38 MAPK decreased significantly (Figure 5(c)). The P38 activator anisomycin was used to demonstrate the direct effect of fucosterol on P38 MAPK/PPARγ. After being treated for 48 h, the protein of cells were extracted to evaluate the expression of P38 MAPK, PPARγ, and RXRα. However, the use of a single drug did not have a significant effect on all the MAPK pathways. Therefore, fucosterol may act by inhibiting P38 MAPK activation, but had no effect on JNK or ERK.

4. Discussion

The incidence of AIP has increased worldwide; thus, it is prudent to explore the potential activity of natural products that have low side effects to develop more effective therapeutic strategies [18–21]. Fucosterol derived from the brown alga *Eisenia bicyclis* is the most abundant phytosterol and has various biological activities, including antioxidant, anticancer, and antidiabetic properties [14]. Recently, fucosterol was found to have an anti-inflammatory effect but its mechanism of liver protection remains unclear [15, 22].

After tail vein injection, ConA can activate T cells and macrophages, exert cytotoxic effects through perforin and granzyme and cause cell death that can be divided into

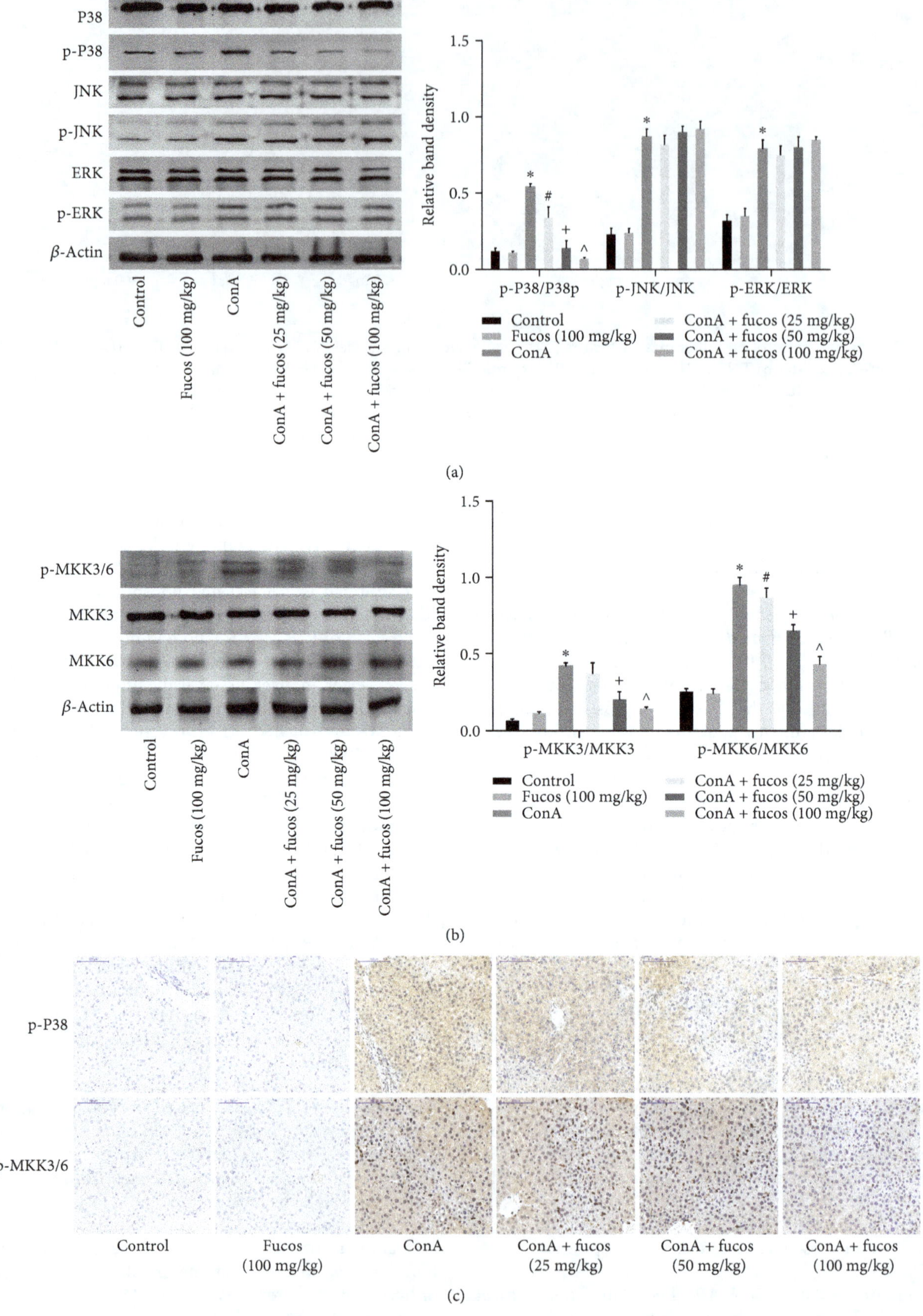

Figure 5: Continued.

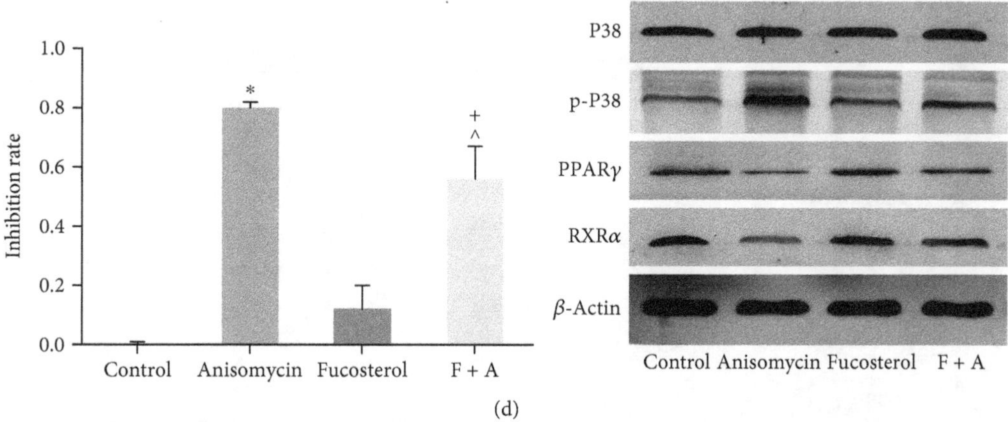

(d)

Figure 5: Effect of fucosterol on MAPK family activation. (a) Western blot and analysis of P38, p-P38, JNK, p-JNK, ERK, and p-ERK. (b) Western blot and analysis of p-MKK3/6, MKK3 and MKK6. (c) Immunohistochemistry was used to detect p-P38 and p-MKK3/6 levels at 8 h. Original magnification: 200x. (d) The proliferation of LO2 with CCK8 assay and Western blot and analysis of P38, p-P38, PPARγ, and RXRα. Data are expressed as mean ± SD ($n = 6$, $^*P < 0.05$ for ConA versus control, $^\#P < 0.05$ for ConA + fucosterol (25 mg/kg) versus ConA, $^+P < 0.05$ for ConA + fucosterol (50 mg/kg) versus ConA + fucosterol (25 mg/kg), and $^\wedge P < 0.05$ for ConA + fucosterol (100 mg/kg) versus ConA + fucosterol (50 mg/kg)).

necrosis, apoptosis, and autophagy according to cell morphology. FasL expression is induced during this process, which mediates TNF-α, IL-6, and IL-1β secretion, causing autophagy-associated necrosis and apoptosis [23–25]. Therefore, if a therapeutic agent could effectively inhibit these three cell death pathways, it could protect liver cells. First, we detected the effect of fucosterol on necrosis. ALT and AST release peaked 8 h after ConA injection, which was explained by the membrane permeability of liver cells that caused ALT and AST release to blood. Fucosterol pretreatment reduced transaminase levels and had a greater effect under higher doses, indicating that the drug can effectively reduce liver cell necrosis. The pathology directly reflects the edema and necrosis in the tissues, and also proves the effect. These results were consistent with the evidence provided by Yoo et al. and Li et al. [16, 26]. Second, we investigated Bcl-2 and Bax expression, which are important indicators of endogenous apoptosis. Bcl-2 and Bax can form homologous or heterologous dimers to regulate apoptosis. Bcl-2, an antiapoptotic protein, showed reduced expression after ConA treatment, while Bax showed increased expression. Fucosterol treatment changed the trend of both these markers [27]. Thus, fucosterol can increase the ratio of Bcl-2/Bax causing decreased Bax/Bax homologous dimers, which normally can lead to cytochrome *c* and AIF release by translocation from the cytosol to mitochondria. At the same time, increased Bcl-2 expression can reduce apoptosis independent of Bax. Pattingre et al. showed that Bcl-2 can downregulate Beclin-1-dependent autophagic cell death [28]. Free Beclin-1 can lead to the conversion of LC3-I to LC3-II, which increases the occurrence of autophagic vesicles and reduces P62 accumulation [29]. Thus, fucosterol can protect liver cells by inhibiting necrosis, apoptosis, and autophagy.

The release of inflammatory factors plays an important role in ConA-induced acute liver injury. Our detection of inflammatory factors showed that the major inducers, such as TNF-α, IL-6, and IL-1β, were markedly decreased in a dose-dependent manner after fucosterol treatment. While, the results from Sun et al. suggested that fucosterol protected HaCaT cells against $CoCl_2$-induced cytotoxicity and inflammatory responses by suppressing HIF1-α [22], Li et al. showed that fucosterol attenuates lipopolysaccharide-induced acute lung injury by inhibiting NF-κB activation [26]. Therefore, we tested whether fucosterol activity in our model was mediated acting on the proinflammatory signaling pathways, such as PPARγ/NF-κB, MAPK, and JAK/STAT. We tested these pathways because Feng et al. provided evidence that many natural products regulate PPARγ [30], and Fuenzalida et al. and Mansour et al. also highlighted the beneficial effects of curcumin and 15-deoxy-Δ12,14-PGJ2, which are mediated by upregulating PPARγ activation [31, 32].

PPARγ is a member of the nuclear transcription factor superfamily that is activated by corresponding ligands and combines with retinoid X receptor (RXR) to form a distinct dimer that regulates transcription [13]. Van Ginderachter et al. and Ricote et al. showed that PPARγ is a negative regulator of macrophage activation [12, 33]. In inflammatory responses, it can bind NF-κB p65/p50 to form an inhibitory transcriptional complex that reduces the expression of related inflammatory factors [6, 11, 34]. Additionally, Ren et al. and Fuenzalida et al. provided evidence that PPARγ upregulates Bcl-2, preventing oxidative stress-induced neuronal and cardiomyocyte degeneration [8, 31]. Our results showed that PPARγ expression and NF-κB p65 activation were increased to different degrees after treatment, indicating that fucosterol might be a potential PPARγ activator. However, there is no evidence that fucosterol binds directly to PPARγ. Based on existing studies, it is believed that MAPK-mediated PPARγ phosphorylation contributes to reduced PPARγ transcriptional activity and, thereby,

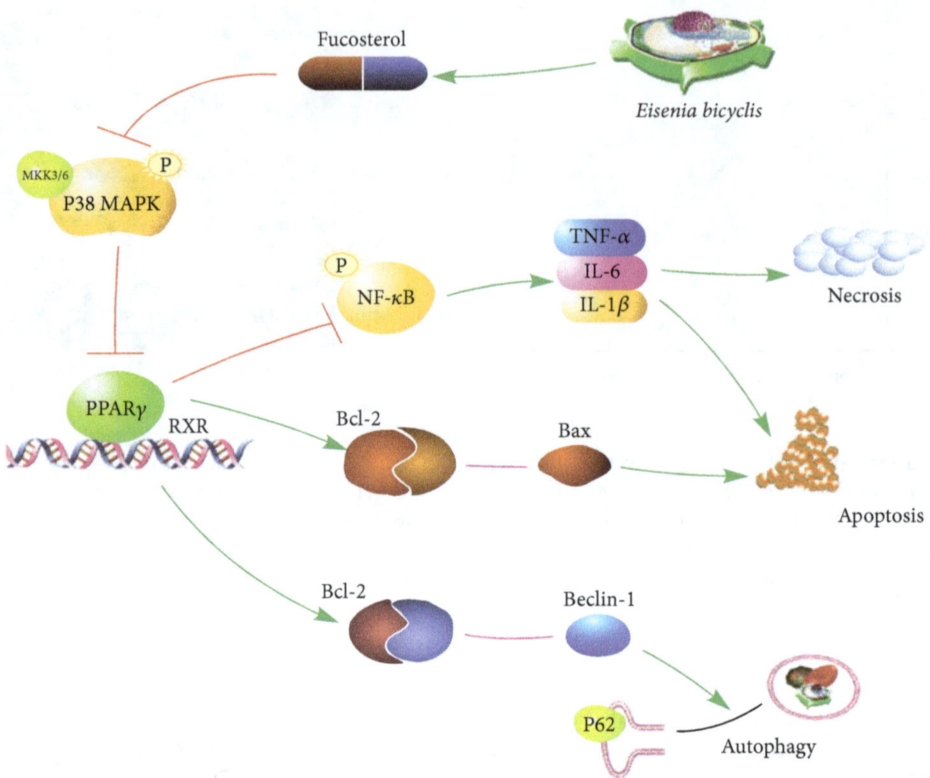

FIGURE 6: Mechanism of fucosterol action. In ConA-induced acute liver injury, fucosterol decreased P38 MAPK phosphorylation and contributed to the increased PPARγ transcriptional activity. Active PPARγ reduced the release of inflammatory factors that cause necrosis and apoptosis by inhibiting the NF-κB pathway. Additionally, Bcl-2, which is upregulated by PPARγ, can combine with Bax and Beclin-1 to reduce apoptosis and autophagy, respectively. Thus, fucosterol attenuates Concanavalin A-induced acute liver injury in mice via the P38 MAPK/PPARγ/NF-κB pathway.

inhibits oxidative injury and inflammation [32, 35]. Fucosterol is associated with the MAPK family [16, 36], therefore, we examined the levels of P38 MAPK, ERK, and JNK phosphorylation. These results showed that although ConA increased the phosphorylation of all three components, fucosterol acted only on the phosphorylation of P38 MAPK in this model (Figure 6). Interestingly, Lee et al. revealed that fucosterol inhibited adipogenesis of 3T3-L1 preadipocytes by modulating FoxO signaling, in which PPARγ was inactivated [37]. These differences could be attributed to the different pathogenesis of the various disease models.

5. Conclusions

Our findings showed that fucosterol alleviated ConA-induced acute liver injury via the P38 MAPK/PPARγ/NF-κB pathway. Our data show that fucosterol attenuated serum liver enzyme levels by inhibiting necrosis and apoptosis in a process mediated by PPARγ activation and NF-κB inhibition, which reduced the release of inflammatory factors. Fucosterol also inhibited apoptosis and autophagy by upregulating Bcl-2 via PPARγ, which reduced the levels of functional Bax and Beclin-1. These findings highlight fucosterol as a promising potential therapeutic agent for AIH.

Authors' Contributions

Wenhui Mo and Chengfen Wang contributed equally to this paper.

Acknowledgments

The research was financially supported by the National Natural Science Foundation of China (Grant nos. 8160472 and 8100466).

References

[1] A. A. Gossard and K. D. Lindor, "Autoimmune hepatitis: a review," *Journal of Gastroenterology*, vol. 47, no. 5, pp. 498–503, 2012.

[2] R. Liberal, C. R. Grant, G. Mieli-Vergani, and D. Vergani, "Autoimmune hepatitis: a comprehensive review," *Journal of Autoimmunity*, vol. 41, pp. 126–139, 2013.

[3] G. Tiegs, J. Hentschel, and A. Wendel, "A T cell-dependent experimental liver injury in mice inducible by concanavalin A," *The Journal of Clinical Investigation*, vol. 90, no. 1, pp. 196–203, 1992.

[4] A. Varthaman, J. Khallou-Laschet, M. Clement et al., "Control of T cell reactivation by regulatory Qa-1-restricted CD8+ T cells," *Journal of Immunology*, vol. 184, no. 12, pp. 6585–6591, 2010.

[5] F. Heymann, K. Hamesch, R. Weiskirchen, and F. Tacke, "The concanavalin A model of acute hepatitis in mice," *Laboratory Animals*, vol. 49, 1_suppl, pp. 12–20, 2015.

[6] M. Chandra, S. Miriyala, and M. Panchatcharam, "PPARγ and its role in cardiovascular diseases," *PPAR Research*, vol. 2017, Article ID 6404638, 10 pages, 2017.

[7] S. Polvani, M. Tarocchi, and A. Galli, "PPARγ and oxidative stress: Con(β) catenating NRF2 and FOXO," *PPAR Research*, vol. 2012, Article ID 641087, 15 pages, 2012.

[8] Y. Ren, C. Sun, Y. Sun et al., "PPAR gamma protects cardiomyocytes against oxidative stress and apoptosis via Bcl-2 upregulation," *Vascular Pharmacology*, vol. 51, no. 2-3, pp. 169–174, 2009.

[9] A. Croasdell, P. F. Duffney, N. Kim, S. H. Lacy, P. J. Sime, and R. P. Phipps, "PPARγ and the innate immune system mediate the resolution of inflammation," *PPAR Research*, vol. 2015, Article ID 549691, 20 pages, 2015.

[10] D. Gomez, N. Munoz, R. Guerrero, O. Acosta, and C. A. Guerrero, "PPARγ agonists as an anti-inflammatory treatment inhibiting rotavirus infection of small intestinal villi," *PPAR Research*, vol. 2016, Article ID 4049373, 17 pages, 2016.

[11] R. Stienstra, C. Duval, M. Muller, and S. Kersten, "PPARs, obesity, and inflammation," *PPAR Research*, vol. 2007, Article ID 95974, 10 pages, 2007.

[12] J. A. Van Ginderachter, K. Movahedi, J. Van den Bossche, and P. De Baetselier, "Macrophages, PPARs, and cancer," *PPAR Research*, vol. 2008, Article ID 169414, 11 pages, 2008.

[13] J. Camps, A. Garcia-Heredia, A. Rull et al., "PPARs in regulation of paraoxonases: control of oxidative stress and inflammation pathways," *PPAR Research*, vol. 2012, Article ID 616371, 10 pages, 2012.

[14] Q. A. Abdul, R. J. Choi, H. A. Jung, and J. S. Choi, "Health benefit of fucosterol from marine algae: a review," *Journal of the Science of Food and Agriculture*, vol. 96, no. 6, pp. 1856–1866, 2016.

[15] H. A. Jung, S. E. Jin, B. R. Ahn, C. M. Lee, and J. S. Choi, "Anti-inflammatory activity of edible brown alga *Eisenia bicyclis* and its constituents fucosterol and phlorotannins in LPS-stimulated RAW264.7 macrophages," *Food and Chemical Toxicology*, vol. 59, pp. 199–206, 2013.

[16] M. S. Yoo, J. S. Shin, H. E. Choi et al., "Fucosterol isolated from *Undaria pinnatifida* inhibits lipopolysaccharide-induced production of nitric oxide and pro-inflammatory cytokines via the inactivation of nuclear factor-κB and p38 mitogen-activated protein kinase in RAW264.7 macrophages," *Food Chemistry*, vol. 135, no. 3, pp. 967–975, 2012.

[17] M. Bozza, J. L. Bliss, R. Maylor et al., "Interleukin-11 reduces T-cell-dependent experimental liver injury in mice," *Hepatology*, vol. 30, no. 6, pp. 1441–1447, 1999.

[18] J. Li, K. Chen, S. Li et al., "Pretreatment with fucoidan from *Fucus vesiculosus* protected against ConA-induced acute liver injury by inhibiting both intrinsic and extrinsic apoptosis," *PLoS One*, vol. 11, no. 4, article e0152570, 2016.

[19] S. Li, Y. Xia, K. Chen et al., "Epigallocatechin-3-gallate attenuates apoptosis and autophagy in concanavalin A-induced hepatitis by inhibiting BNIP3," *Drug Design, Development and Therapy*, vol. 10, pp. 631–647, 2016.

[20] T. Liu, Y. Xia, J. Li et al., "Shikonin attenuates concanavalin A-induced acute liver injury in mice via inhibition of the JNK pathway," *Mediators of Inflammation*, vol. 2016, Article ID 2748367, 14 pages, 2016.

[21] T. Liu, Q. Zhang, W. Mo et al., "The protective effects of shikonin on hepatic ischemia/reperfusion injury are mediated by the activation of the PI3K/Akt pathway," *Scientific Reports*, vol. 7, article 44785, 2017.

[22] Z. Sun, M. A. A. Mohamed, S. Y. Park, and T. H. Yi, "Fucosterol protects cobalt chloride induced inflammation by the inhibition of hypoxia-inducible factor through PI3K/Akt pathway," *International Immunopharmacology*, vol. 29, no. 2, pp. 642–647, 2015.

[23] F. Gantner, M. Leist, A. W. Lohse, P. G. Germann, and G. Tiegs, "Concanavalin A-induced T-cell-mediated hepatic injury in mice: the role of tumor necrosis factor," *Hepatology*, vol. 21, no. 1, pp. 190–198, 1995.

[24] C. Trautwein, T. Rakemann, D. A. Brenner et al., "Concanavalin A-induced liver cell damage: activation of intracellular pathways triggered by tumor necrosis factor in mice," *Gastroenterology*, vol. 114, no. 5, pp. 1035–1045, 1998.

[25] K. Seino, N. Kayagaki, K. Takeda, K. Fukao, K. Okumura, and H. Yagita, "Contribution of Fas ligand to T cell-mediated hepatic injury in mice," *Gastroenterology*, vol. 113, no. 4, pp. 1315–1322, 1997.

[26] Y. Li, X. Li, G. Liu et al., "Fucosterol attenuates lipopolysaccharide-induced acute lung injury in mice," *The Journal of Surgical Research*, vol. 195, no. 2, pp. 515–521, 2015.

[27] L. Ouyang, Z. Shi, S. Zhao et al., "Programmed cell death pathways in cancer: a review of apoptosis, autophagy and programmed necrosis," *Cell Proliferation*, vol. 45, no. 6, pp. 487–498, 2012.

[28] S. Pattingre, C. Bauvy, S. Carpentier, T. Levade, B. Levine, and P. Codogno, "Role of JNK1-dependent Bcl-2 phosphorylation in ceramide-induced macroautophagy," *Journal of Biological Chemistry*, vol. 284, no. 5, pp. 2719–2728, 2009.

[29] C. Gordy and Y. W. He, "The crosstalk between autophagy and apoptosis: where does this lead?," *Protein & Cell*, vol. 3, no. 1, pp. 17–27, 2012.

[30] S. Feng, L. Reuss, and Y. Wang, "Potential of natural products in the inhibition of adipogenesis through regulation of PPARγ expression and/or its transcriptional activity," *Molecules*, vol. 21, no. 10, 2016.

[31] K. Fuenzalida, R. Quintanilla, P. Ramos et al., "Peroxisome proliferator-activated receptor γ up-regulates the bcl-2 anti-apoptotic protein in neurons and induces mitochondrial stabilization and protection against oxidative stress and apoptosis," *Journal of Biological Chemistry*, vol. 282, no. 51, pp. 37006–37015, 2007.

[32] H. H. Mansour, S. M. El Kiki, and S. M. Galal, "Metformin and low dose radiation modulates cisplatin-induced oxidative injury in rat via PPAR-γ and MAPK pathways," *Archives of Biochemistry and Biophysics*, vol. 616, pp. 13–19, 2017.

[33] M. Ricote, A. C. Li, T. M. Willson, C. J. Kelly, and C. K. Glass, "The peroxisome proliferator-activated receptor-γ is a negative regulator of macrophage activation," *Nature*, vol. 391, no. 6662, pp. 79–82, 1998.

[34] Y. Mao, J. Wang, F. Yu et al., "Ghrelin reduces liver impairment in a model of concanavalin a-induced acute hepatitis in mice," *Drug Design, Development and Therapy*, vol. 9, pp. 5385–5396, 2015.

[35] L. Shi, Q. Lin, X. Li et al., "Alliin, a garlic organosulfur compound, ameliorates gut inflammation through MAPK-NF-κB/AP-1/STAT-1 inactivation and PPAR-γ activation," *Molecular Nutrition & Food Research*, vol. 61, no. 9, 2017.

[36] M. S. Kim, G. H. Oh, M. J. Kim, and J. K. Hwang, "Fucosterol inhibits matrix metalloproteinase expression and promotes type-1 procollagen production in UVB-induced HaCAT cells," *Photochemistry and Photobiology*, vol. 89, no. 4, pp. 911–918, 2013.

[37] J. H. Lee, H. A. Jung, M. J. Kang, J. S. Choi, and G. D. Kim, "Fucosterol, isolated from *Ecklonia stolonifera*, inhibits adipogenesis through modulation of FoxO1 pathway in 3T3-L1 adipocytes," *Journal of Pharmacy and Pharmacology*, vol. 69, no. 3, pp. 325–333, 2017.

7

Repeated Autologous Bone Marrow Transfusion through Portal Vein for Treating Decompensated Liver Cirrhosis after Splenectomy

Weiwei Zhang,[1,2] Mujian Teng,[1] Baochi Liu,[2] Qiling Liu,[2] Xin Liu,[2] Yanhui Si,[2] and Lei Li[2]

[1]*Department of Hepatobiliary Surgery, Qianfoshan Hospital Affiliated to Shandong University, Jinan, China*
[2]*Department of General Surgery, Shanghai Public Health Clinical Center, Fudan University, Shanghai, China*

Correspondence should be addressed to Mujian Teng; mujiant66@hotmail.com

Academic Editor: Per Hellström

Objective. This study is aimed at examining the impact of repeated intraportal autologous bone marrow transfusion (ABMT) in patients with decompensated liver cirrhosis after splenectomy. *Methods.* A total of 25 patients with decompensated liver cirrhosis undergoing splenectomy were divided into ABMT and control groups. The portal vein was cannulated intraoperatively using Celsite Implantofix through the right gastroomental vein. Both groups were given a routine medical treatment. Then, 18 mL of autologous bone marrow was transfused through the port in the patients of the ABMT group 1 week, 1 month, and 3 months after laminectomy, while nothing was given to the control group. All patients were monitored for adverse events. Liver function tests, including serum albumin (ALB), alanine aminotransferase (ALT), total bilirubin (TB), prothrombin activity (PTA), cholinesterase (CHE), α-fetoprotein (AFP), and liver stiffness measurement (LSM), were conducted before surgery and 1, 3, and 6 months after surgery. *Results.* Significant improvements in ALB, ALT, and CHE levels and decreased LSM were observed in the ABMT group compared with those in the control group ($P < 0.05$). TB and PTA improved in both groups but with no significant differences between the groups. No significant changes were observed in AFP in the control group, but it decreased in the ABMT group. No major adverse effects were noted during the follow-up period in the patients of either group. *Conclusions.* Repeated intraportal ABMT was clinically safe, and liver function of patients significantly improved. Therefore, this therapy has the potential to treat patients with decompensated liver cirrhosis after splenectomy. This trial was registered with the identification number of ChiCTR-ONC-17012592.

1. Introduction

Liver cirrhosis is an advanced-stage liver disease representing irreversible damage or scarring to the liver and is a major cause of mortality worldwide [1]. Liver transplantation is so far the only effective treatment for decompensated cirrhosis; however, its application is largely restricted by technical difficulties and limited donor sources [2]. Recent advances in stem cell research have prompted the development of stem cell-based therapy in these patients since the stem cells, including bone marrow-derived stem cells, have the capacity for self-renewal and multilineage differentiation [3]. Positive results from stem cell therapy using animal models have led to the evaluation of the feasibility and safety of bone marrow cell (BMC) therapy in patients with chronic liver disease [4–8]. As an accessible source of stem cells, adult human bone marrow contains two major types of stem cells: hematopoietic stem cells (HSCs) and mesenchymal stromal cells (MSCs). HSCs are capable of both self-renewal and differentiation into multiple hematopoietic lineages, while MSCs are nonhematopoietic and represent a minute fraction (0.001%–0.01%) of the total nucleated cell population in the marrow [9].

Previous studies have also shown that transplantation of bone marrow-derived mesenchymal stem cell (BMSC) effectively reduced liver fibrosis and improved liver function by inducing regeneration of the liver in different animal models

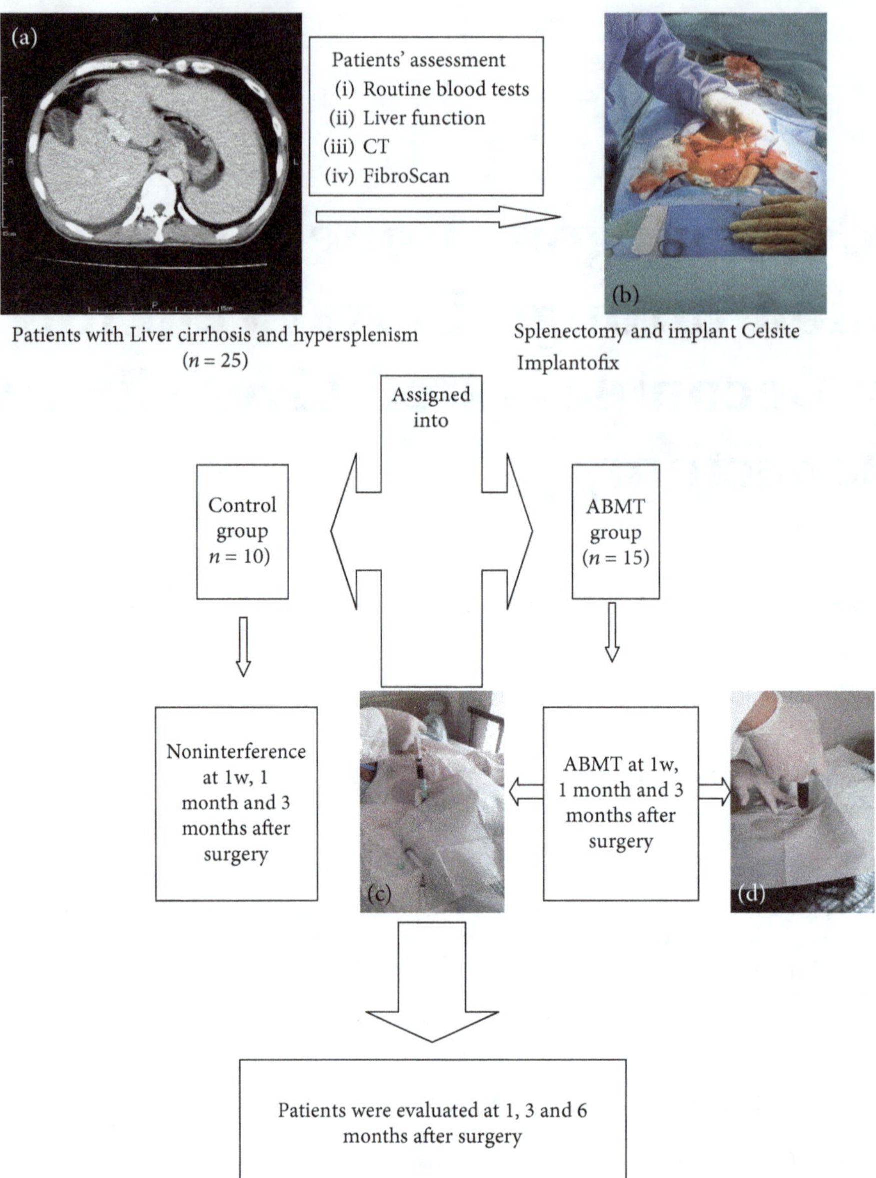

FIGURE 1: Flowchart of the study design. Representative images during the procedure are shown: (a) CT manifestations in patients with liver cirrhosis ($n = 25$), (b) splenectomy and implant using Celsite Implantofix ($n = 25$), (c) bone marrow extraction from the anterior superior iliac spine ($n = 15$), (d) ABMT ($n = 15$).

[10] through the paracrine action of BMSC and fusion with hepatocytes [11, 12]. Nevertheless, cells undergo extensive *in vitro* expansion to obtain a sufficient number of MSCs prior to transplant, increasing the risk for genetic mutations and eventually leading to malignant transformation [13] and decrease of the adipogenic and osteogenic differentiation potential in long-term expanded MSCs [14]. Homing of culture-expanded MSCs is inefficient compared with leukocytes and HSCs due to a lack of relevant cell adhesion and chemokine receptors [15].

It was hypothesized in this study that bone marrow transfusion would improve homing of MSCs and repeated bone marrow transfusion would result in more sustained clinical efficacy and improved liver functions. This exploratory study was therefore designed to investigate the safety and feasibility of the repeated bone marrow transfusion treatment in patients with decompensated liver cirrhosis.

2. Materials and Methods

2.1. Patients. A total of 25 patients with decompensated liver cirrhosis were recruited for this study. All patients attended the Shanghai Public Health Clinical Center, China, from November 2014 to December 2015 and were diagnosed with decompensated liver cirrhosis caused by chronic hepatitis B, hepatitis C, alcoholic cirrhosis, and schistosomiasis cirrhosis. This study was approved by the ethics committee of the Shanghai Public Health Clinical Center, Shanghai, China. This trial was registered with the identification number of ChiCTR-ONC-17012592. All patients provided written

Table 1: Group division.

	Control ($n = 10$)	ABMT ($n = 15$)
Chronic hepatitis B	8	14
Chronic hepatitis C	0	1
Alcoholic cirrhosis	1	0
Schistosomiasis cirrhosis	1	0

informed consent. Patients required splenectomy because of portal hypertension or hypersplenism and met all the following inclusion criteria: age 20–70 years, decompensated liver cirrhosis, abnormal serum albumin (ALB) and/or bilirubin and/or prothrombin time, and no viable hepatocellular carcinoma seen on a computed tomography (CT) scan. The exclusion criteria were evidence of extrahepatic biliary diseases, severe cardiac insufficiency, and no severe diseases such as stroke or myocardial infarction in the last 6 months. All patients were subjected to splenectomy which was performed by laparotomy and associated with nonselective esophagogastric devascularization. During splenectomy, the Celsite Implantofix (B. Braun Medical Inc., France) was implanted in the portal vein through the right gastroomental vein. After surgery, the patients were assigned into two groups: patients who received treatment of autologous bone marrow transfusion (ABMT) and patients who were given nothing (control).

2.2. Bone Marrow Transfusion. Before treatment, all patients underwent upper abdominal vascular enhanced CT examinations to identify the spatial relationship of the portal veins and the hepatic veins and to exclude the possibility of liver tumors. One week after surgery, 36 mL of bone marrow was extracted from the anterior superior iliac spine using a syringe containing heparin in the ABMT group. Then, 18 mL of bone marrow was transfused into the portal vein using Celsite Implantofix in the ABMT group, while nothing was given to the control group. The other 18 mL was analyzed for cell number count, viability, and endotoxin. One month and 3 months after surgery, 18 mL of bone marrow was extracted and transfused directly without analyzed. The stem cell surface markers HLA-DR, CD34, CD45, CD31, CD14, CD19, CD71, CD105, CD73, and CD90 were quantified using appropriate antibodies (Becton Dickinson and Co., NJ, USA) on a fluorescence-activated cell sorting system Gallios (Beckman Coulter, USA).

2.3. Follow-Up. The flowchart of the study design is shown in Figure 1. Briefly, patients were evaluated 1, 3, and 6 months after surgery. Functional liver indices, including ALB, alanine aminotransferase (ALT), total bilirubin (TB), prothrombin activity (PTA), cholinesterase (CHE), and α-fetoprotein (AFP), were used to evaluate the overall condition of patients with decompensated liver cirrhosis. Patients were examined using FibroScan to evaluate liver stiffness measurement (LSM). Treatment effectiveness was defined as a decline in LSM after treatment. The evaluation of liver function ended 6 months after surgery. Adverse effects, such as fever, rash, and nausea, were recorded. Patients' medications except

Table 2: Clinical characteristics of patients.

	Groups		P value
	Control	ABMT	
Sex (male, %)	80%	60%	>0.05
Age (year)	51.29 ± 11.38	45 ± 9.23	>0.05
ALT (U/L)	30.29 ± 15.84	32.42 ± 21.41	>0.05
TB (μmol/L)	28.51 ± 11.91	27.42 ± 20.37	>0.05
PTA (%)	66.29 ± 9.14	56.23 ± 11.27	>0.05
ALB (g/L)	32.64 ± 5.2	32.14 ± 5.46	>0.05
CHE (U/L)	3065 ± 1661	3060 ± 847.9	>0.05
WBC (10^9/L)	2.27 ± 0.71	2.27 ± 1.60	>0.05
RBC (10^9/L)	3.66 ± 0.72	3.19 ± 0.55	>0.05
PLT (10^9/L)	43.11 ± 24.11	44.36 ± 22.01	>0.05
Child–Pugh	7.44 ± 1.23	7.71 ± 1.48	>0.05
LSM (kPa)	22.25 ± 12.78	22.06 ± 13.29	>0.05
AFP (ng/mL)	3.4 ± 2.66	54.68 ± 122.35	>0.05

AFP: α-fetoprotein; ALB: serum albumin; ALT: alanine aminotransferase; CHE: cholinesterase; LSM: liver stiffness measurement; PLT: platelet; PTA: prothrombin activity; RBC: red blood cell; TB: total bilirubin; WBC: white blood cell. Values are mean ± standard deviation.

antiviral therapy were unchanged before and after the therapy and throughout the postoperative follow-up period (except for dosage reduction as a result of improvement in a patient's condition).

2.4. Statistical Analyses. SPSS for Windows version 17.0 software package (SPSS Inc., IL, USA) was used for statistical data analysis. Descriptive statistics were presented as mean ± standard deviation for quantitative variables, whereas qualitative data were expressed as numbers (frequency) and percentages. The changes in liver function parameters relative to baseline 1, 3, and 6 months after treatment were analyzed by multifactor analysis of variance for repeated measures. The chi-square or Fisher's exact test was used for qualitative data. A P value < 0.05 was considered statistically significant. The data used to support the findings of this study are included within this article.

3. Results

3.1. Patient Characteristics. A total of 25 patients (17 men and 8 women) with a mean age of 47.2 ± 10.21 years (range, 28–62) were enrolled in this study and distributed into the control ($n = 10$) and ABMT ($n = 15$) groups. Of the 25 patients included, 22 had hepatitis B cirrhosis, 1 had hepatitis C cirrhosis, 1 had alcoholic cirrhosis, and 1 had schistosomiasis cirrhosis. Group division is shown in Table 1. Demographic and clinical characteristics of the patients are presented in Table 2. At baseline, no significant differences were found between the two groups with regard to age, sex, and levels of ALT, ALB, CHE, TB, PTA, routine blood test (white blood cell (WBC), red blood cell, and platelet (PLT)), LSM, Child–Pugh, and AFP.

3.2. Isolation and Characterization of BMCs. The characteristics of the BMCs isolated from the patients are shown in

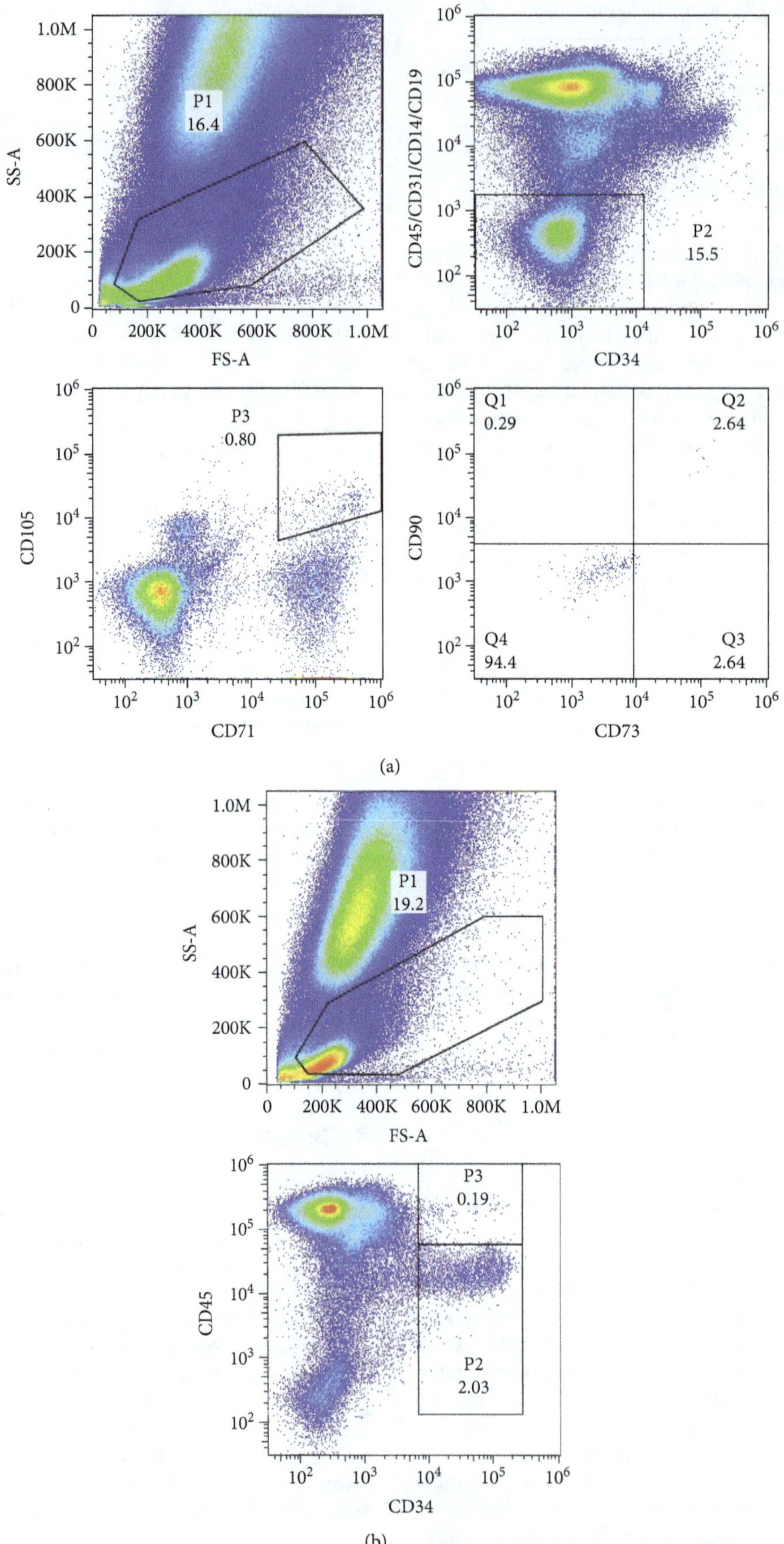

Figure 2: Representative cell surface antigen expression profile of isolated BMCs analyzed by flow cytometry: (a) MSCs, (b) HSCs.

Table 3: The relative percentage of various BM cell populations.

	Statistics %	Cells (18 mL bone marrow)
Hematopoietic stem cells (HSCs)	0.32 ± 0.20	712362.5 ± 493434.1
Mesenchymal stem cells (MSCs)	0.00051 ± 0.00014	1183.75 ± 493.6

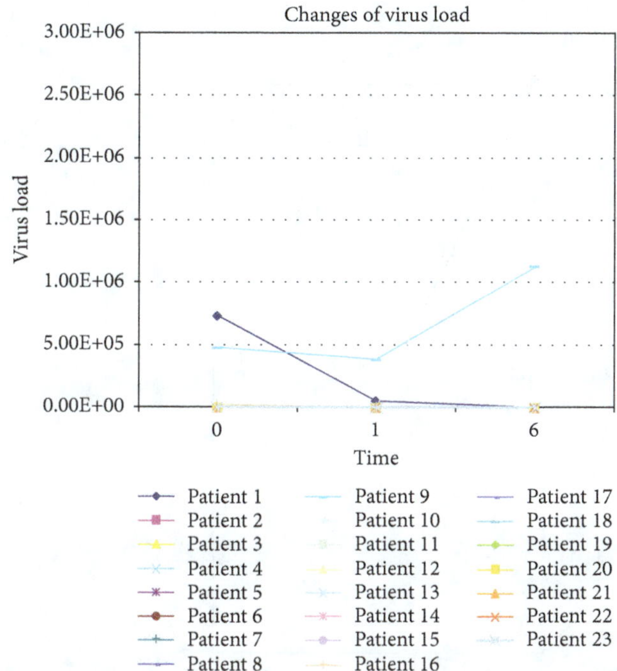

Figure 3: Changes of virus load of patients with decompensated liver cirrhosis caused by chronic hepatitis B and hepatitis C. Patient 9 was with hepatitis C. Patient 1 belonged to the control group, and patient 15 belonged to the AMBT group; the lamivudine had been replaced by entecavir before surgery. Patient 10 belonged to the AMBT group; the lamivudine had been replaced by entecavir in 6 months after surgery. The virus load of the rest of the patients is stable.

Figure 2. Further, 18 mL of autologous bone marrow in which the mean number of infused MSCs was 1183.75 ± 493.6 and the mean number of infused HSCs was 712362.5 ± 493434.14 was transfused in the patients of the ABMT group. The relative percentage of various BM cell populations is shown in Table 3. The isolated BMCs from all patients had a cell viability > 95%. All samples were negative for endotoxin. Isolated MSCs were $CD45^-$, $CD31^-$, $CD14^-$, $CD19^-$, $CD34^-$, $CD105^+$, $CD71^+$, $CD73^+$, and $CD90^+$. Isolated HSCs were $CD45^-$ and $CD34^+$.

3.3. Liver Biochemical Parameters. All patients were followed up for 6 months. All patients with hepatitis B have been treated with antiviral therapy (lamivudine, telbivudine, adefovir dipivoxil, and entecavir) except for one patient who was anti-HBs antibody positive. The patients with hepatitis C have not been treated with antiviral drugs because the antiviral drugs have not been approved by China Food and Drug Administration. In addition to the increase of the viral load in individual patients because of the cause of drug resistance, most of the patients' viral loads are stable. After the increase of the viral load in 3 patients treated by lamivudine, the lamivudine had been replaced by entecavir. Then, the viral load was negative. The changes of the viral load are shown in Figure 3.

The changes in functional liver indices, including ALB, ALT, TB, PTA, and CHE, are shown in Figure 4. In the ABMT group, the LSM decreased effectively and the total effective rate was 80%. In the control group, the total effective rate was 20%. A statistically significant difference was found in the total effective rate between the two groups ($P < 0.05$). The ALT levels in the ABMT group significantly decreased at 6 months, while it increased in the control group. A statistically significant difference was found between the two groups at 6 months (39 ± 27.03 U/L vs. 28 ± 9.22 U/L, $P < 0.05$). The TB levels in the two groups significantly decreased in 6 months but with no statistically significant difference between the two groups (20.5 ± 7.02 vs. 20.24 ± 6.36 mmol/L, $P > 0.05$). The PTA levels greatly increased in both groups after 6 months of treatment relative to baseline. No statistically significant difference was found between the two groups 6 months after treatment (90.14 ± 9.34% vs. 81.15 ± 11.68%, $P > 0.05$). The ALB levels greatly increased in the ABMT group after 6 months of treatment relative to baseline. The mean ALB concentration for patients in the ABMT group was 38.61 ± 4.05 g/L 6 months after treatment versus 33.54 ± 3.37 g/L before treatment ($P < 0.05$). No significant increase was found in the ALB levels in the control group compared with the preoperative levels. A statistically significant difference was found between the two groups ($P < 0.05$) at 6 months. The CHE levels greatly increased in both groups 6 months after treatment relative to baseline and significantly increased in the ABMT group compared with the control group; the difference between the two groups was statistically significant ($P < 0.05$).

3.4. Adverse Effects and Complications. After ABMT into the portal vein using Celsite Implantofix, no bleeding or thrombotic episodes were observed. The AFP levels of the control group had no significant change. However, the AFP levels in the ABMT group decreased. No other adverse effects (such as infection or hypersensitivity) were observed in any of the patients during or after the bone marrow transfusion.

4. Discussion

Patients receiving ABMT demonstrated considerable improvement in their laboratory data, with no procedure-related complications [16]. It is important to treat the causative liver disease, such as viral hepatitis, to maintain the effect

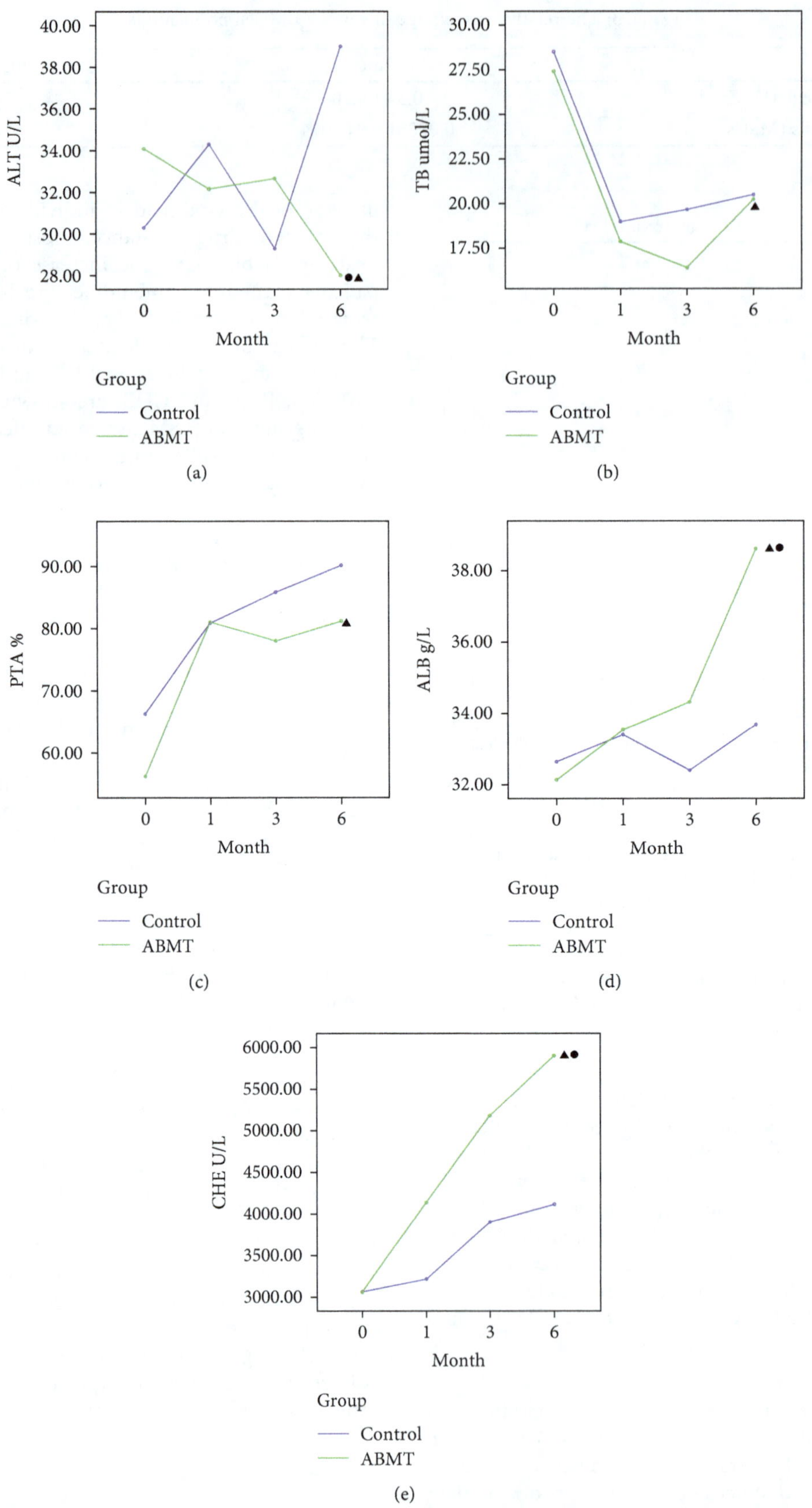

FIGURE 4: Changes in biochemical parameters after splenectomy or combined splenectomy and ABMT therapy in patients with decompensated liver cirrhosis: (a) ALT, (b) TB, (c) PTA, (d) ALB, and (e) CHE. ▲$P < 0.05$ indicates a significant difference versus the baseline value. ●$P < 0.05$ indicates a significant difference between ABMT and control groups.

of such therapies and enhance the resistance of infused cells to viral infection [17] or repeat the injection of stem cells at intervals to achieve sustained response [18].

The ability to isolate the subset of marrow stromal cells with the most extensive replication and differentiation potential would naturally be of utmost importance for both theoretical and applicative reasons. However, identifying the "phenotypic fingerprint" of a stromal stem cell may well be like shooting at a moving target, in that they seem to be constantly changing in response to their microenvironment, both *in vitro* and *in vivo* [19]. Noncultured autologous whole bone marrow was used in this study for the clinical application of liver regeneration therapy. First, no teratoma formation was observed, as seen with embryonic stem cells. Second, these cells were easier to collect compared with the hepatic stem cells in the liver. Moreover, the use of autologous BMC eliminated the problem of potential immunological rejection. With regard to the whole bone marrow, marrow pericytes might be heterogeneous. Some might be recruited during blood vessel formation from resident, preexisting osteogenic cells; others might originate from endothelial cells, and still others might grow from preexisting pericytes during vascular growth. Some would be osteogenic in nature, while others would not [19]. Liver regeneration requires not only hepatic stem cells but also other stromal cells. Therefore, it was proposed that the transplant should be "seeds with the soil," that is, the whole bone marrow transplantation.

Terai et al. have recently shown [8] significant increases in the ALB and total protein levels, an improvement in the Child–Pugh score in all nine patients, and reductions in ascites in six patients with liver cirrhosis after autologous BMC infusion therapy. Gordon et al. [5] also showed that the injection of $CD34^+$ cells into either the portal vein or the hepatic artery improved liver function in patients with liver insufficiency. Noncultured autologous whole bone marrow transfusion (18 mL) was evaluated three times in the present study for treating decompensated liver cirrhosis. 10 patients were treated with nothing and 15 with the bone marrow transfusion. Significant improvements in serum levels of ALT, TB, ALB, PTA, and CHE were observed in patients treated with ABMT. A statistically significant difference was found in ALT, ALB, and CHE between the control and ABMT groups throughout the follow-up period.

Previous studies have shown that splenectomy could improve the liver function. WBC and PLT significantly increased after splenectomy. Serum levels of TB and prothrombin time significantly improved after splenectomy [20]. Significant improvements in the serum levels of ALB, PTA, and CHE were observed in the control group in the present study.

Sandrin et al. [21] had shown that liver stiffness measurements (LSMs) were reproducible, operator-independent and well correlated to fibrosis grade (METAVIR). It is believed that the activation of hepatic stellate cells or myofibroblasts and portal myofibroblasts in the liver leads to the formation and deposition of extracellular matrix, which is the main mechanism of hepatic fibrosis. Oyagi et al. [22] had found that the transplantation of the bone marrow-derived mesenchymal cells (BMMCs) into liver-injured rats significantly suppressed liver fibrosis. In our study, in the ABMT group, the LSM decreased effectively (12 in 15) and the total effective rate was 80%. In the control group, 2 patients were detected with a decrease in LSM in 10 patients. The total effective rate was 20%.

Several possible routes exist for BMC administration, including through the peripheral vein, hepatic artery, or portal vein [8, 23–25]. Celsite Implantofix was implanted in this study in the portal vein through the right gastroomental vein. This method was as simple as the peripheral intravenous infusion, causing almost no risk of operation (such as bleeding and infection); the cost was also relatively low compared with traditional treatment. More importantly, it was much easier to handle than the direct BMC liver transplantation. Further, it was extremely convenient to carry out repeatedly, thereby solving the problem of single BMC transfusion insufficiency.

None of the patients had adverse reactions to ABMT in the present study. The AFP level of two patients in the ABMT group was 435.7 and 149 ng/mL, respectively. No liver cancer was found. The AFP levels decreased after treatment. Moreover, hematopoietic or solid tumors did not develop in the follow-up period of 6 months in the ABMT group.

A small amount of autologous bone marrow was transfused in this study because of the uncertainty in the safety of ABMT and the patient's tolerance of the volume of the extracted bone marrow. However, autologous bone marrow was transfused three times at intervals to achieve a sustained response. The relationship between the volume of the bone marrow transfused and the curative effect will be explored in future studies.

5. Conclusions

In conclusion, repeated autologous whole bone marrow transfusion therapy is promising because it improved the liver function of patients with liver cirrhosis. A larger-scale, randomized, double-blinded study is necessary to demonstrate the full therapeutic value of this protocol. Moreover, the present study was limited by the different etiologies of cirrhosis and baseline patient heterogeneity. Further studies with higher numbers of patients are warranted to better clarify the effect of autologous whole bone marrow transfusion on cirrhosis.

References

[1] S. Friedman and T. Schiano, "Cirrhosis and its sequelae," in *Cecil Textbook of Medicine*, pp. 936-944, Saunders, Philadelphia, PA, USA, 22nd edition, 2004.

[2] M. A. Fink, S. R. Berry, P. J. Gow et al., "Risk factors for liver transplantation waiting list mortality," *Journal of Gastroenterology and Hepatology*, vol. 22, no. 1, pp. 119–124, 2007.

[3] J. D. Sipe, "Tissue engineering and reparative medicine," *Annals of the New York Academy of Sciences*, vol. 961, no. 1, pp. 1–9, 2002.

[4] S. Gaia, A. Smedile, P. Omedè et al., "Feasibility and safety of G-CSF administration to induce bone marrow-derived cells mobilization in patients with end stage liver disease," *Journal of Hepatology*, vol. 45, no. 1, pp. 13–19, 2006.

[5] M. Y. Gordon, N. Levičar, M. Pai et al., "Characterization and clinical application of human CD34$^+$ stem/progenitor cell populations mobilized into the blood by granulocyte colony-stimulating factor," *Stem Cells*, vol. 24, no. 7, pp. 1822–1830, 2006.

[6] A. C. Lyra, M. B. Soares, L. F. da Silva et al., "Feasibility and safety of autologous bone marrow mononuclear cell transplantation in patients with advanced chronic liver disease," *World Journal of Gastroenterology*, vol. 13, no. 7, pp. 1067–1073, 2007.

[7] C. Margini, R. Vukotic, L. Brodosi, M. Bernardi, and P. Andreone, "Bone marrow derived stem cells for the treatment of end-stage liver disease," *World Journal of Gastroenterology*, vol. 20, no. 27, pp. 9098-9105, 2014.

[8] S. Terai, T. Ishikawa, K. Omori et al., "Improved liver function in patients with liver cirrhosis after autologous bone marrow cell infusion therapy," *Stem Cells*, vol. 24, no. 10, pp. 2292–2298, 2006.

[9] M. F. Pittenger, A. M. Mackay, S. C. Beck et al., "Multilineage potential of adult human mesenchymal stem cells," *Science*, vol. 284, no. 5411, pp. 143–147, 1999.

[10] K. A. Cho, G. W. Lim, S. Y. Joo et al., "Transplantation of bone marrow cells reduces CCl4-induced liver fibrosis in mice," *Liver International*, vol. 31, no. 7, pp. 932–939, 2011.

[11] G. Vassilopoulos, P. R. Wang, and D. W. Russell, "Transplanted bone marrow regenerates liver by cell fusion," *Nature*, vol. 422, no. 6934, pp. 901–904, 2003.

[12] P. Zhou, L. Wirthlin, J. McGee, G. Annett, and J. Nolta, "Contribution of human hematopoietic stem cells to liver repair," *Seminars in Immunopathology*, vol. 31, no. 3, pp. 411–419, 2009.

[13] R. P. H. Meier, Y. D. Müller, P. Morel, C. Gonelle-Gispert, and L. H. Bühler, "Transplantation of mesenchymal stem cells for the treatment of liver diseases, is there enough evidence?," *Stem Cell Research*, vol. 11, no. 3, pp. 1348–1364, 2013.

[14] J. Kim, J. W. Kang, J. H. Park et al., "Biological characterization of long-term cultured human mesenchymal stem cells," *Archives of Pharmacal Research*, vol. 32, no. 1, pp. 117-126, 2009.

[15] J. M. Karp and G. S. Leng Teo, "Mesenchymal stem cell homing: the devil is in the details," *Cell Stem Cell*, vol. 4, no. 3, pp. 206-216, 2009.

[16] H. Salama, A. R. N. Zekri, R. Ahmed et al., "Assessment of health-related quality of life in patients receiving stem cell therapy for end-stage liver disease: an Egyptian study," *Stem Cell Research & Therapy*, vol. 3, no. 6, p. 49, 2012.

[17] N. Levičar, M. Pai, N. A. Habib et al., "Long-term clinical results of autologous infusion of mobilized adult bone marrow derived CD34$^+$ cells in patients with chronic liver disease," *Cell Proliferation*, vol. 41, Supplement 1, pp. 115–125, 2008.

[18] A. C. Piscaglia, M. Campanale, A. Gasbarrini, and G. Gasbarrini, "Stem cell-based therapies for liver diseases: state of the art and new perspectives," *Stem Cells International*, vol. 2010, Article ID 259461, 10 pages, 2010.

[19] P. Bianco, M. Riminucci, S. Gronthos, and P. G. Robey, "Bone marrow stromal stem cells: nature, biology, and potential applications," *Stem Cells*, vol. 19, no. 3, pp. 180–192, 2001.

[20] S. H. Kim, D. Y. Kim, J. H. Lim et al., "Role of splenectomy in patients with hepatocellular carcinoma and hypersplenism," *ANZ Journal of Surgery*, vol. 83, no. 11, pp. 865–870, 2013.

[21] L. Sandrin, B. Fourquet, J. M. Hasquenoph et al., "Transient elastography: a new noninvasive method for assessment of hepatic fibrosis," *Ultrasound in Medicine & Biology*, vol. 29, no. 12, pp. 1705–1713, 2003.

[22] S. Oyagi, M. Hirose, M. Kojima et al., "Therapeutic effect of transplanting HGF-treated bone marrow mesenchymal cells into CCl4-injured rats," *Journal of Hepatology*, vol. 44, no. 4, pp. 742–748, 2006.

[23] A. C. Lyra, M. B. P. Soares, L. F. M. da Silva et al., "Infusion of autologous bone marrow mononuclear cells through hepatic artery results in a short-term improvement of liver function in patients with chronic liver disease: a pilot randomized controlled study," *European Journal of Gastroenterology & Hepatology*, vol. 22, no. 1, pp. 33–42, 2010.

[24] T. Saito, K. Okumoto, H. Haga et al., "Potential therapeutic application of intravenous autologous bone marrow infusion in patients with alcoholic liver cirrhosis," *Stem Cells and Development*, vol. 20, no. 9, pp. 1503–1510, 2011.

[25] J. S. am Esch II, W. T. Knoefel, M. Klein et al., "Portal application of autologous CD133$^+$ bone marrow cells to the liver: a novel concept to support hepatic regeneration," *Stem Cells*, vol. 23, no. 4, pp. 463–470, 2005.

8

Sustained Clinical Efficacy and Mucosal Healing of Thiopurine Maintenance Treatment in Ulcerative Colitis

Daniela Pugliese,[1] **Annalisa Aratari**,[2] **Stefano Festa**,[2] **Pietro Manuel Ferraro**,[3] **Rita Monterubbianesi**,[4] **Luisa Guidi**,[1] **Maria Lia Scribano**,[4] **Claudio Papi**,[2] **and Alessandro Armuzzi**[1]

[1]*IBD Unit, Presidio Columbus Fondazione Policlinico Universitario A. Gemelli IRCCS Università Cattolica, Rome 00168, Italy*
[2]*IBD Unit, S. Filippo Neri Hospital, Rome 00135, Italy*
[3]*Nephrology, Presidio Columbus Fondazione Policlinico Universitario A. Gemelli IRCCS Università Cattolica, Rome 00168, Italy*
[4]*IBD Unit, San Camillo Forlanini Hospital, Rome 00152, Italy*

Correspondence should be addressed to Daniela Pugliese; danipug@libero.it

Academic Editor: Vicent Hernández

Background and Aims. Thiopurines are commonly used for treating ulcerative colitis (UC), despite the fact that controlled evidence supporting their efficacy is limited. The aim of this study was to evaluate the long-term outcome of thiopurines as maintenance therapy in a large cohort of UC patients. *Methods.* All UC patients receiving thiopurine monotherapy at three tertiary IBD centers from 1995 to 2015 were identified. The primary endpoint was steroid-free clinical remission. Secondary endpoints were mucosal healing (MH), defined as Mayo endoscopic subscore 0, long-term safety, and predictors of sustained clinical remission. *Results.* We identified 192 patients, contributing a total of 747 person-years of follow-up (median follow-up 36 months, range 1–210 months). Steroid dependency was the most common indication for thiopurine treatment (58%). Steroid-free remission occurred in 45.3% of patients; 36.3% stopped thiopurines because of treatment failure and 18.2% for adverse events or intolerance. The cumulative probability of maintaining steroid-free remission while on thiopurine treatment was 87%, 76%, 67.6%, and 53.4% at 12, 24, 36, and 60 months, respectively. MH occurred in 57.9% of patients after a median of 18 months (range 5–96). No independent predictors of sustained clinical remission could be identified. *Conclusions.* Thiopurines represent an effective and safe long-term maintenance therapy for UC patients.

1. Introduction

Ulcerative colitis (UC) is an inflammatory bowel disease (IBD) needing chronic maintenance therapies in order to prevent symptom relapses and disease progression [1]. Aminosalicylates are the first-line medical option for remission maintenance in the long term for mild to moderate disease [2, 3]. Nevertheless, after a moderate-to-severe disease flare requiring systemic corticosteroids, up to 20% of patients need to escalate therapies because of the development of steroid-dependency and approximately 15% because of steroid-refractoriness [4]. Thiopurines, azathioprine (AZA), and 6-mercaptopurine (6MP) have been considered the reference maintenance treatment for patients with steroid-dependent and steroid-refractory moderate-to-severe UC for many years and are recommended as the first line immunosuppressive therapy by major guidelines [1, 5].

Controlled data supporting the efficacy of thiopurines in UC are limited and are not as robust as in Crohn's disease (CD) [6, 7]. Few old randomized controlled trials (RCTs) addressing AZA and 6MP for the treatment of UC have relevant methodological limitations such as small sample size, inadequate thiopurine dose, heterogeneity of patient populations, limited follow-up, and not well-defined endpoints [8–14]. Despite these limitations, a systematic review and meta-analysis addressing the use of thiopurines in UC concluded that AZA and 6MP are more effective than placebo for the prevention of relapse in UC, with a number needed to treat (NNT) of 5 and an absolute risk reduction (ARR) of 23% compared to placebo [15]. Moreover, the efficacy of thiopurines in UC is supported by several uncontrolled observational studies: a mean efficacy of 65% and 75% for remission induction and maintenance, respectively, has been reported [15]. However, study designs, patients' characteristics, length of follow-up, and endpoints considered are very heterogeneous across studies, making robust conclusions very challenging. Furthermore, mucosal healing (MH) in UC has been poorly investigated with thiopurines, despite the fact that MH has recently emerged as a therapeutic goal in the management of IBDs, both for clinical trials and clinical practice [16].

The aim of this study is to evaluate the long-term effectiveness of thiopurines for maintaining clinical and endoscopic remissions in a large cohort of UC patients in a real-life setting and to explore possible predictors of sustained effectiveness.

2. Patients and Methods

This is an open-label retrospective study of consecutive UC patients treated with thiopurines at three IBD referral centers in Rome, Italy (Presidio Columbus, Fondazione Policlinico Universitario A. Gemelli IRCCS Università Cattolica del Sacro Cuore; S. Filippo Neri Hospital; and San Camillo Forlanini Hospital). Eligible patients included men and women older than 18 years with an established diagnosis of UC, who received maintenance treatment with thiopurine monotherapy from 1995 to 2015. Patients receiving thiopurine monotherapy after a course of anti–tumour necrosis factor (TNF) alpha treatment or after rescue therapy with cyclosporine for severe steroid refractory UC were excluded.

A shared common database was used to collect demographic and clinical data. The following variables were recorded: age at diagnosis, gender, disease duration, disease extent, endoscopic activity, smoking habit, indication for thiopurine treatment, type of thiopurines used (AZA or 6MP), and concomitant medications during induction and maintenance phases. The indications for thiopurine therapy were classified as the following: (1) steroid dependence, (2) maintenance therapy after a severe acute attack responsive to intravenous (iv) steroids, and (3) maintenance therapy for patients with mild to moderate disease with frequent relapses despite optimized treatment with aminosalicylates. Steroid dependency was defined according to the Italian Group for the Study of IBD (IG-IBD) guidelines [5] or as need of at least two steroid courses in the previous year. Patients with two or more clinical relapses in the last year despite appropriate oral and rectal aminosalicylates were considered having frequent relapses. Disease extent was defined according to the Montreal classification [17]; endoscopic activity was evaluated according to the Mayo endoscopic subscore [18]. Baseline endoscopy had to be performed within 3 months before starting thiopurines; follow-up endoscopies were scheduled at variable time points according to clinical judgment. MH was defined as Mayo endoscopic subscore of 0 and assessed for patient achieving sustained steroid-free clinical remission [18]. At the last follow-up visit, data regarding disease activity and whether patients were still on thiopurine maintenance were recorded. The reasons for discontinuation of thiopurines were classified as (1) sustained steroid-free clinical remission; (2) thiopurine failure, defined as clinical relapse requiring therapeutic escalation with corticosteroids and/or biologics or need for colectomy; and (3) intolerance or adverse events (AEs).

The primary endpoint was steroid-free clinical remission, defined as no diarrhea, no haematochezia, and no need of steroids, anti-TNF alpha agents, or surgery during maintenance therapy with thiopurines. Secondary endpoints were the occurrence rate of MH in patients in steroid-free remission and long-term safety. Finally, potential clinical predictors of steroid-free clinical remission and mucosal healing were analysed.

2.1. Statistical Analysis. Data were described using means with standard deviation (SD) and medians with range for continuous data and percentages for discrete data. Cumulative probabilities of continuing thiopurine treatment while in remission and cumulative probability of colectomy in a patient who failed thiopurines were estimated by the Kaplan-Meier method. Associations between clinical variables and treatment efficacy (both for steroid-free remission and mucosal healing) were analysed with logistic regression analysis and expressed as odds ratio (OR) and 95% confidence intervals (95% CI). The following covariates were considered: gender, age, disease duration, disease extension, smoking habit, indication for thiopurine therapy, and concomitant aminosalicylate treatment. A two-tailed p value < 0.05 was regarded as statistically significant. StatsDirect statistical tools (copyright 1990–2001) were used for all calculations.

3. Results

3.1. Baseline Patients' Characteristics. One hundred and ninety-two UC patients (88 male and 104 female) receiving thiopurines as maintenance treatment were enrolled. The demographic and clinical characteristics of patients are summarised in Table 1. Median age at diagnosis was 36 years (range 16–69 years), and the median disease duration was 3.3 years (range 0–31 years). One hundred and seventeen patients (60%) had extensive colitis, and 75 patients (40%) had left-sided disease. Most patients were nonsmokers or former smokers (88%). Steroid dependency was the most common indication for thiopurine treatment (111 of 192 patients, 58%); 36 of 192 patients (19%) received thiopurines following a severe acute attack responsive to intravenous steroids, and 45 of 192 patients (23%) received thiopurines because of frequent clinical relapses despite optimized treatment with aminosalicylates.

At baseline, 148 of 192 patients (77%) were concomitantly treated with corticosteroids. More than 90% of patients received concomitant aminosalicylate maintenance.

AZA was the preferred thiopurine compared to 6MP (90% vs. 10%). All patients received thiopurines at the standard dose of 2.0–2.5 mg/kg for AZA and of 1.0–1.5 mg/kg

Table 1: Demographic and clinical characteristics of patients.

	Patient $n = 192$
Gender n (%)	
Female	104 (54.1)
Male	88 (45.9)
Age, years	
Median (range)	36 (16–69)
Disease duration, years	
Median (range)	3.3 (0–31)
Disease extension n (%)	
Extensive colitis	117 (60)
Left-sided colitis	75 (40)
Mayo endoscopic subscore ∗n (%)	
Mayo 1	16 (9)
Mayo 2	91 (52)
Mayo 3	68 (39)
Smoking habit n (%)	
Yes	23 (12)
No/former smoker	169 (88)
Indication for starting thiopurines n (%)	
Steroid dependency	111 (58)
Maintenance after a severe attack	36 (19)
Frequent relapses	45 (23)
Cotreatment with mesalazine n (%)	175 (91.1)
Duration of thiopurine therapy, months	
Median (range)	36 (1–210)

for 6MP. For both drugs, 50 mg/day was the initial dose progressively increased to the standard dose; dose adjustment was performed during treatment according to clinical judgment. Thiopurine metabolite monitoring, as well as thiopurine methyltransferase (TPMT) activity, was not performed because it is not routinely available in clinical practice in Italy.

Endoscopic data at baseline were available for 175 of 192 patients (91.1%): 91 patients (52%) had moderate endoscopic activity classified as Mayo endoscopic subscore = 2, and 68 patients (39%) had severe endoscopic activity classified as Mayo endoscopic subscore = 3.

3.2. Outcomes. The median follow-up while on thiopurine maintenance was 36 months (range 1–210 months). Participants contributed a total of 747 person-years of follow-up. Overall, 87 of 192 patients (45.3%) achieved steroid-free clinical remission within a median follow-up of 39 months (range 1–210 months). Conversely, 105 of 192 patients (54.6%) withdrew from thiopurines because of treatment failure ($n = 70$, 36.3%) or occurrence of AEs or intolerance ($n = 35$, 18.2%) (Figure 1).

Treatment failure occurred after a median follow-up of 36 months (range 3–173 months), while most patients who discontinued thiopurines for intolerance withdrew the drug within the first year (59%).

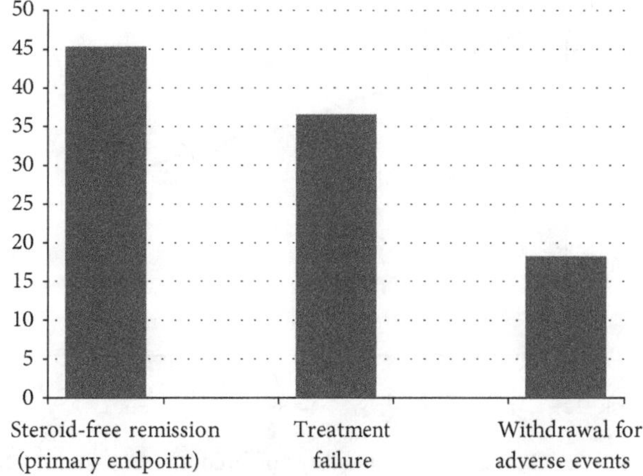

Figure 1: Percentage of patients achieving steroid-free clinical remission and treatment discontinuation for failure and adverse events.

The cumulative probability of maintaining steroid-free remission while on thiopurine treatment was 87%, 76%, 67.6%, and 53.4% at 12, 24, 36, and 60 months, respectively (Figure 2). Among the 87 patients who achieved steroid-free remission, 65 (73.8%) were still on thiopurine therapy at the end of the follow-up, while 22 (25%) were discontinued because of sustained remission after a median length of thiopurine treatment of 39 months (range 14–128 months). Among the 70 patients who were considered treatment failures, 57 (81.4%) received at least one course of systemic corticosteroids, 59 patients (84.2%) escalated to anti-TNF alpha agents, and 15 (21.4%) ultimately required colectomy. The cumulative probability of a course free of colectomy within 5 years after thiopurine failure was 90%, 84.4%, 82.0%, and 67.6% at 12, 24, 36, and 60 months, respectively (Figure 3).

As far as MH is concerned, data are available for a subgroup of 69 of 87 responders, whose baseline and follow-up endoscopy data were available. Follow-up endoscopies were performed after a median time of 18 months (range 5–96 months) after starting thiopurines, according to clinical judgment. Endoscopic activity, expressed as Mayo endoscopic subscore, at baseline and during follow-up is shown in Figure 4. Overall, 40 of 69 patients (57.9%) achieved complete MH while on thiopurine maintenance (Mayo endoscopic subscore = 0).

A logistic regression analysis was performed to explore possible clinical predictors of treatment success. None of the clinical variables included in the model was associated with the probability of steroid-free remission (Table 2) or mucosal healing (data not shown).

3.3. Safety. A total of 45 patients experienced at least one AE related to thiopurine exposure. Overall, 35 patients discontinued thiopurines because of AEs or intolerance. The description and frequency of all AE events in our cohort are reported in Table 3. Gastrointestinal intolerance (including nausea and vomiting) occurred in 13 patients (29%). In 3 patients, switch to 6MP was attempted without success. Thirteen patients (29%) experienced leukopenia (a white blood cell count < 3000/mm), and among them, 10 needed drug

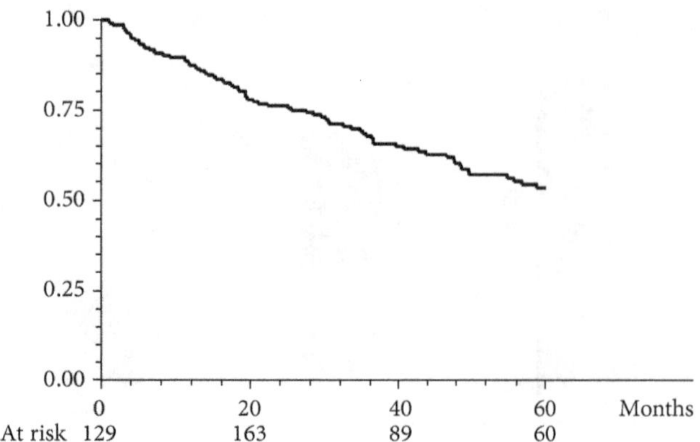

FIGURE 2: Cumulative probability of maintaining steroid-free remission while on thiopurine maintenance in the entire population.

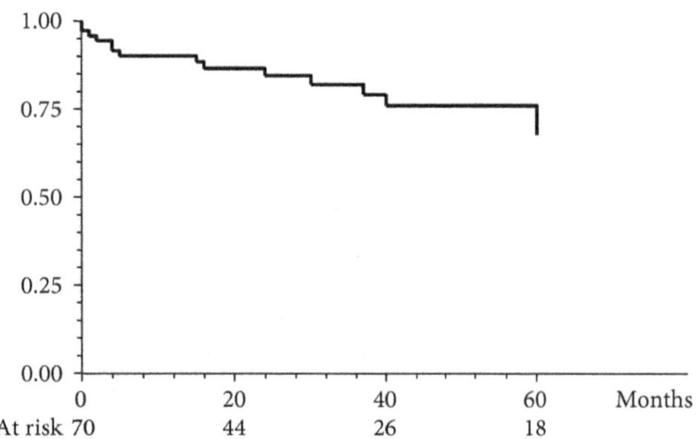

FIGURE 3: Cumulative probability of a course free of colectomy after thiopurine discontinuation for treatment failure.

discontinuation. Elevation of serum transaminases (more than 2–3 times the upper limit of normal) was recorded in 6 patients (13%), and 5 patients were consequently discontinued. No one developed chronic liver disease. In 5 patients (11%), elevation of serum pancreatic enzymes occurred, but only two patients (4%) developed acute pancreatitis requiring hospital admission. Infections were recorded in 14 patients (31%), but only three of them (2 cases of *Listeria monocytogenes* infection and 1 case of Cytomegalovirus colitis) were considered severe and required hospitalization. Two patients (4%) developed malignancies (1 anal cancer and 1 gastric cancer).

4. Discussion

Although thiopurines are widely used as a maintenance treatment in UC and are considered at least as effective as in CD patients [19], controversy still exists regarding their efficacy in maintaining remission in the long term [15]. Evidence-based data supporting the efficacy of AZA and 6MP in UC are limited, and the main evidence comes from observational studies, mainly retrospective. Observational studies report substantial variability in effectiveness of thiopurines in UC, ranging from 40% to 70% [20–26]. However, significant heterogeneity across studies, methodological limitations, small sample size, variable length of follow-up, and different endpoint definitions highlight the uncertainty of the available data.

Our study focuses on the long-term outcome of thiopurine treatment in UC patients in a real-life setting. Although the main limitation of our study is its retrospective design, the large number of patients included and the consistent length of follow-up (760 person-years) are the main strengths. Moreover, we report data addressing MH in a large subgroup of patients, and this represents a peculiarity of our study because thiopurine-induced MH has not been extensively studied and it is usually not assessed in most observational studies [24–26]. Another strength of our study is the strict definition of steroid-free clinical remission, our primary endpoint, that is, the absence of diarrhea and blood in stools, without need of any escalation of therapy, including steroids, anti-TNF alpha agents, or surgery. As previously reported, stool frequency and rectal bleeding alone provide reasonable estimates of disease activity as well as the Mayo scoring system, commonly used in RCTs [27].

MH has been strictly defined as a Mayo endoscopic subscore = 0. Although in several RCTs and cohort experiences MH is usually defined as a Mayo endoscopic subscore ≤ 1 [28], recent observations suggest that there is an improved long-term outcome in patients achieving complete MH (Mayo subscore = 0) compared to patients achieving partial MH (Mayo subscore = 1) [29]. Finally, a survival regression model has been performed to explore possible predictors of sustained efficacy of thiopurines.

Overall results show that approximately 45% of UC patients receiving thiopurines achieve steroid-free remission, 37% fail to respond to thiopurines and need escalation therapy, and less than 20% discontinue the drug because of AEs or intolerance.

Our results suggest a favourable profile of thiopurines in UC in terms of long-term efficacy and safety and are comparable to data recently reported by Sood et al. In their cohort of 255 UC patients, after a median follow-up of 30 months, 60.4% achieved remission, approximately 20% required escalation of therapy, and 30% experienced AEs resulting in thiopurine discontinuation [26]. Other smaller observational studies report comparable results [24, 25]. The probability of achieving steroid-free clinical remission is unpredictable; logistic regression analysis failed to identify any clinical predictor of treatment success confirming previous observations [26]. However, it is interesting to note that early introduction of thiopurines, within the first year after diagnosis, was associated with a reduced probability of achieving steroid-free remission although the data is not statistically significant. We can speculate that patients who require early introduction of thiopurines have a more severe disease onset and a more aggressive early clinical course leading to a worse outcome.

Data concerning endoscopic remission are not available in recently published large series [26]. We have studied the occurrence rate of MH in a subgroup of patients who achieved steroid-free remission and who underwent colonoscopy at

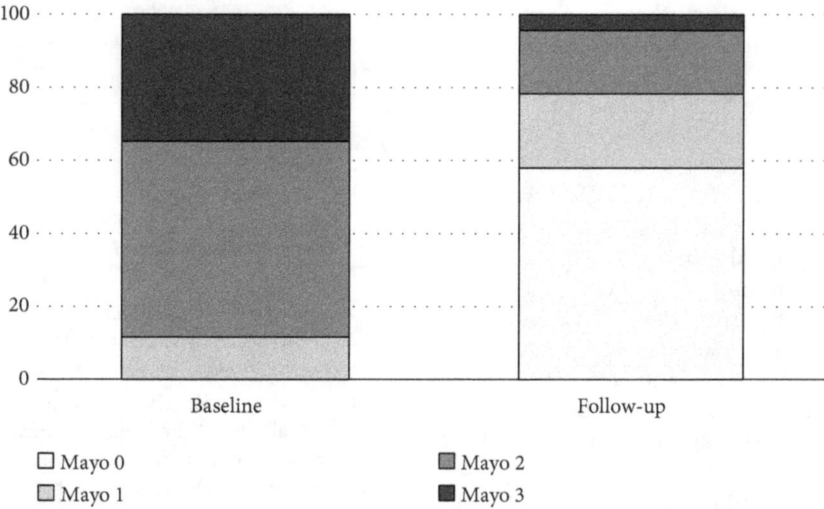

FIGURE 4: Endoscopic activity according to the Mayo endoscopic subscore at baseline and during follow-up in the subgroup of 69 of 87 responders who underwent endoscopy both before starting thiopurines and during follow-up. Mucosal healing (Mayo endoscopic subscore = 0) was achieved in 58% of patients.

TABLE 2: Logistic regression analysis of predictors of steroid-free clinical remission.

Covariates	OR	95% CI	*p* value
Gender (female vs. male)	1.12	0.63–1.98	ns
Age (>40 years vs. <40 years)	0.77	0.42–1.40	ns
Extension (distal colitis vs. extensive colitis)	0.85	0.48–1.49	ns
Smoking habit (yes vs. no/ex)	1.17	0.54–2.53	ns
Starting thiopurine (within 1 year vs. >1 year after diagnosis)	0.48	0.23–1.01	ns
Indication for thiopurine Tx (no steroid dependency vs. steroid dependency)	1.51	0.83–2.73	ns
Concomitant aminosalycilates (no vs. yes)	1.87	0.80–4.39	ns

TABLE 3: Adverse events related to thiopurine exposure.

Type of event	$n = 45$ (%)
Nausea and vomiting	13 (29)
Leukopenia	13 (29)
Elevation of transaminases	6 (13)
Elevation of pancreatic enzymes	3 (6)
Acute pancreatitis	2 (4)
Myalgia	1 (2)
Alopecia	1 (2)
Infections	14 (31)
Serious infections	3 (6)
Malignancy	2 (4)

baseline and after a median of 12 months (range 1–132) after starting thiopurines. Complete endoscopic remission, defined as a Mayo endoscopic subscore = 0, was observed in more than 50% of patients. In recent years, targeting MH is an emerging therapeutic endpoint in the management of UC [16, 30]. MH has been associated to a more favourable outcome in terms of reduction of clinical relapse, steroid needs, hospitalizations, colorectal cancer, and surgery [31]. Although it is commonly accepted that thiopurines are able to induce MH, this effect is slow, the occurrence rate of MH in thiopurine-treated UC has not been systematically investigated, and few data are available. In a recent multicenter retrospective French study on 80 UC patients receiving thiopurine monotherapy, MH (defined as a Mayo endoscopic subscore ≤ 1 and Ulcerative Colitis Endoscopic Index of Severity (UCEIS) < 2) was observed in 43.7% after a mean follow-up of 38 ± 31 months after thiopurine introduction [32]. These findings are similar to our observations.

AEs requiring withdrawal from therapy occurred in 18.2% of patients, a figure similar to that reported in other observational studies [19–24]. However, in other cohort studies, some of which include both CD and UC patients, the occurrence rate of AEs leading to thiopurine discontinuation may be as high as 25–40% [23, 26, 33–35]. In our study, the most common causes of AZA cessation were gastrointestinal symptoms, despite the fact that a slow dose escalation approach was adopted in most patients. A switch to 6MP was attempted in a minority of patients. Myelotoxicity and hepatotoxicity requiring drug discontinuation occurred in about 5% and 3% of patients, respectively. We have no data on TPMT activity and serum thiopurine metabolite concentrations: monitoring metabolites is not a routine practice in Italy, and this approach is not available in most of the hospitals.

In conclusion, in our real-life experience on a large cohort of UC patients, thiopurines are effective for maintaining long-term steroid-free clinical remission and for inducing MH. No predictors of long-term benefit could be identified. Less than 20% of patients discontinue the drug because of AEs or intolerance supporting a favourable benefit/risk profile of thiopurines in UC.

Authors' Contributions

DP, LG, AA (Aratari), RM, MLS, and SF identified eligible patients and collected data; CP and AA (Armuzzi) designed the study design and revised the final manuscript; PMF performed statistical analysis; DP and SF wrote the manuscript.

References

[1] M. Harbord, R. Eliakim, D. Bettenworth et al., "Third European evidence-based consensus on diagnosis and management of ulcerative colitis. Part 2: current management," *Journal of Crohn's and Colitis*, vol. 11, no. 7, pp. 769–784, 2017.

[2] A. C. Ford, K. J. Khan, J. P. Achkar, and P. Moayyedi, "Efficacy of oral vs. topical, or combined oral and topical 5-aminosalicylates, in ulcerative colitis: systematic review and meta-analysis," *American Journal of Gastroenterology*, vol. 107, no. 2, pp. 167–176, 2012.

[3] B. G. Feagan and J. K. Macdonald, "Oral 5-aminosalicylic acid for maintenance of remission in ulcerative colitis," *Cochrane Database of Systematic Review*, vol. 10, article CD000544, 2012Update in Cochrane Database Systematic Review 5:CD000544, 2016.

[4] W. A. Faubion Jr, E. V. Loftus Jr, W. S. Harmsen, A. R. Zinsmeister, and W. J. Sandborn, "The natural history of corticosteroid therapy for inflammatory bowel disease: a population-based study," *Gastroenterology*, vol. 121, no. 2, pp. 255–260, 2001.

[5] P. Gionchetti, F. Rizzello, V. Annese et al., "Use of corticosteroids and immunosuppressive drugs in inflammatory bowel disease: clinical practice guidelines of the Italian Group for the Study of Inflammatory Bowel Disease," *Digestive and Liver Disease*, vol. 49, no. 6, pp. 604–617, 2017.

[6] E. Prefontaine, J. K. Macdonald, and L. R. Sutherland, "Azathioprine or 6-mercaptopurine for induction of remission in Crohn's disease," *Cochrane Database of Systematic Review*, vol. 6, article CD000545, 2010Update in Cochrane Database Systematic Review 4:CD000545, 2013.

[7] N. Chande, P. H. Patton, D. J. Tsoulis, B. S. Thomas, and J. K. MacDonald, "Azathioprine or 6-mercaptopurine for maintenance of remission in Crohn's disease," *Cochrane Database of Systematic Reviews*, vol. 10, article CD000067, 2015.

[8] D. P. Jewell and S. C. Truelove, "Azathioprine in ulcerative colitis: an interim report on a controlled therapeutic trial," *British Medical Journal*, vol. 1, no. 5802, pp. 709–712, 1972.

[9] R. Caprilli, R. Carratù, and M. Babbini, "Double-blind comparison of the effectiveness of azathioprine and sulfasalazine in idiopathic proctocolitis. Preliminary report," *The American Journal of Digestive Diseases*, vol. 20, no. 2, pp. 115–120, 1975.

[10] A. Sood, V. Kaushal, V. Midha, K. L. Bhatia, N. Sood, and V. Malhotra, "The beneficial effect of azathioprine on maintenance of remission in severe ulcerative colitis," *Journal of Gastroenterology*, vol. 37, no. 4, pp. 270–274, 2002.

[11] A. P. Kirk and J. E. Lennard-Jones, "Controlled trial of azathioprine in chronic ulcerative colitis," *British Medical Journal*, vol. 284, no. 6325, pp. 1291-1292, 1982.

[12] A. Sood, V. Midha, N. Sood, and V. Kaushal, "Role of azathioprine in severe ulcerative colitis: one-year, placebo-controlled, randomized trial," *Indian Journal of Gastroenterology*, vol. 19, no. 1, pp. 14–16, 2000.

[13] J. Maté-Jiménez, C. Hermida, J. Cantero-Perona, and R. Moreno-Otero, "6-Mercaptopurine or methotrexate added to prednisone induces and maintains remission in steroid-dependent inflammatory bowel disease," *European Journal of Gastroenterology & Hepatology*, vol. 12, no. 11, pp. 1227–1233, 2000.

[14] S. Ardizzone, G. Maconi, A. Russo, V. Imbesi, E. Colombo, and G. Bianchi Porro, "Randomised controlled trial of azathioprine and 5-aminosalicylic acid for treatment of steroid dependent ulcerative colitis," *Gut*, vol. 55, no. 1, pp. 47–53, 2006.

[15] J. P. Gisbert, P. M. Linares, A. G. McNicholl, J. Maté, and F. Gomollón, "Meta-analysis: the efficacy of azathioprine and mercaptopurine in ulcerative colitis," *Alimentary Pharmacology and Therapeutics*, vol. 30, no. 2, pp. 126–137, 2009.

[16] L. Peyrin-Biroulet, W. Sandborn, B. E. Sands et al., "Selecting Therapeutic Targets in Inflammatory Bowel Disease (STRIDE): determining therapeutic goals for treat-to-target," *American Journal of Gastroenterology*, vol. 110, no. 9, pp. 1324–1338, 2015.

[17] M. S. Silverberg, J. Satsangi, T. Ahmad et al., "Toward an integrated clinical, molecular and serological classification of inflammatory bowel disease: report of a Working Party of the 2005 Montreal World Congress of Gastroenterology," *Canadian Journal of Gastroenterology*, vol. 19, Supplement A, pp. 5A–36A, 2005.

[18] K. W. Schroeder, W. J. Tremaine, and D. M. Ilstrup, "Coated oral 5-aminosalicylic acid therapy for mildly to moderately active ulcerative colitis. A randomized study," *New England Journal of Medicine*, vol. 317, no. 26, pp. 1625–1629, 1987.

[19] J. P. Gisbert, P. Nino, C. Cara, and L. Rodrigo, "Comparative effectiveness of azathioprine in Crohn's disease and ulcerative colitis: prospective, longterm, follow-up study of 394 patients," *Alimentary Pharmacology and Therapeutics*, vol. 28, no. 2, pp. 228–238, 2008.

[20] D. J. Adler and B. I. Korelitz, "The therapeutic efficacy of 6-mercaptopurine in refractory ulcerative colitis," *American Journal of Gastroenterology*, vol. 85, no. 6, pp. 717–722, 1990.

[21] A. J. Lobo, P. N. Foster, D. A. Burke, D. Johnston, and A. T. R. Axon, "The role of azathioprine in the management of ulcerative colitis," *Diseases of the Colon and Rectum*, vol. 33, no. 5, pp. 374–377, 1990.

[22] S. Ardizzone, F. Molteni, V. Imbesi, S. Bollani, and G. Bianchi Porro, "Azathioprine in steroid-resistant and steroid-dependent ulcerative colitis," *Journal of Clinical Gastroenterology*, vol. 25, no. 1, pp. 330–333, 1997.

[23] A. G. Fraser, T. R. Orchard, and D. P. Jewell, "The efficacy of azathioprine for the treatment of inflammatory bowel disease: a 30 year review," *Gut*, vol. 50, no. 4, pp. 485–489, 2002.

[24] A. Lopez-Sanroman, F. Bermejo, E. Carrera, and A. Garcia-Plaza, "Efficacy and safety of thiopurinic immunomodulators (azathioprine and mercaptopurine) in steroid-dependent ulcerative colitis," *Alimentary Pharmacology and Therapeutics*, vol. 20, no. 2, pp. 161–166, 2004.

[25] L. A. Chebli, L. D. de Miranda Chaves, F. F. Pimentel et al., "Azathioprine maintains long-term steroid-free remission through 3 years in patients with steroid-dependent ulcerative colitis," *Inflammatory Bowel Diseases*, vol. 16, no. 4, pp. 613–619, 2010.

[26] R. Sood, S. Ansari, T. Clark, P. J. Hamlin, and A. C. Ford, "Long-term efficacy and safety of azathioprine in ulcerative colitis," *Journal of Crohn's and Colitis*, vol. 9, no. 2, pp. 191–197, 2015.

[27] J. D. Lewis, S. Chuai, L. Nessel, G. R. Lichtenstein, F. N. Aberra, and J. H. Ellenberg, "Use of the noninvasive components of the Mayo score to assess clinical response in ulcerative colitis," *Inflammatory Bowel Diseases*, vol. 14, no. 12, pp. 1660–1666, 2008.

[28] G. D'Haens, W. J. Sandborn, B. G. Feagan et al., "A review of activity indices and efficacy end points for clinical trials of medical therapy in adults with ulcerative colitis," *Gastroenterology*, vol. 132, no. 2, pp. 763–786, 2007.

[29] M. Barreiro-de Acosta, N. Vallejo, D. de la Iglesia et al., "Evaluation of the risk of relapse in ulcerative colitis according to the degree of mucosal healing (Mayo 0 vs 1): a longitudinal cohort study," *Journal of Crohn's and Colitis*, vol. 10, no. 1, pp. 13–19, 2016.

[30] C. Papi and A. Aratari, "Mucosal healing as a treatment for IBD?," *Expert Review of Gastroenterology & Hepatology*, vol. 8, no. 5, pp. 457–459, 2014.

[31] S. C. Shah, J. F. Colombel, B. E. Sands, and N. Narula, "Mucosal healing is associated with improved long-term outcomes of patients with ulcerative colitis: a systematic review and meta-analysis," *Clinical Gastroenterology and Hepatology*, vol. 14, no. 9, pp. 1245–1255.e8, 2016.

[32] C. Prieux-Klotz, S. Nahon, A. Amiot et al., "Rate and predictors of mucosal healing in ulcerative colitis treated with thiopurines: results of a multicentric cohort study," *Digestive Diseases and Sciences*, vol. 62, no. 2, pp. 473–480, 2017.

[33] G. Costantino, F. Furfaro, A. Belvedere, A. Alibrandi, and W. Fries, "Thiopurine treatment in inflammatory bowel disease: response predictors, safety, and withdrawal in follow-up," *Journal of Crohn's and Colitis*, vol. 6, no. 5, pp. 588–596, 2012.

[34] B. Jharap, M. L. Seinen, N. K. H. de Boer et al., "Thiopurine therapy in inflammatory bowel disease patients: analyses of two 8-year intercept cohorts," *Inflammatory Bowel Diseases*, vol. 16, no. 9, pp. 1541–1549, 2010.

9

Magnetic-Guided Capsule Endoscopy in the Diagnosis of Gastrointestinal Diseases in Minors

Yuting Qian, Tingting Bai, Juanjuan Li, Yi Zang, Tong Li, Mingping Xie, Qi Wang, Lifu Wang, and Ruizhe Shen

Department of Gastroenterology, Ruijin Hospital Affiliated to Shanghai Jiaotong University School of Medicine, 197 Second Ruijin Road, Shanghai 200025, China

Correspondence should be addressed to Lifu Wang; lifuwang@sjtu.edu.cn and Ruizhe Shen; srz11009@rjh.com.cn

Academic Editor: Hauke S. Heinzow

Objective. This study aimed at investigating the clinical value of magnetic-guided capsule endoscopy (MGCE) in the diagnosis of gastrointestinal diseases in minors. *Methods.* Eighty-four minor patients hospitalized in the pediatric department at Ruijin Hospital between June 2015 and January 2018 were enrolled for this study. Following bowel preparation, all patients underwent MGCE. The feasibility, safety, diagnostic yield, and sensitivity of MGCE were analyzed. Patients were followed up for more than 2 weeks. *Results.* The main indications for MGCE in minors were Crohn's disease, gastrointestinal bleeding, and abdominal pain. The main causes of gastric disease were gastric inflammatory hyperplasia, exudative gastritis, and polyps. The most common small bowel diseases in minors were Crohn's disease, Henoch-Schonlein purpura, and polyps. The diagnostic yield in the stomach and small intestine was 13.1% and 28.6%, respectively, and the sensitivity was 100% and 96.0%, respectively. No adverse events occurred. *Conclusion.* MGCE is a safe, effective, and well-tolerated procedure with good sensitivity and has a potential clinic value for the diagnosis of gastrointestinal diseases in minors.

1. Introduction

Minor is a special group of patients, whose symptoms and diseases are often different from those of adults, especially for gastrointestinal diseases. In the past 30 years, esophagogastroduodenoscopy (EGD) has been considered as the gold standard for gastric disease investigation but the discomfort limits its use in minors. The appearance of capsule endoscopy (CE) has become a milestone in small bowel examination [1–3]. In 2009, indications of CE have been broadened to patients more than 2 years old by the United States Food and Drug Administration (FDA) and CE is proven safe to pediatrics [4–8]. With the continuous innovation of CE technology, magnetic-guided capsule endoscopy (MGCE) shows its advantages in gastric disease investigation [9–12]. However, there is a lack of the clinical value of magnetic-guided capsule endoscopy in pediatric gastrointestinal diseases. Until now, the decision of the clinical value of MGCE is based on adult research and empirical data based on CE [5, 13, 14]. Therefore, this prospective study aims at investigating the diagnostic value of magnetic-guided capsule endoscopy for minors' gastrointestinal diseases.

2. Materials and Methods

2.1. Study Cohorts. This study recruited patients from 6 to 18 years old hospitalized in the pediatric department from June 2015 to January 2018 at Ruijin Hospital Affiliated to Shanghai Jiaotong University, and the study was approved by the Ruijin Hospital Ethics Committee. Inclusion criteria were IBDU (inflammatory dowel disease unclassified), suspected Crohn's disease, hematemesis, hematochezia, melena, anemia, abdominal pain, diarrhea, abdominal distension, elevated tumor markers, constipation, and dyspepsia. Patients were divided into five groups by complains. The main exclusion criteria were metal implants (cardiac pacemaker, metal valves, metal prosthesis, etc.), impairment of gastrointestinal movement, suspected or diagnosed gastrointestinal obstruction, and history of abdominal surgery. All patients and their guardians were informed of the related process and potential risks during MGCE examination, and all signed consents.

2.2. Magnetic-Guided Capsule Endoscopy System. The NaviCam™ magnetic-guided capsule endoscopy system (Shanghai ANKON Medical Technology Co. Ltd.) was applied in this study. The components included capsule robot, magnetic-guided capsule endoscopy examination bed, translation and rotary table, magnet, console, portable recorder, capsule locator, and ESNavi software. The capsule robot was a capsule-like equipment with the size of 12 mm × 28 mm and took 2 frames per second. The observation view was 140 ± 10°, the working temperature was 20–40°C, and the working time was >8 h. The captured data of the capsule can be instantly transmitted by the data line to the operating table for real-time observation. The activity of the capsule was controlled by the C-arm magnetic field system.

2.3. Preparations. CTE or MRE examination was performed before MGCE examination to exclude intestinal obstruction. Subjects were required to carry out low-residue diet 3 days before the examination. At 8 pm the day before MGCE examination, patients drank polyethylene glycol electrolyte powder (Hengkangzhengqing, Jiangxi Hengkang Pharmaceutical Co. Ltd.) for intestinal cleaning. Patients younger than 10 years old or less than 40 kg took 25 ml/kg laxative, and patients older than 10 years and more than 40 kg took 2000 ml of laxative. On the day of examination, the subjects took 200–300 ml of water at 6 am. 10 ml of simethicone (Bo Xi, Berlin-Chemie AG) was taken 60 min before the examination. All metal belongings were removed (keys, metal dentures, mobile phones, watches, magnetic cards, etc.). Patients were demanded to take in 100 ml to 200 ml before MGCE examination. During the inspection process, if the vision was not clear, patients were asked to continue drinking water until the field of view was satisfied.

2.4. Procedures. The patients put on the portable recorder and lied on the operating bed, then swallowed the capsule robot with 5 ml water through a suction tube. The physician blinded to CTE/MRE result carried out real-time monitoring. During the gastric examination, patients changed positions as ordered for better gastric observation. After finishing gastric investigation, the patients kept walking around and the capsules' location was evaluated 2 h later. Capsule retention in the stomach over 3 hr was applied to the duodenum by a trap under gastroscopy. After 8–12 h, the portable recorder and the suit were recovered and the data of the recorder was exported. Two experienced physicians blinded to each other's results were selected to read the imaging. Different results were finally discussed for agreements. All patients underwent gastroscopy and colonoscopy before or after MGCE examination. Patients with positive findings in the small bowel underwent DBE (Figure 1). Patients were hospitalized for 2–3 days and followed up for more than 2 weeks in order to estimate adverse events.

2.5. Main Outcome Measurements. The main outcome measurements are as follows: (1) gastric examination time; (2) small bowel transit time; (3) the completion rate of stomach examination; (4) the completion rate of small bowel examination (the capsule across the ileocecal valve during examination time); (5) the diagnostic yield (the rate of positive findings) and sensitivity of MGCE in both the stomach and small bowel examinations; and (6) the occurrence of adverse events.

2.6. Statistical Analysis. All the data were represented by mean and standard deviation. Pearson's chi-squared test was used for comparisons of subgroups. Fisher's test was accurately used for a value less than 5. In this study, the p value of a double-tailed case less than 0.05 presented statistically significant differences. All statistical analyses were achieved by IBM SPSS version 2.0.

3. Results

3.1. Study Populations. 84 patients were finally enrolled in this study, with an average age of 12 ± 3.2 years, of which 53 (63.1%) were male. Subgroup I included 35 cases with abdominal pain (41.7%), and the levels of C-reactive protein (CRP) and erythrocyte sedimentation rate (ESR) were 18.6 ± 14.3 mg/l and 20.9 ± 12.7 mm/H, respectively. Subgroup II involved 22 cases with gastrointestinal bleeding: melena (6 patients, 7.1%), hematochezia (6 patients, 7.1%), hematemesis (3 patients, 3.6%), and anemia (7 patients, 8.3%). Patients with anemia had the average hemoglobin of 52.5 ± 14.0 g/l and underwent blood routine, blood smear, hemolytic anemia complete set, and bone wear, but there were no evidences of hematological diseases. They all received blood transfusion. Subgroup III enrolled 8 IBD cases: 6 cases with IBDU (6 patients, 7.1%) and 2 cases with suspected Crohn's disease (2 patients, 2.4%). Subgroup IV involved 3 cases with diarrhea (3.6%); subgroup V included 16 cases with other gastrointestinal discomforts: dyspepsia (12 patients, 14.3%), abdominal distension (2 patients, 2.4%), constipation (1 patient, 1.2%), and high level of CA199 (1 patient, 1.2%). All the patients successfully swallowed the capsule robot without mistaken aspiration. The gastric examination time was 12.1 ± 6.2 min. The mean small intestinal transit time was 248.5 ± 97.7 min. Two patients got metoclopramide to promote gastrointestinal dynamics. A patient's capsule was sent to the duodenum by gastroscopy. All patients completed gastric examination. A case (1.2%) did not complete the small bowel examination and the capsule reached the terminal ileum. During the examination, no patient felt discomfort. All capsules were discharged within two weeks, without capsule retention, intestinal obstruction, perforation, or mistaken aspiration.

3.2. Positive Findings

3.2.1. Positive Findings in the Stomach. Eleven patients had lesions in their stomach (13.1%), including 2 patients (3.6%) with gastric inflammatory hyperplasia, 2 (2.4%) with exudative gastritis, 2 (2.4%) with polyps, 1 (1.2%) with erosive lesions (1, 1.2%), 1 (1.2%) with an ulcer, 1 (1.2%) with

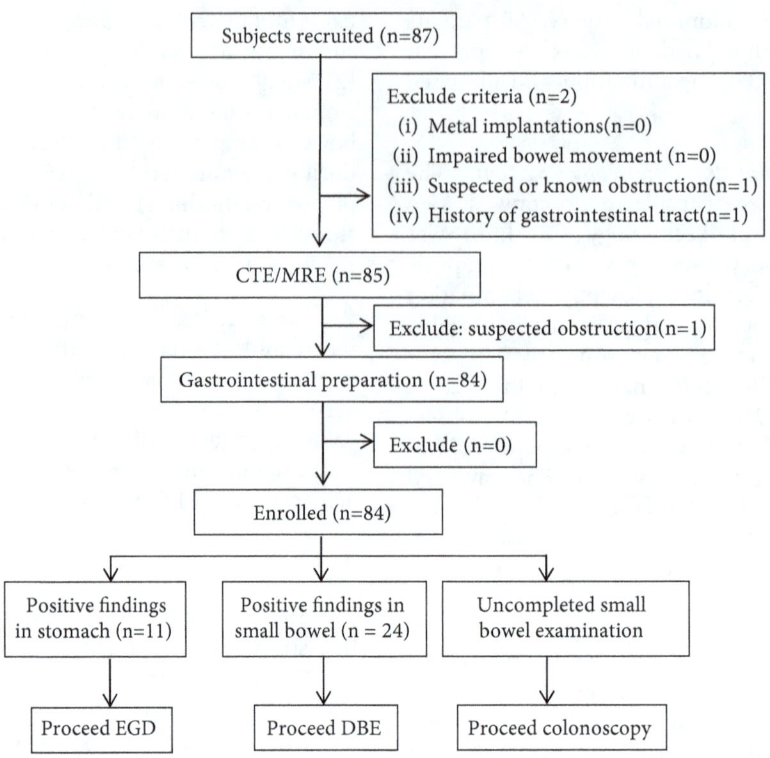

FIGURE 1: Flow chart of the study. EGD: esophagogastroduodenoscopy; DBE: double-balloon enteroscopy.

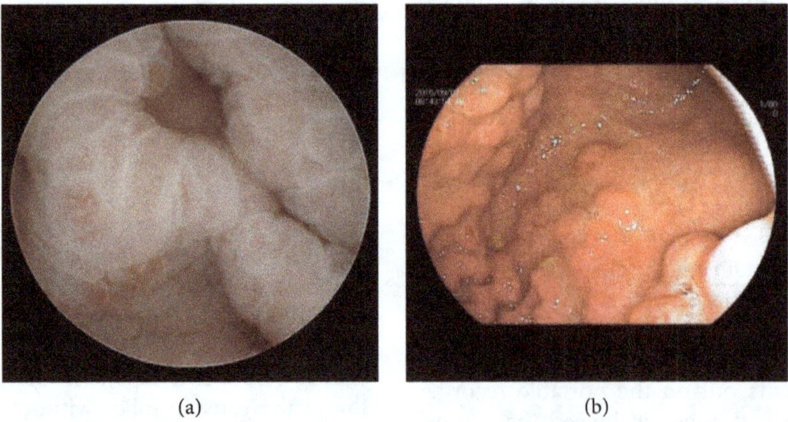

FIGURE 2: Positive findings in the stomach: (a) gastric mucosal nodular change with fold hypertrophy found by magnetic-guided capsule endoscopy; (b) gastric mucosal nodular change with fold hypertrophy verified by gastroscopy.

ectopic pancreas, and 1 (1.2%) with mucosal nodular changes with plica hypertrophy (Figures 2(a) and 2(b)). All lesions were confirmed by gastroscopy. The sensitivity of MGCE was 100%. The patient diagnosed with ectopic pancreas was followed up for 2 years using MGCE with no lesion progression seen.

3.2.2. Positive Findings in the Small Bowel. Of the 84 patients, 25 (29.8%) had positive findings on MGCE and all positive findings were confirmed by DBE. Table 1 shows the positive findings on MGCE in the small intestine subgroups. Crohn's disease (CD) was the most common finding (10 patients, 11.9%) (Figures 3(a), 3(b), and 3(c)), and 9 patients were diagnosed by small bowel imaging including computed tomography enterography (CTE) and magnetic resonance enterography (MRE). All patients received systemic treatments and had symptom relief. Two patients underwent MGCE after 3 and 6 months of step-up treatments; one patient showed mucosal improvement on MGCE, and the other achieved complete mucosal healing. The second most common finding was Henoch-Schonlein purpura (4 patients, 4.8%) for which small bowel imaging was negative. Small intestinal ulcers (3 patients, 3.6%) (Figure 3(d)), intestinal polyposis (3 patients, 3.6%) (Figure 3(e)), vascular malformation (2 patients, 2.4%) (Figure 3(f)), intussusception (1 patient, 1.2%), active bleeding in the jejunum (1 patient,

TABLE 1: Positive findings of MGCE in the small intestine for subgroups ($N = 84$). MGCE: magnetic-guided capsule endoscopy; IBD: inflammatory bowel disease; CD: Crohn's disease; DY: diagnostic yield, the rate of positive findings; VM: vascular malformation.

Subgroups (*N*, DY%)	Purpura	CD	Ulcer	Intussusception	VM	Lymphoma	Bleeding	Polyposis
(I) Abdominal pain (9/35, 25.7)	3	1	2	1	1	1	0	0
(II) Bleeding (7/22, 31.8)	1	1	1	0	1#	0	1	2
(III) IBD (7/8, 87.5)	0	7	0	0	0	0	0	0
(IV) Diarrhea (1/3, 33.3)	0	1	0	0	0	0	0	0
(V) Others ($n = 1/16$, 6.3)	0	0	0	0	0	0	0	1

#Blue rubber bleb nevus syndrome.

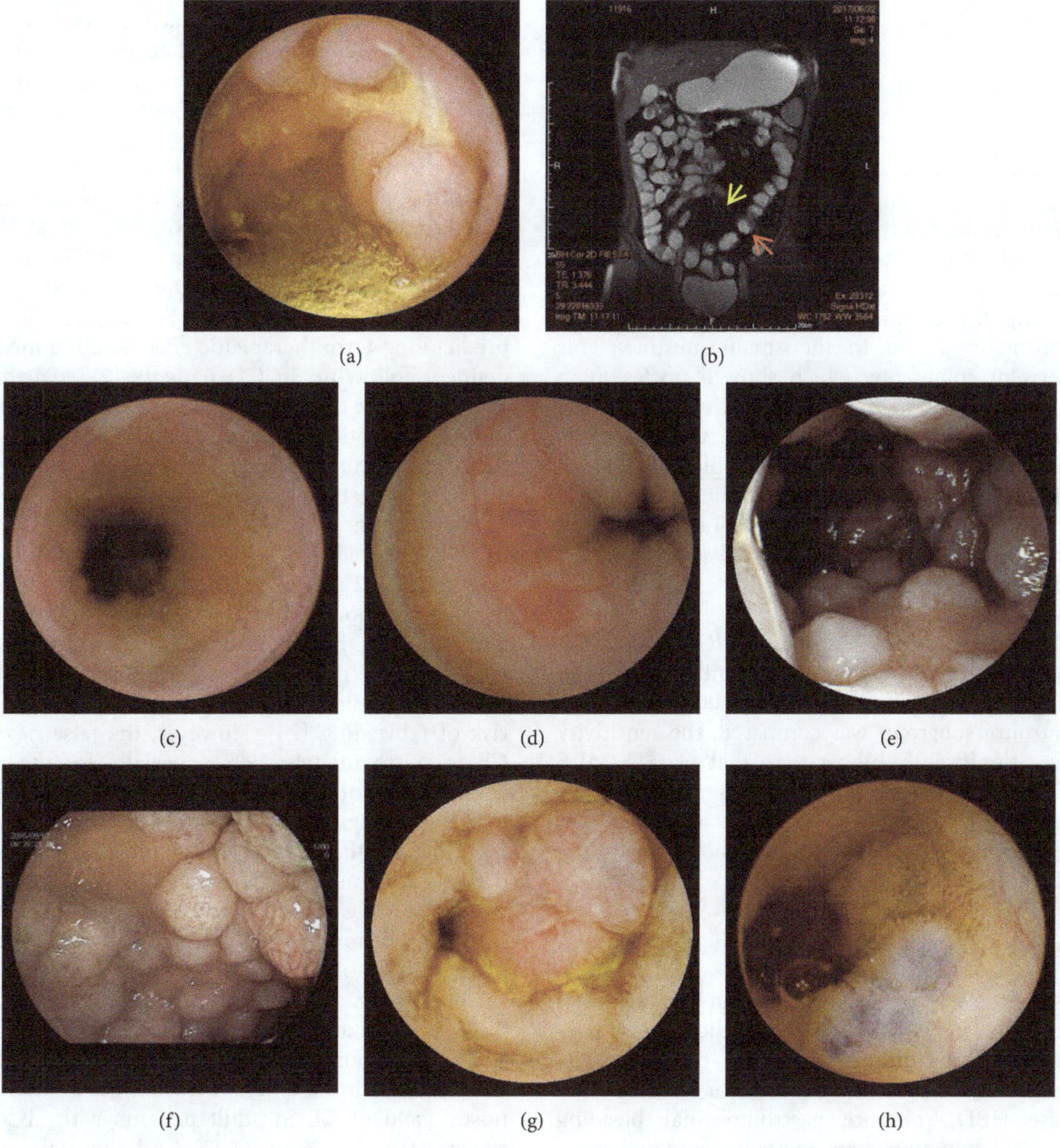

FIGURE 3: Lesions in the small bowel: (a) mucosal hyperplasia with ulceration found by magnetic-guided capsule endoscopy; (b) MRE plain scan, coronal plane, and FIESTA sequence; the red arrow showed the intestinal wall edema and the yellow arrow showed the vascular combs; (c) small bowel stenosis in CD seen by magnetic-guided capsule endoscopy; (e) small bowel ulcer with active bleeding showed by magnetic-guided capsule endoscopy; (f) mucosal segmental nodular change with nodular hypertrophy in the jejunum seen by magnetic-guided capsule endoscopy; (f) mucosal segmental nodular change with nodular hypertrophy in the jejunum verified by double-balloon endoscopy; (g) an adenomatous polyp found by magnetic-guided capsule endoscopy; (h) vascular malformations showed by magnetic-guided capsule endoscopy.

TABLE 2: Comparisons of positive findings on MGCE vs. CTE/MRE ($N = 25$). MGCE: magnetic-guided capsule endoscopy; CTE: computed tomography enterography; MRE: magnetic resonance enterography; VM: vascular malformation.

Positive findings	CE (*N*)	CTE/MRE (*N*)	Confirmed cases (*N*)	Miss rate (%) CE	Miss rate (%) CTE/MRE
Purpura	4	0	4	0	100
CD	10	9	10	0	10
Ulcer	3	0	3	—	—
Intussusception	1	1	1	—	—
VM	2	1	2	—	—
Lymphoma	1	1	1	—	—
Bleeding	1	0	1	—	—
Polyposis	2	0	2	—	—
Enteritis	0	1	1	—	—

1.2%), and non-Hodgkin's lymphoma confirmed by biopsy (Figures 3(g) and 3(h)) were also found on MGCE. In a patient in subgroup I, the capsule did not pass the ileocecal valve during the examining time, but there was no obvious abnormality found in the small intestine. This patient underwent colposcopy which showed no lesion in the terminal ileum. A patient with a negative MGCE was diagnosed with nonspecific enteritis by MRE. Other patients with a negative MGCE underwent other supplemental small intestinal imaging examinations including computed tomography (CT), CTE, MRE, and digital subtraction angiography (DSA). There were no missed diagnoses and no patient was misdiagnosed.

3.2.3. Comparisons of Positive Findings on MGCE and CTE/MRE. The sensitivity of MGCE was significantly higher than that of CTE/MRE (96.0% vs. 52.0%, $p = 0.001$) (Table 2). When the purpura subgroup was compared, the sensitivity of MGCE was significantly higher than that of CTE/MRE (100% vs. 0%,$p = 0.029$). There was no significant difference in sensitivity in the CD subgroup ($p = 0.50$). Other positive findings could not be compared owing to the small sample size.

4. Discussion

The use of small bowel capsule endoscopy in pediatrics has increased since the US FDA extended the indication for capsule endoscopy (CE) to children over 2 years of age in 2009. Currently, in pediatrics, CE is mainly used for inflammatory bowel disease (IBD), obscure gastrointestinal bleeding (OGIB), anemia, abdominal pain, diarrhea, and polyposis [15]. However, in children less than 8 years of age, the incidence of IBD is low, and, as for adults, the main indication for CE is OGIB [14, 16, 17]. Because there is a risk of mistaken aspiration in children, the application of capsule endoscopy in pediatrics remains limited. During the last 10 years, we have accumulated some experience and skill in operating and reading MGCEs in minors, and we found that after scanning the stomach, the MGCE has enough battery power to provide high-quality images while investigating the small bowel in minors. Additionally, the diagnostic yield of MGCE is comparable to ordinary CE in the small intestine. Further, with MGCE, both gastric and small intestinal examination can be performed at the same time, which is well tolerated by minors. However, no studies focusing on this topic have been performed. In this study, with the collaboration of pediatricians, we aimed to investigate the safety, maneuverability, and clinical value of MGCE in the diagnosis of gastrointestinal diseases in minors.

In this study, the sensitivity of MGCE for gastric examination of minors was 100%, which is higher than that in adults (61.9%) [18]. The stomach cavity in a minor has a smaller volume and is softer than that in adults, making a minor's stomach easier to fill with water, which facilitates MGCE navigation. This may explain the high sensitivity found in minors.

In this study, MGCE had a high diagnostic yield of small bowel lesions in the IBD group, which is comparable to that of CE for the small intestine (87.5% vs. 86%) [16]. CE provides evidence for the identification of CD, the reclassification from ulcerative colitis/IBD unclassified to CD, and the adjustment of medical strategy [19, 20]. In addition, CE can predict long-term therapeutic effect and is a means for independent follow-up in CD patients [21]. Furthermore, the MGCE used in this study can help assess gastric involvement in pediatric patients. Therefore, CD could be considered the first indication for MGCE examination in minors.

Gastrointestinal bleeding is another important indication for MGCE. In group II, the diagnostic yield of MGCE is 31.8%. In an adult with OGIB, the diagnostic yield of CE ranges from 32% to 83% [22] and the major causes are vascular malformation, CD, and small bowel tumor [23], which are different from those in minors. In this study, more than 60% of minors with gastrointestinal bleeding had a negative MGCE. In adults, a negative CE provides evidence for a low risk of rebleeding [24]. However, the false negative rate of CE is approximately 19%, especially for the diagnosis of vascular malformation, Meckel's diverticulum, and small intestinal malignant tumor [25]. However, systematic studies focusing on the clinical value of CE in pediatric OGIB patients are limited [2, 5, 13, 26–29] and there are no related studies of MGCE. Therefore, the etiology of gastrointestinal bleeding in minors and the sensitivity, specificity, and predicting factors of MGCE require a study.

Until now, the indications and clinical value of CE in patients with abdominal pain were controversial. In this study, the main causes were Henoch-Schonlein purpura and CD, which are different from those in adults. The diagnostic yield of CE in adult patients with abdominal pain ranges from 20.9% to 24.4%, and the main cause is CD, followed by tumor [30–32]. In this study, the diagnostic yield (25.7%) was slightly higher than that of the adults. The reasons for this could be (1) the patients recruited were hospitalized, and the syndrome may be more severe in them in outpatients; (2) the patients enrolled in this study had elevated C-reactive protein or erythrocyte sedimentation rate, which may be an effective predictor for positive CE findings in patients with abdominal pain [33, 34]; and (3) minors involved in this study had a high incidence of Henoch-Schonlein purpura, which was not frequently found in adult patients. Therefore, large-scale clinical trials confirming the clinical value of MGCE in minors with abdominal pain are still needed.

In the diarrhea subgroup, one patient was diagnosed with CD, and the diagnostic yield of MGCE was higher than that of the adults using CE (33.3% vs. 14%) [35]. Although CE is not recommended as a first-line examination for diarrhea, it facilitates making the diagnosis in 9% of patients with negative conventional endoscopy and imaging examination results [35]. The most common cause is IBD, and hematochezia and hypoalbuminemia on CE are positive predictors for it [36]. There is a lack of clinical studies on CE for patients with dyspepsia, constipation, high level CA 19-9, and abdominal distention, especially in the pediatric population. MGCE may not be suitable for such patients as a first-line procedure, but it remains valuable for suspected IBD in minors.

Currently, CTE and MRE are widely used for diseases of the small intestine, and the diagnostic yield is comparable to that of CE [37, 38]. In this study, MGCE had a better sensitivity than that of CTE and MRE in minors. The possible reasons for this advantage maybe as follows: (1) MGCE is better for scanning the lesions on the mucosal surface, which is where lesions in minors primarily occur; and (2) minors have difficulty cooperating with the CTE and MRE examination processes. However, CTE and MRE can provide supplementary information and, for safety, are still recommended before MGCE in minors to avoid capsule retention.

Swallowing problems in minors during MGCE remains a challenge, especially for patients younger than 8 years of age. We thoroughly explained the procedure process and techniques to the patients and their guardians to comfort them and reduce fear. Patient guidance and encouragement from doctors can help children swallow the capsule smoothly, even for those who are 6 years of age [39]. The overall incidence rate of adverse events is 2% [40], and capsule retention is one of the most common complications, especially for CD patients and patients less than 10 years of age [41]. In children, the high risk of capsule retention may be due to the narrow diameter of the intestinal cavity and the high incidence of CD-related intestinal stenosis. However, during our follow-up period, no adverse events occurred. We consider MGCE to be a safe procedure for minors.

There are some limitations to this study. First, the efficiency of MGCEs in the subgroups could not be compared owing to the small sample size. Second, longer follow-up time is needed to confirm the cure rate, recurrence rate, and accuracy of the original diagnosis. Finally, due to potential swallowing problems, patients less than 6 years of age were not recruited for this study, which may have led to some bias.

5. Conclusion

MGCE is a safe, well-tolerated, and feasible procedure with a high diagnostic yield and sensitivity in minor patients. It has important clinical value and great prospects in the diagnosis of gastrointestinal diseases in minors.

Disclosure

Yuting Qian and Tingting Bai contributed equally to this paper.

Acknowledgments

This work was supported by the National Natural Science Foundation of China (81672719, 81702740).

References

[1] F. Argüelles Arias, E. Donat, I. Fernández-Urien et al., "Guideline for wireless capsule endoscopy in children and adolescents: a consensus document by the SEGHNP (Spanish Society for Pediatric Gastroenterology, Hepatology, and Nutrition) and the SEPD (Spanish Spanish Society for Digestive Diseases)," *Revista Española de Enfermedades Digestivas*, vol. 107, 2015.

[2] S. Oliva, M. Pennazio, S. A. Cohen et al., "Capsule endoscopy followed by single balloon enteroscopy in children with obscure gastrointestinal bleeding: a combined approach," *Digestive and Liver Disease*, vol. 47, no. 2, pp. 125–130, 2015.

[3] K. N. Shim, J. S. Moon, D. K. Chang et al., "Guideline for capsule endoscopy: obscure gastrointestinal bleeding," *Clinical Endoscopy*, vol. 46, no. 1, pp. 45–53, 2013.

[4] C. Dupont-Lucas, M. Bellaïche, O. Mouterde et al., "Capsule endoscopy in children: which are the best indications?," *Archives de Pédiatrie*, vol. 17, no. 9, pp. 1264–1272, 2010.

[5] J. Viala, L. Michaud, M. Bellaiche, and A. Lachaux, "When and how should small-bowel capsule endoscopy be used in children?," *Archives de Pédiatrie*, vol. 24, no. 4, pp. 391–398, 2017.

[6] B. Vadamalayan, M. Hii, J. Kark, and I. Bjarnason, "Feasibility of small bowel capsule endoscopy in children under the age of 4 years: a single centre experience," *Frontline Gastroenterology*, vol. 3, no. 4, pp. 267–271, 2012.

[7] A. Fritscher-Ravens, P. Scherbakov, P. Bufler et al., "The feasibility of wireless capsule endoscopy in detecting small intestinal pathology in children under the age of 8 years: a multicentre European study," *Gut*, vol. 58, no. 11, pp. 1467–1472, 2009.

[8] M. Oikawa-Kawamoto, T. Sogo, T. Yamaguchi et al., "Safety and utility of capsule endoscopy for infants and young children," *World Journal of Gastroenterology*, vol. 19, no. 45, pp. 8342–8348, 2013.

[9] J. F. Rey, H. Ogata, N. Hosoe et al., "Feasibility of stomach exploration with a guided capsule endoscope," *Endoscopy*, vol. 42, no. 07, pp. 541–545, 2010.

[10] P. Swain, A. Toor, F. Volke et al., "Remote magnetic manipulation of a wireless capsule endoscope in the esophagus and stomach of humans (with videos)," *Gastrointestinal Endoscopy*, vol. 71, no. 7, pp. 1290–1293, 2010.

[11] J. Keller, C. Fibbe, F. Volke et al., "Inspection of the human stomach using remote-controlled capsule endoscopy: a feasibility study in healthy volunteers (with videos)," *Gastrointestinal Endoscopy*, vol. 73, no. 1, pp. 22–28, 2011.

[12] Z. Liao, X. D. Duan, L. Xin et al., "Feasibility and safety of magnetic-controlled capsule endoscopy system in examination of human stomach: a pilot study in healthy volunteers," *Journal of Interventional Gastroenterology*, vol. 2, no. 4, pp. 155–160, 2012.

[13] H. Nuutinen, K. L. Kolho, P. Salminen et al., "Capsule endoscopy in pediatric patients: technique and results in our first 100 consecutive children," *Scandinavian Journal of Gastroenterology*, vol. 46, no. 9, pp. 1138–1143, 2011.

[14] N. Zevit and R. Shamir, "Wireless capsule endoscopy of the small intestine in children," *Journal of Pediatric Gastroenterology and Nutrition*, vol. 60, no. 6, pp. 696–701, 2015.

[15] S. A. Cohen and A. I. Klevens, "Use of capsule endoscopy in diagnosis and management of pediatric patients, based on meta-analysis," *Clinical Gastroenterology and Hepatology*, vol. 9, no. 6, pp. 490–496, 2011.

[16] R. A. Enns, L. Hookey, D. Armstrong et al., "Clinical practice guidelines for the use of video capsule endoscopy," *Gastroenterology*, vol. 152, no. 3, pp. 497–514, 2017.

[17] H. Yamamoto, H. Ogata, T. Matsumoto et al., "Clinical practice guideline for enteroscopy," *Digestive Endoscopy*, vol. 29, no. 5, pp. 519–546, 2017.

[18] U. W. Denzer, T. Rösch, B. Hoytat et al., "Magnetically guided capsule versus conventional gastroscopy for upper abdominal complaints: a prospective blinded study," *Journal of Clinical Gastroenterology*, vol. 49, no. 2, pp. 101–107, 2015.

[19] S. B. Min, M. Le-Carlson, N. Singh et al., "Video capsule endoscopy impacts decision making in pediatric IBD: a single tertiary care center experience," *Inflammatory Bowel Diseases*, vol. 19, no. 10, pp. 2139–2145, 2013.

[20] I. M. Gralnek, S. A. Cohen, H. Ephrath et al., "Small bowel capsule endoscopy impacts diagnosis and management of pediatric inflammatory bowel disease: a prospective study," *Digestive Diseases and Sciences*, vol. 57, no. 2, pp. 465–471, 2012.

[21] Y. Niv, "Small-bowel mucosal healing assessment by capsule endoscopy as a predictor of long-term clinical remission in patients with Crohn's disease: a systematic review and meta-analysis," *European Journal of Gastroenterology & Hepatology*, vol. 29, no. 7, pp. 844–848, 2017.

[22] Y. W. Min and D. K. Chang, "The role of capsule endoscopy in patients with obscure gastrointestinal bleeding," *Clinical Endoscopy*, vol. 49, no. 1, pp. 16–20, 2016.

[23] C. S. E. Wang, J. N. Li, Y. N. Wang, H. Yang, and J. M. Qian, "Diagnostic value analysis of capsule endoscopy in obscure gastrointestinal bleeding patients of different ages," *Zhonghua Yi Xue Za Zhi*, vol. 97, no. 36, pp. 2848–2851, 2017.

[24] P. Katsinelos, J. Kountouras, G. Chatzimavroudis et al., "Factors predicting a positive capsule endoscopy in past overt obscure gastrointestinal bleeding: a multicenter retrospective study," *Hippokratia*, vol. 20, no. 2, pp. 127–132, 2016.

[25] C. Van de Bruaene, P. Hindryckx, C. Snauwaert et al., "The predictive value of negative capsule endoscopy for the indication of obscure gastrointestinal bleeding: no reassurance in the long term," *Acta Gastro-Enterologica Belgica*, vol. 79, no. 4, pp. 405–413, 2016.

[26] B. Sahn and S. Bitton, "Lower gastrointestinal bleeding in children," *Gastrointestinal Endoscopy Clinics of North America*, vol. 26, no. 1, pp. 75–98, 2016.

[27] M. Thomson, "Paediatrics: diagnostic yield of paediatric lower gastrointestinal endoscopy," *Nature Reviews Gastroenterology & Hepatology*, vol. 13, no. 7, pp. 382–384, 2016.

[28] P. Katsinelos, G. Lazaraki, A. Gkagkalis et al., "The role of capsule endoscopy in the evaluation and treatment of obscure-overt gastrointestinal bleeding during daily clinical practice: a prospective multicenter study," *Scandinavian Journal of Gastroenterology*, vol. 49, no. 7, pp. 862–870, 2014.

[29] Z. Liao, R. Gao, F. Li et al., "Fields of applications, diagnostic yields and findings of OMOM capsule endoscopy in 2400 Chinese patients," *World Journal of Gastroenterology*, vol. 16, no. 21, pp. 2669–2676, 2010.

[30] M. Xue, X. Chen, L. Shi, J. Si, L. Wang, and S. Chen, "Small-bowel capsule endoscopy in patients with unexplained chronic abdominal pain: a systematic review," *Gastrointestinal Endoscopy*, vol. 81, no. 1, pp. 186–193, 2015.

[31] J. Egnatios, K. Kaushal, D. Kalmaz, and A. Zarrinpar, "Video capsule endoscopy in patients with chronic abdominal pain with or without associated symptoms: a retrospective study," *PLoS One*, vol. 10, no. 4, article e0126509, 2015.

[32] L. Yang, Y. Chen, B. Zhang et al., "Increased diagnostic yield of capsule endoscopy in patients with chronic abdominal pain," *PLoS One*, vol. 9, no. 1, article e87396, 2014.

[33] M. Nakano, S. Oka, S. Tanaka et al., "Indications for small-bowel capsule endoscopy in patients with chronic abdominal pain," *Internal Medicine*, vol. 56, no. 12, pp. 1453–1457, 2017.

[34] P. Katsinelos, K. Fasoulas, A. Beltsis et al., "Diagnostic yield and clinical impact of wireless capsule endoscopy in patients with chronic abdominal pain with or without diarrhea: a Greek multicenter study," *European Journal of Internal Medicine*, vol. 22, no. 5, pp. e63–e66, 2011.

[35] L. C. Fry, E. J. Carey, A. D. Shiff et al., "The yield of capsule endoscopy in patients with abdominal pain or diarrhea," *Endoscopy*, vol. 38, no. 5, pp. 498–502, 2006.

[36] H. J. Song, J. S. Moon, S. R. Jeon et al., "Diagnostic yield and clinical impact of video capsule endoscopy in patients with chronic diarrhea: a Korean multicenter CAPENTRY study," *Gut and Liver*, vol. 11, no. 2, pp. 253–260, 2017.

[37] M. Choi, S. Lim, M. G. Choi, K. N. Shim, and S. H. Lee, "Effectiveness of capsule endoscopy compared with other diagnostic modalities in patients with small bowel Crohn's disease: a meta-analysis," *Gut and Liver*, vol. 11, no. 1, pp. 62–72, 2017.

[38] E. Casciani, G. D. Nardo, S. Chin et al., "MR Enterography in paediatric patients with obscure gastrointestinal bleeding," *European Journal of Radiology*, vol. 93, pp. 209–216, 2017.

[39] B. A. Barth, S. Banerjee, Y. M. Bhat et al., "Equipment for pediatric endoscopy," *Gastrointestinal Endoscopy*, vol. 76, no. 1, pp. 8–17, 2012.

[40] M. Rezapour, C. Amadi, and L. B. Gerson, "Retention associated with video capsule endoscopy: systematic review and meta-analysis," *Gastrointestinal Endoscopy*, vol. 85, no. 6, pp. 1157–1168.e2, 2017, e1152.

[41] Y. J. Lim, O. Y. Lee, Y. T. Jeen et al., "Indications for detection, completion, and retention rates of small bowel capsule endoscopy based on the 10-year data from the Korean capsule endoscopy registry," *Clinical Endoscopy*, vol. 48, no. 5, pp. 399–404, 2015.

Analysis of Prognostic Factors for Resected Synchronous and Metachronous Liver Metastases from Colorectal Cancer

Ilenia Bartolini,[1] Maria Novella Ringressi,[1] Filippo Melli,[1] Matteo Risaliti,[1] Marco Brugia,[2] Enrico Mini,[2] Giacomo Batignani,[1] Paolo Bechi,[1] Luca Boni,[3] and Antonio Taddei[1]

[1]*Department of Surgery and Translational Medicine, University of Florence, AOU Careggi, Largo Brambilla 3, 50134 Florence, Italy*
[2]*Department of Experimental and Clinical Medicine, AOU Careggi, Largo Brambilla 3, 50134 Florence, Italy*
[3]*Clinical Trials Coordinating Center of Istituto Toscano Tumori, AOU Careggi, Largo Brambilla 3, 50134 Florence, Italy*

Correspondence should be addressed to Ilenia Bartolini; ilenia.bartolini@gmail.com

Academic Editor: Chiara Molinari

Background. Surgical treatment is the cornerstone in the management of colorectal cancer (CRC) liver metastases. The aim of this study is to identify clinicopathological factors affecting disease-free (DFS) and overall survival (OS) in patients undergoing potentially curative liver resection for CRC metastasis. *Methods.* All consecutive patients undergoing liver resection for first recurrence of CRC from February 2006 to February 2018 were included. Prognostic impact of factors related to the patient, primary and metastatic tumors, was retrospectively tested through univariate and multivariate analyses. *Results.* Seventy patients were included in the study. Median postoperative follow-up was 37 months (range 1–119). Median DFS and OS were 15.2 and 62.7 months, and 5-year DFS and OS rates were 16% and 53%. In univariate analysis, timing of metastasis presentation/treatment (combined colorectal and liver resection, "bowel first" approach or metachronous presentation) ($p < 0.0001$), ASA score ($p = 0.003$), chemotherapy after liver surgery ($p = 0.028$), T stage ($p = 0.021$), number of resected liver lesions ($p < 0.0001$), and liver margin status ($p = 0.032$) was significantly associated with DFS while peritoneal resection at colorectal surgery ($p = 0.026$), ASA score ($p = 0.036$), extension of liver resection ($p = 0.024$), chemotherapy after liver surgery ($p = 0.047$), and positive nodes ($p = 0.018$) with OS. In multivariate analysis, timing of metastasis presentation/treatment, ASA score, and chemotherapy (before and after liver surgery) resulted significantly associated with DFS and timing of metastasis presentation/treatment, positive nodes, peritoneal resection at colorectal surgery, and surgical approach (open or minimally invasive) of colorectal resection with OS. *Conclusions.* Surgery may provide good DFS and OS rates for CRC liver metastasis. Patient selection for surgery and correct timing of intervention within a multidisciplinary approach may be improved by taking into account negative prognostic factors which stress the importance of systemic therapy.

1. Introduction

Colorectal cancer (CRC) is the third leading cause of cancer-related death in developed countries [1]. The liver is the commonest site of distant spread of CRC, and liver metastases occur in up to 60% of those patients [2, 3].

Surgical treatment is the cornerstone of management of CRC, apart from staging. Nevertheless, some authors believe in a promoting effects of surgery on tumor spread stating that manipulation of the tumor and its vessels may promote tumor spillage, production of growth factors, and reduction of the release of antiangiogenic factors [4, 5]. On the contrary, other authors suggest that removal of at least great majority of tumor burden may reduce proinflammatory effects and the release of circulating malignant cell leading to a better control of metastasizing cells from host immunity [6, 7]. Due to the technical and technological improvements in liver surgery and perioperative care, hepatic resection has become at least a part of the standard of care in metastatic CRC. Indications to liver resection have been widened along the past 3 decades maintaining acceptable morbidity and mortality rates [8]. Nowadays, patients are considered suitable for surgery if all the disease can be resected with negative margins and preserving an adequate liver remnant [9, 10]. Unfortunately, only about 25% of the patients affected meets these criteria [3]. Moreover, a multimodality and multidisciplinary evaluation and treatment, when appropriate, is of paramount importance in this selected group of metastatic patients in order to provide the best chances of cure [11, 12].

In patients fit for surgery, resection may provide 5-year survival rates of 40–74% [9, 11, 12], 10-year survival rates of 16–23%, and a cure rate of 20% [10] compared to a 5-year survival rate of about 5% in case of palliative treatments [3]. On the other hand, recurrence rate is reported to be high (60–80%) with a 10–15% of early recurrence and disease-specific deaths [8].

In order to help in the selection of the more appropriate treatment, some prognostic factors in patients suffering from CRC and metastatic CRC have been identified [2, 3, 8, 10]. The aim of this study is to verify and analyze different factors which may affect disease-free survival (DFS) and overall survival (OS). They are either related to the patient, to the primitive CRC, or liver metastasis in the selected group of patients who underwent liver resection for first and isolated recurrence of colorectal cancer. Its perspective is the identification of the subgroups of patients who could benefit more from surgical resection in order to improve patient selection and the choice of adequate timing for liver resection within a multimodality treatment.

2. Materials and Methods

2.1. Study Design and Patients. From February 2006 to February 2018, all the patients affected by "liver only" first metastasization from CRC who underwent potentially curative surgical resection at the Hepatobiliary Surgery Unit of Careggi Teaching Hospital were included in the study. Patients undergoing intraoperative radiofrequency ablation (RFA) with a curative intent were also included. Patients with a primary rectal squamocellular carcinoma were excluded. Preoperative workup included triple phase-contrast enhanced computed tomography (CT) scan and pancolonoscopy. Liver volume assessment was performed when indicated. Magnetic resonance and positron emission tomography (PET) scan were used to rule out doubtful cases. Intraoperative ultrasound sonography (IOUS) was routinely used during liver surgery. Follow-up was done according to a standardized scheduled program including CT scan or abdominal ultrasound, colonoscopy, and blood test examination. It could be modified according to oncologist's indications. Retrieval of follow-up data was completed including the revision of any available medical records and phone call interviews.

Day of liver surgery was chosen as reference date. Disease-free interval was considered as the time between liver surgery and the diagnosis of any site of recurrence of disease or until the date of death while overall survival was considered as time between the liver surgery and the date of death or the last visit for alive patients. Recurrences were treated with surgery, chemotherapy, radiotherapy, percutaneous treatment, combinations of them, or best supportive care as appropriate.

According to timing of metastasis presentation/treatment, patients were divided into 3 groups: "synchronous combined surgery" that included patients who underwent combined surgery for primary tumor and liver metastasis, "synchronous bowel first" that included patients with metastatic disease from the beginning of their neoplastic history but liver metastases were not treated during colorectal surgery, and "metachronous" that included patients who developed liver metastasis after colorectal cancer surgery. The decision to perform combined or delayed surgery in synchronous presentation with or without any perioperative chemotherapy was discussed during Hospital Tumor Board meetings. Patient's conditions (i.e., comorbidities, bowel obstruction) and wishes, number, dimension, and position of the liver metastases at preoperative examination (confirmed or not at surgery time) were taken into account. Right colon comprehended lesions located from the cecum to transverse; left colon included also lesions located in the rectum. In univariate analysis, converted procedures were grouped with open surgery because this study is not an "intention-to-treat" analysis. Peritoneal resection was defined as any resection of the anterior aspect of the peritoneum macroscopically adherent/infiltrated by the primary tumor. Major hepatectomies were defined as resection of at least 3 segments according to Brisbane's classification [13]. Postoperative complications occurred after hepatic resections were evaluated if classified as at least grade 3 or 4 according to Clavien-Dindo classification [14]. Chemotherapy before and after liver surgery was considered if administered to the patient despite the interruption of the initially scheduled program. The lesion size (maximum diameter for both primary and metastatic tumors) and number of hepatic metastases resected were retrieved from histopathological response. T stage was classified according to American Joint Committee on Cancer (AJCC) TNM staging system, 7th edition definition [15]. Positive liver margins were defined in presence of neoplastic cells within the surface of resected liver.

2.2. Analysis. Patients' data were prospectively collected into a database which was retrospectively reviewed. Continuous variables were reported as median and range while categorical variables were reported as frequency and percentage. Differences between the three groups were analyzed using the Kruskal-Wallis test for continuous variables, while categorical variables were compared using the χ^2 or Fisher exact test when appropriated. Statistical significance was defined as p value ≤ 0.05.

For univariate analysis, estimate of DFS and OS rates was calculated according to the Kaplan-Meier methods and compared using log-rank test. Hazard ratios (HR) and their 95% confidence intervals (CI) were calculated by means of the Cox proportional hazard model. The multivariate Cox regression model was used to evaluate the independent effect on DFS and OS of any factors whose p value was ≤ 0.15 at the univariate analysis. Parameters related to the histopathological response on liver specimens (i.e., number of resected lesions, maximum diameter, and liver margin status) were not considered in multivariate analysis because of their

TABLE 1: Patients' characteristics.

	Synchronous combined surgery ($n = 25$) (35.7%)	Synchronous "bowel first" ($n = 14$) (20%)	Metachronous ($n = 31$) (44.3%)	Total ($n = 70$)	p value
Age (years, range)	68 (34–85)	75 (46–82)	70 (52–85)	69.5 (34–85)	0.730
Sex (n, %)					0.683
Male	15 (60%)	9 (64.3%)	16 (51.6%)	40 (57.1%)	
Female	10 (40%)	5 (35.7%)	15 (48.4%)	30 (42.9%)	
Bowel obstruction (n, %)	5 (20%)	7 (50%)	7 (22.6%)	19 (27.1%)	0.097
Site of primary tumor (n, %)					0.343
Right colon	8 (32%)	2 (14.3%)	11 (35.5%)	21 (30%)	
Left colon	17 (68%)	12 (85.7%)	20 (64.5%)	49 (70%)	
CHT before liver surgery	2 (8%)	11 (78.6%)	20 (64.5%)	33 (47%)	**<0.0001**

CHT = chemotherapy.

TABLE 2: Perioperative results.

	Synchronous combined surgery ($n = 25$) (35.7%)	Synchronous "bowel first" ($n = 14$) (20%)	Metachronous ($n = 31$) (44.3%)	Total ($n = 70$)	p value
Colorectal surgery					
Technique (n, %)					**0.006**
Open	15 (60%)	5 (35.7%)	7 (22.6%)	40 (57.1%)	
Minimally invasive	5 (20%)	9 (64.3%)	17 (54.8%)	31 (44.3%)	
Converted	5 (20%)	0	7 (22.6%)	12 (17.1%)	
Peritoneal resection (n, %)	2 (8%)	1 (7.1%)	2 (6.4%)	5 (7.1%)	1.00
Liver surgery					
ASA (n, %)					0.522
1	3 (12%)	1 (7.1%)	2 (6.4%)	6 (8.6%)	
2	7 (28%)	4 (28.6%)	11 (35.5%)	22 (31.4%)	
3	11 (44%)	6 (42.9%)	17 (54.8%)	34 (48.6%)	
4	4 (16%)	3 (21.4%)	1 (3.2)	8 (11.4)	
Type of surgery (n, %)					**0.024**
Minor/wedge	22 (88%)	7 (50%)	17 (54.8%)	46 (65.7%)	
Major	3 (12%)	4 (28.6%)	10 (32.3%)	17 (24.3%)	
RFA	0	3 (21.4%)	4 (12.9%)	7 (10%)	
Surgery duration (min, range)	300 (170–145)	242.5 (175–369)	230 (50–315)	255 (50–450)	<0.0001
Complications (CD III-IV) (n, %)	3 (12%)	3 (21.4%)	4 (12.9%)	10 (14.3%)	0.743
CHT after liver surgery (n, %)	18 (72%)	4 (28.6%)	17 (54.8%)	39 (55.7%)	**0.032**

ASA = American Society of Anesthesiologists; Minor/wedge = minor hepatectomies/hepatic wedge resections; Major = major hepatectomies; RFA = radiofrequency ablation; CD III-IV = Clavien-Dindo classification grade III-IV; CHT = chemotherapy.

unavailability in the 7 patients who underwent intraoperative curative RFA alone in order to avoid their exclusion from this analysis.

Data were analyzed using the statistical software SAS version 9.2 (SAS Corporation, Cary, NC).

3. Results and Discussion

3.1. Results

3.1.1. Patient Characteristics. Overall, 70 patients were included in the study. Median follow-up was 37 months (range 1–119). In particular, median follow-up among survivors was 48 months (range 2–116). Analyzed patient characteristics are displayed in Table 1. Patients undergoing combined surgery were 25, a two-step surgery was performed in 14 patients, and metachronous presentation of metastases was seen in 31 patients. Age, sex, and primary tumor distribution were similar within these three groups. Chemotherapy before liver surgery was administered in a very low percentage (8%) of "combined surgery" group ($p < 0.0001$).

Perioperative results are shown in Table 2. Open surgery technique ($p = 0.006$) and minor/parenchymal-sparing liver

Table 3: Histopathological results.

	Synchronous combined surgery ($n = 25$) (35.7%)	Synchronous "bowel first" ($n = 14$) (20%)	Metachronous ($n = 31$) (44.3%)	Total ($n = 70$)	p value
Colorectal specimen					
Size (mm, range)	35 (17–130)	54 (25–90)	35 (4–82)	40 (4–130)	**0.024**
T stage* (n, %)					0.065
1-2	2 (8%)	4 (28.6%)	5 (16.1%)	11 (15.7%)	
3	22 (88%)	8 (57.1%)	26 (83.9%)	56 (80%)	
4	1 (4%)	2 (14.3%)	0	3 (4.3%)	
Nodes harvested (n, range)	17 (7–76)	25 (6–48)	26 (9–50)	22 (6–76)	
Positive nodes (n, range)	2 (0–10)	3.5 (0–17)	1 (0–12)	2 (0–17)	0.217
Mucinous histotype	3 (12%)	1 (7.1%)	9 (29%)	13 (18.6%)	0.159
Liver specimen	$n = 25$	$n = 11$	$n = 27$	$n = 63$	
Resected lesions (n, range)	1 (1–11)	2 (1–6)	1 (1–4)	1 (1–11)	0.334
Size (mm, range)	24 (4–50)	35 (15–80)	35 (12–110)	30 (4–110)	**0.005**
Positive margins (n, %)	0	3 (27.3%)	1 (3.7%)	4 (6.35)	**0.015**

*T stage according to TNM definition AJCC 7th edition.

resection ($p = 0.024$) were more frequently applied in "combined surgery" group. ASA score and postoperative complication distribution in the 3 groups were similar with an overall median rate of severe complications after liver surgery of 14.3%. A statistically significant difference in the 3 groups was found for the administration of chemotherapy after liver surgery ($p = 0.032$) with the lowest percentage (28.6%) in "bowel first" group.

Analyzed histopathological results are shown in Table 3. T4 stage ($p = 0.065$) and bigger primary tumors ($p = 0.024$) were more frequently ($p = 0.065$) found in "bowel first" group. Lower median number ($p = 0.334$) and smaller size of liver metastases were reported in "combined surgery" group specimens (24 mm versus 35 mm in the other 2 groups, $p = 0.005$). Higher frequency of positive liver margins ($p = 0.015$) was found in "bowel first" group. Tumor grading was not evaluated since almost all the patients presented a G2 primary tumor. KRAS or BRAF evaluation was not available in 55.7% of the patients; consequently, this variable was not analyzed. However, 24 patients had a RAS wild-type while 15 patients presented a RAS mutation.

3.1.2. Factors Associated with Disease-Free Survival (DFS) and Overall Survival (OS). Recurrence after liver surgery was documented in 46 patients (66%). Early recurrence (within 6 months) occurred in 15 patients (21.4%), recurrence rate within the first year was 37% (26 patients), and no other recurrences were found after the third year from liver surgery. Median time between recurrence and death was 29 months (range 1–89 months). Ninety-day mortality was 1.4%.

Overall, 1-, 3-, and 5-year DFS rates were 59%, 17%, and 16%, respectively, with a median DFS rate of 15.2 months (95% CI 11.2–21.5). Overall, 1-, 3-, and 5-year OS rates were 94%, 68%, and 53%, respectively, with a median OS rate of 62.7 months (95% CI 43.7–67.8).

Results of univariate analysis of factors associated with DFS and OS are shown in Table 4.

Disease presentation and treatment timing (Figure 1) significantly affected DFS ($p < 0.0001$) but not OS ($p = 0.085$). Metachronous group had a median DFS of 23.5 months compared to 14.4 months of DFS for "combined surgery" group and 6 months for "bowel first" group. Compared to "combined surgery group", "bowel first" group had an HR of 3.9 (95% HR CI 1.8–8.2) for DFS.

Surgical approach for colorectal surgery (Figure 2) resulted marginally significant for OS ($p = 0.058$). Compared to open and converted surgery, minimally invasive techniques had an HR of 0.5 (95% HR CI 0.2–1) for OS. Peritoneal resection at colorectal surgery was a negative significant factor for OS ($p = 0.026$) but not for DFS ($p = 0.414$).

ASA score (Figure 3) was significantly associated with both DFS ($p = 0.003$) and OS ($p = 0.036$). Three-year DFS and OS rates for ASA score 1-2 were 38% and 79%, respectively, compared with 6% and 67%, respectively, for ASA score 3 and 0% and 38%, respectively, for ASA score 4.

Extension of hepatic resection (Figure 4) resulted associated with OS ($p = 0.024$) and approached statistical significance in DFS ($p = 0.060$). Patients treated with RF had the worst DFS with 1-year DFS rate of 29% and an HR 2.5 (95% HR CI 1.1–5.7) for DFS if compared to patients treated with wedge/minor hepatic resection. Anyway, 1-year OS for patients treated with RF was 100%. Compared to minor/wedge resections, major hepatectomies had an HR 2.3 (95% HR CI 1.2–4.5) for OS.

Administration of chemotherapy after liver surgery (Figure 5) resulted positively associated with DFS ($p = 0.028$) and OS (0.047). Median time between liver surgery and start of chemotherapy treatment was 6.5 weeks (range 2.1–14.1).

T stage (Figure 6) was found to be a prognostic factor for DFS ($p = 0.002$). T3 stage had an HR 0.65 (95% HR CI 0.3–1.3) for DFS when compared to T1 and 2 stages. Number

TABLE 4: Univariate analysis of factors associated with disease-free and overall survival.

		DFS					OS				
	n	1 y (%)	3 y (%)	5 y (%)	Median (months, CI)	*p* value	1 y (%)	3 y (%)	5 y (%)	Median (months, CI)	*p* value
Timing of metastases presentation/treatment						**<0.0001**					0.085
Synchronous combined	**25**	52	24	20	14.4 (7.2–27.8)		92	66	48	45.3 (31–NE)	
Synchronous "bowel first"	**14**	16	0	0	6 (2–11.4)		84	45	22	23.6 (11.8–70.9)	
Metachronous	**31**	83	19	19	23.5 (14–28.8)		100	78	67	65.7 (58.2–77.2)	
Age						0.648					0.552
<65	**21**	57	14	14	15.2 (7.2–22.1)		100	69	69	67.5 (23.6–77.9)	
≥65	**49**	59	19	16	16.2 (10.4–23.5)		91	68	46	53 (37.9–65.7)	
Sex						0.574					0.929
Male	**40**	59	14	11	16.4 (8.9–21.7)		95	75	57	64.2 (44.4–NE)	
Female	**30**	58	22	22	14 (8.3–23.7)		93	58	49	38.1 (27.1–119.3)	
Bowel obstruction						0.860					0.985
No	**51**	59	17	15	16.4 (10.4–21.7)		92	69	52	62.6 (43.7–70.9)	
Yes	**19**	56	17	0	12.7 (4.2–28.7)		100	64	57	65.7 (21.7–119.3)	
Site of primary tumor						0.488					0.661
Right colon	**21**	60	20	20	16.2 (8.5–29.4)		90	53	41	37.9 (17.1–77.2)	
Left colon	**49**	58	16	13	15.2 (9.4–19.2)		96	74	60	64.7 (44.4–67.8)	
CHT before liver surgery						0.080					0.531
No	**37**	62	23	20	19.2 (8.5–28.7)		92	71	52	62.6 (37.9–77.2)	
Yes	**33**	54	10	10	12.7 (9.4–18)		97	63	58	62.7 (31.1–70.9)	
Colorectal surgery											
Technique						0.885					0.058
Open and converted	**39**	60	15	15	16.2 (8.9–24.8)		92	61	44	45.3 (31.3–67.1)	
Minimally invasive	**31**	57	20	16	15.2 (8.3–23.5)		97	78	72	NE (43.7–NE)	
Peritoneal resection						0.414					**0.026**
No	**65**	60	17	15	16.4 (11.8–21.7)		97	72	56	62.7 (44.3–67.8)	
Yes	**5**	40	20	20	3.3 (1.3–NE)		60	20	20	12.4 (1.3–NE)	
Liver surgery											
ASA						**0.003**					**0.036**
1-2	**28**	73	38	33	21.5 (12.4–67.8)		92	79	62	67.8 (45.3–NE)	
3	**34**	52	6	6	12.6 (7.2–22.4)		97	67	54	62.6 (32–67.1)	
4	**8**	38	0	0	10.9 (1.3–19.2)		88	38	25	20.5 (1.3–NE)	
Type of surgery						0.060					**0.024**
Minor/wedge	**46**	59	22	19	18 (10.4–27.8)		93	69	57	65.7 (43.7–NE)	
Major	**17**	69	13	13	14 (6–21.5)		94	54	34	37.9 (14–62.7)	
RFA	**7**	29	0	0	5 (1.5–18)		100	86	86	62.6 (12.4–119.3)	
Surgery duration						0.999					0.945
<255 min	**34**	67	13	13	18 (12–25)		94	71	55	64.7 (38.1–67.8)	
≥255 min	**36**	51	21	18	12.4 (8.5–21.7)		94	65	51	62.6 (31.1–70.9)	
Complications (CD III-IV)						0.441					0.721
No	**60**	59	18	16	16.2 (10.4–22.1)		95	68	53	62.6 (38.1–67.5)	
Yes	**10**	58	12	12	12.6 (1.3–30.9)		89	67	53	77.2 (9.2–77.2)	
CHT after liver surgery						**0.028**					**0.047**
No	**31**	48	14	9	12 (5–18.1)		90	61	43	53 (19.2–70.9)	
Yes	**39**	67	20	20	18 (11.8–27.8)		97	72	50	67.1 (44.4–70.9)	

Table 4: Continued.

	n	DFS 1 y (%)	DFS 3 y (%)	DFS 5 y (%)	DFS Median (months, CI)	DFS p value	OS 1 y (%)	OS 3 y (%)	OS 5 y (%)	OS Median (months, CI)	OS p value
Colorectal specimen											
Size						0.510					0.188
≤33 mm	**26**	60	8	8	18 (8.9–21.7)		100	79	57	62.7 (45.3–70.9)	
34–49 mm	**20**	69	24	16	23.5 (7.3–29.4)		95	72	64	65.7 (32–119.3)	
≥50 mm	**24**	48	22	22	11.8 (6–15.2)		87	51	40	37.9 (12.6–67.8)	
T stage						**0.002**					0.347
1-2	**11**	51	10	10	12.4 (5–21.6)		90	68	28	53 (6–77.2)	
3	**56**	62	19	17	16.6 (11.8–23.5)		96	68	59	64.7 (43.7–67.7)	
4	**3**	0	0	0	3 (2–3.3)		50	50	50	40 (9.2–70.9)	
Positive nodes						0.098					**0.018**
0	**25**	75	21	21	20.3 (12.4–28.8)		96	86	65	67 (53–119.3)	
1–3	**21**	54	21	16	14.4 (5.8–28.7)		100	83	64	64.7 (37.9–70.9)	
4+	**24**	46	10	10	10.4 (3.6–16.6)		87	37	31	21.7 (14–77.2)	
Mucinous histotype						0.940					0.286
No	**57**	58	17	15	58.2 (38–67)		96	68	50		
Yes	**13**	60	17	17	(9–119.3)		84	67	67		
Liver specimen											
Resected lesions						**0.0001**					0.066
1	**35**	73	26	22	21.6 (15.2–28.7)		91	74	56	64.7 (43.7–77.2)	
2-3	**20**	63	16	16	14.4 (7.3–23.5)		95	60	54	62.7 (21.7–NE)	
4+	**8**	13	0	0	5.7 (1.9–8.5)		100	43	14	27.1 (13.9–38.1)	
Size						0.199					0.088
I tertile	**20**	55	20	15	17.2 (8.5–25)		90	73	50	60.4 (31.3–67.5)	
II tertile	**22**	73	25	25	22.5 (12–28.8)		95	75	60	NE (32–NE)	
III tertile	**21**	57	11	11	12.6 (5–24.8)		94	45	39	31.5 (14–70.9)	
Margin status						**0.032**					0.859
Negative	**59**	63	20	18	16.5 (12–23.5)		100	66	50	58.2 (37.9–67.5)	
Positive	**4**	38	0	0	4.8 (2–15.2)		93	50	50	47.2 (23.6–70.1)	

NE = not evaluable; CHT = chemotherapy; ASA = American Society of Anesthesiologists; Minor/wedge = minor hepatectomies/hepatic wedge resections; Major = major hepatectomies; RFA = radiofreqency ablation; CD III-IV = Clavien-Dindo classification grade III-IV. T stage according to TNM definition AJCC 7th edition.

of positive nodes (Figure 7) was significantly associated with OS ($p = 0.018$). In case of no positive nodes, 3-year OS rate was 86% compared to 83% with 1–3 positive nodes and 37% with at least 4 positive nodes.

Number of liver resected lesions (Figure 8) significantly affected DFS ($p < 0.0001$). For OS, a statistically significant difference was approached ($p = 0.066$). Patients with a single liver metastasis had a 3-year DFS rate of 26% compared to 16% and 0% for patients with 2-3 or 4 or more lesions, respectively. Patients with 4 or more liver lesions had a HR 7.4 (95% HR CI 3–18.4) for DFS when compared to patients with only one liver lesion. Positive liver margins (Figure 9) significatively affected DFS ($p = 0.032$). Patients with positive liver margin had an HR 3.5 (95% HR CI 1–11.6) for DFS if compared to the other patients.

Results of multivariate analysis for DFS and OS are displayed in Tables 5 and 6, respectively. Metachronous presentation, lower ASA score, and administration of chemotherapy (both before and after liver surgery) resulted significantly associated with a longer DFS. Synchronous presentation treated with combined surgery, absence of positive nodes, no peritoneal resection during colorectal surgery, and minimally invasive techniques used to perform colorectal resection were found to be significantly associated with longer OS.

3.2. Discussion. Several prognostic factors for DFS and OS in patients affected by liver metastasis from CRC have been found in this study. Although score systems considering different prognostic factors for CRC already exist [10], this study was conceived to investigate the role of potential prognostic factors related to the patients and either to primary tumor and liver metastasis in a restricted and recently treated cohort of patients. Study group included a consecutive series

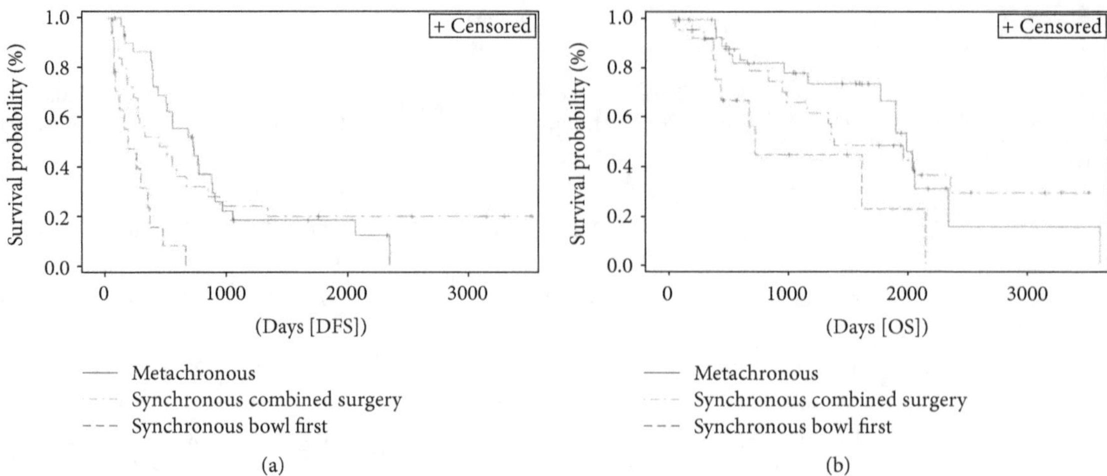

Figure 1: Kaplan-Meier curve of disease-free survival (DFS) ($p < 0.0001$) and overall survival (OS) ($p = 0.085$) stratified by timing of metastases presentation/treatment. Median DFS and OS for patients with synchronous presentation and combined surgery were 14.4 months (95% CI 7.2–27.8) and 45.3 months (95% CI 31–not evaluable [NE]), respectively, versus 6 (95% CI 2–11.4) and 23.6 months (95% CI 11.8–70.9), respectively, for those with synchronous presentation treated with a two-step surgery versus 23.5 (95% CI 14–28.8) and 65.7 months (95% CI 58.2–77.2), respectively, for patients with metachronous presentation.

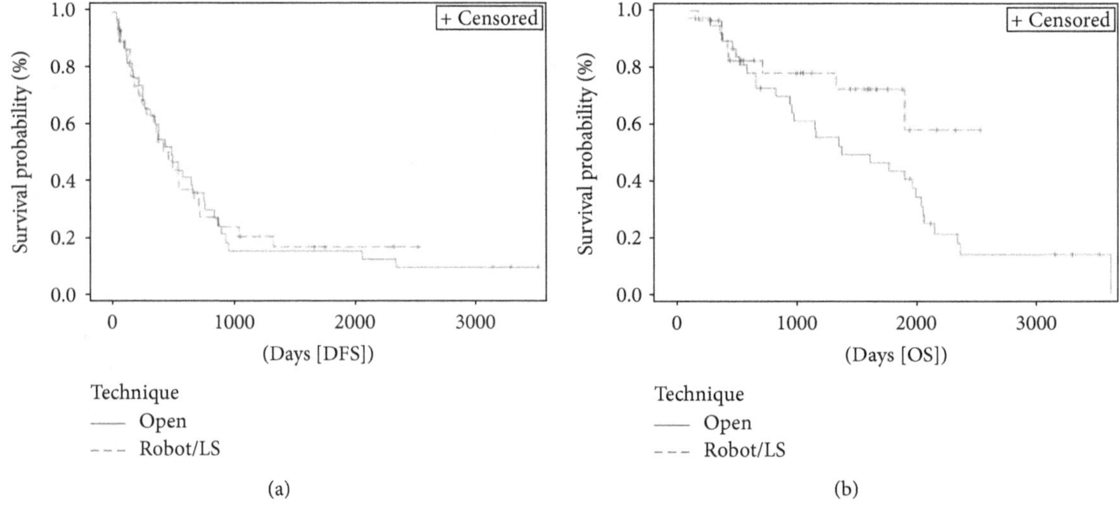

Figure 2: Kaplan-Meier curve of disease-free survival (DFS) ($p = 0.885$) and overall survival (OS) ($p = 0.058$) stratified by technique used to perform colorectal resection. Median DFS and OS for patients undergoing open and converted to open surgery techniques were 16.2 months (95% CI 8.9–24.8) and 45.3 months (95% CI 31.3–67.1), respectively, versus 15.2 (95% CI 8.3–23.5) and NE, respectively, for those undergoing minimally invasive surgery. Open = open surgery approach and "converted to open surgery"; robot/LS = minimally invasive approach including robotic and laparoscopic surgery; NE = not evaluable.

of patients suffering from liver metastasis as first recurrence of disease and undergoing potentially curative resection of liver metastases.

Time of metastatic presentation was a significant prognostic factor in both uni- and multivariate analyses. Patients with synchronous presentation treated with a two-step surgery had the worst prognosis. This group of patients was older, more frequently presenting with bowel obstruction and more comorbidities, with higher percentage of rectal localization of the primary tumor (57% versus 12%) and bigger lesions (median maximum size of 54 mm versus 35 mm). On the contrary, patients undergoing combined surgery received more frequently a parenchymal-sparing operation for smaller and for a median lower number of liver lesions. Obviously, surgery time was significantly longer in "combined surgery" group since surgery included also colorectal resection. However, no negative effects were determined on incidence of postoperative severe complications or on prognosis. Correct timing of resection, especially in synchronous presentation, and unequivocal criteria for surgery are still under debate [3]. In a recently published English population-based study, Vallance et al. [16] demonstrated an increase in number of combined surgery performed along the years, mostly since 2010. Patients fit for surgery, primary

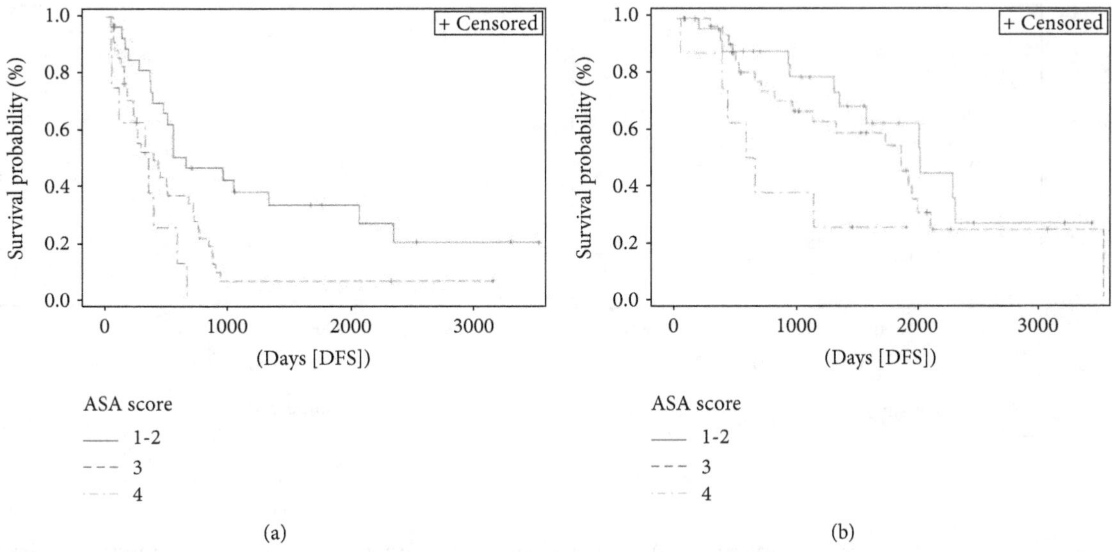

FIGURE 3: Kaplan-Meier curve of disease-free survival (DFS) ($p = 0.003$) and overall survival (OS) ($p = 0.036$) stratified by American Society of Anesthesiologists (ASA) score. Median DFS and OS for patients with ASA score 1-2 were 21.5 months (95% CI 12.4–67.8) and 67.8 months (95% CI 45.3–not evaluable [NE]), respectively, versus 12.6 (95% CI 7.2–22.4) and 62.6 months (95% CI 32–67.1), respectively, for those with ASA score 3 versus 10.9 (95% CI 1.3–19.2) and 20.5 months (95% CI 1.3–NE), respectively, for patients with ASA score 4.

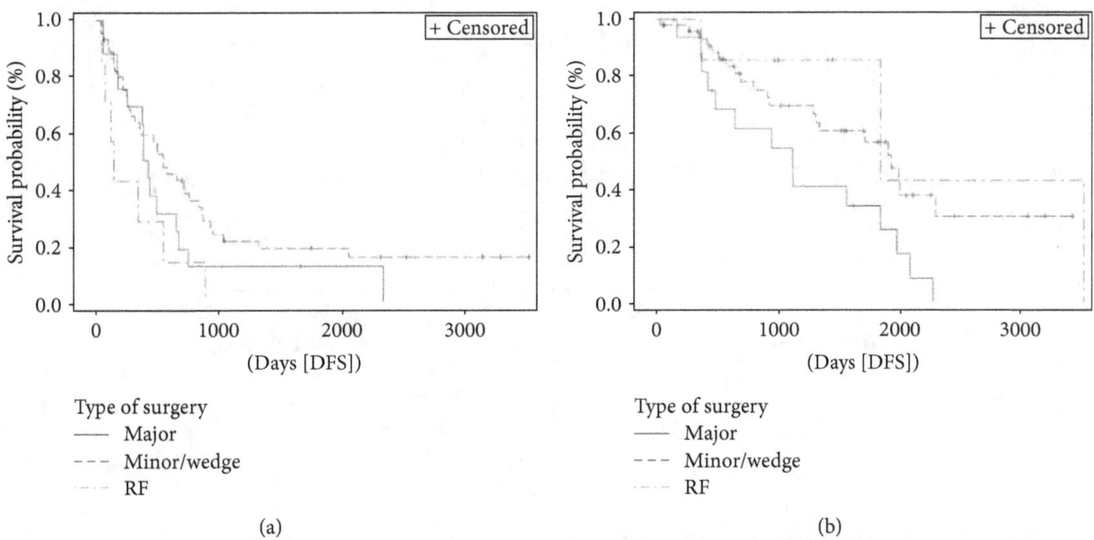

FIGURE 4: Kaplan-Meier curve of disease-free survival (DFS) ($p = 0.060$) and overall survival (OS) ($p = 0.024$) stratified by extension of liver resection. Median DFS and OS for patients undergoing major hepatectomies were 14 months (95% CI 6–21.5) and 37.9 months (95% CI 14–62.7), respectively, versus 18 (95% CI 10.4–27.8) and 65.7 months (95% CI 43.7–NE), respectively, for those undergoing a minor/wedge resections versus 5 (95% CI 1.5–18) and 62.6 months (95% CI 12.4–119.3), respectively, for patients treated with radiofrequency ablation. Major = major hepatectomies; minor/wedge = minor hepatic resection/wedge resection; RF = radiofrequency ablation; NE = not evaluable.

tumor not located in the rectum and superficial and unilobar metastases are the best conditions in which to perform a combined surgery without increase in morbidity and mortality rates [16, 17].

The site of primary tumor did not represent a significant prognostic factor in this series. A slight better prognosis was found for left-sided tumors. On the contrary, recent evidences show a worse prognosis for right colon cancer compared to left colon cancer and the relation between side and genetic alterations, molecular profile, and, consequently, response to chemotherapy [18, 19]. Prognostic relevance of the primary tumor side with a more indolent biology of left-sided cancer was also confirmed in the subgroup of metastatic patients [20, 21]. In the present study, rectal cancer that may have different prognosis was included within left colon group. However, there are previous published reports confirming a better prognosis for patients with liver metastasis from left colon and rectal cancer considered together [3, 22, 23]. Unfortunately, RAS and BRAF status evaluation was unavailable for a great part of this study group

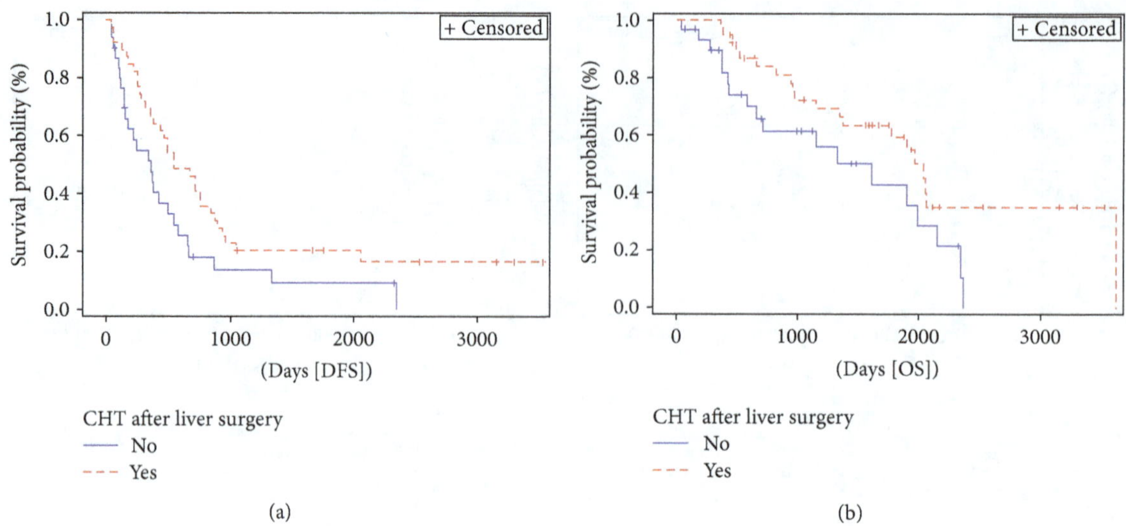

Figure 5: Kaplan-Meier curve of disease-free survival (DFS) ($p = 0.028$) and overall survival (OS) ($p = 0.047$) stratified by administration of chemotherapy after liver surgery. Median DFS and OS for patients not receiving chemotherapy were 12 months (95% CI 5–18.1) and 53 months (95% CI 19.2–70.9), respectively, versus 18 (95% CI 11.8–27.8) and 67.1 months (95% CI 44.4–119.3), respectively, for those receiving chemotherapy. CHT = chemotherapy.

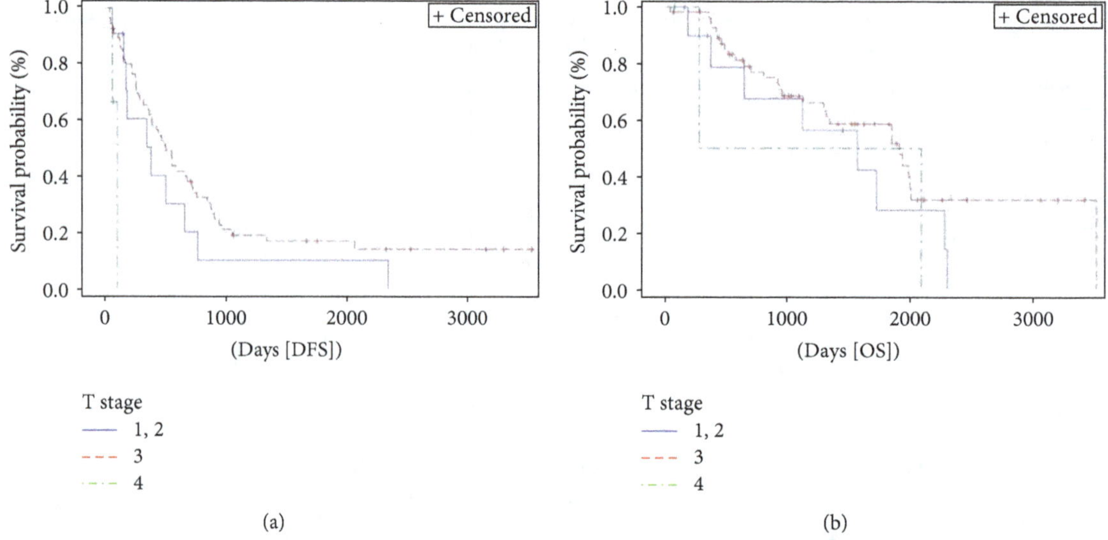

Figure 6: Kaplan-Meier curve of disease-free survival (DFS) ($p = 0.002$) and overall survival (OS) ($p = 0.347$) stratified by T stage*. Median DFS and OS for T1-2 stages were 12.4 months (95% CI 5–21.6) and 53 months (95% CI 6–77.2), respectively, versus 16.6 (95% CI 11.8–23.5) and 64.7 months (95% CI 43.7–67.7), respectively, for T3 stage versus 3 (95% CI 2–3.3) and 40 months (95% CI 9.2–70.9), respectively, T4 stage. *T stage of primary tumor classified according AJCC TNM staging system.

(44.3%) precluding further analysis of this parameter. However, RAS mutation was documented in 15 patients and 10 of them had a left-sided tumor confirming the relevance of molecular feature for the prognosis more than side of the tumor itself.

Technique chosen to perform colorectal surgery was an independent prognostic factor for OS ($p = 0.007$) on multivariate analysis. Advent of minimally invasive surgery was followed by many reports demonstrating at least not inferiority of these new techniques in oncological outcomes [24, 25]. Nevertheless, the well-known advantages in postoperative outcomes of minimally invasive technique with reduction of surgical stress and better preservation of immune system [4], together with lower risk of incisional hernias and adhesions, may explain this benefit in OS rate.

Peritoneal resection at colorectal resection resulted strongly associated with OS rate in both univariate and multivariate analyses even though in the presence of wide 95% confidence intervals. This is consistent with previous findings that peritoneal wound seems to be predictive of the alterations in the immune response more than skin incision [4]. Anyway, the small sample of patients who received a peritoneal resection should lead to a careful and critical analysis of these results.

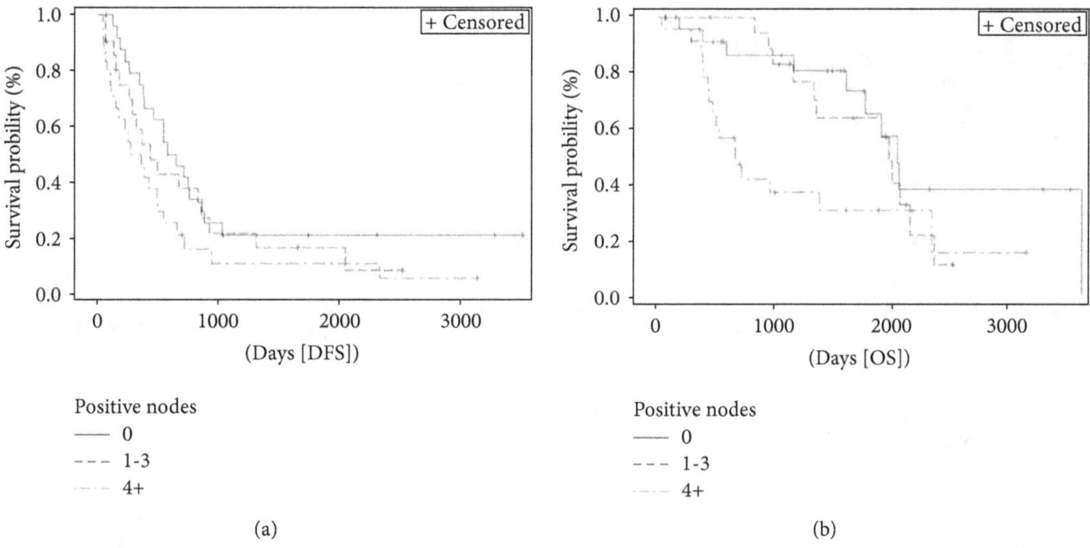

FIGURE 7: Kaplan-Meier curve of disease-free survival (DFS) ($p = 0.098$) and overall survival (OS) ($p = 0.018$) stratified by positive nodes. Median DFS and OS for patients without positive nodes were 20.3 months (95% CI 12.4–28.8) and 67 months (95% CI 53–119.3), respectively, versus 14.4 (95% CI 5.8–28.7) and 64.7 months (95% CI 37.9–70.9), respectively, for those with 1 to 3 positive lymph nodes versus 10.4 (95% CI 3.6–16.6) and 21.7 months (95% CI 14–77.2), respectively, for patients 4 or more positive lymph nodes.

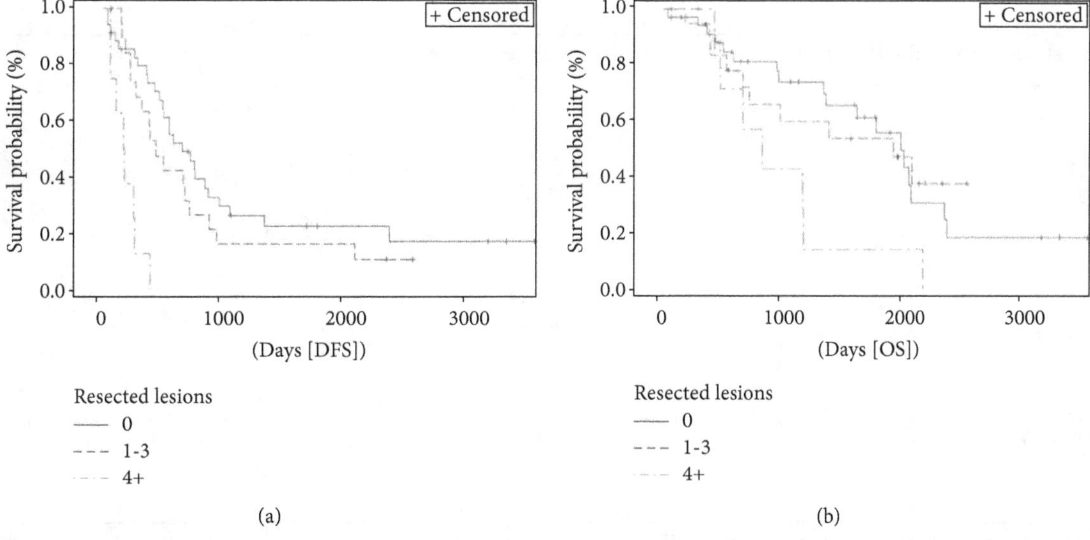

FIGURE 8: Kaplan-Meier curve of disease-free survival (DFS) ($p = 0.0001$) and overall survival (OS) ($p = 0.066$) stratified by number of resected metastatic lesions. Median DFS and OS for patients with 1 metastasis were 21.6 months (95% CI 15.2–28.7) and 64.7 months (95% CI 43.7–77.2), respectively, versus 14.4 (95% CI 7.3–23.5) and 62.7 months (95% CI 21.7–NE), respectively, for those with 2 or 3 metastases versus 5.7 (95% CI 1.9–8.5) and 27.1 months (95% CI 13.9–38.1), respectively, for patients with 4 or more metastases. NE = not evaluable.

ASA score resulted a prognostic factor for DFS in both uni- and multivariate analyses and for OS in univariate analysis. It seems quite obvious that patients in worst conditions may have a worse response against the tumor and have higher chance to die for any cause. Careful selection of ASA 4 patients suitable for surgery is recommended.

In univariate analysis, extension of liver resection approached statistical significance for DFS ($p = 0.060$) and resulted significantly associated with OS ($p = 0.024$). Radiofrequency ablation did not provide equivalent DFS rates when compared to resections. However, beyond intrinsic technical limits, this treatment was used in selected and fragile patients with smaller lesions that may be associated with multiple micrometastasis explaining lower DFS rates consistent with previous literature reports [26]. On the other hand, lesions may be completely treated, and in case of recurrence, procedure may be repeated with a minimum impact on the patients and on liver function explaining encouraging OS rates. Patients undergoing minor hepatic resection or wedge resection had a better prognosis compared to major

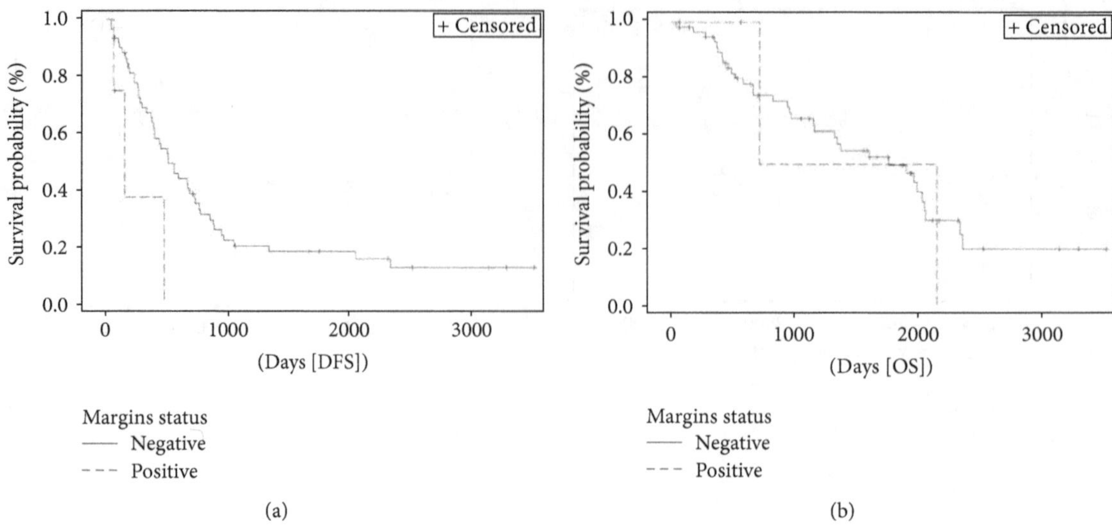

FIGURE 9: Kaplan-Meier curve of disease-free survival (DFS) ($p = 0.032$) and overall survival (OS) ($p = 0.859$) stratified by liver margin status. Median DFS and OS for patients with negative margins were 16.5 months (95% CI 12–23.5) and 58.2 months (95% CI 37.9–67.5), respectively, versus 4.8 (95% CI 2–15.2) and 47.2 months (95% CI 23.6–70.1), respectively, for those having positive margins.

TABLE 5: Multivariate analysis of factors associated with disease-free survival.

	p value	HR	HR and 95% CI
Timing of metastases presentation/treatment	**0.0008**		
Synchronous "combined surgery"	ref	ref	ref
Synchronous "bowel first"	*0.219*	1.9	0.7–5.5
Metachronous	*0.067*	0.5	0.2–1.1
ASA	**0.005**		
1-2	ref	ref	ref
3	*0.001*	2.7	1.5–4.9
4	*0.134*	2.1	0.8–5.5
CHT before liver surgery	**0.027**		
No	ref	ref	ref
Yes	*0.027*	2.5	1.1–5.6
CHT after liver surgery	**0.028**		
No	ref	ref	ref
Yes	*0.028*	0.5	0.2–0.9

ref = reference; ASA = American Society of Anesthesiologists; CHT = chemotherapy.

hepatectomies with a 5-year OS rate of 57% compared to 34%. Parenchymal-sparing operations are becoming the standard of care for CRC liver metastasis even in light of possible liver relapse of disease that may require redo surgery with curative possibilities [27, 28]. Several papers reported the advantages of this technique in terms of reduced postoperative morbidity and some survival benefit with adequate oncological outcomes. In consideration of these results, parenchymal-sparing surgery should be preferred, whenever technically feasible [29, 30].

Chemotherapy before liver surgery resulted a negative prognostic factor for DFS in multivariate analysis in the present study. Vigano et al. [8] proposed to evaluate patient response between end of chemotherapy and liver resection as a "time test" and a prognostic factor suggesting the possibility to exclude from surgery about a 15% of patients who would present early recurrence. However, their findings deserve further evaluations. On the contrary, in this series, administration of chemotherapy after liver surgery resulted a positive prognostic factor for DFS and OS in univariate analysis and for DFS in multivariate analysis. Median time between liver surgery and initiation of chemotherapy was 6.5 weeks (range 2.1–14.1). Obviously, there is a group of patients who could be indicated for adjuvant treatments because of the stage of disease, but they are not considered fit for them. This is mostly related to older age and comorbidities such as previous heart disease. All these factors may be related to the worst OS rate more than chemotherapy itself, coherently with multivariate analysis results. Previously published papers reported improved outcomes after adjuvant

TABLE 6: Multivariate analysis of factors associated with overall survival.

	p value	HR	HR and 95% CI
Timing of metastases presentation/treatment	**0.053**		
Synchronous "combined surgery"	ref	ref	ref
Synchronous "bowel first" surgery"	*0.025*	2.8	1.1–7
Metachronous	*0.895*	1.1	0.5–2.3
Positive nodes	**0.008**		
0	ref	ref	ref
1–3	*0.267*	1.7	0.7–4.4
4+	*0.003*	3.8	1.6–9.1
Peritoneal resection	**0.0003**		
No	ref	ref	ref
Yes	*0.0003*	12.1	3.1–46.7
Technique for colon resection	**0.007**		
Open	ref	ref	ref
Minimally invasive	*0.007*	0.3	0.1–0.7

ref = reference.

chemotherapy without an increase in OS [10, 31] confirming also that elderly patients are often oncologically undertreated [32]. Nevertheless, initiation of chemotherapy within 6–8 weeks is a recognized prognostic factor for OS [33, 34]. Unfortunately, the small sample of patients receiving chemotherapy after surgery in this series precluded a subgroup analysis of the impact of the different chemotherapy regimens and use of molecular targeted therapies.

T stage but not tumor size resulted a prognostic factor for DFS on univariate analysis. While T4 stage resulted associated with very low DFS and OS rates after liver surgery, interestingly, T3 stage had a better prognosis if compared to T1-2 stages. This may be related to the different administrations of chemotherapy being T1-2 stages usually not indicated for chemotherapy. This explanation is consistent with the results of multivariate analysis in which chemotherapy but not T stage resulted independent prognostic factor for DFS. Positive nodes resulted significantly associated with OS in uni- and multivariate analyses. These findings underline the prognostic impact of AJCC TNM classification. Careful selection for liver surgery in patients with a primary tumor T4 stage or N2 is recommended.

Number of resected liver lesions was significantly associated with DFS. On the contrary, size of resected liver lesions did not affect prognosis in this series. Interestingly, intermediate size of liver lesions showed better DFS rates when compared with smaller or bigger lesions. A possible explanation may be that in case of small lesions, presence of multifocal undetectable micrometastases is possible while bigger lesions are related to a huge burden of disease.

Liver margin status was an independent prognostic factor for OS, accordingly to the prognostic importance of at least submillimetric clear margin which has been previously reported [35].

This study has some limitations. It is a retrospective study with the inherent selection bias. It is a small series leading to a careful and critical interpretation of some findings. Nevertheless, because of the small sample available, some variables analyzed were divided into subgroup that may include patients with different prognosis related to that variable (i.e., left colon including rectum or administration of chemotherapy without distinction if a molecular targeted therapy was added or not). A strength of this paper is that a recent series of resected patients has been analyzed, but on the other hand, follow-up period is quite short considering the proposal of at least 10-year follow-up due to the possibility of late recurrence [10]. Furthermore, although follow-up scheduled program was standardized, some patients may be evaluated with a different timing and patient compliance was not always complete. Consequently, date of recurrence may be influenced.

4. Conclusions

In the treatment of liver metastases from CRC, several factors were associated with at least marginal significance with either DFS or OS. Synchronous presentation treated with combined surgery and metachronous presentation, use of a minimally invasive technique in colorectal surgery, no necessity to perform a peritoneal resection in colorectal surgery, minor/wedge liver resection, administration of chemotherapy after liver surgery, T1–3 stages, negative lymph nodes, single liver lesions and negative liver margins were related with better prognosis. Moreover, none of the analyzed factor was associated with a so bad prognosis to contraindicate surgery.

Multimodality and multidisciplinary treatment is of paramount importance to achieve higher cure rates, and in this light, DFS should be the most important parameter to evaluate. Aggressive perioperative systemic treatment may be required in the presence of negative prognostic factors, whenever possible. Nevertheless, patient selection remains challenging and further improvements in prognostication are necessary to identify patients unlikely to benefit from resection.

References

[1] H. J. Bonjer, C. L. Deijen, G. A. Abis et al., "A randomized trial of laparoscopic versus open surgery for rectal cancer," *New England Journal of Medicine*, vol. 372, no. 14, pp. 1324–1332, 2015.

[2] F. Tonelli, F. Leo, S. Nobili, E. Mini, and G. Batignani, "Prognostic factors in primary and iterative surgery of colorectal liver metastases," *Journal of Chemotherapy*, vol. 22, no. 5, pp. 358–363, 2010.

[3] J. Engstrand, H. Nilsson, C. Strömberg, E. Jonas, and J. Freedman, "Colorectal cancer liver metastases - a population-based study on incidence, management and survival," *BMC Cancer*, vol. 18, no. 1, p. 78, 2018.

[4] C. Behrenbruch, C. Shembrey, S. Paquet-Fifield et al., "Surgical stress response and promotion of metastasis in colorectal cancer: a complex and heterogeneous process," *Clinical & Experimental Metastasis*, 2018.

[5] M. Horowitz, E. Neeman, E. Sharon, and S. Ben-Eliyahu, "Exploiting the critical perioperative period to improve long-term cancer outcomes," *Nature Reviews Clinical Oncology*, vol. 12, no. 4, pp. 213–226, 2015.

[6] R. Kim, M. Emi, K. Tanabe, and K. Arihiro, "Tumor-driven evolution of immunosuppressive networks during malignant progression," *Cancer Research*, vol. 66, no. 11, pp. 5527–5536, 2006.

[7] E. Neeman and S. Ben-Eliyahu, "Surgery and stress promote cancer metastasis: new outlooks on perioperative mediating mechanisms and immune involvement," *Brain, Behavior, and Immunity*, vol. 30, pp. S32–S40, 2013.

[8] L. Vigano, S. S. Darwish, L. Rimassa et al., "Progression of colorectal liver metastases from the end of chemotherapy to resection: a new contraindication to surgery?," *Annals of Surgical Oncology*, vol. 25, no. 6, pp. 1676–1685, 2018.

[9] T. M. Pawlik, R. D. Schulick, and M. A. Choti, "Expanding criteria for resectability of colorectal liver metastases," *The Oncologist*, vol. 13, no. 1, pp. 51–64, 2008.

[10] J. M. Creasy, E. Sadot, B. G. Koerkamp et al., "Actual 10-year survival after hepatic resection of colorectal liver metastases: what factors preclude cure?," *Surgery*, vol. 163, no. 6, pp. 1238–1244, 2018.

[11] "NCCN clinical practice guidelines in oncology (NCCN guidelines®) colon cancer," Version 2.2018 — March 14, 2018 https://www.nccn.org/professionals/physician_gls/pdf/colon.pdf.

[12] "NCCN clinical practice guidelines in oncology (NCCN guidelines®) rectal cancer," Version 1.2018 — March 14, 2018 https://www.nccn.org/professionals/physician_gls/pdf/rectal.pdf.

[13] Terminology Committee of the International Hepato-Pancreato-Biliary Association, S. M. Strasberg, J. Belghiti et al., "The Brisbane 2000 terminology of liver anatomy and resections," *HPB*, vol. 2, no. 3, pp. 333–339, 2000.

[14] P. A. Clavien, J. Barkun, M. L. de Oliveira et al., "The Clavien-Dindo classification of surgical complications: five-year experience," *Annals of Surgery*, vol. 250, no. 2, pp. 187–196, 2009.

[15] S. B. Edge and C. C. Compton, "The American Joint Committee on Cancer: the 7th edition of the *AJCC cancer staging manual* and the future of TNM," *Annals of Surgical Oncology*, vol. 17, no. 6, pp. 1471–1474, 2010.

[16] A. E. Vallance, J. van der Meulen, A. Kuryba et al., "The timing of liver resection in patients with colorectal cancer and synchronous liver metastases: a population-based study of current practice and survival," *Colorectal Disease*, vol. 20, no. 6, pp. 486–495, 2018.

[17] P. Gavriilidis, R. P. Sutcliffe, J. Hodson et al., "Simultaneous versus delayed hepatectomy for synchronous colorectal liver metastases: a systematic review and meta-analysis," *HPB*, vol. 20, no. 1, pp. 11–19, 2018.

[18] M. Yahagi, K. Okabayashi, H. Hasegawa, M. Tsuruta, and Y. Kitagawa, "The worse prognosis of right-sided compared with left-sided colon cancers: a systematic review and meta-analysis," *Journal of Gastrointestinal Surgery*, vol. 20, no. 3, pp. 648–655, 2016.

[19] E. Missiaglia, B. Jacobs, G. D'Ario et al., "Distal and proximal colon cancers differ in terms of molecular, pathological, and clinical features," *Annals of Oncology*, vol. 25, no. 10, pp. 1995–2001, 2014.

[20] J. M. Creasy, E. Sadot, B. G. Koerkamp et al., "The impact of primary tumor location on long-term survival in patients undergoing hepatic resection for metastatic colon cancer," *Annals of Surgical Oncology*, vol. 25, no. 2, pp. 431–438, 2018.

[21] J. W. Holch, I. Ricard, S. Stintzing, D. P. Modest, and V. Heinemann, "The relevance of primary tumour location in patients with metastatic colorectal cancer: a meta-analysis of first-line clinical trials," *European Journal of Cancer*, vol. 70, pp. 87–98, 2017.

[22] T. J. Price, C. Beeke, S. Ullah et al., "Does the primary site of colorectal cancer impact outcomes for patients with metastatic disease?," *Cancer*, vol. 121, no. 6, pp. 830–835, 2015.

[23] A. Dupré, H. Z. Malik, R. P. Jones, R. Diaz-Nieto, S. W. Fenwick, and G. J. Poston, "Influence of the primary tumour location in patients undergoing surgery for colorectal liver metastases," *European Journal of Surgical Oncology*, vol. 44, no. 1, pp. 80–86, 2018.

[24] J. F. Salem, S. Gummadi, and J. H. Marks, "Minimally invasive surgical approaches to colon cancer," *Surgical Oncology Clinics of North America*, vol. 27, no. 2, pp. 303–318, 2018.

[25] M. N. Ringressi, L. Boni, G. Freschi et al., "Comparing laparoscopic surgery with open surgery for long-term outcomes in patients with stage I to III colon cancer," *Surgical Oncology*, vol. 27, no. 2, pp. 115–122, 2018.

[26] E. K. Abdalla, J. N. Vauthey, L. M. Ellis et al., "Recurrence and outcomes following hepatic resection, radiofrequency ablation, and combined resection/ablation for colorectal liver metastases," *Annals of Surgery*, vol. 239, no. 6, pp. 818–827, 2004.

[27] Y. Mise, T. A. Aloia, K. W. Brudvik, L. Schwarz, J. N. Vauthey, and C. Conrad, "Parenchymal-sparing hepatectomy in colorectal liver metastasis improves salvageability and survival," *Annals of Surgery*, vol. 263, no. 1, pp. 146–152, 2016.

[28] D. Moris, S. Ronnekleiv-Kelly, A. A. Rahnemai-Azar et al., "Parenchymal-sparing versus anatomic liver resection for colorectal liver metastases: a systematic review," *Journal of Gastrointestinal Surgery*, vol. 21, no. 6, pp. 1076–1085, 2017.

[29] M. Donadon, M. Cescon, A. Cucchetti et al., "Parenchymal-sparing surgery for the surgical treatment of multiple colorectal liver metastases is a safer approach than major hepatectomy not impairing patients' prognosis: a bi-institutional propensity score-matched analysis," *Digestive Surgery*, 2017.

[30] G. Torzilli, L. Viganò, A. Gatti et al., "Twelve-year experience of "radical but conservative" liver surgery for colorectal metas-

tases: impact on surgical practice and oncologic efficacy," *HPB*, vol. 19, no. 9, pp. 775–784, 2017.

[31] B. Nordlinger, H. Sorbye, B. Glimelius et al., "Perioperative FOLFOX4 chemotherapy and surgery versus surgery alone for resectable liver metastases from colorectal cancer (EORTC 40983): long-term results of a randomised, controlled, phase 3 trial," *The Lancet Oncology*, vol. 14, no. 12, pp. 1208–1215, 2013.

[32] A. S. Bojer and O. Roikjær, "Elderly patients with colorectal cancer are oncologically undertreated," *European Journal of Surgical Oncology (EJSO)*, vol. 41, no. 3, pp. 421–425, 2015.

[33] Y. W. Kim, E. H. Choi, B. R. Kim, W. A. Ko, Y. M. Do, and I. Y. Kim, "The impact of delayed commencement of adjuvant chemotherapy (eight or more weeks) on survival in stage II and III colon cancer: a national population-based cohort study," *Oncotarget*, vol. 8, no. 45, pp. 80061–80072, 2017.

[34] S. Nachiappan, A. Askari, R. Mamidanna et al., "The impact of adjuvant chemotherapy timing on overall survival following colorectal cancer resection," *European Journal of Surgical Oncology (EJSO)*, vol. 41, no. 12, pp. 1636–1644, 2015.

[35] E. Sadot, B. G. Koerkamp, J. N. Leal et al., "Resection margin and survival in 2368 patients undergoing hepatic resection for metastatic colorectal cancer: surgical technique or biologic surrogate?," *Annals of Surgery*, vol. 262, no. 3, pp. 476–485, 2015.

11

Prognostic Role of Platelet-to-Lymphocyte Ratio in Hepatocellular Carcinoma with Different BCLC Stages

Wan-fu Lin,[1] **Mao-feng Zhong**,[2] **Yu-ren Zhang**,[1] **Huan Wang**,[1] **He-tong Zhao**,[1] **Bin-bin Cheng**,[1] **and Chang-quan Ling**[1]

[1]*Department of Traditional Chinese Medicine, Changhai Hospital, Second Military Medical University, Shanghai 200433, China*
[2]*Graduate School of Shanghai University of Traditional Chinese Medicine, Shanghai 201203, China*

Correspondence should be addressed to Bin-bin Cheng; cbb8202@126.com and Chang-quan Ling; changquanling@smmu.edu.cn

Academic Editor: Nicola Silvestris

The role of platelet-to-lymphocyte ratio (PLR) in the prognosis of hepatocellular carcinoma (HCC) patients with different Barcelona Clinic Liver Cancer (BCLC) stages remains controversial. This systematic review and meta-analysis aimed to determine the efficacy of PLR on HCC prognosis. Five electronic databases were searched for clinical trials focusing on the role of PLR in the prognosis of HCC. A total of 297 potential studies were initially identified, and 9 studies comprising 2449 patients were finally enrolled to evaluate the association between the pretreatment PLR and clinical outcomes of overall survival (OS), disease-free survival (DFS), and event occurrence in patients with HCC in different BCLC stages. An elevated pretreatment PLR indicated unfavorable worse OS (HR = 1.73; 95% CI: (1.46, 2.04); $P < 0.00001$) and DFS (HR = 1.30; 95% CI: (1.06, 1.60); $P = 0.01$). Subgroup analysis indicated that high PLR indicated poor OS among BCLC-B/C patients without heterogeneity, while PLR in BCLC-A patients indicated high statistical heterogeneity with I^2 value of 78%. As for the correlation between PLR and event occurrence, high PLR was related to poor clinical event occurrence only among BCLC-C patients, though obvious heterogeneity was observed in all different BCLC stages. In conclusion, PLR may be a significant biomarker in the prognosis of HCC in different BCLC stages.

1. Introduction

Inflammation, a protective immune response to harmful stimuli such as pathogens and dead cells, is mounted by the evolutionarily conserved innate immune system with tight regulation of host [1]. Homogeneous inflammation is vital for health; insufficient inflammation may lead to persistent infection of pathogens, while excessive inflammation may cause chronic or systemic inflammatory diseases. Inflammation is linked to a variety of diseases such as Alzheimer's disease, Parkinson's disease, diabetes, and cancer [2, 3]. In 1863, Virchow initially clarified the relation of inflammation and cancer through the theory of leukocyte infiltrates within tumors, which is commonly considered a hallmark of cancer now [4, 5]. Since then, more and more evidences have revealed that inflammatory response correlates closely with tumor progression such as angiogenesis and tumor invasion. It is verified that the invasion and migration of tumor cells correlate closely with inflammation-related cells, including lymphocytes [6], neutrophils [7, 8], and platelets [9]. Classically, platelets are considered as crucial effector cells in hemostasis; however, extensive experiments have also illuminated their potential role in inflammatory responses—they may recognize and kill invading pathogens and also release various mediators modifying immune and endothelial cell responses [10]. Besides, clinical studies have also implied that platelets may lead to tumor growth and metastasis [11], since higher platelet counts were associated with shorter survival time and increased recurrence after treatment in various solid tumors [12, 13]. As a crucial component of host immune surveillance system, lymphocyte plays an important role in patients with various types of

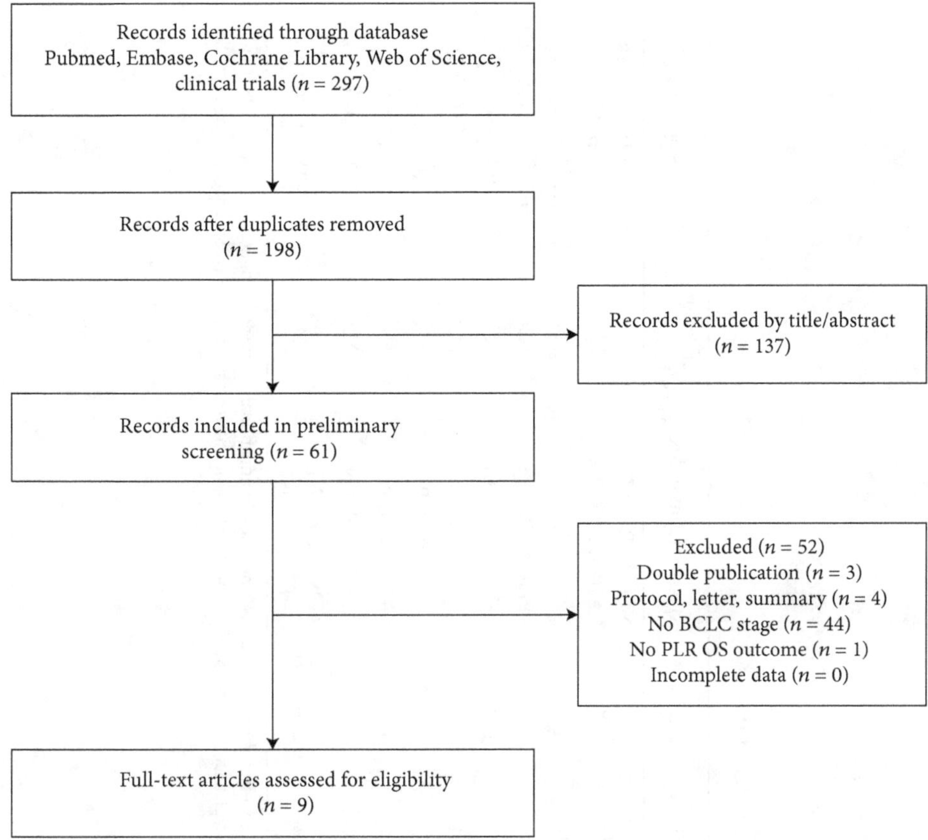

Figure 1: Flow diagram for study identification and inclusion.

malignant neoplasms [14]. Accumulated evidences indicated that tumor-infiltrating lymphocytes may influence disease outcomes of patients with malignant neoplasms [15, 16]—higher platelet counts may indicate a poor prognosis while lymphocyte infiltration around a tumor may associate with a better prognosis; the platelet-to-lymphocyte ratio (PLR) may be a useful index for the prognosis of tumor patients [17, 18].

Hepatocellular carcinoma (HCC) is the second most common cause of cancer-related deaths worldwide and is an aggressive tumor type with poor prognosis [19]. More and more evidences indicate that the occurrence and development of HCC is correlated closely with both inflammation and immunocytes [20, 21]. Recent studies also indicated that PLR may be a potential index for the prognosis of HCC after resection [22], liver transplantation [23], or transarterial chemoembolization (TACE) [24]. However, no agreement is reached among available studies due to small sample size. Thus, we conducted this meta-analysis to evaluate the prognostic role of PLR in different Barcelona Clinic Liver Cancer (BCLC) stages of HCC.

2. Methods

2.1. Information Sources and Search Strategies. Five electronic databases including PubMed, Web of Science, EMBASE, Elsevier, and Cochrane Library were searched for clinical trials in original articles. The last completed database search was undertaken on July 28, 2017. Search terms included "liver cancer," "hepatocellular carcinoma," "hepatoma*," "platelet," "lymphocyte," "platelet to lymphocyte ratio," and "platelet-lymphocyte ratio" title/abstract. References cited in the retrieved articles were also scanned for relevant studies.

The most important inclusive criterion was studies concerning the prognostic role of PLR in HCC. Other eligible criteria include studies with data on BCLC, disease-free survival (DFS), and overall survival (OS). Nonclinical studies, case reports, review articles, editorials, comments, and articles without accessible full text for quality assessment or data extraction were all excluded.

2.2. Data Extraction. The selection of studies was performed independently by 2 reviewers (Wan-fu Lin and Mao-feng Zhong), and the third investigator (Yu-ren Zhang) was consulted to resolve any disagreements. The following data of each included study were collected: the information of authors such as the name and affiliation, year of publication, research time and location, sample size, patients' age, gender, BCLC stage, intervention regimes, inflammation index, time of follow-up, and outcomes of interest. We also contacted the corresponding author if we need more detailed data.

2.3. Quality Appraisal and Risk of Bias. The quality appraisal and risk of bias of each included study were independently evaluated by two reviewers (Huan Wang and He-tong Zhao)

Table 1: Characteristics of the included studies.

Study	Year	Country	Treatment	Study time	Sample size	Mean age (y)	Male	PLR cutoff value	Measurement index	Follow-up (median; months)	BCLC stage of patients
He and Lin et al.	2017	Chinese	TACE	2007.1–2015.7	216	53.05	200	94.62	NLR, PLR, PNI, PI, mGPS, NLR-PLR	14.4	A1 (23); A2 (4); A4 (9); B (98); C (82)
Yang et al.	2017	Chinese	Hepatectomy	2010.4–2013.10	778	51.98	671	150	PLR	NR	0/A (236); B/C (537)
Liu et al.	2016	Chinese	Hepatectomy	2004.7–2011.4	223	54	189	NR	PLR, NLR, APRI	NR	0/A (126); B/C (97)
Casadei et al.	2016	Italy	Sorafenib	2012–2015	56	NR	47	15.0	PLR, NLR, SII	NR	B (13); C (43)
Xue et al.	2016	Chinese	TACE	2007.1–2011.4	178	52.57	154	150	PLR	11.4	B (115); C (63)
Shiozawa et al.	2016	Japan	Sorafenib	2009.6–2015.1	16	67.5	12	ΔPLR% > 20%	NLR, PLR	NR	B (12); C (4)
Chan et al.	2015	Chinese	Hepatectomy	2001.1–2011.11	324	56.8	283	150	PLR, NLR, PNI	NR	A (324)
Xue et al.	2015	Chinese	TACE	2007.1–2011.3	291	53.05	258	150	PLR, NLR, PNI	NR	B (182); C (109)
Ni et al.	2015	Chinese	Hepatectomy	2010.12–2012.1	367	55	308	150 and 300	GPS, mGPS, NLR, PLR, PI, PNI	24	A (244); B (106); C (17)

TACE: transarterial chemoembolization; NR: not reported; NLR: neutrophil-to-lymphocyte ratio; PLR: platelet-to-lymphocyte ratio; PNI: prognostic nutritional index; PI: prognostic index; mGPS: modified Glasgow Prognostic Score; NLR-PLR: neutrophil/platelet-to-lymphocyte ratio; APRI: aspartate aminotransferase/platelet ratio index; SII: systemic immune-inflammation index; GPS: Glasgow Prognostic Score; PI: prognostic index.

Table 2: Quality assessment and risk of bias of the included trials.

Study	Selection				Comparability	Exposure			Score
	1	2	3	4	5	6	7	8	
He and Lin	*	*			*	*	*	*	6
Yang et al.	*	*			*	*	*	*	6
Liu et al.	*	*				*	*	*	5
Casadei et al.	*	*			*	*	*	*	6
Xue et al.	*	*			*	*	*	*	6
Shiozawa et al.	*	*			*	*	*	*	6
Chan et al.	*	*			*	*	*	*	6
Xue et al.	*	*			*	*	*	*	6
Ni et al.	*	*			*	*	*	*	6

*The score of each item.

with Newcastle-Ottawa Quality Assessment Scale (NOS). The scale included 3 parameters of quality: selection, comparability, and outcome assessment, with ranges from 0 to 4, 0 to 1, and 0 to 3 points, respectively. The study with the highest quality may score 9 points. The study with scores ≥ 6 was considered as high quality and scores ≥ 5 as eligible quality. The consensus about the methodological quality of all the studies was achieved since any disagreement between the two reviewers was resolved through discussion.

2.4. Data Synthesis and Analysis. The Review Manager (RevMan, the Cochrane Collaboration, Oxford, UK) version 5.3 was used for data synthesis and analysis. To determine heterogeneity, the chi-squared and I-squared tests were performed. Then, fixed-effect model or random effects model was applied based on the heterogeneity of different trials. Funnel plots and Egger's tests were used to assess the potential publication bias. The main prognosis outcomes were OS, DFS, or recurrence-free survival (RFS). Pooled estimates were expressed as hazard ratios (HR) and 95% confidence interval (CI). $P < 0.05$ with two-side test was considered statistically significant.

3. Results

3.1. Search Results. Two hundred and ninety-seven studies potentially relevant to this research project were initially identified after searching PubMed, Web of Science, EMBASE, Elsevier, and Cochrane Library. After excluding duplicate articles, 198 potentially eligible studies were selected. Of these, 137 studies were excluded after reading the titles and abstracts. The full texts of the remaining 61 studies were carefully screened. Subsequently, 52 papers were further excluded since they did not meet the inclusion criteria. Finally, 9 studies were included in this meta-analysis. The selection process is depicted in Figure 1.

3.2. Characteristics of Included Studies. The 9 included studies were all published between 2015 and 2017 [24–32], among which 7 trials were from China, 1 from Japan, and 1 from Italy. All these trials were retrospective cohort studies with a total of 2449 participants enrolled. Of these included patients, 1692 received hepatic resection, 685 received TACE treatment, and 72 received sorafenib therapy. As for gender, 2122 participants were male (86.65%) compared to 327 female (13.35%), with mean age ranged from 51.98 to 67.5 years. The cases in BCLC stages A, B, and C were 966, 526, and 318, respectively, while 634 participants from 2 trials were not indicated BCLC-B/C clearly, and the remaining 5 participants were not shown BCLC stages. The median follow-up time ranged from 11.4 months to 24 months, excluding 6 studies without exact follow-up time. As for PLR, 8 studies reported a "high" PLR level with survival data, among which the cutoff value of PLR was 150 in 5 included papers and determined using different methods among the other 3 studies. The characteristics of included studies are shown in Table 1.

3.3. Quality Assessment and Risk of Bias of the Included Trials. The quality appraisal and risk of bias of each included review were independently evaluated with Newcastle-Ottawa Quality Assessment Scale, and the result is shown in Table 2. In the table, 1–8 represent the quality indicators from the Newcastle-Ottawa Scale: 1: is the case definition adequate? 2: representativeness of the cases; 3: selection of controls; 4: definition of controls; 5: comparability of cases and controls on the basis of the design or analysis; 6: ascertainment of exposure; 7: same method of ascertainment for cases and controls; 8: nonresponse rate.

All of the 9 papers are eligibility quality studies and 8 of which are considered to show high-quality studies (scores ≥ 6).

3.4. Correlation between PLR and OS. Among all the included trials, 6 studies that reported the relationship between high PLR and OS were selected into this meta-analysis [24–26, 29, 31, 32]. Since the BCLC stages of HCC patients may influence OS significantly, we compared the relationship of PLR and OS among patients with different BCLC stages. The results indicated that in total BCLC stages, the heterogeneity of the high-PLR studies was 10%. Therefore, a random effects model was used for statistical analysis, and the result showed that patients with a high baseline PLR may have a lower OS rate (HR = 1.73; 95% CI: (1.46, 2.04); $P < 0.00001$) (Figure 2(a)). Sensitivity analyses suggested

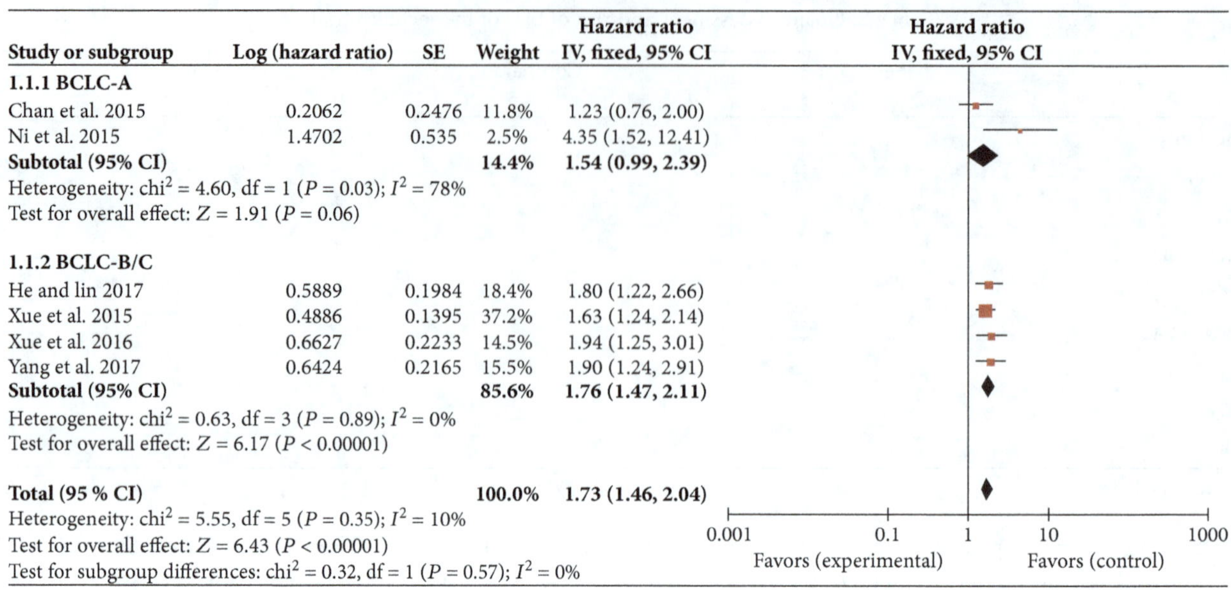

(a)

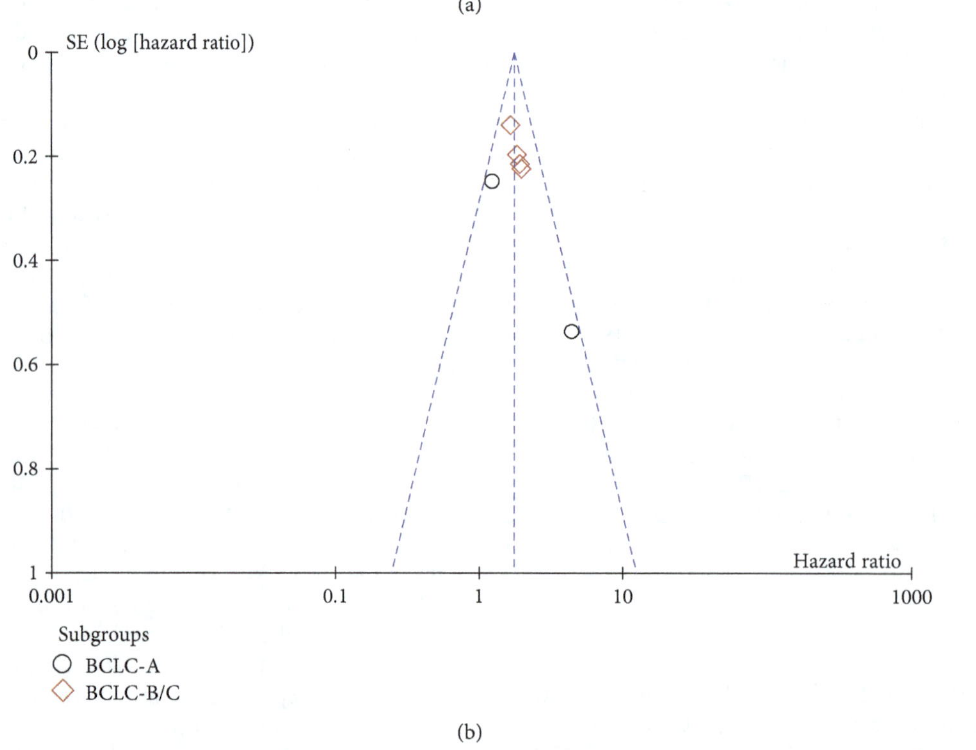

(b)

FIGURE 2: Correlation between platelet-to-lymphocyte ratio and overall survival. (a) Forest plot of comparison of the included trials; (b) funnel plot of comparison of the included trials.

that the pooled effect of the PLR on OS was not affected by changing effect model. The funnel plot was symmetric (Figure 2(b)). For further analysis, we made a reasonable classification of the precise BCLC stage since several trials could not get specific count relationship between the PLR and corresponding BCLC stage in the OS. For example, the study of Ni et al. [32] was considered as BCLC-A subgroup with the larger proportion of BCLC-A patients. Finally, the included studies were divided into BCLC-A subgroup or BCLC-B/C subgroup. The prognostic role of high PLR for OS in different BCLC stages is shown in Figure 2(a). In the BCLC-A subgroup, the result indicated high statistical heterogeneity with an I^2 value of 78% (HR = 1.54; 95% CI: (0.99, 2.39); $P = 0.06$). However, for the BCLC-B/C subgroup, 4 trials showed almost no heterogeneity in the consistency of the trial results ($I^2 = 2\%$). The prognostic role of high PLR for OS was favored with statistically significant (HR = 1.76; 95% CI: (1.47, 2.11); $P < 0.00001$).

3.5. Correlation between PLR and DFS. As another index for the prognosis of HCC patients, DFS was reported in 3 studies [26, 31, 32]. Therefore, the relationship between PLR and

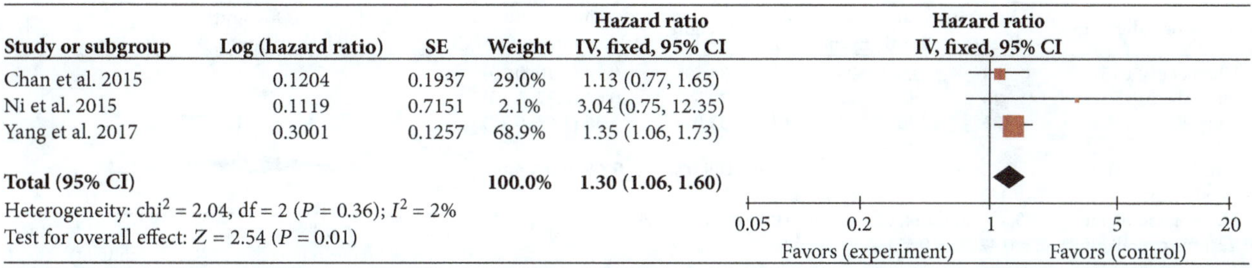

(a)

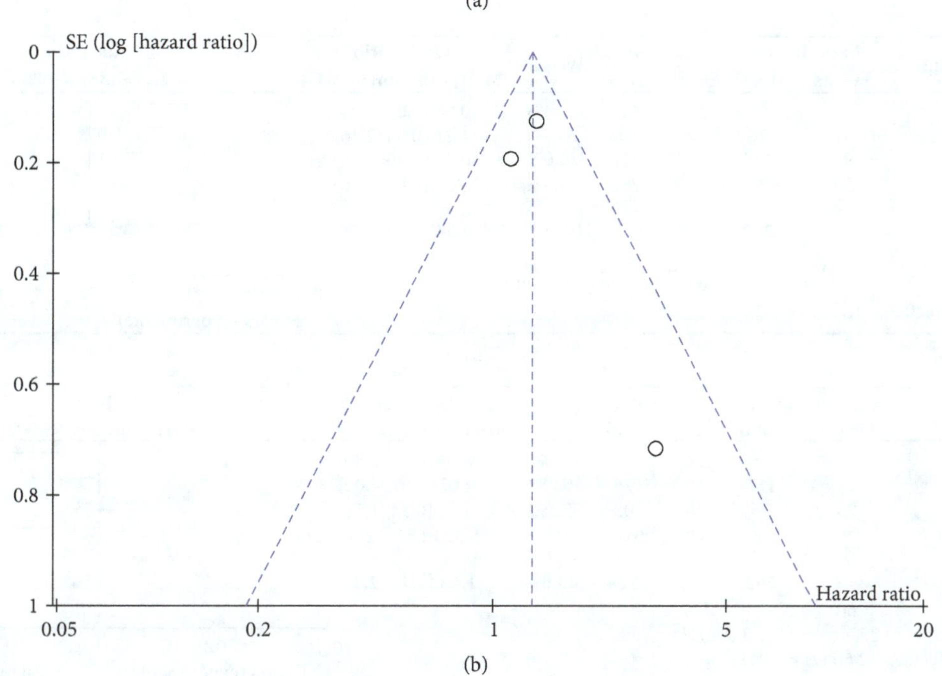

(b)

FIGURE 3: Correlation between platelet-to-lymphocyte ratio and disease-free survival. (a) Forest plot of comparison of the included trials; (b) funnel plot of comparison of the included trials.

DFS of these 3 included studies was analyzed. As shown in Figure 3(a), the result showed mild heterogeneity in the consistency of these trials ($I^2 = 2\%$). Therefore, a random effects model was used for meta-analysis, and the result indicated that patients with high pretreatment PLR had poor DFS (HR = 1.30; 95% CI: (1.06, 1.60); $P = 0.01$). Sensitivity analyses suggested that the pooled effect of PLR on DFS was not affected by changing effect model. The funnel plot was symmetric (Figure 3(b)).

3.6. Correlation between PLR and Event Occurrence. Apart from the main indexes such as OS and DFS observed in these trials, event occurrences such as total bilirubin and alanine transaminase were also indicated in 5 trials [24, 26, 29, 31, 32]. These studies investigated the correlation between PLR and event occurrence. Thus, we further analyze their relationship according to different BCLC stages. As shown in Figures 4(a) and 4(b), the heterogeneity in the results of BCLC-A and BCLC-B was high with an I^2 value of 97% and 87%, respectively. And the test for overall effect indicated no statistical significance ($P > 0.05$). However, for the BCLC-C patients, although obvious heterogeneity was observed in the meta-analysis ($I^2 = 77\%$), the test for overall effect indicated statistical significance ($P = 0.01$), which meant that high PLR may be related to poor clinical event occurrence (Figure 4(c)). Sensitivity analyses suggested that the pooled effect of PLR on event occurrence was affected by changing random effects model. The funnel plot showed that 2 trials were out of the symmetric region (Figure 4(d)).

4. Discussion

As a major health problem, liver cancer is the sixth most common cancer worldwide with approximately 850,000 new cases diagnosed each year and the second leading cause of cancer-related deaths with approximately 800,000 death toll per year. Among all primary liver cancers, HCC constitutes 85–90% [33–35]. However, no standard quantitative biomarkers are perfect enough to assess the clinical outcomes in patients with HCC until now. Considering the reproducible and consistent features of biomarkers, blood parameters such as NLR and PLR may be potential since they are convenient and easy to be acquired during routine clinical practice.

The predicted role of PLR has been studied among various cancers. For example, Zhao et al. [36] evaluated the prognostic significance of PLR in esophageal cancer patients with a total of 6699 patients from 16 studies. The results

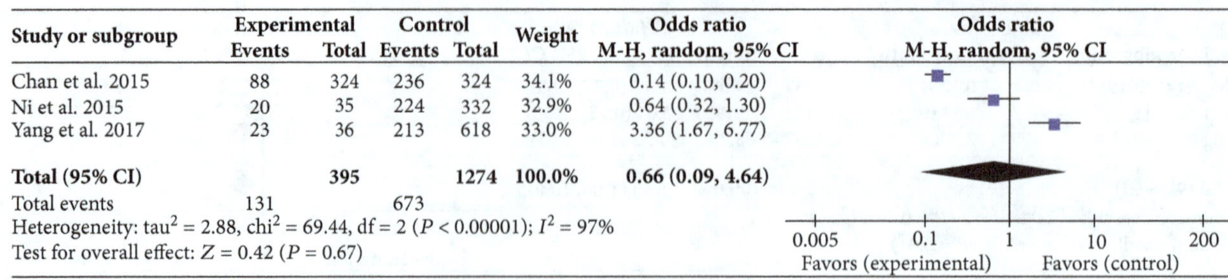

Study or subgroup	Experimental Events	Experimental Total	Control Events	Control Total	Weight	Odds ratio M-H, random, 95% CI
Chan et al. 2015	88	324	236	324	34.1%	0.14 (0.10, 0.20)
Ni et al. 2015	20	35	224	332	32.9%	0.64 (0.32, 1.30)
Yang et al. 2017	23	36	213	618	33.0%	3.36 (1.67, 6.77)
Total (95% CI)		**395**		**1274**	**100.0%**	**0.66 (0.09, 4.64)**
Total events	131		673			

Heterogeneity: $\text{tau}^2 = 2.88$, $\text{chi}^2 = 69.44$, df = 2 ($P < 0.00001$); $I^2 = 97\%$

Test for overall effect: $Z = 0.42$ ($P = 0.67$)

(a)

Study or subgroup	Experimental Events	Experimental Total	Control Events	Control Total	Weight	Odds ratio M-H, random, 95% CI
Yang et al. 2017	4	36	369	618	22.4%	0.08 (0.03, 0.24)
Xue et al. 2016	51	76	64	102	26.3%	1.21 (0.65, 2.26)
Xue et al. 2015	92	115	157	176	26.0%	0.48 (0.25; 0.94)
Ni et al. 2015	12	35	94	332	25.3%	1.32 (0.63, 2.76)
Total (95% CI)		**262**		**1228**	**100.0%**	**0.54 (0.19, 1.52)**
Total events	159		684			

Heterogeneity: $\text{tau}^2 = 0.96$, $\text{chi}^2 = 23.36$, df = 3 ($P < 0.0001$); $I^2 = 87\%$

Test for overall effect: $Z = 1.17$ ($P = 0.24$)

Odds ratio M-H, random, 95% CI: 0.005 0.1 1 10 200 — Favors (experimental) Favors (control)

(b)

Study or subgroup	Experimental Events	Experimental Total	Control Events	Control Total	Weight	Odds ratio M-H, random, 95% CI
Ni et al. 2015	3	35	14	332	6.2%	2.13 (0.58, 7.80)
Xue et al. 2015	23	115	19	176	30.6%	2.07 (1.07, 4.00)
Xue et al. 2016	25	76	38	102	55.5%	0.83 (0.44, 1.54)
Yang et al. 2017	9	36	36	618	7.6%	5.39 (2.36, 12.31)
Total (95% CI)		**262**		**1228**	**100.0%**	**1.63 (1.11, 2.40)**
Total events	60		107			

Heterogeneity: $\text{chi}^2 = 13.25$, df = 3 ($P < 0.004$); $I^2 = 77\%$

Test for overall effect: $Z = 2.50$ ($P = 0.01$)

Odds ratio M-H, random, 95% CI: 0.01 0.1 1 10 100 — Favors (experimental) Favors (control)

(c)

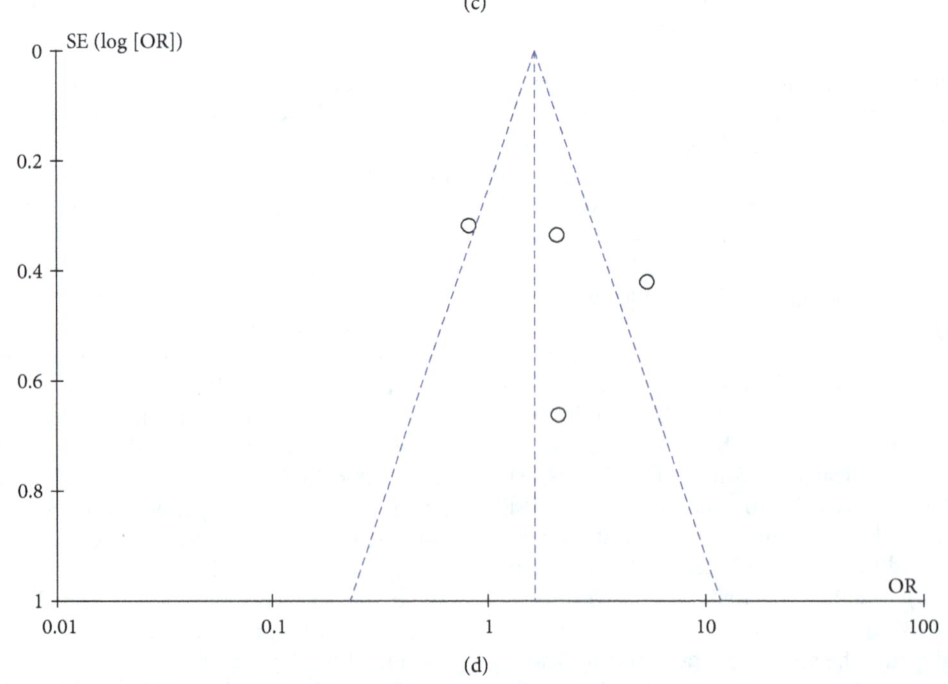

(d)

FIGURE 4: Correlation between platelet-to-lymphocyte ratio and event occurrence. (a) Forest plot of comparison of the included trials of BCLC-A; (b) forest plot of comparison of the included trials of BCLC-B; (c) forest plot of comparison of the included trials of BCLC-C; (d) funnel plot of comparison of the included trials of BCLC-C.

demonstrated that higher PLR predicted poorer OS, DFS, and CFS. Elevated PLR is also negatively related to the OS of patients with urological cancers except bladder cancer [37].

In the present study, we utilized the existing evidence from 9 included studies to obtain the pooled results to evaluate the predicted role of PLR in HCC. The results showed that an elevated pretreatment PLR indicated unfavorable worse OS (HR = 1.73; 95% CI: (1.46, 2.04); $P < 0.00001$) and DFS (HR = 1.30; 95% CI: (1.06, 1.60); $P = 0.01$), although there are several studies that focused on the relationship between PLR and HCC prognosis. For example, Fu et al. retrospectively analyzed the data of 268 patients with operable solitary large HCC and found that PLR combined with microvascular invasion and tumor size could be considered as a score system to predict survival in solitary large HCC. Multivariate analysis showed that PLR is associated with DFS significantly (HR = 1.004, $P = 0.003$), indicating that PLR may be a potential prognostic index for patients with solitary large HCC [38]. The study of He and Lin [25] just focused on HCC patients treated with TACE and recombinant human type-5 adenovirus H101, while Lai et al. [39] focused on the role of PLR in HCC patients after liver transplantation. In spite that Fu et al. [40] investigated the prognostic value of PLR and BCLC stages among HCC patients who underwent hepatectomy, they just concluded that BCLC stage could be considered as an independent predictor of OS and RFS without the relationship of PLR and BCLC stages. In our current meta-analysis, inclusion criteria of every trial were HCC and BCLC staging criteria, not for TNM or other unclear staging criteria. We further analyzed the role of PLR in different BCLC stages. As for the correlation between PLR and OS, high PLR indicating poor OS in BCLC-B/C patients was statistically significant without heterogeneity in the consistency of the trial results, while the result of BCLC-A patients indicated high statistical heterogeneity with an I^2 value of 78%. On the other hand, as for the correlation between PLR and event occurrence, high PLR was related to poor clinical event occurrence in BCLC-C patients only, while obvious heterogeneity was observed in all different BCLC stages. Therefore, more prospective cohort studies should be carried out to explore the prognostic role of PLR in different BCLC stages of HCC. Furthermore, we enrolled HCC patients with various treatments such as TACE, hepatectomy, and sorafenib, which may help to decrease the heterogeneity and extend the use of PLR in HCC patients.

It is also to be noted that several limitations of our study should be carefully considered. Firstly, all the enrolled studies were retrospective, thus some biases, such as information bias, misclassification bias, and selection bias, may have existed in the meta-analysis. Secondly, the sample size in the present study is so small that only 3 trials were enrolled in the analysis of the correlation between PLR and DFS. Thirdly, to unify the statistical method, we adopt univariable HR that might also increase bias into our study. Fourthly, no study mentioned information regarding dropouts, which might have exaggerated the prognostic effects. Finally, platelet and lymphocyte levels are easily influenced by other factors, such as infection, inflammation in other tissues, and medications taken before HCC treatment, and thereby the PLR measurement may be affected.

Taking all of these into consideration, PLR may be considered as a significant biomarker in the prognosis of HCC in different BCLC stages. Compared to other prognostic markers, PLR seems to be an inexpensive, widely-obtained, repeatable, and reliable predictor for HCC patients. HCC patients with high PLR may benefit from modifying inflammatory responses and modulating the immune system. More studies are warranted to draw a more powerful conclusion that may be significant for clinical practice.

Authors' Contributions

Wan-fu Lin, Mao-feng Zhong, and Yu-ren Zhang had the idea and designed the review. They also identified reports and extracted the data. Huan Wang and He-tong Zhao independently evaluated the quality appraisal and risk of bias of each included review. Bin-bin Cheng provided statistical advice. Wan-fu Lin and Mao-feng Zhong checked for statistical inconsistency and interpreted the data. Wan-fu Lin and Yu-ren Zhang drafted the report, and all other authors critically reviewed the article. Chang-quan Ling was responsible for planning and guidance. Wan-fu Lin, Mao-feng Zhong, and Yu-ren Zhang contributed equally to this work.

Acknowledgments

This study was supported by the grants from the National Natural Science Foundation of China (nos. 81430101, 81774077, and 81673655).

References

[1] H. Guo, J. B. Callaway, and J. P. Ting, "Inflammasomes: mechanism of action, role in disease, and therapeutics," *Nature Medicine*, vol. 21, no. 7, pp. 677–687, 2015.

[2] T. Strowig, J. Henao-Mejia, E. Elinav, and R. Flavell, "Inflammasomes in health and disease," *Nature*, vol. 481, no. 7381, pp. 278–286, 2012.

[3] E. Elinav, R. Nowarski, C. A. Thaiss, B. Hu, C. Jin, and R. A. Flavell, "Inflammation-induced cancer: crosstalk between tumours, immune cells and microorganisms," *Nature Reviews Cancer*, vol. 13, no. 11, pp. 759–771, 2013.

[4] J. Pollard, "Bacteria, inflammation and cancer," *Nature Reviews Immunology*, vol. 15, no. 9, p. 528, 2015.

[5] D. Hanahan and R. A. Weinberg, "Hallmarks of cancer: the next generation," *Cell*, vol. 144, no. 5, pp. 646–674, 2011.

[6] C. Criscitiello, V. Bagnardi, G. Pruneri et al., "Prognostic value of tumour-infiltrating lymphocytes in small HER2-positive breast cancer," *European Journal of Cancer*, vol. 87, pp. 164–171, 2017.

[7] C. Hsueh, L. Tao, M. Zhang et al., "The prognostic value of preoperative neutrophils, platelets, lymphocytes, monocytes and calculated ratios in patients with laryngeal squamous cell cancer," *Oncotarget*, vol. 8, no. 36, pp. 60514–60527, 2017.

[8] E. Borazan, A. A. Balik, Z. Bozdag et al., "Assessment of the relationship between neutrophil lymphocyte ratio and prognostic factors in non-metastatic colorectal cancer," *Turkish Journal of Surgery*, vol. 33, no. 3, pp. 185–189, 2017.

[9] L. Repsold, R. Pool, M. Karodia, G. Tintinger, and A. M. Joubert, "An overview of the role of platelets in angiogenesis, apoptosis and autophagy in chronic myeloid leukaemia," *Cancer Cell International*, vol. 17, no. 1, p. 89, 2017.

[10] S. J. Kim, R. P. Davis, and C. N. Jenne, "Platelets as modulators of inflammation," *Seminars in Thrombosis and Hemostasis*, vol. 44, no. 2, pp. 91–101, 2017.

[11] B. Tesfamariam, "Involvement of platelets in tumor cell metastasis," *Pharmacology & Therapeutics*, vol. 157, pp. 112–119, 2016.

[12] D. Buergy, F. Wenz, C. Groden, and M. A. Brockmann, "Tumor–platelet interaction in solid tumors," *International Journal of Cancer*, vol. 130, no. 12, pp. 2747–2760, 2012.

[13] S. S. Andrade, J. T. Sumikawa, E. D. Castro et al., "Interface between breast cancer cells and the tumor microenvironment using platelet-rich plasma to promote tumor angiogenesis - influence of platelets and fibrin bundles on the behavior of breast tumor cells," *Oncotarget*, vol. 8, no. 10, pp. 16851–16874, 2017.

[14] N. Dirican, Y. A. Karakaya, S. Gunes, F. T. Daloglu, and A. Dirican, "Association of intra-tumoral tumour-infiltrating lymphocytes and neutrophil-to-lymphocyte ratio is an independent prognostic factor in non-small cell lung cancer," *The Clinical Respiratory Journal*, vol. 11, no. 6, pp. 789–796, 2017.

[15] N. Lee, L. R. Zakka, M. C. Mihm Jr., and T. Schatton, "Tumour-infiltrating lymphocytes in melanoma prognosis and cancer immunotherapy," *Pathology*, vol. 48, no. 2, pp. 177–187, 2016.

[16] P. P. Santoiemma and D. J. Powell Jr., "Tumor infiltrating lymphocytes in ovarian cancer," *Cancer Biology & Therapy*, vol. 16, no. 6, pp. 807–820, 2015.

[17] S. Diem, S. Schmid, M. Krapf et al., "Neutrophil-to-lymphocyte ratio (NLR) and platelet-to-lymphocyte ratio (PLR) as prognostic markers in patients with non-small cell lung cancer (NSCLC) treated with nivolumab," *Lung Cancer*, vol. 111, pp. 176–181, 2017.

[18] W. Song, C. Tian, K. Wang, R. J. Zhang, and S. B. Zou, "Preoperative platelet lymphocyte ratio as independent predictors of prognosis in pancreatic cancer: a systematic review and meta-analysis," *PloS One*, vol. 12, no. 6, article e0178762, 2017.

[19] H. Dang, A. Takai, M. Forgues et al., "Oncogenic activation of the RNA binding protein NELFE and MYC signaling in hepatocellular carcinoma," *Cancer cell*, vol. 32, no. 1, pp. 101–114.e8, 2017.

[20] K. Jin, T. Li, G. Sanchez-Duffhues, F. Zhou, and L. Zhang, "Involvement of inflammation and its related micro RNAs in hepatocellular carcinoma," *Oncotarget*, vol. 8, no. 13, pp. 22145–22165, 2017.

[21] T. F. Greten, X. W. Wang, and F. Korangy, "Current concepts of immune based treatments for patients with HCC: from basic science to novel treatment approaches," *Gut*, vol. 64, no. 5, pp. 842–848, 2015.

[22] B. K. Goh, J. H. Kam, S.-Y. Lee et al., "Significance of neutrophil-to-lymphocyte ratio, platelet-to-lymphocyte ratio and prognostic nutrition index as preoperative predictors of early mortality after liver resection for huge (≥10 cm) hepatocellular carcinoma," *Journal of Surgical Oncology*, vol. 113, no. 6, pp. 621–627, 2016.

[23] W. Xia, Q. Ke, Y. Wang et al., "Predictive value of pre-transplant platelet to lymphocyte ratio for hepatocellular carcinoma recurrence after liver transplantation," *World Journal of Surgical Oncology*, vol. 13, no. 1, p. 60, 2015.

[24] T. C. Xue, Q. A. Jia, N. L. Ge et al., "The platelet-to-lymphocyte ratio predicts poor survival in patients with huge hepatocellular carcinoma that received transarterial chemoembolization," *Tumour biology*, vol. 36, no. 8, pp. 6045–6051, 2015.

[25] C. B. He and X. J. Lin, "Inflammation scores predict the survival of patients with hepatocellular carcinoma who were treated with transarterial chemoembolization and recombinant human type-5 adenovirus H101," *PloS One*, vol. 12, no. 3, article e0174769, 2017.

[26] H. J. Yang, J. H. Jiang, Q. A. Liu et al., "Preoperative platelet-to-lymphocyte ratio is a valuable prognostic biomarker in patients with hepatocellular carcinoma undergoing curative liver resection," *Tumour Biology*, vol. 39, no. 6, 2017.

[27] Y. Liu, Z. X. Wang, Y. Cao, G. Zhang, W. B. Chen, and C. P. Jiang, "Preoperative inflammation-based markers predict early and late recurrence of hepatocellular carcinoma after curative hepatectomy," *Hepatobiliary & Pancreatic Diseases International*, vol. 15, no. 3, pp. 266–274, 2016.

[28] A. Casadei Gardini, E. Scarpi, L. Faloppi et al., "Immune inflammation indicators and implication for immune modulation strategies in advanced hepatocellular carcinoma patients receiving sorafenib," *Oncotarget*, vol. 7, no. 41, pp. 67142–67149, 2016.

[29] T. C. Xue, N. L. Ge, X. Xu, F. Le, B. H. Zhang, and Y. H. Wang, "High platelet counts increase metastatic risk in huge hepatocellular carcinoma undergoing transarterial chemoembolization," *Hepatology research*, vol. 46, no. 10, pp. 1028–1036, 2016.

[30] K. Shiozawa, M. Watanabe, T. Ikehara et al., "Plasma biomarkers as predictive factors for advanced hepatocellular carcinoma with sorafenib," *Gan to kagaku ryoho. Cancer & chemotherapy*, vol. 43, no. 7, pp. 863–867, 2016.

[31] A. W. Chan, S. L. Chan, G. L. H. Wong et al., "Prognostic nutritional index (PNI) predicts tumor recurrence of very early/early stage hepatocellular carcinoma after surgical resection," *Annals of Surgical Oncology*, vol. 22, no. 13, pp. 4138–4148, 2015.

[32] X. C. Ni, Y. Yi, Y. P. Fu et al., "Prognostic value of the modified Glasgow Prognostic Score in patients undergoing radical surgery for hepatocellular carcinoma," *Medicine*, vol. 94, no. 36, article e1486, 2015.

[33] X. Wang, N. Wang, F. Cheung, L. Lao, C. Li, and Y. Feng, "Chinese medicines for prevention and treatment of human hepatocellular carcinoma: current progress on pharmacological actions and mechanisms," *Journal of Integrative Medicine*, vol. 13, no. 3, pp. 142–164, 2015.

[34] J. M. Llovet, J. Zucman-Rossi, E. Pikarsky et al., "Hepatocellular carcinoma," *Nature reviews Disease primers*, vol. 2, no. 16018, 2016.

[35] X. F. Zhai, Z. Chen, B. Li et al., "Traditional herbal medicine in preventing recurrence after resection of small hepatocellular carcinoma: a multicenter randomized controlled trial," *Journal of integrative medicine*, vol. 11, no. 2, pp. 90–100, 2013.

[36] Q. T. Zhao, X. P. Zhang, H. Zhang, and G. C. Duan, "Prognostic role of platelet to lymphocyte ratio in esophageal cancer: a meta-analysis," *Oncotarget*, vol. 8, no. 67, pp. 112085–112093, 2017.

[37] D. Y. Li, X. Y. Hao, T. M. Ma, H. X. Dai, and Y. S. Song, "The prognostic value of platelet-to-lymphocyte ratio in urological cancers: a meta-analysis," *Scientific Reports*, vol. 7, no. 1, p. 15387, 2017.

[38] J. Y. Shen, C. Li, T. F. Wen et al., "A simple prognostic score system predicts the prognosis of solitary large hepatocellular carcinoma following hepatectomy," *Medicine*, vol. 95, no. 31, article e4296, 2016.

[39] Q. Lai, E. Castro Santa, J. M. Rico Juri, R. S. Pinheiro, and J. Lerut, "Neutrophil and platelet-to-lymphocyte ratio as new predictors of dropout and recurrence after liver transplantation for hepatocellular cancer," *Transplant international*, vol. 27, no. 1, pp. 32–41, 2014.

[40] Y. P. Fu, X. C. Ni, Y. Yi et al., "A novel and validated inflammation-based score (IBS) predicts survival in patients with hepatocellular carcinoma following curative surgical resection: a STROBE-compliant article," *Medicine*, vol. 95, no. 7, article e2784, 2016.

A Retrospective Analysis of Colorectal Serrated Lesions from 2005 to 2014 in a Single Center: Importance of the Establishment of Diagnostic Patterns

Priscilla S. P. Oliveira,[1] **Rita B. Carvalho**,[2] **Daniela O. Magro**,[1] **Michel G. Camargo**,[1,2] **Carlos A. R. Martinez**,[1,2] **and Claudio S. R. Coy**[1,2]

[1]*Department of Surgery, Medical Sciences School, Campinas State University, Campinas 13083-887, Brazil*
[2]*Diagnostic Center of Diseases of the Digestive System-Gastrocentro, Medical Sciences School, Campinas State University, Campinas 13083-878, Brazil*

Correspondence should be addressed to Priscilla S. P. Oliveira; priportel@uol.com.br

Academic Editor: Giovanni D. De Palma

Background. Serrated colorectal lesions are increasingly recognized as an important process in the development of colorectal cancer. Endoscopic and histological diagnosis may be difficult, and knowledge of the serrated lesions is important for the establishment of strategies for treating colorectal lesions. We aimed to analyze serrated lesions diagnosed at a single center and evaluate if there was an increase in their identification over the years. *Design and Setting.* A retrospective analysis of colonoscopy reports was performed at a specialized center from 2005 to 2014. *Methods.* Colonoscopy reports about any resected endoscopic lesions were reviewed and subjected to histological diagnosis from 2005 to 2014. Then, serrated lesions were evaluated based on morphological characterization, location, size, occurrence of synchronous lesions, and the patient's history of colorectal cancer and polyps. *Results.* A total of 2126 colonoscopy examination reports were reviewed, and 3494 lesions were analyzed. On histopathological examination, 1089 (31.2%) were classified as hyperplastic polyps, 22 (0.6%) as sessile serrated adenomas, and 21 (0.6%) as traditional serrated adenomas. There was an increase in the number of cases of sessile and traditional serrated adenomas diagnosed after 2010. Before 2010, two cases of sessile serrated adenomas and seven cases of traditional serrated adenomas were diagnosed; after 2010, 20 cases of sessile serrated adenoma and 14 cases of traditional serrated adenomas were diagnosed. *Conclusion.* There was an increase in the diagnosis of sessile serrated adenomas over the years, which can be attributed to better accuracy in colonoscopy and histological classification.

1. Introduction

Nowadays, owing to the high incidence of and mortality due to colorectal cancer, there is a need for effective prevention strategies. Since fecal occult blood tests are employed for population screening, colonoscopy is regarded as a gold standard procedure owing to its high sensitivity for detecting polyps. Removal of polyps is associated with a decrease in colorectal cancer incidence, and better knowledge of the molecular colorectal cancer-related pathways involved in precancerous lesions is essential to increase their detection as well as to establish better screening programs.

Until 1990, three types of lesions were associated with the development of colorectal neoplasia: tubular adenomas, tubulovillous adenomas, and villous adenomas. They originate from serial gene mutations, particularly the *APC* and *KRAS* genes, and are known as the classical adenoma-to-carcinoma sequence.

Hyperplastic polyps, which are common in the colon and particularly in the rectum, were considered nonneoplastic lesions for several years [1–3]. In 1990, a group of pathologists identified architectural changes similar to those in hyperplastic lesions in a few colorectal adenomas. These were termed as serrated adenomas [4]. Because of their similar architectural appearance and the suggestion that some of these adenomas may develop from initial hyperplastic polyps, a new group of lesions was defined. These lesions display similar histological characteristics and present diagnostic difficulties to pathologists; therefore, establishment of reproducible criteria for their diagnosis was necessary. The classification of the serrated lesions has been modified over the years since 1990 because knowledge regarding histology has increased. The changes in their histological classification brought difficulties in their correct diagnosis. Only in 2010, the World Health Organization published the latest classification where the serrated lesions were differentiated into sessile serrated adenomas or sessile serrated polyps, traditional serrated adenomas, and hyperplastic polyps. This is the classification of choice for these lesions since then [5–8].

Serrated lesions started receiving increased attention after studies demonstrated that they were more frequent in the right colon as well as their association with faster development into carcinoma, when compared to the classical adenoma-to-carcinoma sequence. The epigenetic origin of cancer cells is where alterations result from the hypermethylation of cytosine- and guanine-rich regions, in which a sequence of events may culminate in the inactivation of the *hMLH1* gene. This pathway is associated with the *BRAF* gene mutation, which is mutually exclusive from the *KRAS* gene mutation, which is involved in the so-called "serrated pathway." It is considered the second most common mechanism for the development of colorectal cancer [5, 7–12]. On the other hand, traditional serrated adenomas are now known to be secondary to the *KRAS* gene mutation and can evolve through the classical adenoma-to-carcinoma transition [5–7]. So, traditional serrated adenomas mostly resemble conventional adenomas with respect to the endoscopic appearance and molecular behavior.

Nowadays, there are two aspects that may be related to the lower occurrence of the diagnosis of the serrated lesions, ranging from 0.1% to 14.7%: endoscopic detection and histological criteria for the correct diagnosis and classification [13, 14]. In the Brazilian population, there are no studies that evaluate its prevalence and clinical and endoscopic aspects.

We aimed to evaluate the number of serrated lesions diagnosed before and after 2010, when the current histological classification was developed and established, as well as evaluate its localization, size, and morphological features.

2. Methods

2.1. Study Design. We retrospectively analyzed data from colonoscopies performed at the Gastrocentro of the State University of Campinas (UNICAMP) between January 1, 2005, and December 31, 2014, to determine the number of the serrated lesions diagnosed in this period and if there was an increase in its diagnosis after an increase in the knowledge about this lesion. We also aimed to describe the characteristics of the serrated lesions (morphological characterization, size, and localization) and prevalence of these kinds of lesions regarding all the lesions associated with the development of colorectal neoplasia. Colonoscopies with a positive result for elevated polyps or flat lesions were included. The locations of the lesions were classified as follows: proximal colon (from the cecum to the splenic flexure) and distal colon and rectum (from the splenic flexure to the rectum). Regarding size, the lesion sizes were classified as <10 mm, 10–20 mm, and >20 mm.

The lesions were grouped as conventional adenomas (tubular adenomas, tubulovillous adenomas, and villous adenomas) and serrated lesions (hyperplastic polyps, sessile serrated adenomas, and traditional serrated adenomas). Histological diagnoses were done by different pathologists, and there was no histological review. Usage of histological classification for serrated lesions began in 2005, and the classification has changed over the years. After 2010, the criteria used were those defined by the World Health Organization guidelines, which were issued in that year; these are the same that have been used until today [5].

All colonoscopies were done in the same endoscopy unit but with different endoscopists, and histological diagnoses were analyzed by the Department of Pathology, UNICAMP, using different pathologists but all with experience in the gastrointestinal tract.

2.2. Participants. All colonoscopy reports from patients older than 18 years who had undergone resection of at least one lesion and histological analysis were included. The participants were referred to Gastrocentro (a specialized public unit for gastrointestinal diseases of UNICAMP) from the outpatient units of Hospital de Clinicas-UNICAMP with any indication for colonoscopy. Patients with familial adenomatous polyposis, Lynch syndrome, or hyperplastic polyposis syndrome, with imprecise endoscopic descriptions were excluded. Cases with posterior histological diagnosis revision were also excluded.

2.3. Variables. Indication for colonoscopy, number of lesions per examination, and aspects related to each resected lesion (size, location, and endoscopic appearance) as well as epidemiological criteria (sex and age) were analyzed. The locations of the lesions were classified as follows: proximal colon and distal colon and rectum. Regarding size, the lesions sizes were classified as <10 mm, 10–20 mm, and >20 mm. The Paris Classification was applied for morphological description [15, 16]. The lesions were grouped into conventional adenomas and serrated lesions.

The associations of different types of serrated lesions with conventional adenomas, as well as with other serrated lesion types, were analyzed.

2.4. Data Analysis. The Statistical Package for the Social Sciences (SPSS) software, version 16, (Statistical Package for the Sciences - SPSS Inc., Chicago, IL, USA) was used for descriptive and statistical analyses. The chi-square statistical test was employed, and statistical significance of 5% was considered.

2.5. Ethics. The study protocol was approved by the ethics committee of UNICAMP (number 36002414.0.0000.5404).

3. Results

3.1. Overall Population. Reports of a total of 2126 examinations involving 1772 patients (mean age 61.3 ± 11.5 years) were analyzed. The total number of lesions detected was 3494, from which 1132 (32.4%) were serrated. From 2005 to 2009, 745 examinations with positive results for polyps were performed, and 1381 were performed in the subsequent years ($P < 0.001$). The average number of lesions identified through colonoscopy was 1.65 (1–13), and 761 (35.8%) patients had more than one lesion.

The most common indications for examinations included a history of colorectal cancer and a previous personal history of polyps in the colon and/or rectum (15.9% and 15.1%, respectively). Other indications were a family history of colorectal cancer (2.3%), preoperative evaluation of colorectal cancer (2.1%), unknown (1.6%), and other reasons (64.2%).

The histological type, total number of each lesions, and percentage of the lesion types found via colonoscopies are demonstrated in Table 1.

3.2. Sex and Age. Regarding the diagnosis of serrated lesions, there were no differences between sex and mean age. One woman was found to have a sessile serrated adenoma and a traditional serrated adenoma via the same examination.

The mean age of the patients with sessile serrated adenomas was 62 ± 12.1 years, while that of the patients with traditional serrated adenomas was 60.2 ± 16.6 years.

3.3. Colonoscopy Indication. In eight patients (four with sessile serrated adenomas and four with traditional serrated adenomas), the indication for colorectal cancer was postoperative cancer follow-up findings. Two patients with sessile serrated adenomas had synchronous colorectal adenocarcinoma detected via preoperative colonoscopy. A history of colorectal polyps was observed in two examinations involving sessile serrated adenomas and in six involving traditional serrated adenomas. No patient with a family history of colorectal cancer had lesions with a histological diagnosis of sessile serrated adenoma or traditional serrated adenoma.

3.4. Location, Size, and Morphological Aspects. Most of the sessile serrated adenomas were observed in the proximal colon ($n = 21$, 95.4%), while traditional serrated adenomas were mainly observed in the distal colon and rectum ($n = 13$, 61.9%). One case with a traditional serrated adenoma did not have a descriptive location. Hyperplastic polyps were reported in all segments, with predominance in the distal colon and rectum ($n = 569$, 52.2%), followed by the proximal colon ($n = 208$, 19.1%). The distributions of sessile serrated adenoma and traditional serrated adenoma classified according to size, localization, and morphology are shown in Table 2.

We noted the presence of 15 polyps diagnosed as hyperplastic polyps > 10 mm in the right colon and 6 polyps in the transverse colon.

3.5. Association with Conventional Adenomas. Tubular adenomas were detected in 11 examinations involving sessile serrated adenomas and in six involving traditional serrated adenomas, while tubulovillous adenoma was only detected in one examination involving a sessile serrated adenoma. One patient presented with sessile serrated adenoma, traditional serrated adenoma, and synchronous tubular adenoma.

Table 1: Histological type, total number of each lesion (frequency), and percentage of the lesions found via colonoscopies along with distribution of all the histological types of only serrated lesions.

	n	%
Histological type		
Tubular adenoma	2085	59.7
Hyperplastic polyp	1089	31.2
Tubulovillous adenoma	217	6.2
Adenocarcinoma	46	1.3
Sessile serrated adenoma	22	0.6
Traditional serrated adenoma	21	0.6
Villous adenoma	14	0.4
Total	3494	100
Serrated lesions		
Hyperplastic polyp	1089	96.2
Sessile serrated adenoma	22	1.94
Traditional serrated adenoma	21	1.86
Total	1132	100

3.6. Synchronous Serrated Lesions. Five examinations involving hyperplastic polyps showed concomitant sessile serrated adenomas, and four showed concomitant traditional serrated adenomas. One patient presented with three traditional serrated adenomas in the same examination, and two other patients demonstrated more than one serrated lesion in the same examination (one with two traditional serrated adenomas and the other with one traditional serrated adenoma and one sessile serrated adenoma). An association with cancer was observed in two examinations involving sessile serrated adenomas and in one involving traditional serrated adenoma.

3.7. Absolute Value of Sessile Serrated Adenomas and Traditional Serrated Adenomas. The number of sessile serrated adenomas and traditional serrated adenomas showed a large variation over the study period, with an increase in the last 5 years (Figures 1 and 2).

No case of sessile serrated adenoma or traditional serrated adenoma was diagnosed in 2006 and 2009. After 2010, there was an increase in the number of serrated lesions diagnosed, with an average of 7 lesions per year. Two sessile serrated adenomas and seven traditional serrated adenomas were diagnosed between 2005 and 2009, while 20 sessile serrated adenomas and 14 traditional serrated adenomas were diagnosed between 2010 and 2015, showing a significant increase in the recent years ($P < 0.001$). The relative frequencies of traditional serrated adenomas and sessile serrated adenomas before and after 2010 were 0.8% and 2.3%, respectively.

TABLE 2: Descriptive analysis of serrated lesions. The distribution of the serrated lesions according to their general aspects: the mean age, localization, and size and morphological characteristics.

		Sessile serrated adenoma (SSA)	Traditional serrated adenoma (TSA)
Mean age		62 ± 12.1	60.2 ± 16.6
Location	Proximal colon	21–95.4%	7–33.3%
	Distal colon and rectum	1–4.6%	13–61.9%
	No description	—	1–4.8%
Size	<10 mm	15–68.2%	12–57.1%
	10–20 mm	7–31.8%	5–23.8%
	>20 mm	—	1–4.8%
	No description	—	3–14.3%
Morphology	Sessile	13–59.1%	17–80.9%
	Superficially elevated	9–40.9%	1–4.8%
	Pedunculated	—	2–9.5%
	No description	—	1–4.8%

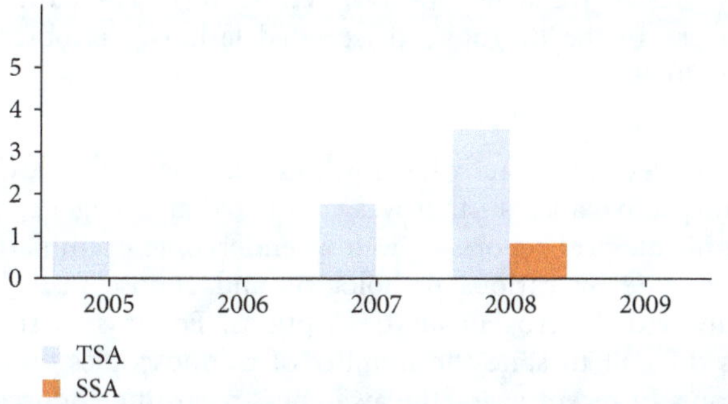

FIGURE 1: Number of sessile serrated adenomas and traditional serrated adenomas from 2005 to 2009 (year; lesions diagnosed—absolute value). One case of traditional serrated adenoma was diagnosed in 2005, two in 2007, and four in 2008. One case of sessile serrated adenoma was diagnosed in 2008.

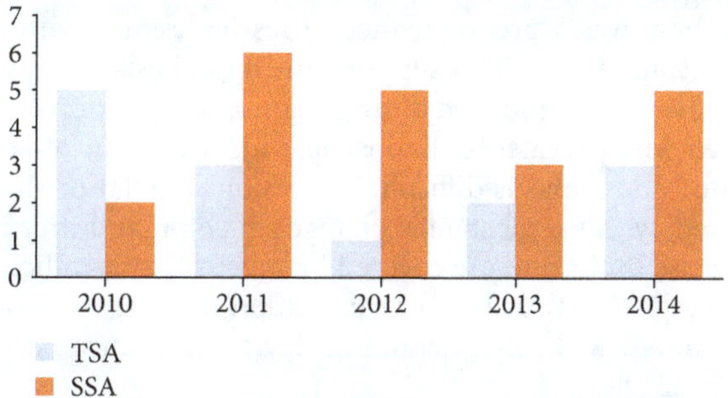

FIGURE 2: Number of sessile serrated adenomas and traditional serrated adenomas from 2010 to 2014 (year; lesions diagnosed—absolute value). Two sessile serrated adenomas were diagnosed in 2010, six in 2011, five in 2012, three in 2013, and five in 2014. The number of traditional adenomas diagnosed was five in 2010, three in 2011, one in 2012, two in 2013, and three in 2014.

4. Discussion

The diagnosis of serrated lesions may be challenging. For many years, serrated lesions were all classified as hyperplastic and nonneoplastic lesions. Today, owing to better knowledge about molecular pathways, the serrated lesions are known to be a more aggressive form of precancerous lesions. Therefore, accurate identification and diagnosis have practical implications in screening for colorectal cancer, and the analysis of a case by case may contribute to better accuracy.

When comparing serrated lesions with other adenomas, the prevalence of hyperplastic polyps in this sample was as expected (i.e., one-third of all polyps). However, when analyzed in comparison with serrated lesions only, hyperplastic polyps were the majority (96.2%). This value was higher than that in the literature, although other studies also found hyperplastic polyps to be the most frequent type (75% of all serrated lesions) [5, 12, 13].

However, the discrepancy in the prevalence of sessile serrated adenomas was high. This sample in this study showed a prevalence of 0.6%, which was close to the minimum values (0.1% to 14.7%), relative to all polyps found in the colon. However, when only serrated lesions were analyzed (1.9%), the prevalence was lower (they are generally estimated to comprise up to 25% of all serrated lesions) [5, 7, 17]. The prevalence of traditional serrated adenomas, which is considered rare, was within the expected range [5, 14, 18].

This large difference in the prevalence of hyperplastic polyps and sessile serrated adenomas between this study and other reports may be explained by the different classifications adopted since the lesions were first discovered. Moreover, studies that evaluated the prevalence of sessile serrated adenomas reported a higher prevalence of sessile serrated adenoma lesions based on histological reviews [4, 6, 9, 13, 18, 19].

Furthermore, the difference between the criteria for the diagnosis of sessile serrated adenomas may have been a confounding factor that affected the different prevalence rates in different studies as more knowledge has been acquired over the years [5, 15, 19, 20].

Since histological aspects of sessile serrated adenomas can cause them to be mistaken for hyperplastic polyps, this may also justify the low prevalence of sessile serrated adenomas compared with hyperplastic polyps. Moreover, the difficulty in the diagnosis of superficial elevated lesions through colonoscopies owing to their endoscopic characteristics may also have contributed to their lower prevalence.

The retrospective design of the study also contributed to this difference. Although the histological and endoscopic examinations were performed at a referral center for gastrointestinal tract pathologies, the examiners could not be selected.

Although there were divergences among published data on the prevalence of sessile serrated adenomas, the same was not true for their location. Sessile serrated adenomas were often observed in the proximal colon, and their appearance (sessile and/or elevated) matched that in the literature. As in other studies, no sessile serrated adenoma was diagnosed in the distal colon and rectum [9, 21]. Traditional serrated adenomas were present in greater numbers in the distal colon and rectum, as was expected.

Regarding the endoscopic aspects of the Paris Classification, there was a predominance of sessile lesions, with only one elevated lesion. This supports the hypothesis that lesions may have gone unnoticed during colonoscopies, contributing to their low prevalence. Endoscopic identification of sessile serrated adenomas is difficult. The lesions are flat or slightly elevated, with no substantial changes in color, and they have imprecise limits and are covered by mucus that is difficult to remove [5, 7, 12]. A better visualization of these lesions can be achieved with high-definition devices and chromoscopy [9, 17, 22, 23].

Another important examination-related aspect that may have contributed to the low prevalence of sessile serrated adenomas is that colorants were not routinely used in the right colon. Despite the importance of their role in the diagnosis of sessile serrated adenomas, there have been no reports on their use in examinations that detected sessile serrated adenomas or hyperplastic polyps > 10 mm in the proximal colon [12, 22].

The difference between the prevalence of serrated lesions in this study and in the published data, as well as the differences in the distribution and macroscopic characteristics, raises questions about the quality of diagnoses and whether there have been any improvements from the increased experience of endoscopic examiners and pathologists. Payne et al. [24] reported an association between the rate of resection of adenomas and the diagnosis of serrated lesions. Therefore, endoscopic examinations performed by more experienced endoscopists will yield a high detection of serrated lesions.

We observed an increase in the number of sessile serrated adenomas and traditional serrated adenomas diagnosed within the last 5 years of the study period. In the last 5 years, there were no changes in the histological classification of the serrated lesions, and the pathologists have more years of experience with these kind of lesions.

Data for this study were collected from one of the region's reference centers for the treatment of colorectal cancer and inflammatory bowel disease. Therefore, most of the patients submitted to colonoscopies presented risk factors for the development of precursor lesions or colorectal cancer, as evidenced by the indications for the examinations. On the other hand, previous data were mostly related to screening tests that were performed in asymptomatic patients [25–28].

A relevant aspect of this study is regarding the occurrence of synchronous lesions. The simultaneous occurrence of conventional adenomas and sessile serrated adenomas or traditional serrated adenomas was 51.28%. Previous reports showed that the presence of conventional adenomas with serrated lesions was uncommon [28].

The prevalence of serrated lesions in this study differed from that in other studies in some ways, since we detected a higher number of hyperplastic polyps and observed very similar distributions between sessile serrated adenomas and traditional serrated adenomas. The increases in the number of examinations performed and in the number of serrated lesions diagnosed were significant; there was an increase in the relative frequency of serrated lesions. Therefore, an increase in the diagnosis of serrated lesions was observed after 2010.

However, this study has some limitations. Our study is a retrospective analysis that was conducted at a single center, but histological reports as well as endoscopic examinations were done by various pathologists and endoscopists, certainly with heterogeneous descriptions. For this reason, it was difficult to state the number of colonoscopies without lesions. In recent years, the awareness regarding endoscopic appearance on serrated lesions particularly in the right colon contributed to better accuracy. Unfortunately, the use of chromoendoscopy or magnification techniques like narrow band imaging was not always employed in the unit of date origin of this study because the heterogeneity of the colonoscopists. Besides that, before 2010, many lesions that are now classified as sessile serrated adenomas were classified as hyperplastic (before the adoption of the criteria for histological classification published by the World Health Organization for serrated lesions in 2010). Hence, we did not review the histological features, which could have influenced the number of the serrated lesions detected.

5. Conclusion

There was an increase in the diagnosis of sessile serrated adenomas after 2010, which can be attributed to better accuracy of colonoscopy and the histological classification.

Acknowledgments

We thank the Graduate Committee of the School of Medical Sciences of the University of Campinas for their support in this study.

References

[1] B. C. Morson, "Precancerous and early malignant lesions of the large intestine," *The British Journal of Surgery*, vol. 55, no. 10, pp. 725–731, 1968.

[2] E. R. Fearon and B. Vogelstein, "A genetic model for colorectal tumorigenesis," *Cell*, vol. 61, no. 5, pp. 759–767, 1990.

[3] E.-Y. K. Choi and H. D. Appelman, "A historical perspective and exposé on serrated polyps of the colorectum," *Archives of Pathology & Laboratory Medicine*, vol. 140, no. 10, pp. 1079–1084, 2016.

[4] T. A. Longacre and C. M. Fenoglio-Preiser, "Mixed hyperplastic adenomatous polyps/serrated adenomas: a distinct form of colorectal neoplasia," *The American Journal of Surgical Pathology*, vol. 14, no. 6, pp. 524–537, 1990.

[5] D. Snover, D. Ahnen, R. Burt, and O. Rea, "Serrated polyps of the colon and rectum and serrated polyposis: WHO classification of tumors," in *Pathology and Genetics. Tumors of Digestive System*, pp. 160–165, Lyon: IARC, 2010.

[6] E. Torlakovic, E. Skovlund, D. C. Snover, G. Torlakovic, and J. M. Nesland, "Morphologic reappraisal of serrated colorectal polyps," *The American Journal of Surgical Pathology*, vol. 27, no. 1, pp. 65–81, 2003.

[7] C. S. Huang, F. A. Farraye, S. Yang, and M. J. O'Brien, "The clinical significance of serrated polyps," *The American Journal of Gastroenterology*, vol. 106, no. 2, pp. 229–240, 2011, quiz 241.

[8] S. Yang, F. A. Farraye, C. Marck, O. Posnik, and M. J. O'Brien, "BRAF and KRAS mutations in hyperplastic polyps and serrated adenomas of the colorectum: relationship to histology and CpG island methylation status," *The American Journal of Surgical Pathology*, vol. 28, no. 11, pp. 1452–1459, 2004.

[9] T. Matsumoto, M. Mizuno, M. Shimizu, T. Manabe, M. Iida, and M. Fujishima, "Serrated adenoma of the colorectum: colonoscopic and histologic features," *Gastrointestinal Endoscopy*, vol. 49, no. 6, pp. 736–742, 1999.

[10] D. C. Snover, "Update on the serrated pathway to colorectal carcinoma," *Human Pathology*, vol. 42, no. 1, pp. 1–10, 2011.

[11] J. R. Jass, V. L. J. Whitehall, J. Young, and B. A. Leggett, "Emerging concepts in colorectal neoplasia," *Gastroenterology*, vol. 123, no. 3, pp. 862–876, 2002.

[12] B. Bordaçahar, M. Barret, B. Terris et al., "Sessile serrated adenoma: from identification to resection," *Digestive and Liver Disease*, vol. 47, no. 2, pp. 95–102, 2015.

[13] M. Bettington, N. Walker, C. Rosty et al., "Critical appraisal of the diagnosis of the sessile serrated adenoma," *The American Journal of Surgical Pathology*, vol. 38, no. 2, pp. 158–166, 2014.

[14] H. Y. Kim, S. M. Kim, J. H. Seo, E. H. Park, N. Kim, and D. H. Lee, "Age-specific prevalence of serrated lesions and their subtypes by screening colonoscopy: a retrospective study," *BMC Gastroenterology*, vol. 14, no. 1, article 82, 2014.

[15] K. J. Spring, Z. Z. Zhao, R. Karamatic et al., "High prevalence of sessile serrated adenomas with BRAF mutations: a prospective study of patients undergoing colonoscopy," *Gastroenterology*, vol. 131, no. 5, pp. 1400–1407, 2006.

[16] "The Paris endoscopic classification of superficial neoplastic lesions: esophagus, stomach, and colon," *Gastrointestinal Endoscopy*, vol. 58, no. 6, pp. S3–S43, 2003.

[17] E. Jaramillo, S. Tamura, and H. Mitomi, "Endoscopic appearance of serrated adenomas in the colon," *Endoscopy*, vol. 37, no. 3, pp. 254–260, 2005.

[18] F.-I. Lu, D. W. van Niekerk, D. Owen, S. P. L. Tha, D. A. Turbin, and D. L. Webber, "Longitudinal outcome study of sessile serrated adenomas of the colorectum: an increased risk for subsequent right-sided colorectal carcinoma," *The American Journal of Surgical Pathology*, vol. 34, no. 7, pp. 927–934, 2010.

[19] K. Abdeljawad, K. C. Vemulapalli, C. J. Kahi, O. W. Cummings, D. C. Snover, and D. K. Rex, "Sessile serrated polyp prevalence determined by a colonoscopist with a high lesion detection rate and an experienced pathologist," *Gastrointestinal Endoscopy*, vol. 81, no. 3, pp. 517–524, 2015.

[20] B.-M. Wang, H.-L. Cao, X. Chen et al., "Detection rate, distribution, clinical and pathological features of colorectal serrated polyps," *Chinese Medical Journal*, vol. 129, no. 20, pp. 2427–2433, 2016.

[21] P. Ponugoti, J. Lin, R. Odze, D. Snover, C. Kahi, and D. K. Rex, "Prevalence of sessile serrated adenoma/polyp in hyperplastic appearing diminutive rectosigmoid polyps," *Gastrointestinal Endoscopy*, vol. 85, no. 3, pp. 622–627, 2017.

[22] J. Pohl, A. Schneider, H. Vogell, G. Mayer, G. Kaiser, and C. Ell, "Pancolonic chromoendoscopy with indigo carmine versus standard colonoscopy for detection of neoplastic lesions: a randomised two-centre trial," *Gut*, vol. 60, no. 4, pp. 485–490, 2011.

[23] T. Morita, S. Tamura, J. Miyazaki, Y. Higashidani, and S. Onishi, "Evaluation of endoscopic and histopathological features of serrated adenoma of the colon," *Endoscopy*, vol. 33, no. 9, pp. 761–765, 2001.

[24] S. R. Payne, T. R. Church, M. Wandell et al., "Endoscopic detection of proximal serrated lesions and pathologic identification of sessile serrated adenomas/polyps vary on the basis of center," *Clinical Gastroenterology and Hepatology*, vol. 12, no. 7, pp. 1119–1126, 2014.

[25] D. Li, C. J. Jin, C. McCulloch et al., "Association of large serrated polyps with synchronous advanced colorectal neoplasia," *The American Journal of Gastroenterology*, vol. 104, no. 3, pp. 695–702, 2009.

[26] A. Buda, M. De Bona, I. Dotti et al., "Prevalence of different subtypes of serrated polyps and risk of synchronous advanced colorectal neoplasia in average-risk population undergoing first-time colonoscopy," *Clinical and Translational Gastroenterology*, vol. 3, no. 1, p. e6, 2012.

[27] C. Macaron, H. T. Vu, R. Lopez, R. K. Pai, and C. A. Burke, "Risk of metachronous polyps in individuals with serrated polyps," *Diseases of the Colon & Rectum*, vol. 58, no. 8, pp. 762–768, 2015.

[28] C. J. Kahi, K. C. Vemulapalli, D. C. Snover, K. H. Abdel Jawad, O. W. Cummings, and D. K. Rex, "Findings in the distal colorectum are not associated with proximal advanced serrated lesions," *Clinical Gastroenterology and Hepatology*, vol. 13, no. 2, pp. 345–351, 2015.

13

10Fr S-Type Plastic Pancreatic Stents in Chronic Pancreatitis Are Effective for the Treatment of Pancreatic Duct Strictures and Pancreatic Stones

Ken Ito, Naoki Okano, Seiichi Hara, Kensuke Takuma, Kensuke Yoshimoto, Susumu Iwasaki, Yui Kishimoto, and Yoshinori Igarashi

Division of Gastroenterology and Hepatology, Toho University Omori Medical Center, Tokyo, Japan

Correspondence should be addressed to Ken Ito; ken.itou@med.toho-u.ac.jp

Guest Editor: Khalid M. Khan

Aim. Endoscopic pancreatic stenting for refractory pancreatic duct strictures associated with impacted pancreatic stones in chronic pancreatitis cases has yielded conflicting results. We retrospectively evaluated the efficacy of endoscopic treatment in chronic pancreatitis patients with pancreatic duct strictures. *Methods.* Pancreatic sphincterotomy, dilatation procedures, pancreatic brush cytology, and pancreatic juice cytology were routinely performed, and malignant diseases were excluded. After gradual dilatation, a 10 Fr plastic pancreatic stent was inserted. The stents were replaced every 3 months and removed after the strictures were dilated. Statistical analyses were performed to determine the risk of main pancreatic duct restenosis. *Results.* Endoscopic pancreatic stents were successfully placed in 41 of a total of 59 patients (69.5%). The median duration of pancreatic stenting was 276 days. Pain relief was obtained in 37 of 41 patients (90.2%). Seventeen patients (41.5%) had recurrence of main pancreatic duct stricture, and restenting was performed in 16 patients (average placement period 260 days). During the follow-up period, pancreatic cancer developed in three patients (5.1%). Multivariate analysis revealed that the presence of remnant stones after stenting treatment was significantly associated with a higher rate of main pancreatic duct restenosis ($p = 0.03$). *Conclusion.* The use of 10 Fr S-type plastic pancreatic stents with routine exchange was effective for both short-term and long-term outcomes in chronic pancreatitis patients with benign pancreatic duct strictures and impacted pancreatic stones.

1. Introduction

Chronic pancreatitis is a progressive, irreversible inflammatory disease characterized by pain, which is the symptom that requires treatment in most cases [1]. This disease is thought to be caused by increased pressure within the pancreatic ductal system and/or pancreatic parenchyma, secondary to the outflow obstruction of the main pancreatic duct (MPD) [2].

It has been reported that endoscopic pancreatic duct stenting provides both short-term and long-term relief from persistent or relapsing pain in severe chronic pancreatitis with distal ductal strictures and proximal dilation [3–8].

Several stents of various shapes and diameter have been used for endoscopic pancreatic stenting (EPS) [4–7, 9–14]. In consideration of the migration of the pancreatic stent, a polyethylene straight-type PS (Amsterdam type) [5], with 1 cm interval side holes, were the common PS for endoscopic pancreatic stenting [5]. We had an experience of using Amsterdam-type PS with a case of back pain from the early stage, in which we were forced to remove and exchange in the early timing. So, we started and preferred to use a polyolefin elastomer material with double-bended type (S shape) [15–17], which was a more soft material and suitable at the main pancreatic duct. This is the first reason we only use S-type pancreatic stent in our Hospital.

In addition, endoscopic pancreatic stenting in Japan has been approved for medical health insurance coverage in April 2012, and at that time, only S-type plastic pancreatic stent (Olympus Co.) was the only plastic stent which was funded by the national medical insurance in Japan. From these two reasons, we evaluated the efficacy of approved medical health insurance coverage pancreatic stents. The

European Society of Gastrointestinal Endoscopy (ESGE) Clinical Guideline recommended the use of 10 Fr diameter plastic stents in chronic pancreatitis associated with severe strictures [18]. S-type plastic stents have proven to be safe and efficient for the treatment of pancreatic duct strictures by EPS [12, 13, 19, 20]. MPD obstruction has been reported to be caused by strictures (47%), stones (18%), or a combination of both (32%) in most patients [4, 6, 7, 10, 13, 21]. The combination of extracorporeal shock wave lithotripsy (ESWL) and EPS is considered to be the treatment modality for ameliorating pain in patients with chronic pancreatitis [4, 7, 17, 22–29]. However, only a few cases of severe pancreatic duct strictures with impacted pancreatic stones in patients using 10 Fr S-type plastic pancreatic stents (plastic PS) have been reported so far. The present study retrospectively evaluated the short-term and long-term efficacies and outcomes of using 10 Fr S-type plastic PS for the treatment of pancreatic duct strictures and impacted pancreatic stones in patients with chronic pancreatitis.

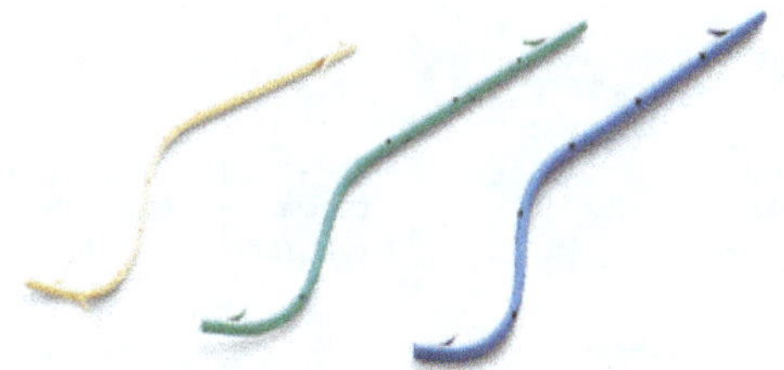

From left to right, 7 Fr (yellow), 8.5 Fr (green), 10 Fr (blue).

FIGURE 1: Devices of pancreatic stents.

2. Methods

2.1. Patients. From May 2005 to November 2013, 148 chronic pancreatitis and pancreatolithiasis patients were treated by endoscopic stone extraction and ESWL at Toho University Omori Medical Center, Tokyo, Japan. Among them, 59 patients, who underwent 10 Fr S-type pancreatic stent placement and were followed up for over 12 months, were selected for evaluation in the present study.

Adaptation for EPS was based on clinical symptoms (e.g., abdominal pain), presence of pancreatic duct stones in the Santorini or Wirsung ducts, detection of upstream MPD dilatation by diagnostic imaging (ultrasonography, contrast enhanced computed tomography (CT), and magnetic resonance cholangiopancreatography), and the presence or absence of abdominal complaints with exacerbation of glucose tolerance and diabetic mellitus.

EPS was not funded by the national medical insurance of Japan until April 2012; therefore, this study was conducted with the approval of the Toho University Omori Medical Center's Institutional Review Board and in accordance with the Declaration of Helsinki. Clinicopathological data were obtained from patients' medical records. Written informed consent was obtained from each patient before the procedures.

2.2. EPS Equipment and Procedures. All procedures were performed with a TJF240 or TJF260V duodenoscope (Olympus Co., Tokyo, Japan). Endoscopic pancreatic sphincterotomy (EPST) has consistently been performed before MPD stenting [21]. When selective MPD cannulation was difficult, precutting was performed with EPST as a secondary procedure [30]. After identification of the pancreatic duct stricture via pancreatography, a guidewire was negotiated through its tail, as close as possible to the MPD, and dilatation was attempted.

Routine pancreatic cytology was performed before commencing with the dilatation procedure to confirm the absence of malignancy in the MPD stricture. Although we typically used 0.035-inch Revowave standard-type and Revowave hard-type guidewires (Piolax Medical Devices Inc., Kanagawa, Japan), a 0.025-inch VisiGlide or VisiGlide 2 guidewire (Olympus Co.) was also used in patients with severe strictures. Similarly, despite the use of a dilation catheter (SBDC; Cook Co., Winston-Salem, NC, USA) or a 6 mm diameter balloon catheter for endoscopic pancreatic duct dilation (EPDBD: MaxPass; Olympus Co.) for stricture dilation before stenting, a Soehendra stent retriever (SSR; Cook Co.) was used as an alternative device to dilate the more challenging strictures [31–33]. Pancreatic duct stones have been effectively treated by a combination therapy of both EL and ESWL as a first-line treatment method [34]. ESWL was first started with an electromagnetic lithotripter (Lithoskop; Siemens AG, Munich, Germany); a wire-guided basket (FG-V436P Tetra-V wire-guided basket; Olympus Co.) was then introduced after ESWL fragmentation of the ductal stones. In instances where ESWL was unsuccessful, electrohydraulic lithotripsy (EHL) was performed as a second attempt using the 10 Fr SpyGlass Direct Visualization system (Boston Scientific, Natick, MA). An S-type plastic PS (Olympus Co.) was used for the MPD stricture (Figure 1). A pancreatic stent of adequate diameter (7 or 8.5 Fr) and length (4, 6, or 8 cm) was used during stone fragmentation. In cases where pancreatic stenting was unsuccessful owing to large stone burden, a 5 Fr ENPD (Cook Co.) was temporarily placed until fragmentation had occurred. After the residual stones were almost crushed by ESWL, they were removed endoscopically, and a 10 Fr S-type plastic PS was finally inserted into the exposed MPD stricture. Follow-up data were collected after the placement of the 10 Fr stent. EPS exchange and pancreatic duct brush cytology were performed every 3 months during the duration of stent application. Additional stone extraction was performed in the presence of small stones that remained in the MPD.

Finally, the dilation effect was revealed after repeated stent exchanges for at least 3 months to 1 year, wherein the pancreatic stent was removed and the patient was followed up in the outpatient department. Patients presenting with no improvement in pain symptoms after the stent-placement procedures were referred to the surgeon. In cases where malignancy was revealed by cytology, the stenting therapy was interrupted and appropriate treatment (surgery or chemotherapy) was initiated. Stent reinsertion was performed in patients with pain relapse, MPD restenosis, and stone recurrence after stent removal. These algorithms are shown in Figure 2.

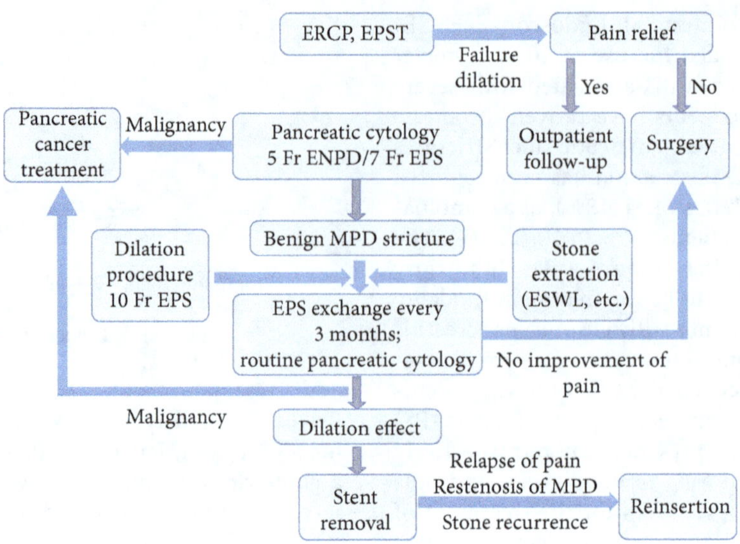

FIGURE 2: Algorithm of the treatments.

2.3. Postprocedural Evaluation and Patient Follow-Up. Clinical outcomes were evaluated according to the following parameters: technical success of stent placement, number of stent exchanges, placement periods, effect of pain relief, adverse events, coexisting rates of malignant disease, and both restenosis as well as restenting rates. The risk factors for MPD restenosis were as follows: alcohol as an etiology of chronic pancreatitis, resumption of alcohol after stent removal, continued smoking habit, presence of single or multiple stones, retention of stones after stent removal, recurrence of stones during the stenting treatment, and stricture at the body of MPD or Santorini duct. In addition to these factors, re-stricture during stenting treatment, re-stricture with diffuse pancreatic stones, and the presence of re-strictures and diffuse stones due to alcohol consumption are also considered as risk factors for pancreatic cancer.

2.4. Definition of Events. The primary study outcome was pain relief (control) and dilation during both short-term and long-term evaluation of the clinical success. The secondary outcome was defined by the diagnosis of malignancy following cytology during stent exchange and restenosis after the stent-free term.

Short-term and long-term periods were set for each of the two groups, the stent-placement success group and the stent-placement failure group. For the success group, short-term was defined as the period when the first repeat EPS was placed, whereas long-term was defined as the period when the stent was removed after the first repeat stent exchange session. In the stent placement failure group, short-term was defined as the period during which the first admission attempting to place the EPS (actually, it only displays the clinical outcomes) was performed, whereas long-term was defined as the period after the admission term of the first failure attempt of the EPS placement.

2.5. Statistical Analysis. Statistical analysis was performed using SPSS for Windows, version 11.0J (SPSS Inc., Chicago, IL). Absolute numbers and percentages as well as median (with interquartile range) are computed to describe patients' age, stent-placement periods, number of stent exchanges, and follow-up periods. Categorical values were compared by chi-square test, and continuous variables were compared using Mann-Whitney *U* tests. Univariate logistic regression analysis was performed to identify risk factors associated with MPD restenosis and pancreas cancer. Factors with $p < 0.05$ were retained for multiple logistic regression analysis, and those demonstrating statistical significance ($p < 0.05$) on a multivariate analysis were considered verifiable predictive factors.

3. Results

3.1. Patient Characteristics. The characteristics of the 59 patients in this study are presented in Table 1. This study included 47 males and 12 females, with an age range of 25–81 years (median, 56 years). The etiology of chronic pancreatitis was alcohol abuse in 51 patients, idiopathic in seven, and iatrogenic in one patient. Severe strictures were located in the head (48), body (6), genu (3), and the Santorini duct (2) of the patients. All patients had pancreatic stones in the MPD (a single stone in 16 patients and multiple stones in 43 patients). There were 53 smokers and six nonsmokers.

3.2. Short-Term Outcomes during Plastic PS Placement. Table 2 summarizes the short-term outcomes during EPS placement. The stents were successfully placed in 41 of 59 patients (69.5%). The median duration of pancreatic stenting was 276 days (range, 30–589 days). In total, 169 pancreatic stents were placed during this study, and PPS placement was performed approximately 1–16 times (median, 4 times) during the stenting session. The median number of times endoscopic retrograde cholangiopancreatography (ERCP) was performed from the first ERCP until 10 Fr plastic PS placement was 3.5. Thirty-seven (90.2%) of 41 patients who received EPS placement achieved pain relief. However, 15

Table 1: Patient characteristics.

	N
Gender, male/female	47/12
Age, median (ranges)	56 (25–81)
Etiology	
Alcoholic (%)	51 (86.4)
Not alcoholic (%)	8 (13.6)
(Idiopathic/iatrogenic)	(7/1)
Stricture location	
Head/body/head + body/Santorini duct	48/6/3/2
Pancreatic stone location	
Single/diffuse	16/43
Smoke, yes/no	53/6

patients (83.3%) in the EPS-failure group also achieved pain relief indicating no difference when compared with the EPS placement group. Among the 18 patients without EPS placement, 10 followed ESWL, four underwent observation at the outpatient department, and four presented with continuing abdominal complaints requiring surgical treatment. The reasons for plastic PS placement failure in the 18 patients included inability to properly cannulate MPD with EPST (10 patients) and inadequate pancreatic stone lithotripsy (eight patients). However, successful stone extraction was obtained in four patients, whereas in 14 patients the extraction proved to be a failure revealing significant differences between the two groups. EPST or precut was performed in all patients. The precut technique was performed in four out of 41 patients (9.8%) in the EPS-success group, and in 15 of the 18 patients (83.3%) in the EPS-failure group. For MPD dilation, SSR was effective in 24 patients (58.5%) because of the presence of severe strictures. Stent-related complications occurred in seven (3.6%) patients. Plastic PS had to be removed in three patients because of continuing abdominal pain. Furthermore, three out of four stent-occlusion cases resulted in severe complications; one patient presented with pancreatic abscess, one with colon fistula, which was treated under observation, while the third patient presented with splenic abscess, which was subsequently treated by percutaneous drainage. All the three aforementioned patients had multiple diffuse stones in the tail of the MPD.

Table 2: Short-term outcomes: during EPS placement.

	Success	Failure	p value
Results (%)	41 (69.5)	18 (30.5)	
Stent placement period, median	276	—	
(ranges)	(30–589)	—	
Exchanges, total	169	—	
No. of exchange, median (ranges)	4 (1–16)		
EPS placement; Santorini duct/Wirsung duct	3/38	—	
No. of times of ERCP until the 10 Fr EPS placement, median	3.5	—	
[1]Pain relief (%)	37 (90.2)	15 (83.3)	0.19
Additional treatment			
None	11	4	
Surgery	0	4	
ESWL	30	10	
Reasons for failure			
Lithotripsy failure (ESWL, EHL)	—	8	
Deep cannulation failure	—	10	
[1]Stone location			
Single stone/multiple stones	12/29	5/13	0.62
[1]Stone extraction results (%)	37 (90.2)	4 (0.22)	<0.01[2]
EPST/precut	37/4	3/15	
PD dilation procedure device			
SSR	24 (58.5)	0	
SBDC	14 (34.1)	1	
EPDBD	3 (7.3)	17	
Complications			
Abdominal pain after stent placement	3	0	
Stent occlusion (complications pancreatitis/pancreatic abscess/ colon-fistula/splenic abscess)	4 (1/1/1/1)	0	
Dislocation			
EPST hemorrhage	1	0	
Pancreatitis	3	1	
(Post-ERCP/post-ESWL/ post-EHL)	2	3	
GW perforation	(0/1/1)	(1/0/2)	
Pseudocyst rupture	1 0	3 1	

[1]p values: chi-square test. [2]Statistically significant. SSR: Soehendra stent retriever catheter; SBDC: Soehendra biliary balloon dilator; EPDBD: endoscopic pancreatic duct balloon dilation.

3.3. Long-Term Outcomes. Table 3 shows the long-term follow-up outcomes of the 59 patients. The median follow-up periods were 27 months after EPS insertion and 36 months in the EPS-failure group, indicating no differences between the two groups. Recurrence of MPD stricture was observed in 17 (41.5%) of the 41 patients. The median re-stricture time after removal of the first EPS was 191 (58–919) days. Re-stricture was observed in seven patients as a result of retention of MPD stones. Furthermore, exacerbation of chronic pancreatitis was noted because of resumption of alcohol in four patients and the recurrence of stones in two other patients. Sixteen patients (39.0%) received restenting (second placement), and the median period of these EPS placements was 260 (113–759) days. During this follow-up period, pancreatic cancer had developed in 3 (7.3%) patients, which was diagnosed 211 days after the first stent removal. Pancreatic duct cytology was performed in one patient after abdominal CT, whereas the two other patients were diagnosed by pancreatic duct cytology during routine stent exchange. One patient with pharyngeal

Table 3: Long-term outcomes after stent removal.

Events	EPS success	EPS failure	p value
N	41	18	—
[1]Follow-up periods (month, median)	26.0	36.0	0.20
Location of stricture			
Head/body/head + body/dorsal-duct	12/1/2/2	15/3/0/0	
MPD restenosis (%)	17 (41.5)	—	—
[2]Time to restenosis (days, median)	191		
Causes of restenosis			
Remaining stones (%)	7 (17.1)		
Resumption of alcohol (%)	4 (9.8)		
Major papilla restenosis (%)	3 (7.3)		
Recurrence of stones (%)	2 (4.9)		
Restenting (%)	16 (39.0)	—	
Re-placement period (days, median)	260		
Complications			
Pancreatic abscess	1 (36)	0	
Papillary restenosis	1 (359)	0	
Liver abscess	1 (37)	0	
[3]Coexisting malignant disease (%)	3 (5.9)	1 (2.9)	0.64
Pancreatic cancer (%)	3 (5.9)	0	
(Diagnosed day after 1st EPST, median)	(211)	—	
Pharyngeal cancer (%)	0	1 (2.9)	
(Diagnosed day after 1st EPST, median)	—	(1613)	

[1]p values: Mann-Whitney U test. The following month was counted after the first performance of EPST. [2]Counted from the EPS removal day when MPD dilation effect was revealed. [3]p values: chi-square test.

cancer was diagnosed 1613 days after the first ERCP. Plastic PS placement had failed, but fortunately, pain relief was achieved after precut addition. After pain relief, upper esophagogastroduodenoscopy and abdominal CT were performed every year at the outpatient department.

3.4. Risk Factors for MPD Restenosis and Factors of Pancreas Cancer. Tables 4 and 5 show the risk factors for MPD restenosis. Among the seven risk factors revealed by univariate analysis, "remaining stones after stent removal" and "stricture at the body of the MPD" were found to be associated with MPD restenosis. In the multivariate analysis, "remaining stones after stent removal" was identified as an independent factor of MPD restenosis. No significant risk factors for pancreatic cancer were observed in this study (Table 6).

4. Discussion

In the present study, we retrospectively evaluated the usefulness and long-term outcomes of chronic pancreatitis with MPD strictures and pancreatic stones. 10 Fr S-type plastic PS were successfully placed in 69.5% of 59 patients in this study. The success rates of EPS placements have been reported to range from 85%–98% [4–6], which is higher than that observed in the present study (69.5%). However, contrary to previous reports [35], most patients in this study (11 of 14 patients with 10 Fr S-type plastic PS and stone extraction failure) presented with diffuse pancreatic stones. These findings suggest that the inclusion of patients with diffuse pancreatic stones along with MPD obstruction had a negative influence on the technical success and may be responsible for the low clinical success rates. Immediate pain relief was obtained in 37 of the 41 patients (90.2%) with 10 Fr S-type plastic PS placement, which is in agreement with previously published reports where the placement of stents has been reported to be followed immediately by pain relief in approximately 65%–95% patients [4–7, 10, 13, 14, 36]. As observed in the present study, it takes several sessions of ERCP to place a 10 Fr plastic PS in the duct. Impacted pancreatic stones (diffuse or large) or severe PD strictures inhibit deep pancreatic cannulation, and it is challenging to place a 10 Fr S-type plastic PS during the first session. However, it is important to place a small-diameter stent early in the session to decompress the dilated MPD [8]. Pain relief is expected to be achieved in the early session, after which stone fragmentation and removal of MPD obstruction are performed followed by the placement of the 10 Fr S-type plastic PS over several steps. Furthermore, it is important to traverse the MPD obstruction using several guidewires; stricture-dilation procedures using SSR have proven to be useful in previous studies [32, 33]. In the present study, SSR was utilized in 58.6% patients with MPD strictures, indicating its usefulness as one of the key facilitators in MPD dilatation.

In addition, this study shows that the EPST or precutting techniques used in the EPS failure cases were effective in relieving pain. In one of our previous reports, we have shown that MPD hypertension is decreased by using either one of these techniques, leading to a reduction in abdominal pain [34]. Placement of stents is a relatively easy, acceptable, safe, and effective procedure, which can be used to alleviate the symptoms of chronic pancreatitis rapidly.

On the other hand, complications including stent occlusion and migration usually occur during the early phase after stent placement [37, 38]. Fortunately, no migration was noted within the duration of stent application in the present study; however, three patients presented with severe complications after stent occlusion. One patient presented with a pancreatic abscess, while another presented with a colon fistula, which was treated by observation. In addition, there was one case of splenic abscess, which was treated by percutaneous drainage. All three patients presented with diffuse multiple stones in the tail of the MPD. In our experience, the immediate complications of endoscopic stenting were mild, transient, and easily managed.

Statistical results of the present retrospective study revealed that "remaining stones during stent treatment" was the main factor for restenosis. There may also have been residual stones in the branch ducts in spite of cleaning the MPD during the stone retrieval treatments [35]. As

TABLE 4: Risk factors for MPD restenosis (univariate analysis).

	Restenosis (+)	Restenosis (−)	OR (95% CI)	p
[1]Alcohol etiology of chronic pancreatitis +/−	16/2	20/3	1.2 (0.18–8.07)	0.62
[1]Resumption of alcohol after stent removal +/−	4/13	1/23	7.07 (0.71–70.19)	0.08
[1]Continued smoke +/−	17/0	22/2	—	—
[1]Single/multiple stones	5/13	6/15	1.04 (0.26–4.21)	0.95
[1]Remaining stones after stent removal +/−	6/12	1/22	11.1 (1.18–102.38)	[2]**0.02**
[1]Recurrence of stones during stenting treatment +/−	3/14	0/22	—	—
[1]Stricture at the body of MPD +/−	5/12	1/21	0.11 (0.01–1.09)	[2]**0.04**

[1]Unordered categorical variables. [2]Statistically significant.

TABLE 5: Risk factors for MPD restenosis (multivariate).

	Restenosis (+)	Restenosis (−)	OR (95% CI)	p
[1]Remaining stones after stent removal +/−	6/12	1/22	11.44 (1.22–107.4)	[2]**0.03**
[1]Associated body of MPD strictures +/−	5/12	1/21	0.17 (0.02–1.88)	0.14

[1]Unordered categorical variables. [2]Statistically significant.

TABLE 6: Risk factors for pancreatic cancer (univariate analysis).

	Coexist cancer (+)	Coexist cancer (−)	OR (95% CI)	p
Alcohol etiology of chronic pancreatitis +/−	3/0	33/5	—	—
Resumption of alcohol after stent removal +/−	0/3	3/35	—	—
Continued smoking +/−	3/0	35/3	—	—
Single/multiple stones	2/1	26/10	0.77 (0.06–9.45)	0.84
Remaining stones after stent removal +/−	0/3	31/7	—	—
Re-stricture during stenting treatment +/−	0/3	17/21	—	—
Re-stricture with diffuse pancreatic stone +/−	0/3	12/26	—	—
Re-stricture, diffuse stone with an alcohol etiology +/−	0/3	12/26	—	—

many rates of diffuse stones were included in this study, the presence of stones in the side branches of the MPD must be taken into consideration after stent removal for long-term results.

In contrast to the study by Talamini et al., other studies including the present one found that neither resumption of alcohol consumption nor smoking after stent removal was associated with a significant increase in the rate of MPD restenosis [39]. Thus, the influence of tobacco use and alcohol consumption on MPD restenting outcome is still open to debate [5, 6, 39].

Despite the nearly statistically significant ($p = 0.08$) association between resumption of alcohol consumption after stent removal and MPD restenosis, a potentially important observation in this study is that alcohol prohibition should be continued not only throughout the duration of stent application but afterwards as well. Only two patients (4.9%) were able to abstain from smoking in this study. In future, we intend to evaluate the outcomes of MPD restenosis during smoking abstinence.

Importantly, the possibility of comorbid pancreatic cancer must also be considered during long-term EPS follow-up. Whereas most pancreatic duct strictures that occur during chronic pancreatitis are benign, a suspicion of malignancy requires prompt action involving surgical treatment rather than endoscopic stenting. All malignant cases were diagnosed by pancreatic brushing cytology in this study. Interestingly, MPD re-stricture did not aid in suspecting cases of malignancy; it was difficult to detect the presence of malignancy in two patients using imaging techniques such as enhanced CT and MRCP. Instead, the condition was diagnosed by routine pancreatic duct cytology. Previous studies have reported difficulties in diagnosing pancreatic malignancies arising in preexisting chronic pancreatitis [40, 41]. These facts indicate that in addition to cautious imaging follow-up, routine cytology must be performed after the treatment procedures.

The appropriate diameter as well as the duration of placement of the stents have not been determined in the present study. The use of the 10 Fr S-type plastic PS, which was replaced every 3 months, proved to be beneficial for the patients in this study; hence, this could be considered as the first line of treatment for both short-term and long-term endoscopic pancreatic stenting.

However, in this study, we experienced a serious complication concerning stent occlusion due to the presence of diffuse stones that remain in the tail of the MPD. Therefore, alternative methods such as multiple plastic stents and self-expandable covered metallic stents, as well as other surgical treatments, should also be thoroughly discussed for the treatment of refractory MPD strictures [42–46]. Further extensive studies involving pancreatic stents are required in future. In long-term stent application, it is important not to continue with the placement of an endoscopic stent in refractory cases in order to prevent pancreatic dysfunction and the development of pancreatic cancer. Therefore, it is important not to stick to the endoscopic stent placement in refractory cases, recurring pancreatitis exacerbation, and long-term stent application.

The current study is associated with some limitations. Since it is a study in a few cases (small sample size), there are some limitations in referring in this discussion. This was a retrospective and single-center study and limited external validity to this study; therefore, the possibility of unintentional selection bias cannot be fully excluded. Multivariate analysis data for risk of MPD restenosis (OR and 95% CI) was wide, and risk factors of pancreas cancer were not assessed in this study. This might have affected the outcome of small samples, so the results of this analysis cannot be generalized to other geographical regions of the world.

Despite this limitation, some factors indicated the statistical significance of the outcomes. Our explanatory analysis proceeded the use of 10 Fr S-type plastic pancreatic stents with routine exchange or both short-term and long-term outcomes in chronic pancreatitis patients with benign pancreatic duct strictures and impacted pancreatic stones, and this research is thought to lead to the next study. Therefore, our findings need to be confirmed in a prospective study.

In conclusion, we herein demonstrate that using 10 Fr S-type plastic PS with routine exchange is effective for both short-term and long-term outcomes. It is effective and useful in chronic pancreatitis patients with benign pancreatic duct strictures and impacted pancreatic stones.

Additional Points

Core Tips. 10 Fr S-type plastic pancreatic stents are effective for the treatment of pancreatic duct strictures and pancreatic stones in chronic pancreatitis.

Ethical Approval

The study protocol was in accordance with the Declaration of Helsinki 1975, as revised in 2013, and was approved by the ethics committee of our facility (25-83). Written informed consent was obtained from all participants. This manuscript has not been published in any language, in whole or in part, and is not under consideration for publication elsewhere.

Authors' Contributions

The format of this section will be as follows: Ito K designed the research and wrote the manuscript, Okano N and Igarashi Y designed the research, and Hara S, Takuma K, Yoshimoto K, Iwasaki S, and Kishimoto Y performed the research and collected the data.

Acknowledgments

We thank the paramedical, medical, and endoscopy staff at the Division of Gastroenterology and Hepatology of the Department of the Internal Medicine, Toho University, for making this study possible. I wish to thank Professor Yoshitaka Murakami (Department of Medical Statistics, Toho University) and Dr Yoshinori Kikuchi (Division of Gastroenterology and Hepatology, Toho University Omori Medical Center) for the advice about statistical research. We also wish to thank the paramedical, medical, and endoscopy staff at the Division of Gastroenterology and Hepatology of the Department of the Internal Medicine, Toho University, for making this study possible.

References

[1] K. Mergener and J. Baillie, "Chronic pancreatitis," *The Lancet*, vol. 350, no. 9088, pp. 1379–1385, 1997.

[2] M. L. Steer, I. Waxman, and S. Freedman, "Chronic pancreatitis," *The New England Journal of Medicine*, vol. 332, no. 22, pp. 1482–1490, 1995.

[3] K. Huibregtse, B. Schneider, A. A. Vrij, and G. N. J. Tytgat, "Endoscopic pancreatic drainage in chronic pancreatitis," *Gastrointestinal Endoscopy*, vol. 34, no. 1, pp. 9–15, 1988.

[4] M. Cremer, J. Deviere, M. Delhaye, M. Baize, and A. Vandermeeren, "Stenting in severe chronic pancreatitis: results of medium-term follow-up in seventy-six patients," *Endoscopy*, vol. 23, no. 3, pp. 171–176, 1991.

[5] K. F. Binmoeller, P. Jue, H. Seifert, W. C. Nam, J. Izbicki, and N. Sochendra, "Endoscopic pancreatic stent drainage in chronic pancreatitis and a dominant stricture: long-term results," *Endoscopy*, vol. 27, no. 9, pp. 638–644, 1995.

[6] T. Ponchon, R. M. Bory, F. Hedelius et al., "Endoscopic stenting for pain relief in chronic pancreatitis: results of a standardized protocol," *Gastrointestinal Endoscopy*, vol. 42, no. 5, pp. 452–456, 1995, 8566637.

[7] M. E. Smits, S. M. Badiga, E. A. J. Rauws, G. N. J. Tytgat, and K. Huibregtse, "Long-term results of pancreatic stents in

chronic pancreatitis," *Gastrointestinal Endoscopy*, vol. 42, no. 5, pp. 461–467, 1995.

[8] J. Deviere, M. Delhaye, and M. Cremer, "Pancreatic duct stones management," *Gastrointestinal Endoscopy Clinics of North America*, vol. 13, no. 2, pp. 86–93, 1998.

[9] D. E. Morgan, J. K. Smith, K. Hawkins, and C. M. Wilcox, "Endoscopic stent therapy in advanced chronic pancreatitis: relationships between ductal changes, clinical response, and stent patency," *The American Journal of Gastroenterology*, vol. 98, no. 4, pp. 821–826, 2003, 12738462.

[10] G. C. Vitale, K. Cothron, E. A. Vitale et al., "Role of pancreatic duct stenting in the treatment of chronic pancreatitis," *Surgical Endoscopy*, vol. 18, no. 10, pp. 1431–1434, 2004.

[11] N. Eleftheriadis, F. Dinu, M. Delhaye et al., "Long-term outcome after pancreatic stenting in severe chronic pancreatitis," *Endoscopy*, vol. 37, no. 3, pp. 223–230, 2005.

[12] T. Ukita, A. Moriyama, A. Tada et al., "Successful management of postoperative pancreatic fistula by application of constructed S-type pancreatic stent after operation for abnormal biliary-pancreatic junction," *Endoscopy*, vol. 35, no. 3, p. 253, 2003, 12584651.

[13] T. Ishihara, T. Yamaguchi, K. Seza, H. Tadenuma, and H. Saisho, "Efficacy of s-type stents for the treatment of the main pancreatic duct stricture in patients with chronic pancreatitis," *Scandinavian Journal of Gastroenterology*, vol. 41, no. 6, pp. 744–750, 2006.

[14] A. Weber, J. Schneider, B. Neu et al., "Endoscopic stent therapy for patients with chronic pancreatitis: results from a prospective follow-up study," *Pancreas*, vol. 34, no. 3, pp. 287–294, 2007, 17414050.

[15] P. A. Testoni, "Endoscopic stenting in benign pancreatic diseases," *Journal of Oncology Practice*, vol. 8, 1 Supplement, pp. 141–150, 2007.

[16] T. Ukita, "Pancreatic stenting for the preservation of pancreatic function in chronic pancreatitis with stricture," *Digestive Endoscopy*, vol. 15, no. 2, pp. 108–112, 2003.

[17] Y. Igarashi, K. Ito, T. Mimura et al., "Endoscopic pancreatic drainage," *Gastroenterological Endoscopy*, vol. 46, no. 12, pp. 2582–2588, 2004.

[18] J. M. Dumonceau, M. Delhaye, A. Tringali et al., "Endoscopic treatment of chronic pancreatitis: European Society of Gastrointestinal Endoscopy (ESGE) Clinical Guideline," *Endoscopy*, vol. 44, no. 08, pp. 784–800, 2012, 22752888.

[19] Y. Fukuda, T. Tsuyuguchi, Y. Sakai, S. Tsuchiya, and H. Saisyo, "Diagnostic utility of peroral cholangioscopy for various bile-duct lesions," *Gastrointestinal Endoscopy*, vol. 62, no. 3, pp. 374–382, 2005, 16111955.

[20] H. E. Adamek, R. Jakobs, A. Buttmann, M. U. Adamek, A. R. J. Schneider, and J. F. Riemann, "Long term follow up of patients with chronic pancreatitis and pancreatic stones treated with extracorporeal shock wave lithotripsy," *Gut*, vol. 45, no. 3, pp. 402–405, 1999.

[21] M. J. Farnbacher, S. Mühldorfer, M. Wehler, B. Fischer, E. G. Hahn, and H. T. Schneider, "Interventional endoscopic therapy in chronic pancreatitis including temporary stenting: a definitive treatment?," *Scandinavian Journal of Gastroenterology*, vol. 41, no. 1, pp. 111–117, 2006.

[22] H. Grimm, W. H. Meyer, V. C. Nam, and N. Soehendra, "New modalities for treating chronic pancreatitis," *Endoscopy*, vol. 21, no. 02, pp. 70–74, 1989, 2707174.

[23] M. Delhaye, A. Vandermeeren, M. Baize, and M. Cremer, "Extracorporeal shock-wave lithotripsy of pancreatic calculi," *Gastroenterology*, vol. 102, no. 2, pp. 610–620, 1992, 1732129.

[24] H. T. Schneider, A. May, J. Benninger et al., "Piezoelectric shock wave lithotripsy of pancreatic duct stones," *The American Journal of Gastroenterology*, vol. 89, no. 11, pp. 2042–2048, 1994, 7942733.

[25] M. Delhaye, M. Arvanitakis, G. Verset, M. Cremer, and J. Devière, "Long-term clinical outcome after endoscopic pancreatic ductal drainage for patients with painful chronic pancreatitis," *Clinical Gastroenterology and Hepatology*, vol. 2, no. 12, pp. 1096–1106, 2004, 15625655.

[26] T. Rösch, S. Daniel, M. Scholz et al., "Endoscopic treatment of chronic pancreatitis: a multicenter study of 1000 patients with long-term follow-up," *Endoscopy*, vol. 34, no. 10, pp. 765–771, 2002.

[27] A. Gabbrielli, M. Pandolfi, M. Mutignani et al., "Efficacy of main pancreatic-duct endoscopic drainage in patients with chronic pancreatitis, continuous pain, and dilated duct," *Gastrointestinal Endoscopy*, vol. 61, no. 4, pp. 576–581, 2005.

[28] D. L. Cahen, D. J. Gouma, Y. Nio et al., "Endoscopic versus surgical drainage of the pancreatic duct in chronic pancreatitis," *The New England Journal of Medicine*, vol. 356, no. 7, pp. 676–684, 2007.

[29] J. M. Dumonceau, G. Costamagna, A. Tringali et al., "Treatment for painful calcified chronic pancreatitis: extracorporeal shock wave lithotripsy versus endoscopic treatment: a randomised controlled trial," *Gut*, vol. 56, no. 4, pp. 545–552, 2007.

[30] Y. W. Joo, J. H. Yoon, S. C. Cho et al., "Endoscopic pancreatic sphincterotomy: indications and complications," *The Korean Journal of Internal Medicine*, vol. 24, no. 3, pp. 190–195, 2009.

[31] J. J. Ziebert and J. A. DiSario, "Dilation of refractory pancreatic duct strictures: the turn of the screw," *Gastrointestinal Endoscopy*, vol. 49, no. 5, pp. 632–635, 1999.

[32] T. H. Baron and D. E. Morgan, "Dilation of a difficult benign pancreatic duct stricture using the Soehendra stent extractor," *Gastrointestinal Endoscopy*, vol. 46, no. 2, pp. 178–180, 1997.

[33] B. Brand, F. Thonke, S. Obytz et al., "Stent retriever for dilation of pancreatic and bile duct strictures," *Endoscopy*, vol. 31, no. 2, pp. 142–145, 1999.

[34] K. Ito, Y. Igarashi, N. Okano et al., "Efficacy of combined endoscopic lithotomy and extracorporeal shock wave lithotripsy, and additional electrohydraulic lithotripsy using the SpyGlass direct visualization system or X-ray guided EHL as needed, for pancreatic lithiasis," *BioMed Research International*, vol. 2014, Article ID 732781, 8 pages, 2014.

[35] N. Sasahira, M. Tada, H. Isayama et al., "Outcomes after clearance of pancreatic stones with or without pancreatic stenting," *Journal of Gastroenterology*, vol. 42, no. 1, pp. 63–69, 2007.

[36] J. Boursier, V. Quentin, V. le Tallec et al., "Endoscopic treatment of painful chronic pancreatitis: evaluation of a new flexible multiperforated plastic stent," *Gastroentérologie Clinique et Biologique*, vol. 32, no. 10, pp. 801–805, 2008.

[37] S. O. Ikenberry, S. Sherman, R. H. Hawes, M. Smith, and G. A. Lehman, "The occlusion rate of pancreatic stents," *Gastrointestinal Endoscopy*, vol. 40, no. 5, pp. 611–613, 1994.

[38] M. J. Farnbacher, R. E. Voll, R. Faissner et al., "Composition of

clogging material in pancreatic endoprostheses," *Gastrointestinal Endoscopy*, vol. 61, no. 7, pp. 862–866, 2005.

[39] G. Talamini, C. Bassi, M. Falconi et al., "Pain relapses in the first 10 years of chronic pancreatitis," *American Journal of Surgery*, vol. 171, no. 6, pp. 565–569, 1996.

[40] A. Fritscher-Ravens, L. Brand, W. T. Knofel et al., "Comparison of endoscopic ultrasound-guided fine needle aspiration for focal pancreatic lesions in patients with normal parenchyma and chronic pancreatitis," *The American Journal of Gastroenterology*, vol. 97, no. 11, pp. 2768–2775, 2002.

[41] M. Topazian, H. Aslanian, and D. Andersen, "Outcome following endoscopic stenting of pancreatic duct strictures in chronic pancreatitis," *Journal of Clinical Gastroenterology*, vol. 39, no. 10, pp. 908–911, 2005.

[42] G. Costamagna, M. Bulajic, A. Tringali et al., "Multiple stenting of refractory pancreatic duct strictures in severe chronic pancreatitis: long-term results," *Endoscopy*, vol. 38, no. 03, pp. 254–259, 2006.

[43] P. Eisendrath and J. Deviere, "Expandable metal stents for benign pancreatic duct obstruction," *Gastrointestinal Endoscopy Clinics of North America*, vol. 9, no. 3, pp. 547–554, 1999.

[44] D. H. Par k, M. H. Kim, S. H. Moon, S. S. Lee, D. W. Seo, and S. K. Lee, "Feasibility and safety of placement of a newly designed, fully covered self-expandable metal stent for refractory benign pancreatic ductal strictures: a pilot study (with video)," *Gastrointestinal Endoscopy*, vol. 68, no. 6, pp. 1182–1189, 2008.

[45] S. H. Moon, M. H. Kim, D. H. Park et al., "Modified fully covered self-expandable metal stents with antimigration features for benign pancreatic-duct strictures in advanced chronic pancreatitis, with a focus on the safety profile and reducing migration," *Gastrointestinal Endoscopy*, vol. 72, no. 1, pp. 86–91, 2010.

[46] K. Okushima, J. Yoshino, K. Inui, H. Miyoshi, and Y. Nakamura, "Short-term metal stenting for treatment of main pancreatic duct strictures associated with chronic pancreatitis," *Digestive Endoscopy*, vol. 17, no. 3, pp. 230–234, 2005.

14

Helicobacter pylori Eradication in Idiopathic Thrombocytopenic Purpura

Bum Jun Kim,[1,2] Hyeong Su Kim,[1] Hyun Joo Jang,[3] and Jung Han Kim[1]

[1]*Division of Hemato-Oncology, Department of Internal Medicine, Kangnam Sacred-Heart Hospital, Hallym University Medical Center, Hallym University College of Medicine, Seoul, Republic of Korea*
[2]*Department of Internal Medicine, National Army Capital Hospital, The Armed Forces Medical Command, Sungnam, Gyeonggi-do, Republic of Korea*
[3]*Division of Gastroenterology, Department of Internal Medicine, Dongtan Sacred-Heart Hospital, Hallym University Medical Center, Hallym University College of Medicine, Hwasung, Gyeonggi-do, Republic of Korea*

Correspondence should be addressed to Hyun Joo Jang; jhj1229@hallym.or.kr and Jung Han Kim; harricil@hallym.or.kr

Academic Editor: Maria P. Dore

Objective. Several recent reviews of published studies have shown that the eradication of *H. pylori* infection in patients with ITP improved thrombocytopenia in about half of the cases. However, most included studies were observational case series. We performed the first meta-analysis of randomized trials to gain a better insight into the effect of *H. pylori* eradication in ITP patients. *Methods.* A systematic computerized search of the electronic databases including PubMed, EMBASE, Google Scholar, and Cochrane Library (up to December 2017) was conducted. *Results.* From six studies, a total of 241 patients (125 in eradication group and 116 in control group) were included in the meta-analysis. Patients in the eradication group showed significantly higher overall platelet response rate than those in the control group (odds ratio = 1.93, 95% confidence interval: 1.01–3.71, $P = 0.05$). In the subgroup analysis, however, children in the eradication group failed to show statistically better response rate than those in the noneradication group (odds ratio = 1.80, 95% confidence interval: 0.88–3.65, $P = 0.11$). *Conclusions.* This meta-analysis indicates that *H. pylori* eradication has a significant therapeutic effect in patients with ITP. Considering the intrinsic limits in the design and sample size of the included studies, however, large randomized controlled trials are warranted to validate the therapeutic impact of *H. pylori* eradication in adults as well as children with ITP.

1. Introduction

Idiopathic or immune thrombocytopenic purpura (ITP) is an autoimmune-mediated acquired bleeding disorder of children as well as adults. It is characterized by the destruction of host platelet caused by anti-platelet antibodies [1]. However, the mechanisms that trigger the development of platelet auto-antibodies remain poorly understood. Persistent thrombocytopenia for more than 6 or 12 months defines the chronic form of ITP [2, 3]. ITP is typically a diagnosis of exclusion, made by clinicians after ruling out other possible etiologies. ITP can be a primary disease or secondary to a variety of etiologies including bacterial or viral infection, autoimmune disease, or neoplasm [1–3].

Helicobacter pylori (H. pylori) is the most common microbial pathogen that colonizes in the mucosal layer of the stomach. It is causally associated with a variety of gastrointestinal disorders including chronic gastritis, gastric mucosal atrophy, peptic ulcer, gastric mucosa-associated lymphoid tissue lymphoma, and gastric adenocarcinoma [4, 5]. A pathophysiologic link between ITP and *H. pylori* infection was initially proposed in 1998 by Gasbarrini et al. who reported a significant increase of platelet count after bacterial eradication in 8 of 11 ITP patients infected with *H. pylori* [6]. Although the pathogenesis of *H. pylori*-associated ITP is still uncertain, several studies have suggested that *H. pylori* virulence factor, cytotoxin-associated gene A (CagA), stimulates the development of anti-CagA antibodies (Abs) that cross-react with platelet surface antigens (Ags), resulting in thrombocytopenia [7–9]. Many studies have reported that *H. pylori* eradication led to an increase of platelet counts and even a regression of ITP [10–18]. As other studies have failed to demonstrate the beneficial effect of bacterial eradication in ITP [19–21], however, there is a debate as to whether the eradication of *H. pylori* in chronic ITP is effective in increasing platelet counts or not.

Several recent reviews of previously published studies have shown that the eradication of *H. pylori* infection in patients with chronic ITP improved thrombocytopenia in about half of the cases [22–24]. The metaregression model revealed that the success of bacterium eradication was highly significant as an explanatory variable for increase of platelet count [22]. However, most studies included were observational case series [22–24], which might subject the results to possible bias. In addition, several recent randomized trials in adults or children showed the inconsistent effect of bacterium eradication on platelet recovery in ITP patients infected with *H. pylori* [16–21]. Therefore, we performed this meta-analysis of randomized trials to gain a better insight into the effect of *H. pylori* eradication in ITP patients.

2. Materials and Methods

2.1. Publication Searching Strategy. The current study was conducted according to the preferred reporting items for systematic reviews and meta-analyses (PRISMA) guidelines [25, 26]. A systematic computerized search of the electronic databases including PubMed, EMBASE, Google Scholar, and Cochrane Library (up to December 2017) was performed. The search used the following keywords variably combined: "*Helicobacter pylori*," "*H. pylori*," "thrombocytopenia," "idiopathic thrombocytopenic purpura," "immune thrombocytopenic purpura," and "ITP." The related article function in PubMed was used to identify all relevant articles. In addition, the bibliographic references of all retrieved studies and reviews were evaluated for additional eligible articles.

2.2. Inclusion Criteria. We only included randomized controlled trials in this meta-analysis. Retrospective or observational case control studies were excluded. Eligible studies should meet the following inclusion criteria: (i) patients with a diagnosis of chronic ITP according to the American Society of Hematology (ASH) guidelines [2]; (ii) *H. pylori* infection documented by reliable tests such as ^{13}C-urea breath test (UBT), serologic test for antibody to *H. pylori*, stool antigen test, or histology of gastric mucosal biopsies; (iii) randomization of ITP patients infected with *H. pylori* to either bacterial eradication or noneradication; (iv) providing treatment outcomes (platelet counts or response rate) of these two groups. Reports published only in abstract form were not considered eligible.

2.3. Data Extraction. Two reviewers (BJK and HJJ) independently screened relevant studies and extracted the data from each eligible study. If these two authors did not agree, the other investigator (JHK) was consulted to resolve the disagreement through discussion.

The following data were extracted from the included studies: the first author, year of publication, country, number of patients, demographics (age, gender), detecting methods for *H. pylori* infection, duration of ITP, treatment, platelet counts (before and after treatment) or treatment outcomes, and relapse rate.

2.4. Quality Assessment. The methodological quality of the randomized trials was scored using the Jadad five-item scale, taking into account randomization, double-blinding process, and withdrawals [27]. The final score ranged from 0 to 5, with low-quality studies having a score ≤ 2 and high-quality studies having a score of ≥ 3.

2.5. Statistical Analyses. We chose to record the overall response rate (ORR) as primary assessment criteria. The odds ratios (ORs) and 95% confidence intervals (CIs) for ORR were calculated indirectly from original articles. The effect size of ORR was pooled through OR and its 95% CI. The heterogeneity across studies was estimated by the Q statistics and I^2 inconsistency test. The fixed-effect model (Mantel–Haenszel method) was used for pooling homogeneous outcomes ($P \geq 0.1$ and $I^2 \leq 50\%$), and the random-effect model (DerSimonian–Laird method) was selected if significant heterogeneity was observed ($P < 0.1$ and $I^2 > 50\%$).

The RevMan version 5.3 was used to combine the data. The plots show a summary estimate of the results from all the studies combined. The size of the squares represents the estimate from each study, reflecting the statistical "weight" of the study. Outcomes are provided as forest plots with diamonds representing the estimate of the pooled effect and the width of diamond implying its precision. The line of no effect is number one for binary outcomes, which depicts statistical significance if not crossed by the diamond [28]. The OR > 1.0 implies better response for patients receiving the eradication treatment of *H. pylori* infection.

The possibility of publication bias was assessed with a visual inspection of the graphical funnel plot [29]. The statistical methods for detecting funnel plot asymmetry were the rank correlation tests of Begg and Mazumdar and Egger's regression asymmetry test [29, 30]. Statistical significance was considered for a P value of less than 0.05 for the summary estimate of OR and publication biases.

3. Results

3.1. Results of Search. A total of 157 potentially relevant articles were initially found, but 111 of them were excluded after careful screening of the titles and abstracts. We retrieved 46 articles for full-text evaluation and further excluded 40 by the inclusion criteria. Finally, 6 studies were included in the meta-analysis [16–21]. Figure 1 shows the search flow diagram of this meta-analysis.

3.2. Characteristics of the Included Studies. Table 1 summarizes the main characteristics and treatment outcomes of the six studies. Four studies were conducted in children [18–21] and the remaining 2 in adults [16, 17]. The most common detection method for *H. pylori* infection was UBT [16, 18–21]. The prevalence of *H. pylori* infection ranged

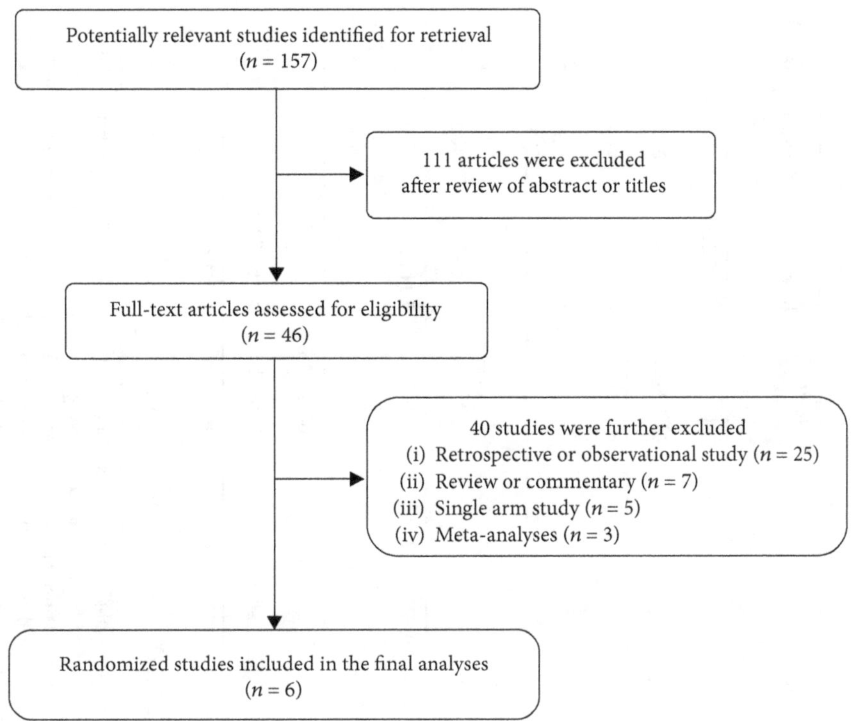

FIGURE 1: Flow diagram of search process.

from 25.9% [21] to 73.9% [20]. Bacterium eradication consisted of standard triple therapy including clarithromycin, amoxicillin, and proton-pump inhibitor (PPI) (omeprazole or lansoprazole) for 7–14 days. Except for one study [16], patients in the control arms were usually treated with corticosteroid (prednisone or prednisolone) or PPI alone.

3.3. Platelet Response to Treatment. In most studies, complete response (CR) was defined as the achievement of a platelet count more than 150×10^9/L [16, 18–21]. However, the threshold for partial response (PR) varied among studies although platelet count with a net increase of greater than 30×10^9/L was most commonly adopted [17, 18, 20, 21] (Table 1). We defined the ORR by adding CR rate and PR rate. The ORR varied from 14.3% [19] to 88.2% [18] in the eradication arms and from 0% [16] to 88.1% [18] in the noneradication arms.

3.4. Quality of the Included Studies. The Jadad scores for the 6 randomized studies was 2 or less. The studies announced that patients were randomly assigned by concealed allocation, but no more information on the method to generate the sequence of randomization was available.

3.5. Therapeutic Effect of H. pylori Eradication: Meta-Analysis. From the six studies, a total of 241 patients (125 in the eradication group and 116 in the control group) were included in the meta-analysis of ORs for ORR. The fixed-effect model was selected because there was no significant heterogeneity among studies ($X^2 = 4.11$, $P = 0.53$, $I^2 = 0\%$). Patients in the eradication group showed significantly higher ORR than those in the control group (OR = 1.93, 95% CI: 1.01–3.71, $P = 0.05$) (Figure 2(a)).

In the subgroup analysis, children in the eradication group failed to show statistically higher ORR than those in the noneradication group (OR = 1.80, 95% CI: 0.88–3.65, $P = 0.11$) (Figure 2(b)). There was no significant heterogeneity among studies ($X^2 = 1.38$, $P = 0.71$, $I^2 = 0\%$), and the fixed-effect model was used for pooling the data.

3.6. Publication Bias. Begg's funnel plot and Egger's test indicated no evidence of substantial publication bias for ORR (Begg's $P = 0.452$, Egger's $P = 0.465$) (Figure 3).

4. Discussion

Despite the findings indicating that *H. pylori* infection plays an etiological role in ITP, several randomized trials to date have shown the inconsistent results in the effect of bacterium eradication. In this meta-analysis of 6 randomized trials, we evaluated the therapeutic effect of *H. pylori* eradication in patients with ITP. Our results indicate that bacterium eradication has a significant impact on platelet recovery in ITP.

ITP is considered an organ-specific autoimmune disease. It is mediated by anti-platelet Abs that bind to host platelets and megakaryocytes, accelerating platelet destruction by the reticuloendothelial system [31]. The auto-Abs primarily target platelet surface glycoproteins such as GP IIb/IIIa and GP Ib. Although the triggering factors for ITP are obscure, bacterial or viral infections are known to be associated with the development of ITP, indicating that infectious agents may play a critical role in the pathogenesis of a particular subset of ITP [32].

Table 1: Summary of the six included studies.

First author (year) Country [ref]	Number of ITP pts	Detection of Hp infection	Number of Hp (+) pts	Randomization	Number of pts	M/F	Mean age (yr) (SD or range)	Duration of ITP (yr)	Platelet at enrollment ($\times 10^9$/L)	Platelet after 6 mo of Tx ($\times 10^9$/L)	Response[‡] (CR + PR)	Relapse at 1 year	Jadad score
Suzuki (2005) Japan [16]	36	UBT or histology	25 (69.4%)	Eradication	13	5/8	57.4 ± 15.0	5.8 ± 7.2	54.7 ± 26.9	114.5 ± 90.5	6 (46.2%)	NA	2
				Noneradication (observation)	12	5/7	56.2 ± 7.8	4.6 ± 5.2	48.4 ± 22.1	48.1 ± 26.0	0 (0%)	NA	
Tsutsumi (2005) Japan [17]	25	Anti-Hp antibody	17 (68%)	Eradication	9	2/7	60.3	NA	NA	NA	6 (66.7%)	2 (33.3%)	2
				Noneradication (PPI)	8	3/5	63.3	NA	NA	NA	5 (62.5%)	2 (40%)	
Li (2009) China [18]	NA	UBT	93	Eradication + PD	51	27/24	6.7 ± 2.4	NA	NA	NA	45 (88.2%)	11 (21.6%)	1
				Noneradication (PD)	42	22/20	5.8 ± 2.7	NA	NA	NA	37 (88.1%)	17 (40.5%)	
Treepongkaruna (2009) Thailand [19]	55	UBT	16 (29.1%)	Eradication + PD	7	3/4	11.0	3.4 (1.7–6.9)	23.0 (3.0–84.0)	NA	1 (14.3%)	NA	2
				Noneradication (PD)	9(8)*	4/5	10.8	5.1 (1.2–9.5)	34.0 (3.0–86.0)	NA	1 (12.5%)	NA	
Tang (2013) China [20]	92	UBT	68 (73.9%)	Eradication ± PD	34	NA	NA (child)	NA	14.8 ± 0.4	160.4 ± 1.0	26 (76.5%)	NA	2
				Noneradication (±PD)	34	NA	NA (child)	NA	15.1 ± 0.3	80.6 ± 1.1	20 (58.8%)	NA	
Brito (2015) Brazil [21]	85	UBT or stool Ag test	22 (25.9%)	Eradication ± PD	11	6/5	12.7 (4.9–17.5)	5 (1–8)	35.0 (1–145)	128 ± 73	7 (63.6%)	NA	2
				Noneradication (±PD)	11	5/6	10.5 (5.8–17.7)	3 (0.7–11)	47 (8–139)	63 ± 44	4 (36.4%)	NA	

ITP: idiopathic or immune thrombocytopenia purpura; Hp: *Helicobacter pylori*; UBT: ^{13}C-urea breath test; pts: patients; yr: years; mo: months; SD: standard deviation; PPI: proton-pump inhibitor, PD: prednisone or prednisolone; Tx: treatment; CR: complete platelet response; PR: partial platelet response; NA: not available. *One patient was withdrawn due to massive gastrointestinal bleeding, requiring high-dose prednisolone. ‡Overall response criteria: Suzuki: platelet count increased by more than 50×10^9/L 6 months after eradication therapy; Tsutsumi: platelet count with a net increase greater than 30×10^9/L or a 50% increase in platelet count with a net increase of 10×10^9/L but less than 30×10^9/L; Li: platelet count with a net increase greater than 30×10^9/L; Treepongkaruna: platelet count more than 100×10^9/L sustaining for at least 3 months; Tang: platelet count more than 50×10^9/L or platelet count with a net increase greater than 30×10^9/L; Brito: platelet increase greater than $20–30 \times 10^9$/L.

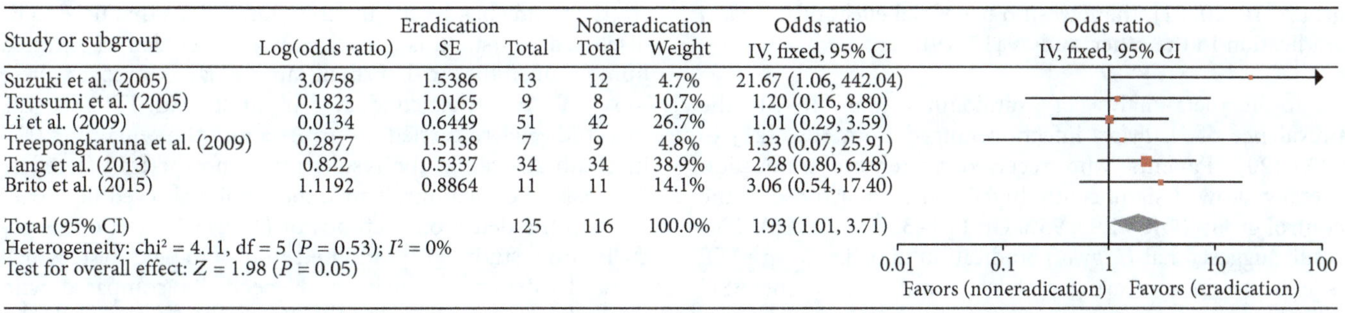

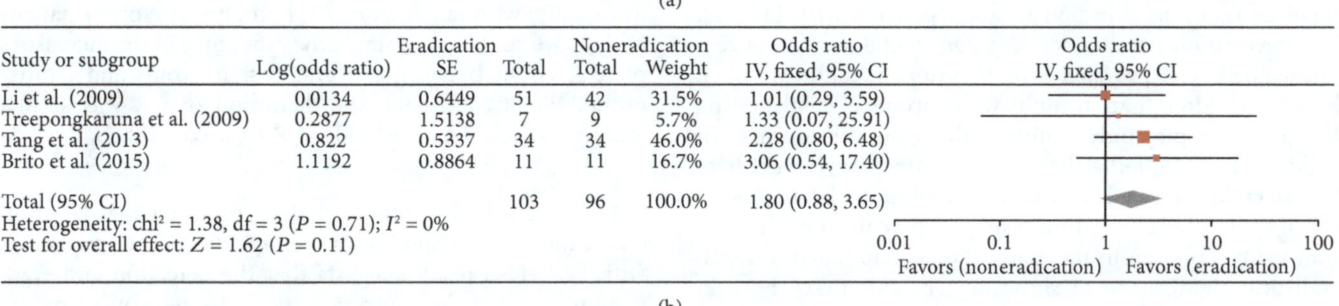

FIGURE 2: Forest plots of odds ratios for overall platelet response rates in all patients (a) and in children (b).

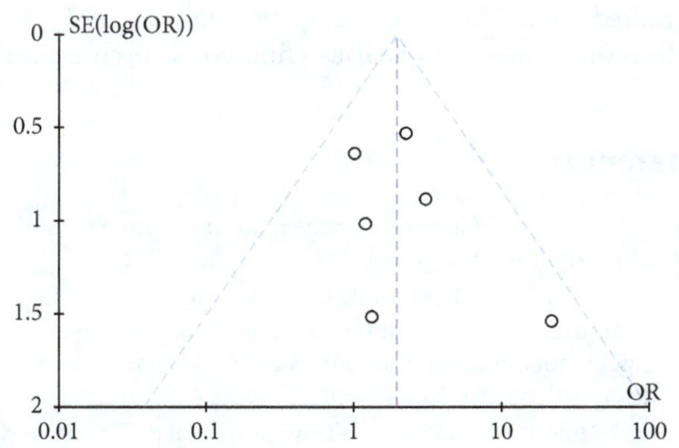

FIGURE 3: Funnel plot for publication bias regarding overall response rates.

Since the first report in 1998 [6], the accumulating data have indicated that *H. pylori* may contribute to the pathogenesis of chronic ITP [7, 9, 31–34]. In addition, numerous clinical studies have reported that *H. pylori* eradication resulted in an increase of platelet counts in ITP [10–18]. Various mechanisms have been proposed for the role of *H. pylori* in chronic ITP: the production of Ag-specific Abs that are cross-reactive with platelet surface glycoproteins (GP IIb/IIIa or GP Ib) due to molecular mimicry increased plasmacytoid dendritic cell numbers and variable host immune response to virulence factors such as vacuolating-associated cytotoxin gene A (VacA) and CagA [7, 9, 33, 34]. A recent study in China reported that the FcγRIIB expression on circulating monocytes is downregulated in *H. pylori*-infected ITP patients [35]. Therefore, *H. pylori* infection may play an important role in the development of ITP by activating the Fcγ receptor of monocytes/macrophages through downregulation of the inhibitory receptor FcγRIIB. Despite mounting evidence of the association of *H. pylori* and ITP, published studies are inconclusive due to the scarcity of controlled clinical trials to date and some reports presenting conflicting results [16–21]. Moreover, empirical treatment of *H. pylori* in children with ITP remains controversial [36, 37]. Therefore, validating the therapeutic effects of *H. pylori* eradication has a critical impact on clinical diagnosis and treatment of ITP.

In the previous systemic reviews, the pooled prevalence of *H. pylori* infection in ITP ranged from 58% [38] to 65% [23]. The first meta-analysis by Franchini et al. reviewed 17 studies with 788 ITP patients, including 494 infected with *H. pylori* [22]. There was a statistically significant difference in the increase of platelet count in patients for whom *H. pylori* eradication was successful, compared with untreated patients (weighted mean difference (WMD) of 40.77×10^9/L, 95% CI: 20.92–60.63) and those who failed eradication (WMD of 52.16×10^9/L, 95% CI: 27.79–64.91). Another systemic review with a meta-analysis of 1555 patients with ITP from 25 studies reported the weighted mean CR (platelet count more than 100×10^9/L) of 42.7% and ORR (platelet count $\geq 30 \times 10^9$/L and at least doubling of basal platelet count) of 50.3% after successful eradication of *H. pylori* [23]. In addition, the most recent systemic review by Frydman et al. confirmed that eradication treatment in *H. pylori*-positive adult ITP patients resulted in about a 50% CR rate [24]. These findings indicate the beneficial effect of bacterium eradication in ITP patients infected with *H. pylori*. Except for one [16], however, almost all articles included in those reviews were retrospective or observational studies [22–24]. Thereafter, five more randomized trials were conducted in adult or children ITP patients [17–21]. While three studies observed a significant difference in the platelet response between the eradication group and noneradication group [16, 20, 21], there was no beneficial effect of *H. pylori* eradication in the other studies [17–19].

In this meta-analysis of 6 randomized trials [16–21], the prevalence of *H. pylori* infection ranged from 30% [21] to 74% [20]. Patients who received bacterium eradication therapy showed significantly higher ORR than those in the control group (OR = 1.93, 95% CI: 1.01–3.71, $P = 0.05$). This result suggests that *H. pylori* eradication in patients with ITP is effective in increasing platelet count. The recent ASH guidelines have recommended the examination and treatment of *H. pylori* infection in adult patients with ITP [2]. However, routine testing for *H. pylori* in children is not recommended. The prevalence of *H. pylori* infection is much lower in children than in adults with chronic ITP, suggesting that *H. pylori* play only a minor role in the development of childhood ITP [39]. Platelet responses after *H. pylori* eradication in children were highly variable and inconsistent among studies [18–21, 39–41]. In the subgroup analysis of the current study, children in the eradication group failed to reach statistical significance to show higher ORR than those in the control group (OR = 1.80, 95% CI: 0.88–3.65, $P = 0.11$). However, the subgroup analysis included only 4 studies with a small number of patients. Therefore, this finding seems not sufficient to determine the therapeutic efficacy of *H. pylori* eradication in childhood ITP. Larger randomized trials are necessary to confirm the beneficial role of *H. pylori* eradication in childhood ITP.

A number of questions regarding the eradication of *H. pylori* infection in ITP still remain to be resolved, including the difference of efficacy among countries, factors predicting the platelet response, and mechanisms responsible for therapeutic effect associated with *H. pylori* eradication [39]. There was a great variability in the platelet responses of *H. pylori* eradication between Western and Eastern series [23]. Studies from Japan tended toward better response rates (28%–100%) than those from USA, Spain, and Mexico (<20%). The reason for such variability among countries is not clear, but geographic differences in the epidemic *H. pylori* strains may, at least in part, account for the difference in the platelet responses. The frequency of CagA-positive strains varies among geographic locations. Eastern Asian *H. pylori* strains have been found as more pathogenic, correlating with an increased development of gastric adenocarcinoma in *H. pylori*-positive patients in East Asia [42, 43]. The majority of *H. pylori* strains detected in East Asia express CagA, whereas the proportion of CagA-positive *H. pylori* strains in Western countries was much lower [44]. Immune response to CagA protein may be associated with improved platelet count after *H. pylori* eradication in patients with ITP [7–9]. Takahashi et al. observed that the level of anti-CagA Ab in the platelet eluates declined in three patients showing CR after eradication [7]. Kodama et al. reported that reduction in the anti-CagA antibody titer after eradication therapy was significantly greater in responders than in non-responders [9]. These findings suggest that anti-CagA Ab titer may be a biomarker to determine who is indicated for bacterium eradication among patients with ITP.

Our study has several inherent limitations that need to be discussed. First, this meta-analysis included a limited number of studies with a small sample size. Moreover, there were only two trials conducted in adults with ITP. Second, five studies were carried out in Asia and the remaining trial in South Africa. So the results might not be transferred to Caucasian populations. Third, the studies showed heterogeneity in the detection methods of *H. pylori* infection. Especially one study [17] adopted the serologic test which showed inferior sensitivity and specificity compared with other diagnostic methods [45]. Fourth, most studies had a low quality with Jadad score ≤ 2. Fifth, because of the paucity of data, we could not evaluate the difference in the increase of platelet count between the eradication group and control group. Finally, although the definition of CR was similar among studies, the threshold for PR varied a little.

In conclusion, our meta-analysis indicates that *H. pylori* eradication has a significant therapeutic effect in patients with ITP. This result suggests that the detection and eradication of *H. pylori* infection need to be considered in patients with chronic ITP. Taking into account the intrinsic limits in the design and sample size of the included studies, however, large randomized controlled trials are warranted to validate the therapeutic impact of *H. pylori* eradication in adults as well as children with chronic ITP.

References

[1] C. E. Neunert, "Current management of immune thrombocytopenia," *Hematology*, vol. 2013, pp. 276–282, 2013.

[2] J. N. George, S. H. Woolf, G. E. Raskob et al., "Idiopathic thrombocytopenic purpura: a practice guideline developed by explicit methods for the American Society of Hematology," *Blood*, vol. 88, no. 1, pp. 3–40, 1996.

[3] C. Neunert, W. Lim, M. Crowther et al., "The American Society of Hematology 2011 evidence-based practice guideline for immune thrombocytopenia," *Blood*, vol. 117, no. 16, pp. 4190–4207, 2011.

[4] S. Suerbaum and P. Michetti, "Helicobacter pylori infection," *The New England Journal of Medicine*, vol. 347, no. 15, pp. 1175–1186, 2002.

[5] Y.-I. Kim, S.-J. Cho, J. Y. Lee et al., "Effect of Helicobacter pylori eradication on long-term survival after distal gastrectomy for gastric cancer," *Cancer Research and Treatment*, vol. 48, no. 3, pp. 1020–1029, 2016.

[6] A. Gasbarrini, F. Franceschi, R. Tartaglione, R. Landolfi, P. Pola, and G. Gasbarrini, "Regression of autoimmune thrombocytopenia after eradication of Helicobacter pylori," *The Lancet*, vol. 352, no. 9131, p. 878, 1998.

[7] T. Takahashi, T. Yujiri, K. Shinohara et al., "Molecular mimicry by Helicobacter pylori CagA protein may be involved in the pathogenesis of H. pylori-associated chronic idiopathic thrombocytopenic purpura," *British Journal of Haematology*, vol. 124, no. 1, pp. 91–96, 2004.

[8] F. Franceschi, N. Christodoulides, M. H. Kroll, and R. M. Genta, "Helicobacter pylori and idiopathic thrombocytopenic purpura," *Annals of Internal Medicine*, vol. 140, no. 9, pp. 766-767, 2004.

[9] M. Kodama, Y. Kitadai, M. Ito et al., "Immune response to CagA protein is associated with improved platelet count after Helicobacter pylori eradication in patients with idiopathic thrombocytopenic purpura," *Helicobacter*, vol. 12, no. 1, pp. 36–42, 2007.

[10] R. Stasi, Z. Rossi, E. Stipa, S. Amadori, A. C. Newland, and D. Provan, "Helicobacter pylori eradication in the management of patients with idiopathic thrombocytopenic purpura," *The American Journal of Medicine*, vol. 118, no. 4, pp. 414–419, 2005.

[11] T. Inaba, M. Mizuno, S. Take et al., "Eradication of Helicobacter pylori increases platelet count in patients with idiopathic thrombocytopenic purpura in Japan," *European Journal of Clinical Investigation*, vol. 35, no. 3, pp. 214–219, 2005.

[12] D. Veneri, M. Krampera, and M. Franchini, "High prevalence of sustained remission of idiopathic thrombocytopenic purpura afterHelicobacter pylorieradication: A long-term follow-up study," *Platelets*, vol. 16, no. 2, pp. 117–119, 2009.

[13] N. Rostami, M. Keshtkar-Jahromi, M. Rahnavardi, M. Keshtkar-Jahromi, and F. S. Esfahani, "Effect of eradication of Helicobacter pylori on platelet recovery in patients with chronic idiopathic thrombocytopenic purpura: a controlled trial," *American Journal of Hematology*, vol. 83, no. 5, pp. 376–381, 2008.

[14] G. Emilia, M. Luppi, P. Zucchini et al., "Helicobacter pylori infection and chronic immune thrombocytopenic purpura: long-term results of bacterium eradication and association with bacterium virulence profiles," *Blood*, vol. 110, no. 12, pp. 3833–3841, 2007.

[15] H. Kim, CoOperative Study Group A for Hematology (COSAH), W.-S. Lee et al., "Efficacy of Helicobacter pylori eradication for the 1st line treatment of immune thrombocytopenia patients with moderate thrombocytopenia," *Annals of Hematology*, vol. 94, no. 5, pp. 739–746, 2015.

[16] T. Suzuki, M. Matsushima, A. Masui et al., "Effect of Helicobacter pylori eradication in patients with chronic idiopathic thrombocytopenic purpura-a randomized controlled trial," *The American Journal of Gastroenterology*, vol. 100, no. 6, pp. 1265–1270, 2005.

[17] Y. Tsutsumi, H. Kanamori, H. Yamato et al., "Randomized study of Helicobacter pylori eradication therapy and proton pump inhibitor monotherapy for idiopathic thrombocytopenic purpura," *Annals of Hematology*, vol. 84, no. 12, pp. 807–811, 2005.

[18] C. X. Li, D. J. Liu, C. Q. Pan, X. F. Sang, and X. Li, "Effect of Helicobacter pylori eradication on childhood acute idiopathic thrombocytopenic purpura," *Nan Fang Yi Ke Da Xue Xue Bao*, vol. 29, no. 6, pp. 1243-1244, 2009.

[19] S. Treepongkaruna, N. Sirachainan, S. Kanjanapongkul et al., "Absence of platelet recovery following Helicobacter pylori eradication in childhood chronic idiopathic thrombocytopenic purpura: a multi-center randomized controlled trial," *Pediatric Blood & Cancer*, vol. 53, no. 1, pp. 72–77, 2009.

[20] Y. Tang, S. C. Wang, L. J. Wang, Y. Liu, H. Y. Wang, and Z. J. Wang, "Clinical significance of Helicobacter pylori in children with idiopathic thrombocytopenic purpura," *Zhongguo Shi Yan Xue Ye Xue Za Zhi*, vol. 21, no. 2, pp. 419–421, 2013.

[21] H. S. H. Brito, J. A. P. Braga, S. R. Loggetto, R. S. Machado, C. F. H. Granato, and E. Kawakami, "Helicobacter pyloriinfection & immune thrombocytopenic purpura in children and adolescents: a randomized controlled trial," *Platelets*, vol. 26, no. 4, pp. 336–341, 2015.

[22] M. Franchini, M. Cruciani, C. Mengoli, G. Pizzolo, and D. Veneri, "Effect of Helicobacter pylori eradication on platelet count in idiopathic thrombocytopenic purpura: a systematic review and meta-analysis," *Journal of Antimicrobial Chemotherapy*, vol. 60, no. 2, pp. 237–246, 2007.

[23] R. Stasi, A. Sarpatwari, J. B. Segal et al., "Effects of eradication of Helicobacter pylori infection in patients with immune thrombocytopenic purpura: a systematic review," *Blood*, vol. 113, no. 6, pp. 1231–1240, 2009.

[24] G. H. Frydman, N. Davis, P. L. Beck, and J. G. Fox, "Helicobacter pylori eradication in patients with immune thrombocytopenic purpura: a review and the role of biogeography," *Helicobacter*, vol. 20, no. 4, pp. 239–251, 2015.

[25] D. Moher, A. Liberati, J. Tetzlaff, D. G. Altman, and PRISMA Group, "Preferred reporting items for systematic reviews and meta-analyses: the PRISMA statement," *Annals of Internal Medicine*, vol. 151, no. 4, pp. 264–9, W64, 2009.

[26] N. Panic, E. Leoncini, G. de Belvis, W. Ricciardi, and S. Boccia, "Evaluation of the endorsement of the preferred reporting items for systematic reviews and meta-analysis (PRISMA) statement on the quality of published systematic review and meta-analyses," *PLoS One*, vol. 8, no. 12, article e83138, 2013.

[27] A. R. Jadad, R. A. Moore, D. Carroll et al., "Assessing the quality of reports of randomized clinical trials: is blinding necessary?," *Controlled Clinical Trials*, vol. 17, no. 1, pp. 1–12, 1996.

[28] N. J. Wald and J. P. Bestwick, "Presentation of meta-analysis plots," *Journal of Medical Screening*, vol. 22, no. 1, pp. 49–51, 2015.

[29] J. A. C. Sterne, A. J. Sutton, J. P. A. Ioannidis et al., "Recommendations for examining and interpreting funnel plot asymmetry in meta-analyses of randomised controlled trials," *BMJ*, vol. 343, no. jul22 1, article d4002, 2011.

[30] M. Egger, G. D. Smith, M. Schneider, and C. Minder, "Bias in meta-analysis detected by a simple graphical test," *BMJ*, vol. 315, no. 7109, pp. 629–634, 1997.

[31] R. Stasi, "Immune thrombocytopenia: pathophysiologic and clinical update," *Seminars in Thrombosis and Hemostasis*, vol. 38, no. 5, pp. 454–462, 2012.

[32] R. Stasi, F. Willis, M. S. Shannon, and E. C. Gordon-Smith, "Infectious causes of chronic immune thrombocytopenia," *Hematology/Oncology Clinics of North America*, vol. 23, no. 6, pp. 1275–1297, 2009.

[33] A. Saito, A. Yokohama, Y. Osaki et al., "Circulating plasmacytoid dendritic cells in patients with primary and Helicobacter pylori-associated immune thrombocytopenia," *European Journal of Haematology*, vol. 88, no. 4, pp. 340–349, 2012.

[34] K. Satoh, T. Hirayama, K. Takano et al., "VacA, the vacuolating cytotoxin of Helicobacter pylori, binds to multimerin 1 on human platelets," *Thrombosis Journal*, vol. 11, no. 1, p. 23, 2013.

[35] Z. Wu, J. Zhou, P. Prsoon, X. Wei, X. Liu, and B. Peng, "Low expression of FCGRIIB in macrophages of immune thrombocytopenia-affected individuals," *International Journal of Hematology*, vol. 96, no. 5, pp. 588–593, 2012.

[36] T. Kühne and P. Imbach, "Management of children and adolescents with primary immune thrombocytopenia: controversies and solutions," *Vox Sanguinis*, vol. 104, no. 1, pp. 55–66, 2013.

[37] M. Ferrara, L. Capozzi, and R. Russo, "Effect ofHelicobacter pylorieradication on platelet count in children with chronic

idiopathic thrombocytopenic purpura," *Hematology*, vol. 14, no. 5, pp. 282–285, 2013.

[38] M. Franchini and D. Veneri, "Helicobacter pylori infection and immune thrombocytopenic purpura: an update," *Helicobacter*, vol. 9, no. 4, pp. 342–346, 2004.

[39] M. Kuwana, "Helicobacter pylori-associated immune thrombocytopenia: clinical features and pathogenic mechanisms," *World Journal of Gastroenterology*, vol. 20, no. 3, pp. 714–723, 2014.

[40] G. Russo, V. Miraglia, F. Branciforte et al., "Effect of eradication of Helicobacter pylori in children with chronic immune thrombocytopenia: a prospective, controlled, multicenter study," *Pediatric Blood & Cancer*, vol. 56, no. 2, pp. 273–278, 2011.

[41] G. Loffredo, M. G. Marzano, R. Migliorati et al., "The relationship between immune thrombocytopenic purpura and Helicobacter pylori infection in children: where is the truth?," *European Journal of Pediatrics*, vol. 166, no. 10, pp. 1067-1068, 2007.

[42] O. Matsunari, S. Shiota, R. Suzuki et al., "Association between Helicobacter pylori virulence factors and gastroduodenal diseases in Okinawa, Japan," *Journal of Clinical Microbiology*, vol. 50, no. 3, pp. 876–883, 2012.

[43] M. Hatakeyama, "Oncogenic mechanisms of the Helicobacter pylori CagA protein," *Nature Reviews Cancer*, vol. 4, no. 9, pp. 688–694, 2004.

[44] R. Suzuki, S. Shiota, and Y. Yamaoka, "Molecular epidemiology, population genetics, and pathogenic role of Helicobacter pylori," *Infection, Genetics and Evolution*, vol. 12, no. 2, pp. 203–213, 2012.

[45] R. P. H. Logan and M. M. Walker, "ABC of the upper gastrointestinal tract: epidemiology and diagnosis of Helicobacter pylori infection," *BMJ*, vol. 323, no. 7318, pp. 920–922, 2001.

15

Diverse Expression of IL-32 in Diffuse and Intestinal Types of Gastric Cancer

Mladen Pavlovic,[1] Nevena Gajovic,[2] Milena Jurisevic,[3] Slobodanka Mitrovic,[4] Gordana Radosavljevic,[2] Jelena Pantic,[2] Nebojsa Arsenijevic,[2] and Ivan Jovanovic[2]

[1]*Department of Surgery, Faculty of Medical Sciences, University of Kragujevac, Serbia*
[2]*Center for Molecular Medicine and Stem Cell Research, Faculty of Medical Sciences, University of Kragujevac, Serbia*
[3]*Department of Pharmacy, Faculty of Medical Sciences, University of Kragujevac, Serbia*
[4]*Department of Pathology, Faculty of Medical Sciences, University of Kragujevac, Serbia*

Correspondence should be addressed to Nevena Gajovic; gajovicnevena@yahoo.com

Academic Editor: Mitsuro Kanda

Introduction. Gastric cancer (GC) represents one of the most common cancers worldwide, frequently diagnosed at advanced stages with poor prognosis, indicating on need for new diagnostic and prognostic markers. The aim of the study was to determine the expression of IL-32, proinflammatory and angiogenic mediators, in patients with diffuse and intestinal gastric cancer and the relationship with clinicopathological aspects. *Material and Methods.* The tissue samples of diffuse and intestinal types of tumor of 70 patients with gastric cancer were analyzed. Expression of IL-32, VEGF, IL-17, and CD31 was measured by immunohistochemistry. *Results.* IL-32 expression was significantly lower in tissue samples from patients with diffuse type of gastric cancer that is also a severe and more progressive form (TNM stages III and IV, poor histological differentiation, and higher nuclear grade III). Expression of IL-17 was also decreased in patients with diffuse type of gastric cancer. Microvascular density was diminished in diffuse type of gastric cancer. *Conclusions.* Downregulated expression of IL-32 in tumor tissue of patients with diffuse type of gastric cancer may implicate on its role in limiting ongoing proinflammatory and proangiogenic processes. This emphasizes on unrecognized role of IL-32 in biology of diffuse type of gastric cancer.

1. Introduction

Gastric cancer is the fourth most common type of cancer and the second cause of cancer-related deaths after lung cancer [1, 2]. The various incidence of gastric cancer among population is considered to be mainly associated with variations in diet [3, 4]. The poor prognosis of this type of tumor is mainly because of late diagnosis and because the early stages do not give any clinical manifestations.

One of the most widely used histological classification of gastric cancer is based on Lauren's criteria, in which gastric adenocarcinoma is a heterogeneous disease histologically divided into intestinal, diffuse, mixed, and indeterminate subtypes [4, 5] and can be anatomically classified as proximal or distal type of tumor [2, 6]. These two types of tumors differ in morphology, epidemiology, progression pattern, genetic basis, and clinical manifestations. Intestinal tumor cells are often adhesive metastatic cells that usually form tubular or glandular structures [1, 7, 8]. Intestinal type of gastric cancer spreads via lymphatic or vascular vessels, and the lesions are irregularly straggled. Diffuse gastric cancer consists of nonadhesive cells that predominantly infiltrate stroma, that is not characteristic of intestinal form. The fact that diffuse type of gastric cancer mainly invades peritoneum cavity is one of the main reasons for shorter duration of disease and poor prognosis [7, 9, 10].

Inflammation and angiogenesis are important factors for carcinogenesis that have big impact on progression and invasion of tumor cells [11–13]. Numerous investigations have revealed various molecular and cellular pathways that are vital for linking inflammation and cancer [13–15]. The effect of immune cells on tumor cells partly depends on the production of cytokines, chemokines, growth factors, and reactive oxygen species [16].

One of the most intriguing among numerous cytokines that has role in both hallmarks of cancer is recently described interleukin 32. IL-32 induces the production of proinflammatory cytokines and also directly affects the development and maturation of specific immune cells [17, 18]. IL-32 is also involved in numerous inflammatory and infectious diseases, including rheumatoid arthritis, chronic obstructive pulmonary disease, mycobacterium tuberculosis infections, and inflammatory bowel disease [19–23]. Regarding the role of this cytokine in tumor biology, it is diverse and opposite. This is mainly due to different isoforms that are located in tumor tissue. Expression of this cytokine in tumor tissue is, in most cases, higher than that in peritumoral or normal tissue and has a prognostic significance; the higher expression usually is strongly correlated with worse prognosis and more progressive form of disease [24, 25]. Some literature data showed antitumorigenic effect of this cytokine [26]. Its role in tumor angiogenesis is still controversial and less defined.

There are almost no data about the role and expression pattern of this cytokine in different histological forms of gastric cancer and intestinal and diffuse type of gastric cancer. The aim of this study is to reveal some data about expression and possible role in gastric carcinogenesis, especially in these two tumor types: diffuse and intestinal gastric cancer.

2. Material and Methods

2.1. Ethic Approvals. The study was conducted at the Center for Abdominal Surgery, Center for Pathology, Clinical Center of Kragujevac, and Center for Molecular Medicine and Stem Cell Research, Faculty of Medical Sciences, University of Kragujevac, Serbia. All patients gave their informed consent. Ethical approvals were obtained from relevant Ethics Committees of the Clinical Center of Kragujevac, Kragujevac, Serbia, and Faculty of Medical Sciences, University of Kragujevac, Serbia (number 01-11478). All research procedures were made according to the *Principles of Good Clinical Practice* and the Declaration of Helsinki.

2.2. Patients. The study included 70 patients with gastric cancer. The diagnosis of gastric cancer was based on gastroscopic and histopathological criteria. The study excludes patients with no well-defined pathology, inadequate clinical document, or with previously diagnosed gastric cancer who were treated with radiation and chemotherapy. In the present study, we analyzed clinical data about age, gender, pathologic reports (nuclear grade and well/moderate/poor differentiation), and clinical stage by TNM (tumor, nodes, and metastasis) of patients with gastric cancer. Well-differentiated and moderately differentiated tumors (well/moderate) were defined as low-grade lesions, whereas poorly differentiated tumors (poor) were defined as high-grade lesions according to the WHO guidelines [27]. Grading was based on the evaluation of the worst area, excluding areas of focal dedifferentiation present at the invasive margin of the tumor [28]. Poorly differentiated tumors have repeatedly been shown to behave more aggressively than well-/moderately differentiated carcinomas in multivariate analysis [28]. The classification of nuclear grade of tumor tissue (I + II and III + IV) was based on the evaluation of the size and shape of the nucleus in tumor cells and the percentage of tumor cells that are in the process of dividing or growing [29].

2.3. Immunohistochemical Staining of VEGF, IL-32, IL-17, and CD31. Paraffin-embedded samples were consecutively cut to a thickness of 4–5 μm. Each section was deparaffinized and rehydrated with graded ethanol. Antigen retrieval was performed by microwave heating for 20 minutes in 10 mM sodium citrate buffer (pH 6.0). Activity of endogenous peroxidase was blocked with a 3% hydrogen peroxide solution for 10 min at room temperature. After washing with PBS, slides were incubated with mono/polyclonal antibodies against VEGF (ab16883, Abcam, Cambridge, UK, at a 1 : 200 dilution), IL-32 (ab37158, Abcam, Cambridge, UK, at 10 μg/ml), IL-17 (ab79056, Abcam, Cambridge, UK, at a 1 : 100 dilution), and CD31 (ab79056, Abcam, Cambridge, UK, at a 1 : 200 dilution) for 60 min in a humid chamber, respectively. Sections were washed in PBS three times and then incubated with anti-rabbit/mouse secondary antibody, respectively, for 15 min at room temperature. Immunostaining was performed using the Envision system with diaminobenzidine (DakoCytomation, Glostrup, Denmark). Finally, the signal was developed with 3,3-diaminobenzidine tetrahydrochloride (DAB), and all of the slides were counterstained with hematoxylin. Negative controls were treated in the same way with the primary antibodies omitted. Positive controls consisted of tissue known to contain the protein of interest [30]. An Olympus microscope (BX50 model) equipped with a digital camera was used to prepare microphotographs with magnifications of 200x or 400x.

2.4. IHC Scoring. Two independent pathologists investigated all tissue specimens. The tissue samples were analyzed using semiquantitative modified scoring system, according to the percentage of tumor tissue stained with IL-32 and intensity of staining [25, 31]. The IHC score was calculated by addition of the percentage of positively stained cells to the staining intensity. The percentage of positive cells ranged between 0 and 3, i.e., 0, if less than 10% of tumor cells were stained; 1, if 10–25% of tumor cells were stained; 2, if 25–50% were positive; and 3, if >50% were positive. The staining intensity was scored as 0 for negative, 1 for weak, 2 for moderate, and 3 for strong intensity. The IHC score was ranged between 0 and 6.

VEGF scoring was calculated according to the presence, intensity, and percent of positive cells, as previously described [30, 31]. Brown or brown-yellow staining in the cell membrane or cytoplasm was considered as positive. The negative controls were unstained. The number of positive cells in 500 tumor cells was counted within 3 randomly selected high-power fields (×400). Four grades were defined according to the percentage of positively stained cells: 0, no immunopositive cells; 1, <25% immunopositive cells; 2, 25–50% immunopositive cells; 3, >50% immunopositive cells. Four grades were defined according to color-staining

TABLE 1: Baseline characteristics of patients with intestinal and diffuse type of GC.

	Gastric cancer		p
	Intestinal type ($n = 50$)	Diffuse type ($n = 20$)	
Gender (male/female)	41/9	8/12	0.025
Age (mean (range))	75.07 (54–92)	65.20 (55–79)	0.005
TNM classification (I and II/III and IV)	30/20	6/14	0.045
Nuclear grade (I/II/III)	4/35/11	0/0/20	0.001
Histological differentiation rate (well/moderate/poor)	11/26/13	0/0/20	0.001
Blood vessel invasion (absent/present)	37/13	8/12	0.011

intensity: 0, no color; 1, weak, pale yellow; 2, medium brown; 3, strong, dark brown.

Two independent pathologists considered CD-31-positive single endothelial cells or CD-31-positive clusters of endothelial cells as a microvessel. At first, slides were examined at an original magnification of 40x. Three "hot spots" (areas with the highest microvessel density) from each slide were identified and these are as were photographed by a digital camera at an original magnification of 200x. The area of this histological field was 0.704 μm. MVD (microvessel/HPF) and the number of microvessels evaluated according to Weidner et al. (1991). MVD of the specimen was estimated as a mean of MVD in three histological fields.

Expression of IL-17 was localized in the cytoplasm of mononuclear cells. Light microscopic analysis was performed by manually counting positively stained cells in 3 separate areas of intratumoral regions under 400x high-power magnifications [32].

2.5. Statistical Analysis. The data were analyzed using the commercially available SPSS 20.0 software. The results were reported as mean and standard error of mean (SEM). Results were analyzed using the Student's t-test for independent samples if the data had normal distribution or Mann–Whitney U test for data without normal distribution. Spearman's correlation assessed the possible relationship between the IL-32 expression and histological form of gastric cancer. Strength of correlation was defined as negative or positive weak (−0.3 to −0.1 or 0.1 to 0.3), moderate (−0.5 to −0.3 or 0.3 to 0.5), or strong (−1.0 to −0.5 or 1.0 to 0.5). Statistical significance was set at $p < 0.05$.

3. Results

Seventy patients with gastric cancer were enrolled in this study. Clinical and pathologic characteristics of these patients are presented in Table 1. Patients with gastric cancer were divided in two groups on the basis of type of tumor: diffuse form and intestinal form of gastric cancer. Significant difference was observed in gender distribution ($p = 0.025$). Histopathological analysis confirmed that 12 female patients had diagnosed diffuse type of gastric cancer while 41 male patients had intestinal form of gastric cancer (41 males and 8 females). Moreover, significant difference was observed in age between patients with diffuse (mean age 65.2 ± 2.72) and intestinal type of gastric cancer (mean age 75.07 ± 1.13). Patients with diagnosed intestinal form of gastric cancer were significantly greater ($p = 0.005$) in comparison to patients with diffuse form of tumor (Table 1).

3.1. More Severe and Aggressive Disease Associated to Diffuse Form of Tumor. Patients with different forms of gastric cancer were divided into two categories on the basis of TNM stage of disease: I + II and III + IV. As shown in Table 1, patients with diffuse form of tumor appear to have an advanced TNM stage of disease (TNM stage III + IV) ($p = 0.045$), while patients with intestinal form of gastric cancer mostly had localized tumor (TNM stage I + II).

Patients with diffuse form of gastric cancer appeared to have higher nuclear grade ($p = 0.001$), while patients with intestinal form of gastric cancer mostly had lower nuclear grade (Table 1).

Further, we analyzed patients with different forms of gastric cancer, according to histological differentiation rate: well/moderate and poor. Majority of patients with diffuse form of cancer had poor tumor tissue differentiation ($p = 0.001$), while patients with intestinal form of gastric cancer had mostly better tumor tissue differentiation (Table 1). According to results from Table 1, TNM classification and nuclear and histological grade suggested that patients with diffuse type of gastric cancer have more severe form of disease compared to patients with intestinal form of tumor.

3.2. Lower Expression of IL-32 Associated to Diffuse Form of Gastric Cancer. The results have shown that majority of patients with diffuse type of gastric cancer had score 4 or less, while most of the patients with intestinal form of tumor had score 4 or higher ($p = 0.001$; Figure 1(a), right panel). Within patients with diffuse type of gastric cancer, IL-32 score 2 was recorded for 40% of patients, while IL-32 score 2 was recorded for 3% of patients with intestinal type of gastric cancer (Figure 1(a), left panel). Moreover, Spearman's correlation test revealed that higher expression of IL-32 negatively correlates with more severe diffuse form of gastric cancer ($r = -0.367$; $p = 0.002$).

3.3. Lower Microvascular Density and IL-17 Expression in Diffuse Form of Gastric Cancer. Immunohistochemistry results have shown that patients with diffuse form of tumor have significantly lower MVD in comparison to patients with intestinal type of gastric cancer ($p = 0.009$), suggesting on dramatically less level of angiogenesis in diffuse form of gastric cancer (Figure 2(a)).

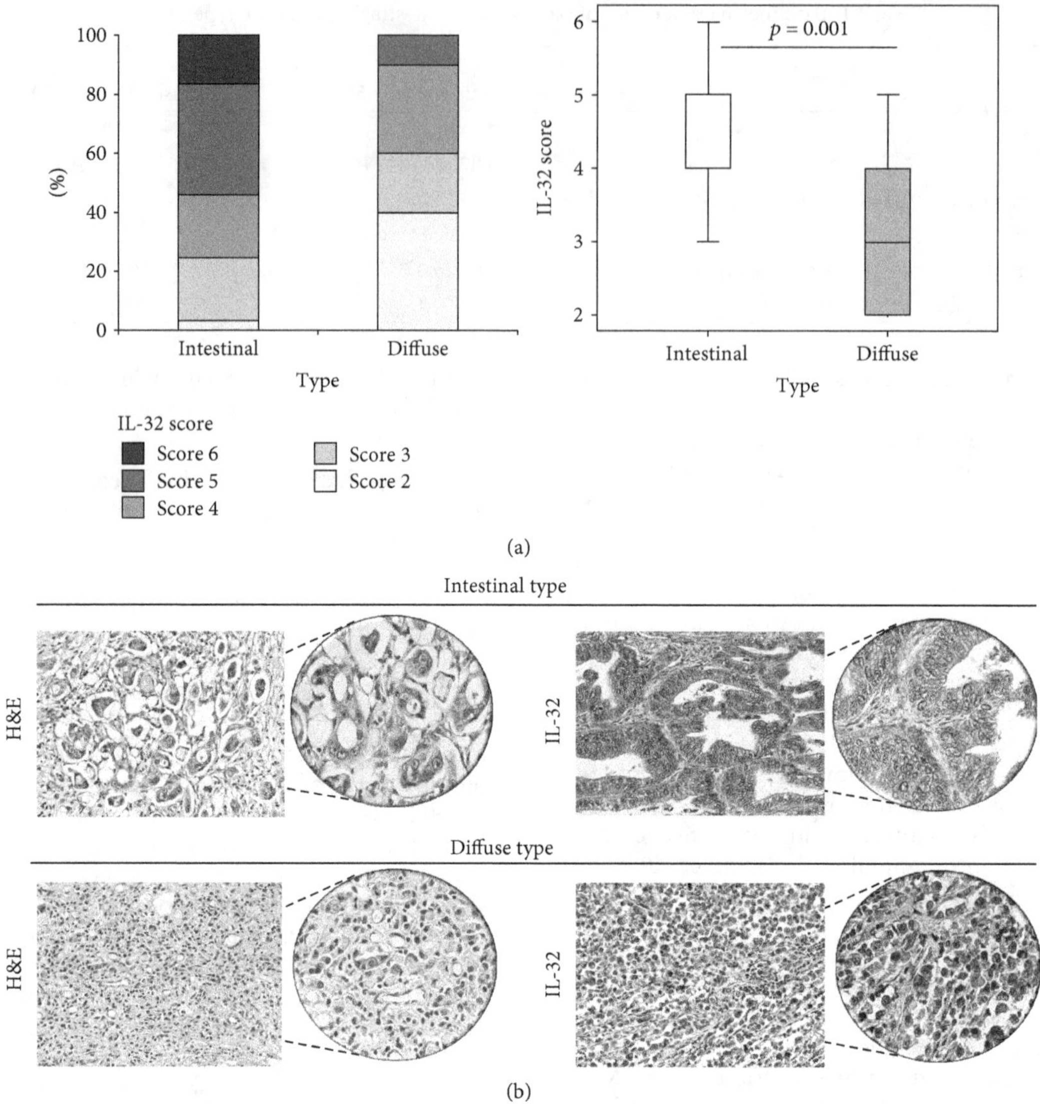

FIGURE 1: IL-32 score in patients with intestinal and diffuse form of gastric cancer. (a) Patients with diffuse type of cancer had IL-32 score 4 or less, while patients with intestinal type had IL-32 score 4 or higher. Significantly lower IL-32 score in patients with diffuse type in comparison to patients with intestinal type of gastric cancer ($p = 0.001$). p values were assessed by Student's unpaired t-test. (b). H&E staining of representative tumor tissue of intestinal and diffuse type of gastric cancer. Representative IL-32 staining in patients with intestinal and diffuse type of gastric cancer (200 and 400x magnification).

There was no statistical difference in VEGF expression between patients with diffuse and intestinal type of gastric cancer (Figure 3(b)). Analyses of IL-17 expression have revealed that patients with diffuse form of gastric cancer had significantly lower expression of this cytokine in comparison to patients with intestinal tumor form ($p = 0.029$; Figure 3(a)).

4. Discussion

Gastric cancer is one of the most frequently diagnosed malignancies and the second cause of cancer-related death in population [2]. According to Lauren's classification as well as the World Health Organization, there are two major histological entities of gastric cancer: intestinal and diffuse type [33, 34]. *Helicobacter pylori* infection; *Helicobacter pylori*-associated chronic gastritis, atrophy, and intestinal metaplasia; lifestyle; and diet are the main risk factors for the development of intestinal type of gastric cancer [35, 36]. On the contrary, diffuse type of this tumor is more frequently linked to with genetic mutations [2]. Intestinal type of gastric cancer consists of tubular or glandular metaplastic cell formations, while poorly differentiated diffuse form of tumor is usually formed of cells without gland formation, with the presence of signet ring cells and mucin [37, 38]. Our results have shown that diffuse form of cancer dominated in younger female patients while intestinal form of gastric cancer was more frequent in elder male patients (Table 1). Moreover, TNM classification, nuclear grade, and histological score clearly suggested that diffuse form of cancer is more severe than intestinal form (Table 1). These results are in line with previous reports

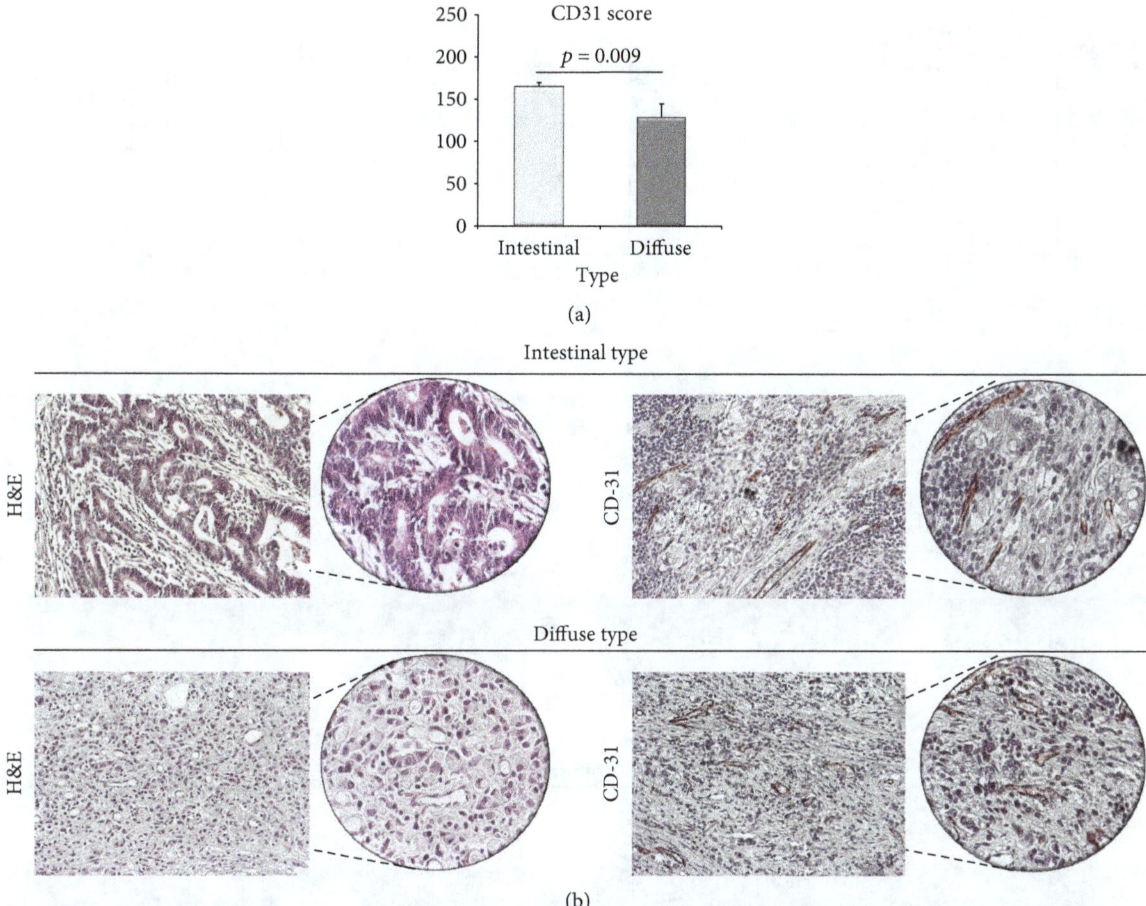

FIGURE 2: Microvascular density of intestinal and diffuse form of gastric cancer. (a) MVD was significantly lower in patients with diffuse form compared to patients with intestinal form of gastric cancer ($p = 0.009$). p values were assessed by Mann–Whitney rank sum test. (b) H&E staining of representative tumor tissue of intestinal and diffuse type of gastric cancer. Representative sections demonstrate MVD in tumor tissue of patients with intestinal and diffuse type of gastric cancer (200 and 400x magnification).

claiming that intestinal gastric cancer most commonly occurs in elderly male patients and exhibits a longer course and better prognosis, while diffuse form is often associated with younger age, predominantly in younger women with worse prognosis [9, 38].

In order to investigate potential biological role of IL-32 in obvious difference in severeness of diffuse form of gastric cancer in comparison to intestinal form, we have analyzed the expression of IL-32 in tumor tissue. Our results revealed higher IL-32 expression in patients with diffuse type of gastric cancer in comparison to intestinal form of tumor. It has been reported that systemic concentration of IL-32 is significantly increased in patients with gastric cancer in comparison to healthy control [24]. Ishigami et al. have shown that tumor depth and lymph node metastases as well as lymphatic and venous invasion developed more frequently in IL-32-positive gastric cancer [39]. Earlier study also confirmed that expression of IL-32 in patients with gastric cancer positively correlated with poor prognosis. Moreover, IL-32 by promoting production of MMP2, MMP9, IL-8, and VEGF facilitates invasion as well as migration of tumor cells [40]. Interestingly, all the data refer to intestinal type of gastric cancer.

The degree of microvascular density in tumor is nowadays assessed by CD31 protein expression. Platelet/endothelial cell adhesion molecule-1 (PECAM-1) or CD31 is a multifunctional molecule involved in different processes like platelet biology, signal transduction, transendothelial migration of leukocytes, and inflammation as well as endothelial cell biology [41]. Moreover, CD31 plays an important role in tumor biology in few ways. It is one of the most abundant junctions set deep between endothelial cells, thus supporting the integrity of endothelial membrane and regulating leukocyte migration and vascular permeability [41, 42]. Our results have revealed that diffuse form of gastric cancer had significantly lower MVD in comparison to intestinal form of tumor. Previous reports have suggested that intestinal form of gastric cancer spreads predominantly in the liver via direct hematogenous way, while diffuse gastric cancer is more invasive and gives metastatic lesions directly in peritoneal cavity. The reason for this different way of spreading tumors is the fact that intestinal form is more dependent on angiogenesis in comparison to diffuse form of tumor [43]. In line with the previous findings are our results suggesting that decreased MVD reflects less degree of angiogenesis in diffuse form in comparison to intestinal form of gastric cancer.

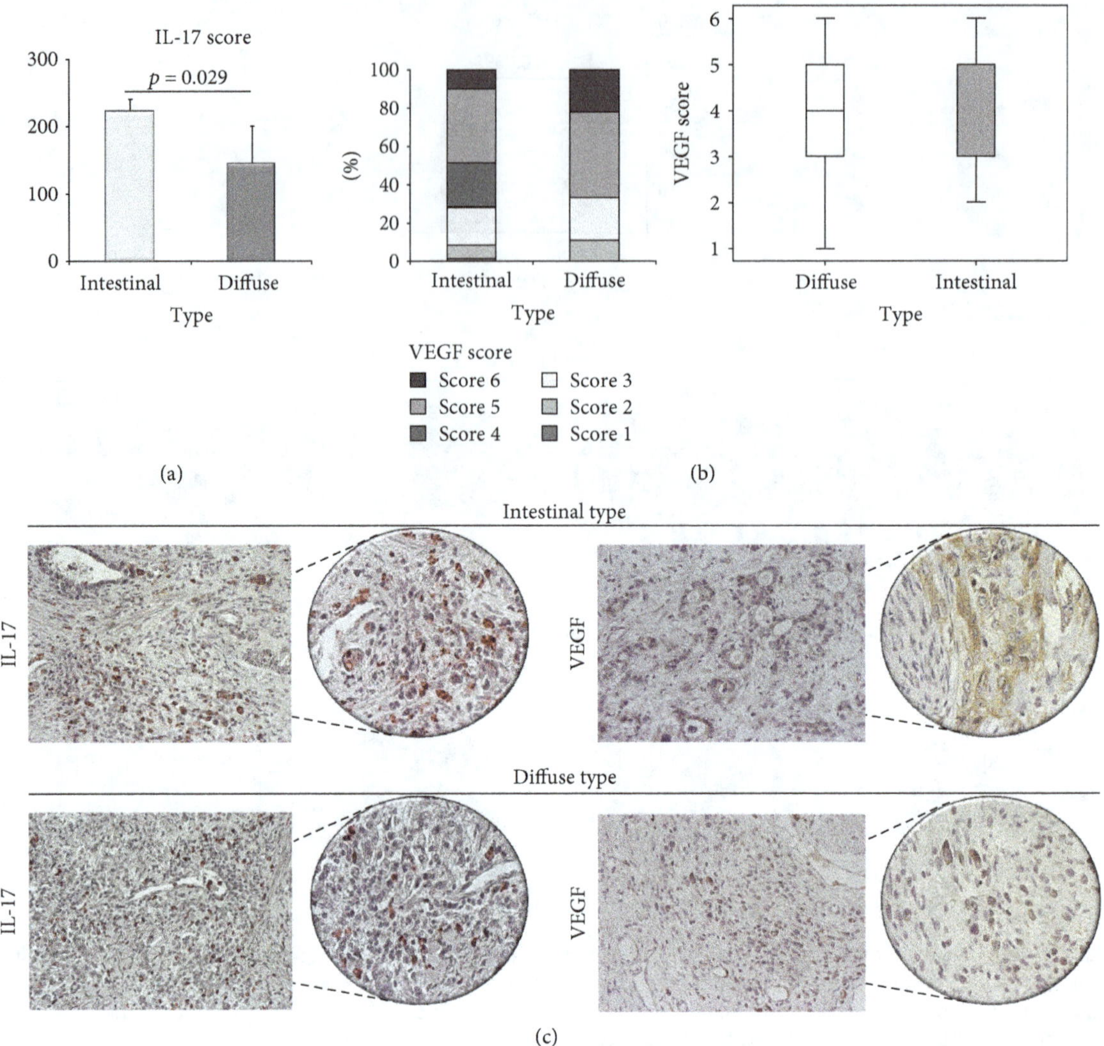

FIGURE 3: Immunohistochemical analysis of IL-17 and VEGF in patients with intestinal and diffuse form of gastric cancer. (a) Significantly lower IL-17 score in patients with diffuse type in comparison to patients with intestinal type of gastric cancer ($p = 0.029$). (b) No statistical significance in VEGF score between patients with diffuse form and intestinal form of gastric cancer ($p > 0.05$). p values were assessed by Mann–Whitney rank sum test. (c) Representative IL-17 and VEGF staining in tumor tissue of patients with intestinal and diffuse type of gastric cancer (200 and 400x magnification).

As the reason for this significant difference in microvascular density can be the presence or absence of different pro-/antiangiogenic markers, in the continuation of our research, we have focused on analyzing expression of these factors in diffuse and intestinal form of gastric cancer. First, we have analyzed expression of vascular endothelial growth factor (VEGF), which is one of the most potent proangiogenic factors. VEGF is an endothelial cell-specific mitogen which is important for endothelial cell survival, proliferation, and migration [44, 45]. The main sources of this factor are various cell types such as tumor cells, macrophages, or platelets [46]. Abundant expression of VEGF has an important role in the pathogenesis of cancer, proliferation of tumor cells, and the development of metastatic lesions [47, 48]. However, we have not found significant difference between expression of VEGF in diffuse and intestinal form of gastric cancer. This result suggests that difference in microvascular density between diffuse and intestinal type of gastric cancer is not caused by VEGF.

IL-17 is a cytokine produced mainly by Th17 cells, although other types of cells such as $\gamma\delta$ T lymphocytes and type 3 innate lymphoid cells can also be important sources of this cytokine [49]. Previous reports suggested that IL-17 is abundantly expressed in different forms of tumors and that its concentration positively correlates with VEGF expression in tumors [50]. Moreover, Iida et al. have shown that patients whose infiltrates in gastric cancers had increased number of Th17 cells with increased expression of IL-17 and IL-23 mRNA had more invasive form of tumors [32]. Our analyses of IL-17 expression in gastric cancer have showed that patients with diffuse form of tumor had significantly lower expression of this cytokine compared to patients with intestinal form of the tumor (Figure 3(a)). This result is in line with previous studies suggesting that IL-17 has an important role as a proangiogenic factor [51]. Moreover, significant lower

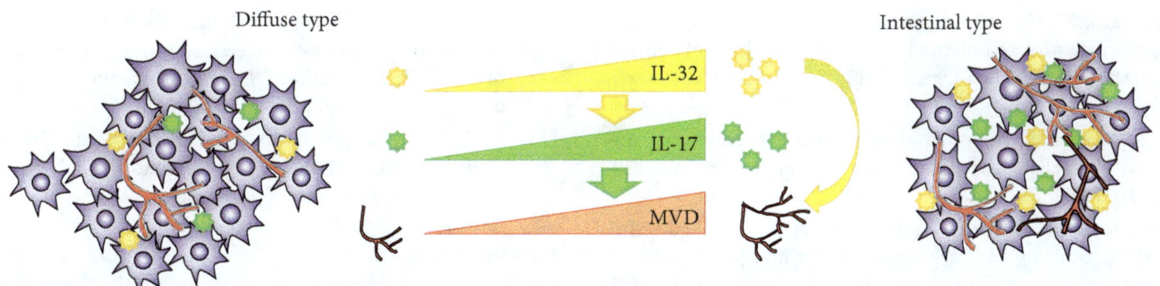

Figure 4: Schematic diagram describing mechanism responsible for IL-32-mediated suppression of angiogenesis in diffuse type of gastric cancer. IL-32 directly and indirectly, through the suppression of IL-17, reduces angiogenesis and subsequent microvascular density, which in turn attenuates hematogenous metastasis of diffuse type of gastric cancer.

expression of IL-17 and no detectable difference in VEGF expression suggest that diminished IL-17 may cause reduce angiogenesis and subsequent milder microvascular density in diffuse type of gastric cancer.

According to the presented data, it appears that decreased expression of IL-32 may inhibit production of proinflammatory and proangiogenic factor IL-17 and thus suppresses formation of new blood vessels which in turn results in diminished hematogenous metastatic potential of diffuse form of cancer (Figure 4).

5. Conclusions

In summary, decreased local presence of IL-32, reflected through a lower expression, in diffuse type of gastric cancer patients, with a higher nuclear grade, poor tumor tissue differentiation, and advanced TNM stage of disease, may be considered as a sign of the tumor's malignant progression and, consequently, of a poor prognosis for patients. This finding throws a new light on the role of IL-32 in biology of diffuse form of gastric cancer.

Acknowledgments

The authors thank Aleksandar Ilic for the excellent technical assistance. This work was supported by grants from the Serbian Ministry of Science and Technological Development (175071 and 175069), Serbia, and from the Faculty of Medical Sciences, University of Kragujevac (Project JP 15/16), Serbia.

References

[1] Y. C. Chen, W. L. Fang, R. F. Wang et al., "Clinicopathological variation of Lauren classification in gastric cancer," *Pathology and Oncology Research*, vol. 22, no. 1, pp. 197–202, 2016.

[2] B. Hu, N. El Hajj, S. Sittler, N. Lammert, R. Barnes, and A. Meloni-Ehrig, "Gastric cancer: classification, histology and application of molecular pathology," *Journal of Gastrointestinal Oncology*, vol. 3, no. 3, pp. 251–261, 2012.

[3] S. Liu, F. Feng, G. Xu et al., "Clinicopathological features and prognosis of gastric cancer in young patients," *BMC Cancer*, vol. 16, no. 1, p. 478, 2016.

[4] J. H. Pyo, S. Ahn, H. Lee et al., "Clinicopathological features and prognosis of mixed-type T1a gastric cancer based on Lauren's classification," *Annals of Surgical Oncology*, vol. 23, no. S5, pp. 784–791, 2016.

[5] F. Berlth, E. Bollschweiler, U. Drebber, A. H. Hoelscher, and S. Moenig, "Pathohistological classification systems in gastric cancer: diagnostic relevance and prognostic value," *World Journal of Gastroenterology*, vol. 20, no. 19, pp. 5679–5684, 2014.

[6] J. Shi, Y. Qu, and P. Hou, "Pathogenetic mechanisms in gastric cancer," *World Journal of Gastroenterology*, vol. 20, no. 38, pp. 13804–13819, 2014.

[7] S. Susman, R. Barnoud, F. Bibeau et al., "The Lauren classification highlights the role of epithelial-to-mesenchymal transition in gastric carcinogenesis: an immunohistochemistry study of the STAT3 and adhesion molecules expression," *Journal of Gastrointestinal and Liver Diseases*, vol. 24, no. 1, pp. 77–83, 2015.

[8] L. J. Xiao, E. H. Zhao, S. Zhao et al., "Paxillin expression is closely linked to the pathogenesis, progression and prognosis of gastric carcinomas," *Oncology Letters*, vol. 7, no. 1, pp. 189–194, 2014.

[9] M. Z. Qiu, M. Y. Cai, D. S. Zhang et al., "Clinicopathological characteristics and prognostic analysis of Lauren classification in gastric adenocarcinoma in China," *Journal of Translational Medicine*, vol. 11, no. 1, p. 58, 2013.

[10] M. Cislo, A. A. Filip, G. J. Arnold Offerhaus et al., "Distinct molecular subtypes of gastric cancer: from Laurén to molecular pathology," *Oncotarget*, vol. 9, no. 27, pp. 19427–19442, 2018.

[11] W. Lin and M. Karin, "A cytokine-mediated link between innate immunity, inflammation, and cancer," *The Journal of Clinical Investigation*, vol. 117, no. 5, pp. 1175–1183, 2007.

[12] G. Landskron, M. De La Fuente, P. Thuwajit, C. Thuwajit, and M. A. Hermoso, "Chronic inflammation and cytokines in the tumor microenvironment," *Journal of Immunology Research*, vol. 2014, Article ID 149185, 19 pages, 2014.

[13] D. W. Beury, K. H. Parker, M. Nyandjo, P. Sinha, K. A. Carter, and S. Ostrand-Rosenberg, "Cross-talk among myeloid-derived suppressor cells, macrophages, and tumor cells impacts the inflammatory milieu of solid tumors," *Journal of Leukocyte Biology*, vol. 96, no. 6, pp. 1109–1118, 2014.

[14] G. Di Caro, M. Carvello, S. Pesce et al., "Circulating inflammatory mediators as potential prognostic markers of human colorectal cancer," *PLoS One*, vol. 11, no. 2, article e0148186, 2016.

[15] S. E. Erdman and T. Poutahidis, "Cancer inflammation and regulatory T cells," *International Journal of Cancer*, vol. 127, no. 4, pp. 768–779, 2010.

[16] M. Jovanovic, N. Gajovic, N. Zdravkovic et al., "Fecal galectin-3: a new promising biomarker for severity and progression of colorectal carcinoma," *Mediators of Inflammation*, vol. 2018, Article ID 8031328, 11 pages, 2018.

[17] B. Khawar, M. H. Abbasi, and N. Sheikh, "A panoramic spectrum of complex interplay between the immune system and IL-32 during pathogenesis of various systemic infections and inflammation," *European Journal of Medical Research*, vol. 20, no. 1, p. 7, 2015.

[18] P. Felaco, M. L. Castellani, M. A. De Lutiis et al., "IL-32: a newly-discovered proinflammatory cytokine," *Journal of Biological Regulators & Homeostatic Agents*, vol. 23, no. 3, pp. 141–147, 2009.

[19] M. El-Far, P. Kouassi, M. Sylla, Y. Zhang, A. Fouda, T. Fabre et al., "Proinflammatory isoforms of IL-32 as novel and robust biomarkers for control failure in HIV-infected slow progressors," *Scientific Reports*, vol. 6, no. 1, article 22902, 2016.

[20] G. Mabilleau and A. Sabokbar, "Interleukin-32 promotes osteoclast differentiation but not osteoclast activation," *PLoS One*, vol. 4, no. 1, article e4173, 2009.

[21] M. Shioya, A. Nishida, Y. Yagi et al., "Epithelial overexpression of interleukin-32alpha in inflammatory bowel disease," *Clinical and Experimental Immunology*, vol. 149, no. 3, pp. 480–486, 2007.

[22] M. Kudo, E. Ogawa, D. Kinose et al., "Oxidative stress induced interleukin-32 mRNA expression in human bronchial epithelial cells," *Respiratory Research*, vol. 13, no. 1, p. 19, 2012.

[23] M. G. Netea, T. Azam, E. C. Lewis et al., "Mycobacterium tuberculosis induces interleukin-32 production through a caspase- 1/IL-18/interferon-γ-dependent mechanism," *PLoS Medicine*, vol. 3, no. 8, article e277, 2006.

[24] E. H. Seo, J. Kang, K. H. Kim et al., "Detection of expressed IL-32 in human stomach cancer using ELISA and immunostaining," *Journal of Microbiology and Biotechnology*, vol. 18, no. 9, pp. 1606–1612, 2008.

[25] L. A. B. Joosten, B. Heinhuis, M. G. Netea, and C. A. Dinarello, "Novel insights into the biology of interleukin-32," *Cellular and Molecular Life Sciences*, vol. 70, no. 20, pp. 3883–3892, 2013.

[26] H.-M. Yun, J. H. Oh, J.-H. Shim et al., "Antitumor activity of IL-32β through the activation of lymphocytes, and the inactivation of NF-κB and STAT3 signals," *Cell Death & Disease*, vol. 4, no. 5, article e640, 2013.

[27] S. R. Hamilton and L. A. Aaltonen, "Pathology and genetics: tumours of the digestive system," in *World Health Organization Classification of Tumours*, pp. 103–143, IARC, Lyon, France, 3rd edition, 2000.

[28] G. Lanza, L. Messerini, R. Gafa, and M. Risio, "Colorectal tumors: the histology report," *Digestive and Liver Disease*, vol. 43, Supplement 4, pp. S344–S355, 2011.

[29] S. B. Edge and C. C. Compton, "The American Joint Committee on Cancer: the 7th edition of the AJCC cancer staging manual and the future of TNM," *Annals of Surgical Oncology*, vol. 17, no. 6, pp. 1471–1474, 2010.

[30] E. Lastraioli, L. Boni, M. R. Romoli et al., "VEGF-a clinical significance in gastric cancers: immunohistochemical analysis of a wide Italian cohort," *European Journal of Surgical Oncology*, vol. 40, no. 10, pp. 1291–1298, 2014.

[31] M. Raica, L. Mogoantă, A. M. Cîmpean et al., "Immunohistochemical expression of vascular endothelial growth factor (VEGF) in intestinal type gastric carcinoma," *Romanian Journal of Morphology and Embryology*, vol. 49, no. 1, pp. 37–42, 2008.

[32] T. Iida, M. Iwahashi, M. Katsuda et al., "Tumor-infiltrating CD4+ Th17 cells produce IL-17 in tumor microenvironment and promote tumor progression in human gastric cancer," *Oncology Reports*, vol. 25, no. 5, pp. 1271–1277, 2011.

[33] P. Lauren, "The two histological main types of gastric carcinoma: diffuse and so-called intestinal-type carcinoma. An attempt at a histo-clinical classification," *Acta Pathologica Microbiologica Scandinavica*, vol. 64, no. 1, pp. 31–49, 1965.

[34] F. Petrelli, R. Berenato, L. Turati et al., "Prognostic value of diffuse versus intestinal histotype in patients with gastric cancer: a systematic review and meta-analysis," *Journal of Gastrointestinal Oncology*, vol. 8, no. 1, pp. 148–163, 2017.

[35] M. Yaghoobi, R. Bijarchi, and S. A. Narod, "Family history and the risk of gastric cancer," *British Journal of Cancer*, vol. 102, no. 2, pp. 237–242, 2010.

[36] P. Sipponen, M. Kekki, and M. Siurala, "Atrophic chronic gastritis and intestinal metaplasia in gastric carcinoma. Comparison with a representative population sample," *Cancer*, vol. 52, no. 6, pp. 1062–1068, 1983.

[37] Y. Adachi, K. Yasuda, M. Inomata, K. Sato, N. Shiraishi, and S. Kitano, "Pathology and prognosis of gastric carcinoma: well versus poorly differentiated type," *Cancer*, vol. 89, no. 7, pp. 1418–1424, 2000.

[38] J. Ma, H. Shen, L. Kapesa, and S. Zeng, "Lauren classification and individualized chemotherapy in gastric cancer," *Oncology Letters*, vol. 11, no. 5, pp. 2959–2964, 2016.

[39] S. Ishigami, T. Arigami, Y. Uchikado et al., "IL-32 expression is an independent prognostic marker for gastric cancer," *Medical Oncology*, vol. 30, no. 2, p. 472, 2013.

[40] C.-Y. Tsai, C.-S. Wang, M.-M. Tsai et al., "Interleukin-32 increases human gastric cancer cell invasion associated with tumor progression and metastasis," *Clinical Cancer Research*, vol. 20, no. 9, pp. 2276–2288, 2014.

[41] P. Lertkiatmongkol, D. Liao, H. Mei, Y. Hu, and P. J. Newman, "Endothelial functions of platelet/endothelial cell adhesion molecule-1 (CD31)," *Current Opinion in Hematology*, vol. 23, no. 3, pp. 253–259, 2016.

[42] J. R. Privratsky and P. J. Newman, "PECAM-1: regulator of endothelial junctional integrity," *Cell and Tissue Research*, vol. 355, no. 3, pp. 607–619, 2014.

[43] Y. Kitadai, "Angiogenesis and lymphangiogenesis of gastric cancer," *Journal of Oncology*, vol. 2010, Article ID 468725, 8 pages, 2010.

[44] B. Sennino, F. Kuhnert, S. P. Tabruyn et al., "Cellular source and amount of vascular endothelial growth factor and platelet-derived growth factor in tumors determine response to angiogenesis inhibitors," *Cancer Research*, vol. 69, no. 10, pp. 4527–4536, 2009.

[45] N. Ferrara, K. Houck, L. Jakeman, and D. W. Leung, "Molecular and biological properties of the vascular endothelial growth

factor family of proteins," *Endocrine Reviews*, vol. 13, no. 1, pp. 18–32, 1992.

[46] A. M. Duffy, D. J. Bouchier-Hayes, and J. H. Harmey, "Vascular endothelial growth factor (VEGF) and its role in non-endothelial cells: autocrine signalling by VEGF," in *Madame Curie Bioscience Database*, Landes Bioscience, Austin, TX, USA, 2013.

[47] D. I. R. Holmes and I. Zachary, "The vascular endothelial growth factor (VEGF) family: angiogenic factors in health and disease," *Genome Biology*, vol. 6, no. 2, p. 209, 2005.

[48] Y. Takahashi, Y. Kitadai, C. D. Bucana, K. R. Cleary, and L. M. Ellis, "Expression of vascular endothelial growth factor and its receptor, KDR, correlates with vascularity, metastasis, and proliferation of human colon cancer," *Cancer Research*, vol. 55, no. 18, pp. 3964–3968, 1995.

[49] C. E. Sutton, L. A. Mielke, and K. H. G. Mills, "IL-17-producing $\gamma\delta$ T cells and innate lymphoid cells," *European Journal of Immunology*, vol. 42, no. 9, pp. 2221–2231, 2012.

[50] B. Pan, J. Shen, J. Cao et al., "Interleukin-17 promotes angiogenesis by stimulating VEGF production of cancer cells via the STAT3/GIV signaling pathway in non-small-cell lung cancer," *Scientific Reports*, vol. 5, no. 1, 2015.

[51] M. Numasaki, J.-I. Fukushi, M. Ono et al., "Interleukin-17 promotes angiogenesis and tumor growth," *Blood*, vol. 101, no. 7, pp. 2620–2627, 2003.

16

Clinical Overview of GIST and Its Latest Management by Endoscopic Resection in Upper GI

Cicilia Marcella[1], **Rui Hua Shi**[1], **and Shakeel Sarwar**[2]

[1]*Department of Gastroenterology, Southeast University Affiliated Zhongda Hospital, Nanjing 210009, China*
[2]*Department of Orthopedics, Southeast University Affiliated Zhongda Hospital, Nanjing 210009, China*

Correspondence should be addressed to Rui Hua Shi; ruihuashi@126.com

Academic Editor: Haruhiko Sugimura

Aims. To review the clinical presentation, diagnosis, assessment of risk of malignancy, and recent advances in management (mainly focusing on the role of endoscopic resection) of gastrointestinal stromal tumors (GISTs) in upper GI. *Method*. We searched Embase, Web of science, and PubMed databases from 1993 to 2018 by using the following keywords: "gastrointestinal stromal tumors," "GIST," "treatment," and "diagnosis." Additional papers were searched manually from references of the related articles. *Findings*. The improvement of endoscopic techniques in treating upper gastrointestinal subepithelial tumors especially gastrointestinal tumors has reduced the need for invasive surgery in patients unfit for surgery. Many studies have concluded that modified endoscopic treatments are effective and safe. These treatments permit minimal tissue resection, better dissection control, and high rates of en bloc resection with an acceptable rate of complications.

1. Introduction

Gastrointestinal stromal tumors (GISTs) are the most common mesenchymal subepithelial tumor (SET). They occur in the stomach (60–70%), small intestine (20–30%), duodenum (4-5%), rectum (4-5%), colon (<2%), and esophagus (<1%) [1–3]. They are rarely found in the peritoneum, mesentery, and omentum [4]. GISTs have been proved to arise from the smooth muscle pacemaker interstitial cell of Cajal (ICC) which has a function of coordinating gut motility [5] and peristalsis. GISTs demonstrate a higher incidence rate in men and among blacks, and most patients are between 40 and 80 years old at the time of diagnosis, with a median age of 63 years [6].

Prompt treatment of upper GISTs is very crucial. According to the latest guidelines of NCCN, ESMO, and Japan, a GIST less than 2 cm with no signs of malignancy may be managed with active surveillance. A small tumor size does not exclude the malignant potential in a GIST. Thus, despite the size, the patient should be told about the possibility of malignancy. Many studies have proved the feasibility and safety of endoscopic approaches in treating upper GISTs. These procedures include endoscopic band ligation (EBL), endoscopic submucosal excavation (ESE), endoscopic submucosal dissection (ESD), endoscopic mucosal dissection (EMD), endoscopic submucosal tunnel dissection (ESTD), submucosal tunneling endoscopic resection (STER), endoscopic full-thickness resection (EFTR), laparoscopic endoscopic cooperative surgery (LECS), nonexposed endoscopic wall-inversion surgery (NEWS), and a combination of laparoscopic and endoscopic approaches to neoplasia with a nonexposed technique (CLEAN-NET). We will discuss all the above procedures in this review along with their respective steps. We will also discuss the clinical presentation, malignant potential, and diagnosis of GISTs through imaging and pathology.

2. Clinical Presentation, Imaging, and Pathological Diagnosis

The symptoms of GISTs are nonspecific and depend on the size and location [7]. Many small GISTs (<2 cm) are usually found parenthetically by endoscopy or imaging, since many of them show no symptoms [8]. The most common symptom is gastrointestinal (GI) bleeding, which is present in approximately 50% of the patients, followed by abdominal pain (20–50%) and GI obstruction (10–30%). Other symptoms include melena, hematemesis, fullness, and palpable mass. GISTs that are located in the proximal stomach may lead to dysphagia, while tumors located in the pylorus may present as gastric outlet obstruction [9, 10]. GISTs can be a part of a syndrome called Carney's triad (gastric GIST, pulmonary chondroma, and paraganglioma) or neurofibromatosis type 1 (mostly spindle cell GIST) [11]. GISTs frequently metastasize to the liver and rarely spread to the regional lymph node or other extra-abdominal organs [12].

An initial investigation should include a detailed history and thorough physical examination, followed by imaging studies to both assess the extent of the primary tumor and evaluate the presence of metastatic disease. According to the latest NCCN guidelines, a CT (computed tomography) scan of the abdomen/pelvis is the initial workup for the evaluation, staging, and monitoring of treatment response in a GIST. GISTs typically showed a well-defined soft tissue of relatively low density, which is homogenous on a contrast-enhanced CT scan (Figure 1). On MRI, GISTs typically showed a well-defined, low to intermediate signal intensity on T1-weighted images and high signal intensity on T2-weighted images.

GISTs under endoscopic procedure typically form a well-delineated spherical or hemispheric mass, arising mostly from the muscularis propria (MP) layer beneath the mucosa and pushing it to the lumen to form a smooth contoured elevation (Figure 2). GISTs are usually well circumscribed and surrounded by a pseudocapsule which contributes to the indications for complete resection in endoscopic enucleation.

The pathological diagnosis of a GIST is determined by morphology and immunohistochemical (IHC) findings. The most important one is KIT (CD117), a tyrosine kinase inhibitor which is a transmembrane protein that stimulates cell proliferation and inhibits apoptosis. It presents in almost 95% of GISTs [13]. CD34 expression was also considered to be the most valuable marker before the recognition of the CD117 antibody, and it presents in between 40% and 82% of GISTs [14]. Thus, CD34 expression was accepted as a diagnostic supportive "marker" until now. CD117 can help in distinguishing GISTs from other gastrointestinal mesenchymal tumors, since it is not expressed in smooth muscle or neural tumors [15]. However, some may show CD117 negative, typically the PDGFRα (platelet-derived growth factor α) mutant or wild types. Thus, DOG1 is added as an alternative marker as a supplement in diagnosing GISTs [16]. The 3 main morphological types of GISTs include spindle cell type (70%), epithelioid cell type (20%), and mixed type (10%), which is highly malignant.

3. Malignant Potential

Assessing the malignant potential in GIST patients is crucial for deciding the next step in treatment. The prognosis of a GIST is highly associated with mitotic count, tumor size, tumor necrosis, anatomical location, invasive growth, and

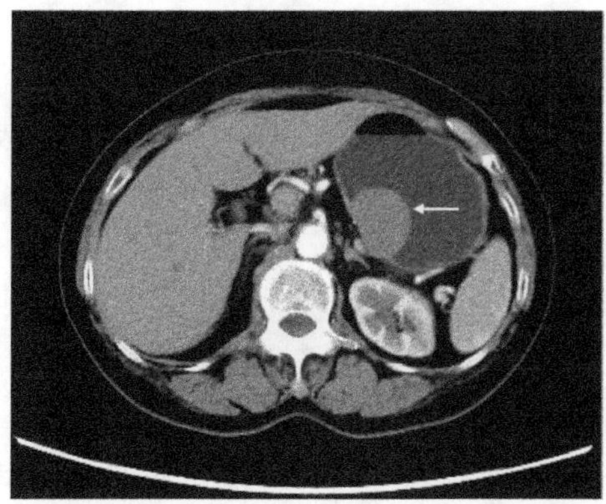

FIGURE 1: An approximately 3.9*2.8 cm gastrointestinal tumor on the lesser curvature of the stomach body seen on enhanced CT imaging (white arrow).

expression of Ki-67 and PCNA index [17, 18]. Tumors with a size greater than 10 cm showing calcifications, irregular margins, heterogeneity, lobulation, and ulceration, along with extraluminal and mesenteric fat infiltration, are more likely to be associated with metastasis [19]. The chart in Figure 3 shows the gastric predictors in assessing the malignant potential of a GIST, according to the latest national comprehensive cancer network (NCCN) guidelines. As shown in the chart, the vertical axis stands for the metastatic rate (%) and the horizontal axis stands for the tumor size (cm) as well as the 2 series for mitotic rate (/50 HPFs). Gastric GISTs with a size of ≤10 cm and having ≤5 mitoses per 50 HPFs have a low malignancy potential [2]. Overall, tumors < 5 cm, and especially <2 cm, have a lower risk of metastasis, in contrast to tumors >5 cm, and especially >10 cm, which have a higher risk of metastasis. For the mitotic rate of <5 mitoses/50 HPF, there is a lower risk of metastasis, compared to those tumors with mitotic rates > 5/50 HPF. Mitotic rates > 10/50 HPF indicate a higher risk of metastasis [20]. These two factors are independent but mutually influential predictors, and are thus added in the NIH guidelines. However, the diagnosis and prediction of the malignant potential of GIST are still difficult.

4. Role of Endoscopy in GIST Patient

Endoscopy has been used worldwide for many purposes. The widespread application of endoscopy and endoscopic ultrasound (EUS) has led to the detection of many early-stage upper GISTs, giving a chance of complete resection. Many authors have claimed that EUS is the most appropriate method for esophagogastric submucosa tumors. A GIST on EUS will appear as hypoechoic, inhomogeneous, anechoic, or having a high echo (when tumors are malignant), and it is commonly located in the third and fourth layer, and rarely in the second layer [21]. EUS may also be used for the prediction of malignancy as well [15]. Palazzo et al. [22] concluded that EUS features suggestive of malignancy include enlarged lymph nodes, size greater than 4 cm, irregular margins, and the presence of cystic spaces within the mass. For a tumor of larger size, EUS can be very useful in differentiating a submucosal tumor

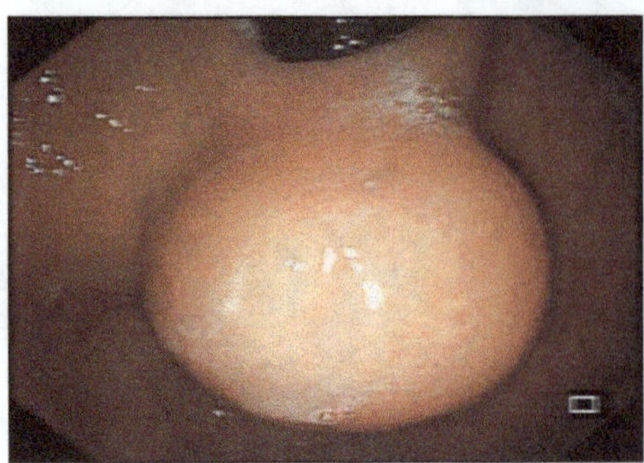

FIGURE 2: A large gastrointestinal tumor located in the lower part of the cardia seen under endoscopy forming a smooth contoured elevation.

(SMT) from extrinsic compression, with 92% sensitivity and 100% specificity [23].

According to their location in the gastric wall, GISTs are classified into 4 types: type 1 (very narrow connection with the MP layer which protrudes into the lumen), type 2 (wide connection with the MP which protrudes into the lumen at an obtuse angle), type 3 (located in the middle of the gastric wall), and type 4 (protrudes into the serosal side of the gastric wall) [24]. Endoscopic enucleation is best suitable for types 1 and 2. Endoscopic enucleation include EBL, ESD, EMD, ESTD, and STER. Types 3 and 4 are commonly resected by other techniques such as EFTR and more advanced methods of endoscopic and laparoscopic combination techniques, such as LECS, NEWS, and CLEAN-NET. The summaries of the included studies reporting relevant outcomes are shown in Tables 1 and 2.

4.1. Endoscopic Band Ligation. EBL was first applied for treating esophageal varices [25]. Later on, it was applied for treating gastrointestinal superficial lesions. For the very first time, Sun et al. [26] concluded that EBL was an effective and safe method for treating small GISTs. 96.6% (28/29) of the cases were resected completely, with a low complication rate (3.4%, 1/29) and recurrence rate (3.4%, 1/29). In this procedure, the tumor was first aspirated with a transparent cap and then ligated with the band. EUS was used to confirm that the hypoechoic mass had been completely confined by the band. The overlying mucosa and submucosal layer were then cut, thus dissecting the tumor. Many authors have demonstrated the safety and efficacy of EBL for gastric GIST [27, 28]. The hurdles of EBL are the limited size of the tumor (≤12 mm) that can be resected due to the size of the transparent cap, and EBL is suitable only for GISTs located in the superficial MP layer [29]. However, EBL is rarely used now to treat GISTs.

4.2. Endoscopic Submucosal Dissection. ESD has been used to remove an SMT, including a GIST. The ESD standard procedure is as follows: identifying and marking the lesion boundaries, injecting a solution (a mixture of normal saline, epinephrine, and indigo carmine dye) into the submucosal layer, initial incision of the mucosa and submucosa layer, and dissecting the tumor (Figure 4). ESD allows a larger resectable size and a higher en bloc resection rate when compared with EBL. He et al. [30] demonstrated that ESD is effective, safe, and feasible in treating large-sized GISTs. A total of 31 patients underwent an ESD for larger-sized GISTs (mean size 2.7 ± 0.72 cm). The results showed favorable outcomes, although 6 patients had intraoperative perforations and were successfully managed endoscopically, with no further surgery required.

Many studies have also demonstrated that ESD is safe and effective when compared to conventional surgical approaches (open or laparoscopic). Soh et al. [31] retrospectively analyzed the comparison of ESD (55 patients) and surgery (27patients) in treating gastric subepithelial tumors (SETs). This proved that ESD is an efficient treatment for gastric SETs with the advantages of shorter hospital stays and lower hospital costs when compared with surgery. Meng et al. [32] evaluated a total of 115 SMT patients who underwent either an ESD (68/115) or laparoscopic wedge resection (LWR) (47/115). Results showed that for tumors < 2 cm and between 2 and 5 cm, ESD was associated with a shorter mean operation time, less blood loss, shorter length of hospital stays and lower cost. It also concluded that ESD can achieve the same rates of en bloc resection and complete resection compared with LWR.

4.3. Endoscopic Muscularis Dissection. EMD was first introduced by Liu et al. [33] as a new endoscopic technique for resecting tumors originating from the MP layer. The procedure includes injecting a solution (a mixture of epinephrine and normal saline) into the submucosal layer, marking the tumor, incising the overlying mucosa to expose the tumor, dissecting the submucosa and muscular tissue around the lesion to better reveal the tumor, and dissecting the tumor. The study included 31 patients (14 = esophageal tumor, 17 = gastric tumor). It achieved 97% (30/31) of complete resections, and the perforation rate was 13% (4/31). Thus, EMD can be a treatment of choice in treating patients with upper-GI subepithelial tumors originating from the MP.

4.4. Endoscopic Submucosal Tunneling. Peroral endoscopic submucosal tumor resection (POET) was first developed by Inoue et al. [34] to treat esophageal or cardia subepithelial tumors. The research concluded that the procedure is feasible for selected submucosal tumors with a size of up to 4 cm. The POET procedure for resecting SETs is referred to as submucosal tunneling endoscopic resection (STER) or endoscopic submucosal tunnel dissection (ESTD). The standard procedures include injecting a solution into the submucosal layer, creating a submucosal tunnel 5 cm above the tumor, dissecting the overlying mucosa or submucosa, dissecting the tumor from the muscular layer, retrieving the specimen, and closing the entry mucosa orifice with hemostatic clips [35–38]. POET is efficient for resecting SETs located at the esophagogastric junction and in the esophagus, which is believed to be a difficult site for laparoscopic wedge resection [39]. It also possesses numerous advantages compared to other surgical procedures, including a shorter hospital stay, lower cost, perseverance of mucosal integrity, faster healing rate, and

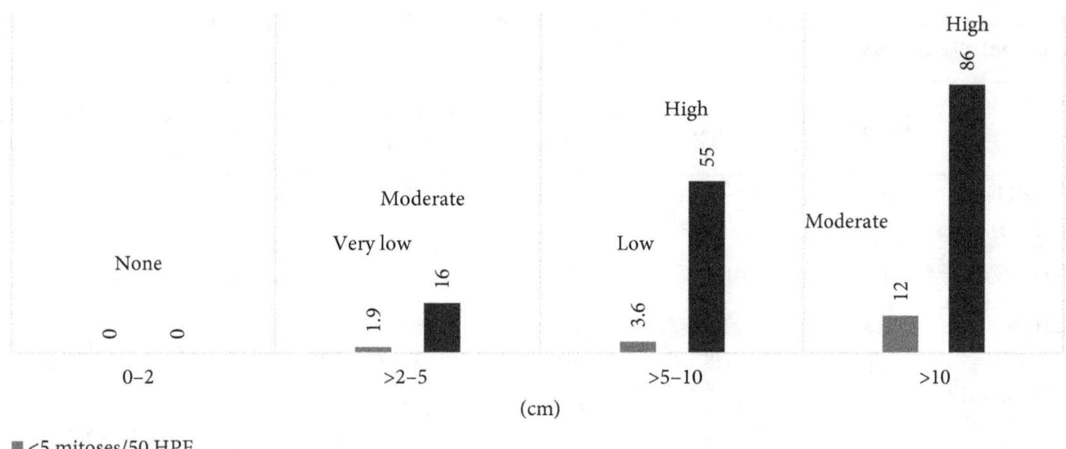

FIGURE 3: Gastric GISTs: risk assessment of malignant potential.

TABLE 1: Relevant outcomes of the endoscopic enucleation procedure for gastrointestinal subepithelial tumors.

Study	n, GIST[1]	Method	Mean tumor size (mm)	Mean procedure time (min)	Complete resection rate (%)	Complication (%)	Mean follow-up (mo), recurrence
Sun et al. [26] (2007)	29, 29	EBL	8.0 (body) 9.0 (fundus) 11.0 (cardia)	—	96.0	3.4	41, 1
Nan et al. [28] (2014)	192, 177	EBL	8.0	—	100	1.0	—
He et al. [30] (2013)	31, 31	ESD	27.0	70.2	100	29.0	14.3, 0
Meng et al. [32] (2016)	68, 49	ESD	25.8	99.3[2]	98.5	11.8	12.9, 0
	47, 31	LWR	37.1	125.2[2]	100	23.4	11.1, 0
Liu et al. [33] (2012)	31, 16	EMD	22.1	76.8	97	12.9	17.7, 0
Ye et al. [35] (2014)	85, 19	STER	19.2	57.2	100	4.7	8.0, 0
Gong et al. [36] (2012)	12, 7	ESTD	19.5	48.3	83.3	16.7	—
Chen et al. [37] (2015)	180, 28	STER	26.0 (median)	45 (median)	90.6	8.3	36 (median), 0
Li et al. [38] (2015)	32, 11	STER	23.0	51.8	100	43.8	28.0, 0

[1]Total number of pathologically diagnosed GIST. [2]Mean procedure time for GIST with a size of 20–50 mm. EBL = endoscopic band ligation; ESD = endoscopic submucosal dissection; LWR = laparoscopic wedge resection; EMD = endoscopic muscularis dissection; STER = submucosal tunneling endoscopic resection; ESTD = endoscopic submucosal tunnel dissection.

decreased risk of gastrointestinal tract leakage and consequent infection [40–42]. POET limitations include the challenge of performing the procedure in the fundus and upper greater curvature of the stomach, and lesions larger than 4 cm are difficult to retrieve perorally.

4.5. Endoscopic Full-Thickness Resection. Suzuki and Ikeda [43] were the first to develop an EFTR technique. Many researches have claimed that the EFTR is a technique of choice for SETs originating from the MP layer. Zhou et al. [44] and Feng et al. [45] demonstrated a successful EFTR procedure without laparoscopic assistance on 26 (16/26 were GISTs) and 48 (43/48 were GISTs) gastric SMTs, respectively. Both claimed to have a 100% complete resection rate with no complications or recurrences in follow-up. The standard procedure includes marking the lesion and injecting a solution (a mixture of normal saline, 1% indigo carmine, and epinephrine) into the submucosal layer, circumferential incision around the lesion in the MP layer, incising the serosal layer to generate active perforation, removing the tumor with its adjacent tissues by snare, and closing the perforated gastric wall with endoscopic clips and endoloop ligature (extra closing device) [46]. Schmidt et al. [47] recommended a method called "suture first, cut later"; whereby a new suturing device is used to suture beneath the tumor after the resection is performed. This method has an advantage of resecting relatively large tumors (±4 cm), regardless of their location. Kappelle et al. [48] reported an EFTR technique using a new flat-based Padlock over-the-scope (OTS) clip for tumors < 2 cm in the gastric wall (7/13) and duodenum (6/13). A total of 13 SETs (2 GISTs) were selected. From the result, the feasibility and effectiveness of achieving 100% R0 resection can be concluded, although several cases (duodenum) were complicated by (micro)perforations. Furthermore, EFTR required the creation of a pseudoperforation, which can increase the risk of intraperitoneal tumor seeding when the pseudocapsule is not intact. Thus, more studies on a larger scale are

Table 2: Relevant outcomes of the endoscopic full-thickness resection and endoscopic-laparoscopic cooperative procedure for gastrointestinal subepithelial tumors.

Study	*n*, GIST[1]	Method	Mean tumor size (mm)	Mean procedure time (min)	Complete resection rate (%)	Complication (%)	Mean follow-up (mo), recurrence
Zhou et al. [44] (2011)	26, 16	EFTR	28.0	105.0	100	0	8.0, 0
Feng et al. [45] (2014)	48, 43	EFTR	15.9	59.7	100	1.0	6.0–24 (range), 0
Kappelle et al. [48] (2017)	13, 2	EFTR[2]	11.0	—	84.6	38.5	3.0–6.0 (range), 0
Ye et al. [46] (2014)	51, 30	EFTR	24.0	52.0	98.0	0	22.4, 0
Hiki et al. [49] (2008)	7, 7	LECS	46.0	169.0	100	0	—
Namikawa and Hanazaki [50] (2015)	8, 8	LECS	31.0	213.0	100	0	—
Mitsui et al. [52] (2011)	6, 5	NEWS	34.8	273.5	100	0	8, 0
Goto et al. [53] (2016)	20, —[3]	NEWS	—[3]	213.5	100	5.0	10.1, 0
Nabeshima et al. [54] (2015)	2, 2	CLEAN-NET	37.5	165.0[4]	100	0	—
Hajer et al. [56] (2018)	10, 4	NEWS	32.7	99	100	20	—
	2, 2	CLEAN-NET	37.5	150	100	0	

[1]Total number of pathologically diagnosed GIST. [2]EFTR using a new flat-based over-the-scope clip. [3]Data unavailable due to limited access. [4]One case underwent CLEAN-NET and cholecystectomy procedure. EFTR = endoscopic full-thickness resection; LECS = laparoscopic endoscopic cooperative surgery; NEWS = nonexposed endoscopic wall-inversion surgery; CLEAN-NET = endoscopic approaches to neoplasia with nonexposed technique.

needed to standardize this technique and skilled endoscopists are required to reduce the risk of intraperitoneal infection caused by inadequate mucosal suturing.

4.6. Laparoscopic Endoscopic Cooperative Surgery. LECS in GISTs is a technique that was first performed by Hiki et al. [49] in 2008. This technique is believed to minimize the dissection of the normal gastric wall with minimal gastric transformation when compared with laparoscopic wedge resection (LWR). The study analyzed 7 patients (6/7 GISTs) with a median tumor size of 4.6 cm. Results showed no intraoperative or postoperative complications. Initially, the tumor location is identified by endoscopy and laparoscopy. Argon plasma coagulation (APC) is used to mark the tumor edge followed by injecting 10% glycerin into the submucosal layer. An insulated tip (IT) knife is used to incise three-fourths of the marked area of the tumor. Subsequent laparoscopic dissection of the seromuscular layer is achieved by making a pseudoperforation, and dissection is done by an ultrasonically activated device. The incision line is sealed with laparoscopic stapling devices. LECS is best suited for gastric GISTs originating from the intramural MP layer [24]. Namikawa and Hanazaki [50] concluded that full-thickness excision using the LECS method is a promising procedure in the treatment of GISTs < 5 cm, with the advantages of reduction in the resected area and lower estimated blood loss when compared to LWR.

4.7. Nonexposed Endoscopic Wall-Inversion Surgery. NEWS was invented in 2010 by Goto et al. [51] to avoid the inevitable intraperitoneal seeding caused by the EFTR technique. The procedure includes endoscopically marking the edge of the lesion, laparoscopically marking the serosal side opposite the mucosal marking, endoscopically injecting a hyaluronate solution into the submucosal layer, laparoscopically incising the circumferential seromuscular layer, pushing and inverting the dissected lesion into the lumen, laparoscopically suturing the seromuscular defect, and finally achieving complete resection by ESD around the lesion. With NEWS, full-thickness resection is achieved without exposing the gastric cavity, thus reducing the subsequent recurrence of peritoneal tumor seeding. Many studies have shown the feasibility of this procedure. However, this procedure is only for lesions less than 3 cm, due to its limitations in retracting the lesion transorally [52, 53].

4.8. Combination of Laparoscopic and Endoscopic Approaches to Neoplasia with Nonexposure Technique. CLEAN-NET was first developed by Inoue et al. [55] in 2012, based on a method called "suture first, cut later". This method permits a full-thickness resection without exposing the gastric lumen to the peritoneal space, thus avoiding peritoneal seeding [54]. The standard procedure includes indicating and injecting a solution into the submucosal layer around the lesion endoscopically, dissecting the seromuscular layer laparoscopically (leaving the mucosa intact), pulling the lesion outwards by sutures placed at the lesion laparoscopically, and achieving complete resection by closing the defect with a laparoscopic stapling device [56]. Its advantages over the NEWS technique lies in the larger size that can be resected using the CLEAN-NET technique (>4 cm). The tumor located on the posterior wall can be very challenging when removed endoscopically [56]. Moreover, this technique is difficult for large intraluminal protrusions, which make it difficult to place the stapling device. Secondly, the accuracy of mucosal resection is lower when compared to the NEWS technique, since the incision line is determined from the serosal side [57].

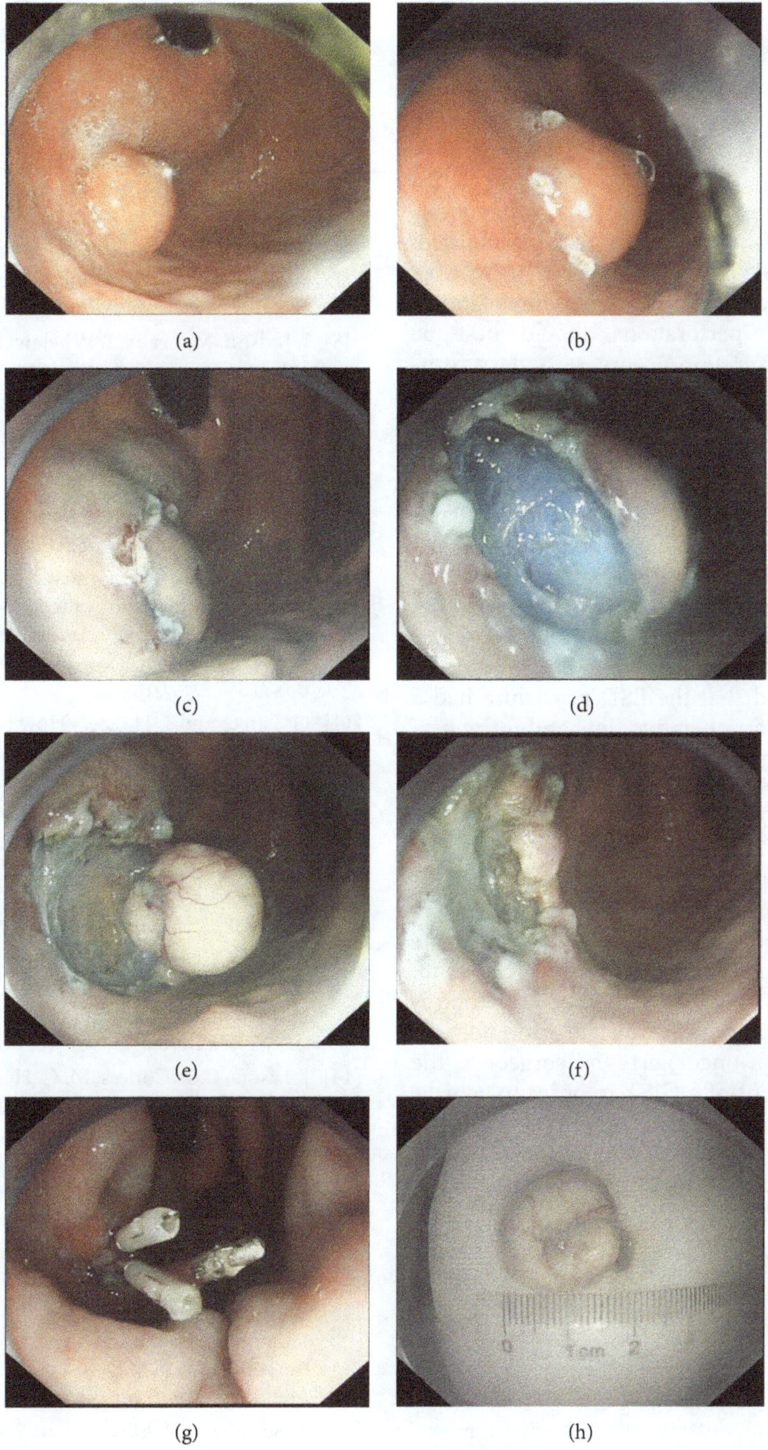

FIGURE 4: Endoscopic submucosal dissection. (a) A 2*2 cm subepithelial tumor located in the gastric fundus. (b) Marking the lesion boundaries. (c) Incision of the tumor was made after lifting the submucosa layer by injecting a mixed solution into the submucosa layer. (d–f) Tumor is resected. (g) Endoscopic clips were used to close the wound. (h) The resected specimen.

5. Follow-up

The guidelines of the NCCN recommended an abdominal and pelvic CT scan every 3-6 mo for 3–5 years and an annual postoperative follow-up, whereas for very small tumors (<2 cm), less frequent observation is acceptable. Incompletely resected tumors or the presence of metastasis mandate an abdominal and pelvic CT scan every 3–6 mo. CT or MRI may be used to determine the progression, while PET/CT can be considered when CT or MRI is ambiguous. To assess unresectable, recurrent, and metastatic disease, as well as the response to preoperative imatinib treatment, an abdominal and pelvic CT scan or MRI is indicated every 8–12 weeks.

6. Conclusion

With an improvement in the knowledge of the pathogenesis of GISTs, accurate diagnosis and treatment can be achieved. Endoscopic treatment of GISTs for the upper GI is feasible and safe, with a relatively acceptable rate of complications. Major complications like perforations should best be avoided. Meanwhile, if perforation occurs, secondary complications like intraperitoneal infection and emphysema should be prevented. Nowadays, newly developed endoscopic procedures are challenging conservative surgery. Although surgery remains the standard therapy for primary and localized GISTs [58], many studies have proved that a minimally invasive treatment by endoscopy is feasible and safe in upper GISTs with sizes of <5 cm. Surgery is associated with higher morbidities and mortalities, and it impairs a patient's quality of life afterwards. A study by Yin et al. [59] proposed 3 different minimally invasive procedures for GISTs ≤ 5 cm. It showed that the ESD procedure had a significant difference in mean operative time and intraoperative bleeding when compared to laparoscopic resection (LAP) and LECS procedure ($P < 0.001$). The mean operative times of ESD, LECS, and LAP were 32.96 ± 11.76 min, 65.33 ± 20.57 min, and 81.67 ± 22.49 min, respectively, while the volumes of mean intraoperative blood loss were 6.98 ± 3.58 ml, 20.00 ± 13.50 ml, and 19.50 ± 11.55 ml, respectively. Thus, the endoscopic approach definitely has some benefits over laparoscopic or open surgery to some limit. The treatment of upper GIST by the endoscopic method is still controversial. A team approach involving an endoscopist, pathologist, radiologist, oncologist, and surgeon is the optimum in the management of a GIST in order to achieve R0 complete resection with minimal complications. However, more studies with relatively long-term outcomes should be carried out and conclusions about the oncological feasibility of endoscopic treatments should be made.

References

[1] D. Machado-Aranda, M. Malamet, Y. J. Chang et al., "Prevalence and management of gastrointestinal stromal tumors," *The American Surgeon*, vol. 75, no. 1, pp. 55–60, 2009.

[2] M. Miettinen and J. Lasota, "Gastrointestinal stromal tumors: pathology and prognosis at different sites," *Seminars in Diagnostic Pathology*, vol. 23, no. 2, pp. 70–83, 2006.

[3] R. P. DeMatteo, J. S. Gold, L. Saran et al., "Tumor mitotic rate, size, and location independently predict recurrence after resection of primary gastrointestinal stromal tumor (GIST)," *Cancer*, vol. 112, no. 3, pp. 608–615, 2008.

[4] J. D. Reith, J. R. Goldblum, R. H. Lyles, and S. W. Weiss, "Extragastrointestinal (soft tissue) stromal tumors: an analysis of 48 cases with emphasis on histologic predictors of outcome," *Modern Pathology*, vol. 13, no. 5, pp. 577–585, 2000.

[5] L. G. Kindblom, H. E. Remotti, F. Aldenborg, and J. M. Meis-Kindblom, "Gastrointestinal pacemaker cell tumor (GIPACT): gastrointestinal stromal tumors show phenotypic characteristics of the interstitial cells of Cajal," *The American Journal of Pathology*, vol. 152, no. 5, pp. 1259–1269, 1998.

[6] T. Tran, J. A. Davila, and H. B. El-Serag, "The epidemiology of malignant gastrointestinal stromal tumors: an analysis of 1,458 cases from 1992 to 2000," *American Journal of Gastroenterology*, vol. 100, no. 1, pp. 162–168, 2005.

[7] S. E. Steigen and T. J. Eide, "Gastrointestinal stromal tumors (GISTs): a review," *APMIS*, vol. 117, no. 2, pp. 73–86, 2009.

[8] I. Judson, M. Leahy, J. Whelan et al., "A guideline for the management of gastrointestinal stromal tumour (GIST)," *Sarcoma*, vol. 6, no. 3, 87 pages, 2002.

[9] M. Miettinen, L. H. Sobin, and J. Lasota, "Gastrointestinal stromal tumors of the stomach: a clinicopathologic, immunohistochemical, and molecular genetic study of 1765 cases with long-term follow-up," *The American Journal of Surgical Pathology*, vol. 29, no. 1, pp. 52–68, 2005.

[10] A. M. Briggler, R. P. Graham, G. F. Westin et al., "Clinicopathologic features and outcomes of gastrointestinal stromal tumors arising from the esophagus and gastroesophageal junction," *Journal of Gastrointestinal Oncology*, vol. 9, no. 4, pp. 718–727, 2018.

[11] G. Lanke and J. H. Lee, "How best to manage gastrointestinal stromal tumor," *World Journal of Clinical Oncology*, vol. 8, no. 2, p. 135, 2017.

[12] G. D. Demetri, M. von Mehren, C. R. Antonescu et al., "NCCN Task Force report: update on the management of patients with gastrointestinal stromal tumors," *Journal of the National Comprehensive Cancer Network*, vol. 8, Supplement 2, pp. S-1–S-41, 2010.

[13] L. R. de Oliveira das Neves, C. T. F. Oshima, R. Artigiani-Neto, G. Yanaguibashi, L. G. Lourenço, and N. M. Forones, "Ki67 and p53 in gastrointestinal stromal tumors—GIST," *Arquivos de Gastroenterologia*, vol. 46, no. 2, pp. 116–120, 2009.

[14] J. Lasota, C. L. Corless, M. C. Heinrich et al., "Clinicopathologic profile of gastrointestinal stromal tumors (GISTs) with primary KIT exon 13 or exon 17 mutations: a multicenter study on 54 cases," *Modern Pathology*, vol. 21, no. 4, pp. 476–484, 2008.

[15] M. Sarlomo-Rikala, A. J. Kovatich, A. Barusevicius, and M. Miettinen, "CD117: a sensitive marker for gastrointestinal stromal tumors that is more specific than CD34," *Modern Pathology*, vol. 11, no. 8, pp. 728–734, 1998.

[16] B. Güler, F. Özyılmaz, B. Tokuç, N. Can, and E. Taştekin, "Histopathological features of gastrointestinal stromal tumors and the contribution of DOG1 expression to the diagnosis," *Balkan Medical Journal*, vol. 32, no. 4, pp. 388–396, 2015.

[17] T. Seidal and H. Edvardsson, "Expression of c-kit (CD117) and Ki67 provides information about the possible cell of origin and clinical course of gastrointestinal stromal tumours," *Histopathology*, vol. 34, no. 5, pp. 416–424, 1999.

[18] M. B. Amin, C. K. Ma, M. D. Linden, J. J. Kubus, and R. J. Zarbo, "Prognostic value of proliferating cell nuclear antigen index in gastric stromal tumors: correlation with mitotic count and clinical outcome," *American Journal of Clinical Pathology*, vol. 100, no. 4, pp. 428–432, 1993.

[19] G. J. C. Burkill, M. Badran, O. al-Muderis et al., "Malignant gastrointestinal stromal tumor: distribution, imaging features, and pattern of metastatic spread," *Radiology*, vol. 226, no. 2, pp. 527–532, 2003.

[20] E. C. H. Lai, S. H. Y. Lau, and W. Y. Lau, "Current management of gastrointestinal stromal tumors—a comprehensive review," *International Journal of Surgery*, vol. 10, no. 7, pp. 334–340, 2012.

[21] T. Nishida, N. Kawai, S. Yamaguchi, and Y. Nishida, "Submucosal tumors: comprehensive guide for the diagnosis and therapy of gastrointestinal submucosal tumors," *Digestive Endoscopy*, vol. 25, no. 5, pp. 479–489, 2013.

[22] L. Palazzo, B. Landi, C. Cellier, E. Cuillerier, G. Roseau, and J. P. Barbier, "Endosonographic features predictive of benign and malignant gastrointestinal stromal cell tumours," *Gut*, vol. 46, no. 1, pp. 88–92, 2000.

[23] D. Oğuz, L. Filik, E. Parlak et al., "Accuracy of endoscopic ultrasonography in upper gastrointestinal submucosal lesions," *Turkish Journal of Gastroenterology*, vol. 15, no. 2, pp. 82–85, 2004.

[24] H. H. Kim, "Endoscopic treatment for gastrointestinal stromal tumor: advantages and hurdles," *World Journal of Gastrointestinal Endoscopy*, vol. 7, no. 3, p. 192, 2015.

[25] H. M. El-Newihi and J. L. Achord, "Emerging role of endoscopic variceal band ligation in the treatment of esophageal varices," *Digestive Diseases*, vol. 14, no. 3, pp. 201–208, 1996.

[26] S. Sun, N. Ge, C. Wang, M. Wang, and Q. Lü, "Endoscopic band ligation of small gastric stromal tumors and follow-up by endoscopic ultrasonography," *Surgical Endoscopy and Other Interventional Techniques*, vol. 21, no. 4, pp. 574–578, 2007.

[27] G. Nan, S. Siyu, S. Shiwei, W. Sheng, and L. Xiang, "Hemoclip-reinforced and EUS-assisted band ligation as an effective and safe technique to treat small GISTs in the gastric fundus," *The American Journal of Gastroenterology*, vol. 106, no. 8, pp. 1560-1561, 2011.

[28] G. Nan, S. Siyu, W. Sheng, L. Xiang, and G. Jintao, "The role of hemoclips reinforcement in the ligation-assisted endoscopic enucleation for small GISTs in gastric fundus," *BioMed Research International*, vol. 2014, Article ID 247602, 5 pages, 2014.

[29] Y. Tan, L. Tan, J. Lu, J. Huo, and D. Liu, "Endoscopic resection of gastric gastrointestinal stromal tumors," *Translational Gastroenterology and Hepatology*, vol. 2, no. 12, p. 115, 2017.

[30] Z. He, C. Sun, Z. Zheng et al., "Endoscopic submucosal dissection of large gastrointestinal stromal tumors in the esophagus and stomach," *Journal of Gastroenterology and Hepatology*, vol. 28, no. 2, pp. 262–267, 2013.

[31] J. S. Soh, J. K. Kim, H. Lim et al., "Comparison of endoscopic submucosal dissection and surgical resection for treating gastric subepithelial tumours," *Scandinavian Journal of Gastroenterology*, vol. 51, no. 5, pp. 633–638, 2016.

[32] F. S. Meng, Z. H. Zhang, Y. Y. Hong et al., "Comparison of endoscopic submucosal dissection and surgery for the treatment of gastric submucosal tumors originating from the muscularis propria layer: a single-center study (with video)," *Surgical Endoscopy and Other Interventional Techniques*, vol. 30, no. 11, pp. 5099–5107, 2016.

[33] B. R. Liu, J. T. Song, B. Qu, J. F. Wen, J. B. Yin, and W. Liu, "Endoscopic muscularis dissection for upper gastrointestinal subepithelial tumors originating from the muscularis propria," *Surgical Endoscopy and Other Interventional Techniques*, vol. 26, no. 11, pp. 3141–3148, 2012.

[34] H. Inoue, H. Ikeda, T. Hosoya et al., "Submucosal endoscopic tumor resection for subepithelial tumors in the esophagus and cardia," *Endoscopy*, vol. 44, no. 3, pp. 225–230, 2012.

[35] L. P. Ye, Y. Zhang, X. L. Mao, L. H. Zhu, X. Zhou, and J. Y. Chen, "Submucosal tunneling endoscopic resection for small upper gastrointestinal subepithelial tumors originating from the muscularis propria layer," *Surgical Endoscopy*, vol. 28, no. 2, pp. 524–530, 2014.

[36] W. Gong, Y. Xiong, F. Zhi, S. Liu, A. Wang, and B. Jiang, "Preliminary experience of endoscopic submucosal tunnel dissection for upper gastrointestinal submucosal tumors," *Endoscopy*, vol. 44, no. 3, pp. 231–235, 2012.

[37] T. Chen, P. H. Zhou, Y. Chu et al., "Long-term outcomes of submucosal tunneling endoscopic resection for upper gastrointestinal submucosal tumors," *Annals of Surgery*, vol. 265, no. 2, pp. 363–369, 2017.

[38] Q. L. Li, W. F. Chen, C. Zhang et al., "Clinical impact of submucosal tunneling endoscopic resection for the treatment of gastric submucosal tumors originating from the muscularis propria layer (with video)," *Surgical Endoscopy*, vol. 29, no. 12, pp. 3640–3646, 2015.

[39] V. W. Y. Wong, O. Goto, H. Gregersen, and P. W. Y. Chiu, "Endoscopic treatment of subepithelial lesions of the gastrointestinal tract," *Current Treatment Options in Gastroenterology*, vol. 15, no. 4, pp. 603–617, 2017.

[40] N. Eleftheriadis, "Submucosal tunnel endoscopy: peroral endoscopic myotomy and peroral endoscopic tumor resection," *World Journal of Gastrointestinal Endoscopy*, vol. 8, no. 2, p. 86, 2016.

[41] J. Lu, X. Lu, T. Jiao, and M. Zheng, "Endoscopic management of upper gastrointestinal submucosal tumors arising from muscularis propria," *Journal of Clinical Gastroenterology*, vol. 48, no. 8, pp. 667–673, 2014.

[42] L. Wang, W. Ren, Z. Zhang, J. Yu, Y. Li, and Y. Song, "Retrospective study of endoscopic submucosal tunnel dissection (ESTD) for surgical resection of esophageal leiomyoma," *Surgical Endoscopy*, vol. 27, no. 11, pp. 4259–4266, 2013.

[43] H. Suzuki and K. Ikeda, "Endoscopic mucosal resection and full thickness resection with complete defect closure for early gastrointestinal malignancies," *Endoscopy*, vol. 33, no. 5, pp. 437–439, 2001.

[44] P. H. Zhou, L. Q. Yao, X. Y. Qin et al., "Endoscopic full-thickness resection without laparoscopic assistance for gastric submucosal tumors originated from the muscularis propria," *Surgical Endoscopy*, vol. 25, no. 9, pp. 2926–2931, 2011.

[45] Y. Feng, L. Yu, S. Yang et al., "Endolumenal endoscopic full-thickness resection of muscularis propria-originating gastric submucosal tumors," *Journal of Laparoendoscopic & Advanced Surgical Techniques*, vol. 24, no. 3, pp. 171–176, 2014.

[46] L. P. Ye, Z. Yu, X. L. Mao, L. H. Zhu, and X. B. Zhou, "Endoscopic full-thickness resection with defect closure using clips and an endoloop for gastric subepithelial tumors arising from the muscularis propria," *Surgical Endoscopy*, vol. 28, no. 6, pp. 1978–1983, 2014.

[47] A. Schmidt, M. Bauder, B. Riecken, D. von Renteln, H. Muehleisen, and K. Caca, "Endoscopic full-thickness resection of gastric subepithelial tumors: a single-center series," *Endoscopy*, vol. 47, no. 2, pp. 154–158, 2015.

[48] W. F. W. Kappelle, Y. Backes, G. D. Valk, L. M. G. Moons, and F. P. Vleggaar, "Endoscopic full-thickness resection of gastric and duodenal subepithelial lesions using a new, flat-based over-the-scope clip," *Surgical Endoscopy*, vol. 32, no. 6, pp. 2839–2846, 2018.

[49] N. Hiki, Y. Yamamoto, T. Fukunaga et al., "Laparoscopic and endoscopic cooperative surgery for gastrointestinal stromal tumor dissection," *Surgical Endoscopy and Other Interventional Techniques*, vol. 22, no. 7, pp. 1729–1735, 2008.

[50] T. Namikawa and K. Hanazaki, "Laparoscopic endoscopic cooperative surgery as a minimally invasive treatment for gastric submucosal tumor," *World Journal of Gastrointestinal Endoscopy*, vol. 7, no. 14, pp. 1150–1156, 2015.

[51] O. Goto, T. Mitsui, M. Fujishiro et al., "New method of endoscopic full-thickness resection: a pilot study of non-exposed endoscopic wall-inversion surgery in an ex vivo porcine model," *Gastric Cancer*, vol. 14, no. 2, pp. 183–187, 2011.

[52] T. Mitsui, K. Niimi, H. Yamashita et al., "Non-exposed endoscopic wall-inversion surgery as a novel partial gastrectomy technique," *Gastric Cancer*, vol. 17, no. 3, pp. 594–599, 2014.

[53] O. Goto, H. Takeuchi, M. Sasaki et al., "Laparoscopy-assisted endoscopic full-thickness resection of gastric subepithelial tumors using a nonexposure technique," *Endoscopy*, vol. 48, no. 11, pp. 1010–1015, 2016.

[54] K. Nabeshima, M. Tomioku, K. Nakamura, and S. Yasuda, "Combination of laparoscopic and endoscopic approaches to neoplasia with non-exposure technique (CLEAN-NET) for GIST with ulceration," *Tokai Journal of Experimental and Clinical Medicine*, vol. 40, no. 3, pp. 115–119, 2015.

[55] H. Inoue, H. Ikeda, T. Hosoya et al., "Endoscopic mucosal resection, endoscopic submucosal dissection, and beyond: full-layer resection for gastric cancer with nonexposure technique (CLEAN-NET)," *Surgical Oncology Clinics of North America*, vol. 21, no. 1, pp. 129–140, 2012.

[56] J. Hajer, L. Havlůj, A. Whitley, and R. Gürlich, "Non-exposure endoscopic-laparoscopic cooperative surgery for stomach tumors: first experience from the Czech Republic," *Clinical Endoscopy*, vol. 51, no. 2, pp. 167–173, 2018.

[57] N. Hiki, S. Nunobe, T. Matsuda, T. Hirasawa, Y. Yamamoto, and T. Yamaguchi, "Laparoscopic endoscopic cooperative surgery," *Digestive Endoscopy*, vol. 27, no. 2, pp. 197–204, 2015.

[58] T. Nishida, J. Y. Blay, S. Hirota, Y. Kitagawa, and Y. K. Kang, "The standard diagnosis, treatment, and follow-up of gastrointestinal stromal tumors based on guidelines," *Gastric Cancer*, vol. 19, no. 1, pp. 3–14, 2016.

[59] X. Yin, Y. Yin, H. Chen et al., "Comparison analysis of three different types of minimally invasive procedures for gastrointestinal stromal tumors ≤5 cm," *Journal of Laparoendoscopic & Advanced Surgical Techniques*, vol. 28, no. 1, pp. 58–64, 2018.

17

Diminished DEFA6 Expression in Paneth Cells Is Associated with Necrotizing Enterocolitis

Laszlo Markasz,[1] Alkwin Wanders,[2] Laszlo Szekely,[3] and Helene Engstrand Lilja[1]

[1]*Department of Women's and Children's Health, Uppsala University, Uppsala, Sweden*
[2]*Department of Biomedical Sciences, Umeå University, Umeå, Sweden*
[3]*Department of Laboratory Medicine, Division of Pathology, Karolinska Institute, Stockholm, Sweden*

Correspondence should be addressed to Laszlo Markasz; laszlo.markasz@kbh.uu.se

Academic Editor: Stephen Fink

Background. Necrotizing enterocolitis (NEC) is the most common gastrointestinal disorder in premature infants with a high morbidity and mortality. Paneth cell dysfunction has been suggested to be involved in the pathogenesis of NEC. Defensin alpha-6 (DEFA6) is a specific marker for Paneth cells acting as part of the innate immunity in the human intestines. The aim of this study was to investigate the expression of DEFA6 in infants with NEC. *Materials and Methods.* Infants who underwent bowel resection for NEC at level III NICU in Sweden between August 2004 and September 2013 were eligible for the study. Macroscopically vital tissues were selected for histopathological evaluation. All infants in the control group underwent laparotomy and had ileostomy due to dysmotility, and samples were taken from the site of the stoma. DEFA6 expression was studied by immunohistochemistry. Digital image analysis was used for an objective and precise description of the samples. *Results.* A total of 12 infants were included in the study, eight with NEC and four controls. The tissue samples were taken from the colon ($n = 1$), jejunum ($n = 1$), and ileum ($n = 10$). Both the NEC and control groups consisted of extremely premature and term infants (control group: 25–40 gestational weeks, NEC group: 23–39 gestational weeks). The postnatal age at the time of surgery varied in both groups (control group: 4–47 days, NEC group: 4–50 days). DEFA6 expression in the NEC group was significantly lower than that in the control group and did not correlate with gestational age. *Conclusion.* The diminished DEFA6 expression in Paneth cells associated with NEC in this study supports the hypothesis that alpha-defensins are involved in the pathophysiology of NEC. Future studies are needed to elucidate the role of alpha-defensins in NEC aiming at finding preventive and therapeutic strategies against NEC.

1. Introduction

Necrotizing enterocolitis (NEC) is a serious gastrointestinal disorder that affects 10–15 percent of premature infants with a birth weight under 1500 g [1]. The mortality rates are up to 50% for infants requiring surgery [2]. Morbidity includes poor neurodevelopmental outcome and short bowel syndrome [3].

Current evidence suggests a multifactorial cause of NEC [1]. Prematurity is the main risk factor, presumably due to immaturity of gastrointestinal motility, intestinal barrier function, and immune defence. Other contributing factors are thought to be genetic predisposition, enteral feeding, intestinal ischemia, and colonization with pathogenic bacteria [1, 4]. The condition is an inflammation in the intestines related to a harmful overreaction of the immature immune system to some insults [4]. The histological appearance shows bacterial invasion of the epithelia and early signs of necrosis of the enterocytes at the top of some villi [5].

Paneth cells are specialized epithelia that play a major role in the innate immune response [6]. They protect intestinal stem cells from pathogens, stimulate stem cell differentiation, and assist in repairing the intestine. The stem cell compartment is located at the base of the crypts, in the small intestine interspersed by Paneth cells [7]. Paneth cells act through the production of antimicrobial proteins/peptides

[8]. The principal antimicrobial peptides, the alpha-defensins DEFA5 and DEFA6, differ in function [9]. DEFA6 shows weak activity against bacteria [10], and its antimicrobial function is activated by reducing milieu as a one-step mechanism by getting the more hydrophobic [11]. DEFA6 may have a key role in protecting the small intestine against invasion by diverse enteric pathogens through self-assembled peptide nanonets [12].

DEFA5 and DEFA6 mRNA levels are detectable at 13.5–17 weeks of gestation in the small intestine but with markedly diminished expression until the middle of the third trimester [13]. Enteric DEFA5 and DEFA6 mRNA levels are significantly lower in fetus and term newborns than in adults, and there are fewer numbers of Paneth cells in the crypts in extreme prematures than in term newborns and adults [13].

Recent studies suggest a key role for Paneth cells in the pathophysiology of NEC [5, 14–16]. The pathogenesis of NEC and inflammatory bowel Crohn's disease show many similarities [5, 17]. In Crohn's, the production of both DEFA5 and DEFA6 by Paneth cells is reduced [18]. Current knowledge of alpha-defensins in NEC is scanty, and the results seem to be controversial [19–21]. A better understanding of NEC is crucial to developing prevention and treatment strategies.

The aim of the study was to investigate the expression of DEFA6 in infants with NEC.

2. Materials and Methods

2.1. Study Population. Infants who underwent bowel resection for NEC at level III NICU in Sweden between August 2004 and September 2013 were eligible for the study (Table 1). The study protocol was approved by the Regional Ethical Review Board, and written informed consent was obtained from the parents.

Oral feeding with breast milk was started within two hours after birth in premature infants both in the control and the NEC groups. NEC was diagnosed by radiological and clinical features and staged according to the criteria of Bell et al. [22]. NEC diagnosis was confirmed during surgery and by histopathological evaluation. Infants with NEC were treated with broad-spectrum antibiotics, and enteral feeding was ceased prior to surgery. Infants with NEC underwent bowel resection, and an enterostomy was created. Those samples that represented macroscopically vital tissue, from ends of the resected intestine, were selected for further histopathological evaluation, and samples with complete mucosal erosion were excluded.

The controls all presented with delay to pass meconium, abdominal distention, and bilious vomiting, and they underwent laparotomy between four and 47 days of life and an ileostomy was created. Samples from the controls used for staining were taken from the site of the stoma. Three of the controls had transient functional immaturity of the intestine, and they were successfully managed with a temporary ileostomy (Table 1). Colonic biopsies in these three controls revealed the presence of immature ganglion cells, and ileal biopsies from the stoma showed the presence of normal ganglion cells. The fourth control was later diagnosed with pseudoobstruction and has still an ileostomy.

2.2. Intestinal Tissue Samples and Immunohistochemistry. We performed both the immunohistochemistry and the image analysis blindly. All samples were sectioned and stained on the same occasion for comparable analysis. Intestinal tissues were fixed in 4% formaldehyde in PBS for 24 h at 4°C. Embedded samples were sectioned (3 μm) and mounted on SuperFrost slides. Samples were deparaffinized through a graded series of xylol-ethanol. To determine the Paneth cell-specific expression of DEFA6, immunohistochemistry was performed by the Benchmark Ultra system (Ventana) and the ultraView Universal DAB Detection Kit (Ventana) and even counterstaining with hematoxylin-eosin was carried out. Tissue sections were incubated with a polyconal rabbit anti-DEFA6 antibody (Prestige Antibodies® Powered by Atlas Antibodies, 1 : 800 dilution) after antigen retrieval in the CC2 buffer (Ventana) for 36 min. Negative control sections were prepared by performing immunostaining procedures without adding primary antibodies. Representative sections were digitally scanned with a 3DHISTECH scanner. The images were exported in TIFF format (10x magnification) with the virtual microscope software Panoramic Viewer (3DHISTECH).

2.3. Image Analysis. ImageJ (freeware) was used for semiautomatic image analysis. The color detection of DAB staining was performed by the IHC Toolbox plugin in ImageJ, which can be effectively used to analyze samples stained by immunohistochemistry [23]. The model for color detection of brown pixels (which corresponded to the DAB staining and the level of DEFA6 expression) was adjusted specifically for the present project. The specificity of color detection was controlled visually. Working with image stacks during the evaluation process allowed the analysis to be made comparable between images. After color detection of DAB staining, the RGB color images were converted to 8-bit files. Inversion of the pixel intensity values resulted in higher pixel intensity corresponding to higher DEFA6 expression. The workflow is presented in Figures 1(a)–1(e). Before analysis, the same threshold window was set on each image in order to filter unspecific too high and/or too low pixel values. Besides the advantages of the method, even some limitations could be considered: the antigen retrieval process and the staining process are not easy to standardize and both can influence DAB intensity. Thus, the measured intensity levels in different studies are not directly comparable if they are performed at different time points.

2.4. DEFA6 Expression. Comparison of the general expression in the tissue was difficult since the height of the mucosa showed variations between patients. A solution was to measure the DAB-stained area as we hypothesized that the staining was homogeneous and had the same intensity for all the samples. We generated an even more standardized process, which showed DEFA6 expression for each μm length of the mucosa. The mucosal part of the sections was selected manually as the region of interest (ROI) (Figure 1(b)), and the size

Table 1: Study population.

Patient code	Diagnosis	Tissue origin	Gestational age at birth (weeks + days)	Birth weight (grams)	Gestational age at surgery (weeks + days)	Postnatal age at surgery (days)	Gender
12244-04_B1	NEC	Ileum	27 + 6	1438	28 + 4	5	Male
9589-10_B	NEC	Ileum	23 + 2	585	30 + 3	50	Male
12106-10_C	NEC	Ileum	26 + 2	1025	27 + 1	6	Male
18596-11_L	NEC	Colon	39 + 0	2360	39 + 4	4	Male
23543-11_B	NEC	Ileum	29 + 2	1225	29 + 6	4	Male
6126-12_A	NEC	Jejunum	26 + 2	912	31 + 0	33	Male
6436-13_C	NEC	Ileum	24 + 1	597	25 + 6	12	Female
33-04_B	NEC	Ileum	34 + 3	2300	35 + 2	6	Female
13749-07_A	Dysmotility	Ileum	36 + 4	3075	39 + 6	23	Male
3267-13	Dysmotility	Ileum	25 + 6	622	31 + 1	37	Female
315-10_1	Dysmotility	Ileum	40 + 4	4320	41 + 1	4	Female
873-12_5	Dysmotility	Ileum	25 + 0	870	31 + 5	47	Female

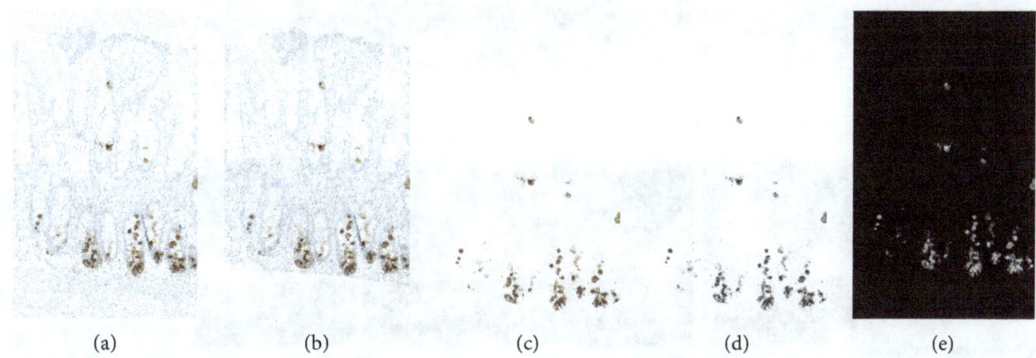

Figure 1: Image processing: DAB staining detection. (a) Original image—RGB color. (b) Selection of the mucosa as the region of interest (ROI). (c) IHC Toolbox plugin in ImageJ selects color, representing DAB staining. (d) Conversion of an RGB image to an 8-bit image (the lowest pixel intensity represents the highest DEFA6 expression and vice versa). (e) Inversion of pixel intensity values results in the highest pixel intensity corresponding to the highest DEFA6 expression.

of the area and the total DAB intensity of ROI were measured by ImageJ.

$$\text{"Length" of mucosa in the ROI} = \frac{\text{Area of ROI}}{\text{Mean height of mucosa}},$$

$$\frac{\text{DEFA6 expression}}{\mu\text{m}} = \frac{\text{Total DAB intensity of ROI}}{\text{"Length" of mucosa in the ROI } (\mu\text{m})}. \tag{1}$$

We calculated the mean value of the mucosal height (μm) for each section from ten representative sites measured by the Panoramic Viewer software. Length in μm could be converted into pixels and vice versa. The "length" of the mucosa part in the ROI is calculated by dividing the area in pixels with the height of the mucosa.

2.5. Statistics. Statistics were assessed in Microsoft Excel by two-sample t-test. A P value of <0.05 was considered to be statistically significant.

3. Results and Discussion

3.1. Study Population. A total of 12 infants were included in the study, eight with NEC and four controls. Patient characteristics are shown in Table 1. The tissue samples were taken from the colon ($n = 1$), jejunum ($n = 1$), and ileum ($n = 10$). Both the NEC and control groups consisted of extremely premature and term infants (control group: 25–40 gestational weeks, NEC group: 23–39 gestational weeks). The postnatal age at the time of surgery varied in both groups (control group: 4–47 days, NEC group: 4–50 days).

3.2. Tissue Characteristics and DEFA6 Expression. Searching in the database of the Human Protein Atlas revealed that DEFA6 is a highly specific marker for Paneth cells with exclusive expression in the intestine in adults [24].

The height of the mucosa varied highly in patients independently of the origin of the tissue or the indication for operation. No correlation between the height of the mucosa and the level of DEFA6 expression or gestational age could be seen (data not shown).

We found Paneth cells in all samples (Figure 2), even in the colon tissue (Figure 2, F). The tissue samples showed

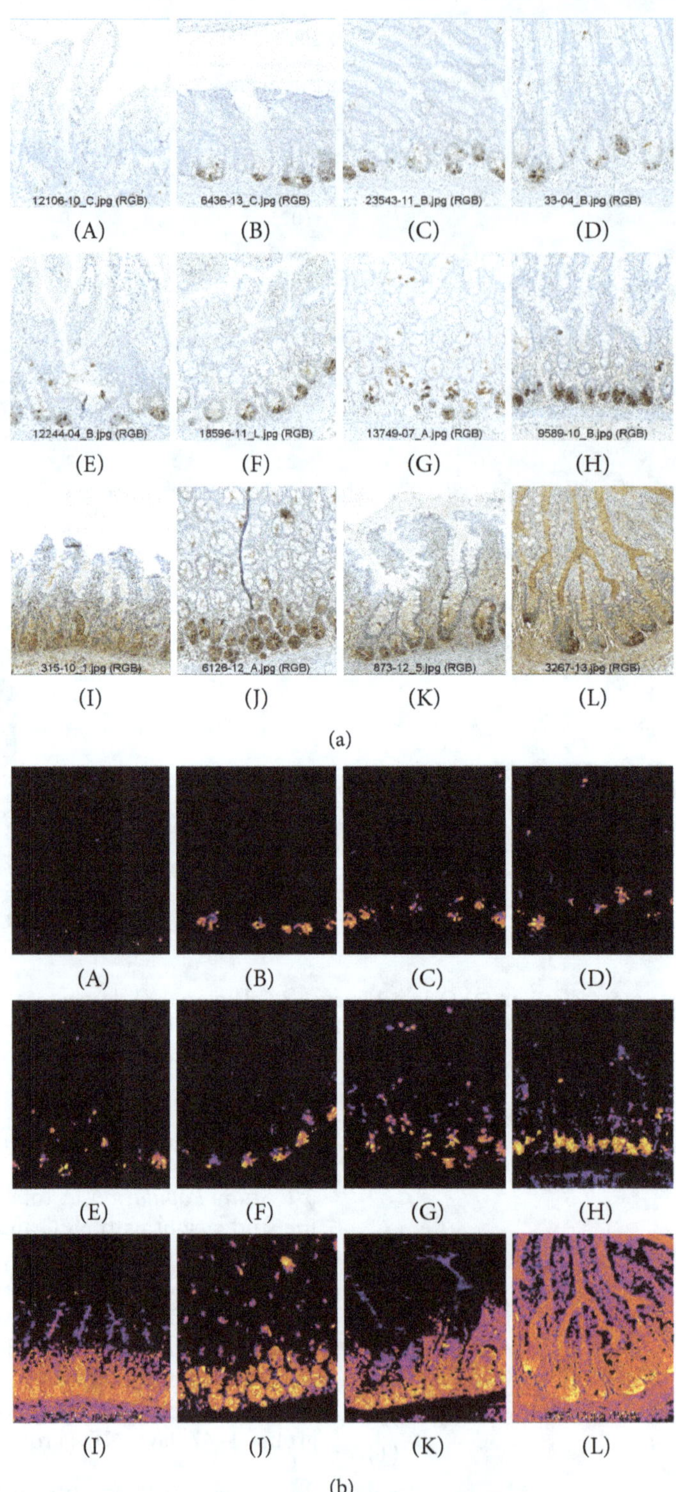

FIGURE 2: DEFA6 expression in the study material. (a) Increasing order of DEFA6 expression in patients. NEC group: A–F, H, and J; control group: G, I, K, L. (b) The lookup tables of images represent the distribution levels of DEFA6, visualized by colors (A–L). Extracellular DEFA6 expression appears in cases of higher general DEFA6 levels (H–L).

different levels of DEFA6 expression (Figure 3). Tissue samples may have varying water content that can influence DAB staining levels; therefore, we performed measurements on the DAB-covered area as well. DEFA6 expression was significantly lower in the NEC group than in the control group, independently of how we evaluated the DAB staining (DEFA6 expression/μm mucosa ($P = 0.019$) or percent area of the mucosa with DEFA6 expression ($P = 0.003$)) (Figure 3). The DEFA6 expression in the NEC group remained low and did not correlate with gestational age;

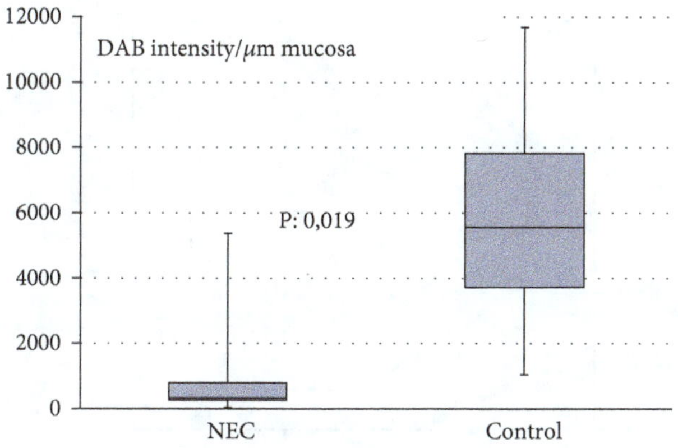

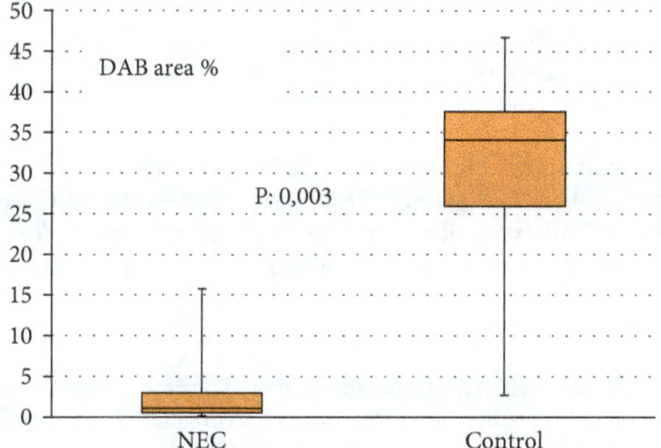

FIGURE 3: DEFA6 expression in the NEC group and the control group. Significant differences in DEFA6 expression irrespective of the evaluating method.

however, higher DEFA6 expression appeared in premature controls (Figure 4).

We were not able to estimate the objective count of Paneth cells due to the confluence of DAB staining in the sections with higher DEFA6 expression. However, the general impression suggests lower Paneth cell density in the NEC group (Figure 2).

3.3. Discussion. In the present study, we found a diminished DEFA6 expression in Paneth cells from infants with NEC compared to controls. Paneth cells and their main products, alpha-defensins, have been well studied in the development of Crohn's disease in adults [7, 16]. In Crohn's, the production of DEFA5 and DEFA6 by Paneth cells was reduced [15], which results in a defective antimicrobial shield and dysfunction of the mucosal barrier [9]. In premature infants, the diminished expression of DEFA5 and DEFA6 may result in higher risk of infection and inflammation. Although recent studies have suggested a Paneth cell dysfunction in NEC [5, 11–13], studies in alpha-defensin DEFA5 and DEFA6 expression in NEC patients are restricted to two previous reports [20, 21]. They investigated the mRNA levels of DEFA5 and DEFA6 and protein level of only DEFA5 but not DEFA6 [20, 21]. An explanation to the absence of studies in DEFA6 protein levels in NEC might be that the reliable commercial antibody for immunohistochemistry was not previously available. The use of immunohistochemistry in our study enabled structural evaluations. The disadvantage of this method is that it detects the actual protein levels, which may not correlate with mRNA levels in case of circumstances with enhanced protein degradation.

Salzman et al. found elevated DEFA5 and DEFA6 mRNA levels in infants with NEC compared with five near-term controls (four patients with intestinal atresia and one with meconium ileus) [20]. Intracellular peptide levels in NEC did not coincide with the elevation in mRNA. Puiman et al. found decreased DEFA5 protein expression in NEC patients [21]. The control group consisted of various diagnoses, namely, intestinal atresia, volvulus, gastroschisis, cloacal malformation, milk curd obstruction, Meckel's diverticulum, and ileus. The comparison with results of other studies is complicated by methodological heterogeneity and variation in gestational age between study populations and variation in diagnosis in the control groups [20, 21]. Nevertheless, similar to our results, alteration in the expression of alpha-defensins DEFA5 and DEFA6 seems to be associated with NEC [20, 21].

The number of Paneth cells [25] and the enteric expression of alpha-defensins in the fetus are low [13]; however, the production after birth is inducible by multiple factors. Both intraluminal bacteria and lipopolysaccharide can stimulate Paneth cell secretion, as well as cholinergic agonists and feeding [25–28]. This corresponds to our observation that DEFA6 expression was high in our fed extremely premature controls. An interpretation of our observations is that the DEFA6 expression is initially low at birth, inducible, and increasing in healthy individuals but remains low in patients who develop NEC.

Interestingly, we found Paneth cell metaplasia in a colonic tissue sample with NEC. This phenomenon has been previously reported in inflammatory bowel disease [29]. Puiman et al. described metaplastic Paneth cells in post-NEC stricture colon samples but not in NEC samples. They suggested that chronic inflammation caused Paneth cell metaplasia [21].

The strength of this study was that it was one of the two studies in DEFA6 expression and NEC. Moreover, we described the setup of a reliable semiquantitative method to study the expression of DEFA6.

The limitations of our study were the small sample size and the fact that the numbers of age-matched control patients were limited since material collection from a healthy control group was not feasible due to ethical reasons. The same problem appeared in previous studies of DEFA5 and DEFA6 where patients with various diagnoses such as volvulus, gastroschisis, small intestinal atresia, and ileus were included as controls [20, 21].

4. Conclusions

The diminished DEFA6 expression in Paneth cells associated with NEC in this study supports the hypothesis that alpha-defensins are involved in the pathophysiology of NEC. Future studies are needed to elucidate the role of alpha-

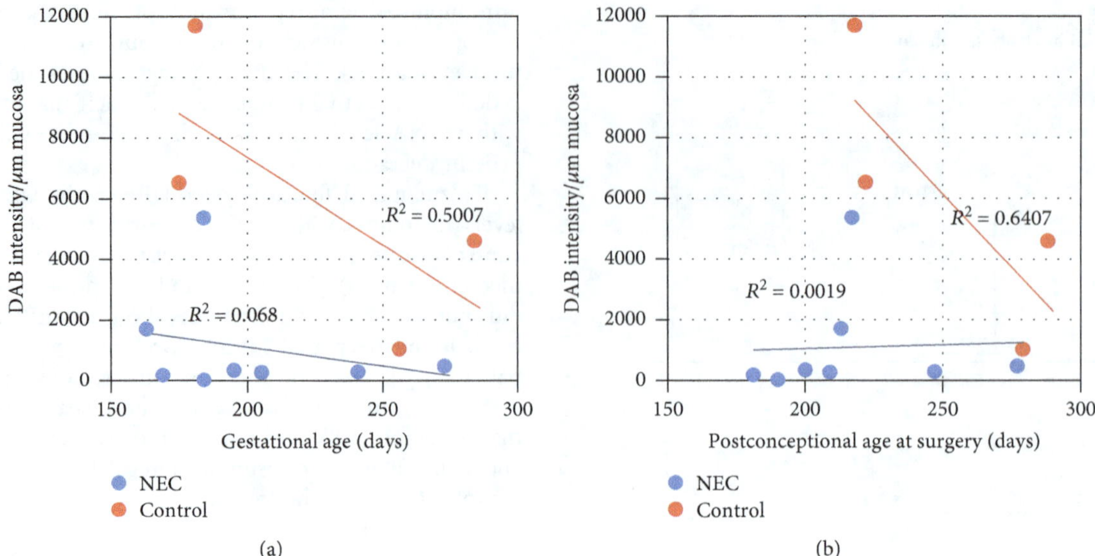

FIGURE 4: Relationship between DEFA6 expression and age. (a) Control patients showed higher level of DEFA6 expression and negative correlation between DEFA6 expression and gestational age. Premature controls had the highest DEFA6 level. Most of the NEC patients showed low DEFA6 expression. No correlation could be confirmed between DEFA6 expression and gestational age in the NEC group. (b) The phenomenon above was more pronounced between DEFA6 expression and postconceptional age at surgery (maturation level). corr: 0.03 (NEC group), corr: −0.74 (control group).

defensins in NEC aiming at finding preventive and therapeutic strategies against NEC.

Acknowledgments

This work was supported by funding from H.R.H. Crown Princess Lovisa's Association for Paediatric Health Care/ Foundation Axel Tielman's Memorial Fund.

References

[1] J. Neu and W. A. Walker, "Necrotizing enterocolitis," *The New England Journal of Medicine*, vol. 364, no. 3, pp. 255–264, 2011.

[2] R. Sharma, J. J. Tepas III, M. L. Hudak et al., "Portal venous gas and surgical outcome of neonatal necrotizing enterocolitis," *Journal of Pediatric Surgery*, vol. 40, no. 2, pp. 371–376, 2005.

[3] D. Duro, L. A. Kalish, P. Johnston et al., "Risk factors for intestinal failure in infants with necrotizing enterocolitis: a Glaser Pediatric Research Network study," *The Journal of Pediatrics*, vol. 157, no. 2, pp. 203–208.e1, 2010.

[4] L. Berman and R. L. Moss, "Necrotizing enterocolitis: an update," *Seminars in Fetal & Neonatal Medicine*, vol. 16, no. 3, pp. 145–150, 2011.

[5] S. J. McElroy, M. A. Underwood, and M. P. Sherman, "Paneth cells and necrotizing enterocolitis: a novel hypothesis for disease pathogenesis," *Neonatology*, vol. 103, no. 1, pp. 10–20, 2013.

[6] J. Paneth, "About the secreting cells in the small intestinal epithelium," *Arch Mikroskop Anat*, vol. 31, pp. 113–191, 1888.

[7] N. Barker, J. H. van Es, J. Kuipers et al., "Identification of stem cells in small intestine and colon by marker gene *Lgr5*," *Nature*, vol. 449, no. 7165, pp. 1003–1007, 2007.

[8] A. J. Ouellette, "Defensin-mediated innate immunity in the small intestine," *Best Practice & Research Clinical Gastroenterology*, vol. 18, no. 2, pp. 405–419, 2004.

[9] P. Chairatana, H. Chu, P. A. Castillo, B. Shen, C. L. Bevins, and E. M. Nolan, "Proteolysis triggers self-assembly and unmasks innate immune function of a human α-defensin peptide," *Chemical Science*, vol. 7, no. 3, pp. 1738–1752, 2016.

[10] B. Ericksen, Z. Wu, W. Lu, and R. I. Lehrer, "Antibacterial activity and specificity of the six human α-defensins," *Antimicrobial Agents and Chemotherapy*, vol. 49, no. 1, pp. 269–275, 2005.

[11] B. O. Schroeder, D. Ehmann, J. C. Precht et al., "Paneth cell α-defensin 6 (HD-6) is an antimicrobial peptide," *Mucosal Immunology*, vol. 8, no. 3, pp. 661–671, 2015.

[12] H. Chu, M. Pazgier, G. Jung et al., "Human α-defensin 6 promotes mucosal innate immunity through self-assembled peptide nanonets," *Science*, vol. 337, no. 6093, pp. 477–481, 2012.

[13] E. B. Mallow, A. Harris, N. Salzman et al., "Human enteric defensins. Gene structure and developmental expression," *Journal of Biological Chemistry*, vol. 271, no. 8, pp. 4038–4045, 1996.

[14] M. A. Underwood, "Paneth cells and necrotizing enterocolitis," *Gut Microbes*, vol. 3, no. 6, pp. 562–565, 2012.

[15] F. H. Heida, G. Beyduz, M. L. C. Bulthuis et al., "Paneth cells in the developing gut: when do they arise and when are they immune competent?," *Pediatric Research*, vol. 80, no. 2, pp. 306–310, 2016.

[16] S. M. Tanner, T. F. Berryhill, J. L. Ellenburg et al., "Pathogenesis of necrotizing enterocolitis," *The American Journal of Pathology*, vol. 185, no. 1, pp. 4–16, 2015.

[17] É. Tremblay, M.-P. Thibault, E. Ferretti et al., "Gene expression profiling in necrotizing enterocolitis reveals pathways common to those reported in Crohn's disease," *BMC Medical Genomics*, vol. 9, no. 1, article 6, 2016.

[18] M. Gersemann, J. Wehkamp, K. Fellermann, and E. F. Stange, "Crohn's disease-defect in innate defence," *World Journal of Gastroenterology*, vol. 14, no. 36, pp. 5499–5503, 2008.

[19] M. A. Underwood and C. L. Bevins, "Defensin-barbed innate immunity: clinical associations in the pediatric population," *Pediatrics*, vol. 125, no. 6, pp. 1237–1247, 2010.

[20] N. H. Salzman, R. A. Polin, M. C. Harris et al., "Enteric defensin expression in necrotizing enterocolitis," *Pediatric Research*, vol. 44, no. 1, pp. 20–26, 1998.

[21] P. J. Puiman, N. Burger-van Paassen, M. W. Schaart et al., "Paneth cell hyperplasia and metaplasia in necrotizing enterocolitis," *Pediatric Research*, vol. 69, no. 3, pp. 217–223, 2011.

[22] M. J. Bell, J. L. Ternberg, R. D. Feigin et al., "Neonatal necrotizing enterocolitis: therapeutic decisions based upon clinical staging," *Annals of Surgery*, vol. 187, no. 1, pp. 1–7, 1978.

[23] J. Shu, G. E. Dolman, J. Duan, G. Qiu, and M. Ilyas, "Statistical colour models: an automated digital image analysis method for quantification of histological biomarkers," *BioMedical Engineering OnLine*, vol. 15, no. 1, article 46, 2016.

[24] "Tissue expression of DEFA6- Summary-The Human Protein Atlas," November 2017, https://www.proteinatlas.org/ENSG00000164822-DEFA6/tissue.

[25] K. Lewin, "The Paneth cell in health and disease," *Annals of the Royal College of Surgeons of England*, vol. 44, no. 1, pp. 23–37, 1969.

[26] T. Peeters and G. Vantrappen, "The Paneth cell: a source of intestinal lysozyme," *Gut*, vol. 16, no. 7, pp. 553–558, 1975.

[27] X. D. Qu, K. C. Lloyd, J. H. Walsh, and R. I. Lehrer, "Secretion of type II phospholipase A2 and cryptdin by rat small intestinal Paneth cells," *Infection and Immunity*, vol. 64, no. 12, pp. 5161–5165, 1996.

[28] M. M. Wieck, C. R. Schlieve, M. E. Thornton et al., "Prolonged absence of mechanoluminal stimulation in human intestine alters the transcriptome and intestinal stem cell niche," *Cellular and Molecular Gastroenterology and Hepatology*, vol. 3, no. 3, pp. 367–388.e1, 2017.

[29] M. Tanaka, H. Saito, T. Kusumi et al., "Spatial distribution and histogenesis of colorectal Paneth cell metaplasia in idiopathic inflammatory bowel disease," *Journal of Gastroenterology and Hepatology*, vol. 16, no. 12, pp. 1353–1359, 2001.

18

Endoscopic Mucosal Resection Performed Underwater for Nonampullary Duodenal Epithelial Tumor: Evaluation of Feasibility and Safety

Goro Shibukawa,[1] Atsushi Irisawa,[1] Ai Sato,[1] Yoko Abe,[1] Akane Yamabe,[1] Noriyuki Arakawa,[1] Yusuke Takasaki,[1] Takumi Maki,[1] Yoshitsugu Yoshida,[1] Ryo Igarashi,[1] Shogo Yamamoto,[1] Tsunehiko Ikeda,[1] and Hiroshi Hojo[2]

[1]*Department of Gastroenterology, Aizu Medical Center, Fukushima Medical University, Aizuwakamatsu, Japan*
[2]*Department of Pathology, Aizu Medical Center, Fukushima Medical University, Aizuwakamatsu, Japan*

Correspondence should be addressed to Atsushi Irisawa; irisawa@fmu.ac.jp

Academic Editor: Mattia Berselli

Objectives. Recently, opportunities to encounter superficial nonampullary duodenal epithelial tumor (SNADET) have increased. EMR and ESD are performed to treat SNADET. However, the rate of perforation is higher than that of other gastrointestinal lesions, regardless of which method is used. Underwater EMR (UW-EMR) is immersion treatment of SNADET, which has low risk of perforation and can remove lesions safely and completely. In the present study, we retrospectively investigated patients in whom UW-EMR was performed to evaluate the feasibility and safety of UW-EMR for the treatment of SNADET. *Methods.* The primary endpoint was to evaluate the feasibility of UW-EMR for the treatment of SNADET, and secondary objective was to determine the operation's safety. *Results.* There were 14 participants, with a total of 16 lesions, who underwent UW-EMR between August 2015 and December 2017. Histological heteromorphism revealed that seven patients had low-grade adenoma, seven had high-grade adenoma, and two had adenocarcinoma. En bloc resection was performed in 14 lesions. In two patients, nodular lesions were observed in the scar and biopsy confirmed recurrences. There were no serious adverse events including bleeding or perforation. *Conclusions.* UW-EMR may be a safe and effective treatment method for SNADET, if its therapeutic indication is adequately considered.

1. Introduction

The incidence of all cancers of the small intestine, including superficial nonampullary duodenal epithelial tumor (SNADET), is remarkably lower than that of other gastrointestinal cancers, such as cancers of the stomach and large intestine [1]. The duodenum has more nonneoplastic lesions than other organs, and the incidence of malignancy among neoplastic lesions appears to be low. However, there has been a recent trend, starting in the 1970s, showing an increase in the incidence of malignancy among neoplastic lesions [2]. In addition, duodenal cancer is often detected at an advanced stage; the 5-year survival rate is less than 30%, and the prognosis is regarded as the worst among all small intestinal cancers [3].

In recent years, opportunities to encounter duodenal tumors have increased because of the popularization of endoscopy for upper gastrointestinal tract screening. However, no definite guidelines have been established regarding the indication of endoscopic therapy for duodenal tumor and selection of treatment strategy because of the low frequency of the procedure being performed.

Endoscopic mucosal resection (EMR) and endoscopic submucosal dissection (ESD) are performed to treat SNADET. However, because the duodenal muscularis propria is extremely thin, the rate of intraoperative or delayed perforation is higher than that of other gastrointestinal lesions, regardless of which method is used. Therefore, these techniques may not be suitable for use as standard treatments [4].

Binmoeller et al. [5, 6] developed the underwater EMR (UW-EMR), in which the EMR is performed while immersed in water. It has been reported that immersion treatment of a superficial tumor of the duodenum, which has a thin wall, and the large intestine, has an extremely low risk of perforation and lesions can be removed safely and completely. Because the muscular layer develops its weight by filling the lumen with water and the mucosal surface swells because of immersion, it is believed that the possibility of gripping the muscular layer at the time of snaring during EMR is extremely low. In the present study, we retrospectively investigated patients in whom UW-EMR was performed to evaluate the feasibility and safety of UW-EMR for treatment of SNADET.

2. Patients and Methods

2.1. Study Design. This was a retrospective study investigating the use of UW-EMR for treatment of SNADET. The primary endpoint was to evaluate the feasibility of UW-EMR for treatment of SNADET, and secondary objective was to determine the operation's safety. This study was reviewed and approved by the Institutional Review Board of Fukushima Medical University and conducted in accordance with the human and ethical principles of research set forth in the Declaration of Helsinki.

2.2. Patients. There were 14 participants, with a total of 16 lesions, who underwent UW-EMR in our department for the treatment of SNADETs between August 2015 and December 2017. The mean age of patients was 61.9 years, and the male to female ratio was 9 to 5. For treatment indication, irrespective of morphology (elevation/depression), the invasion depth was diagnosed endoscopically as an intramucosal tumor, and the size for inclusion was set to 20 mm or less. We set the exclusion criteria as follows: pregnancy, coagulopathy (international normalised ratio > 2.0, platelets < 70 × 100/L), previous endoscopic or surgical treatment of SNADET, and neoplastic lesions that do not meet the inclusion criteria.

2.3. Endoscopic Procedures

2.3.1. Equipment. The endoscopes used were the GIF-HQ290, GIF-Q260, GIF-H290, and GIF-H290Z (Olympus Co., Tokyo, Japan), and the primary snare used was Captivator™ II (elliptical, 13 mm in diameter) (Boston Scientific Japan, Tokyo, Japan). However, depending on the size of the tumor to be treated, the Captivator™ II (elliptical, 27 mm in diameter) and Dualoop 33-16 (elliptical, 16 mm in diameter) (Medico's Hirata Inc., Osaka, Japan) or SD-7P-1 (semicircular, diameter of 23 mm) (Olympus Co., Tokyo, Japan) were used. VAIO 200S (ERBE Co. Ltd., Tuebingen, Germany) was used as the high-frequency generator, and the settings were as follows: Endocut-Q, effect 3, incision time two, incision interval three.

2.3.2. Techniques. UW-EMR was performed using the following procedures (schema was drawn as Figure 1):

(1) The procedures were performed with the patient under sedation. Midazolam was used as the primary sedative (0.15 to 0.30 mg/kg was initially injected intravenously and, if necessary, half of the initial dose or the same amount was further administered), and when sedation was poor or the state of disinhibition due to midazolam use was noted, propofol (0.5 mg/kg/10 s) was also appropriately used in combination.

(2) The endoscope was inserted into the duodenum with the patient in the left lateral decubitus position. After confirming the known tumor (Figure 2), slightly warm distilled water was injected into the duodenal lumen from the accessory channel, and the tumor was completely submerged (Figure 3(a)). If the stagnation of the distilled water in the duodenal lumen was poor when the patient was in the left lateral decubitus position, the position of the patient was changed to supine/abdominal position, so that favorable stagnation of distilled water could be obtained.

(3) The tumor was observed in underwater immersion and we observed until the lesion was slightly bulging from the mucosal surface (Figure 3(b)).

(4) The snare was opened during underwater immersion and was subsequently pressed against the lesion site to confirm that the entire lesion entered the snare, and the lesion was strangulated. Resnaring was performed to confirm that the duodenal muscularis propria was not gripped, and the lesion was excised using an incision wave (Figure 4(a)). Furthermore, the boundary between the tumor and the normal mucosal surface became morphologically clear because of the bulging of the lesion, and because the resected range was clearly observed together with the lens effect of the filled distilled water, preoperative marking was not performed.

(5) After resection, the presence or absence of any remnant of the tumor was confirmed, and when the remnant was confirmed, additional resection was continued using UW-EMR.

(6) After final resection, it was endoscopically confirmed that there were no remnants, and then the resected surface was stitched using a hemoclip (Figure 4(b)). If bleeding continued, even after clip plication, it was treated using cauterization by argon plasma coagulation (APC) and local injection of hypertonic saline epinephrine solution, as appropriate.

(7) On the day after treatment, the presence or absence of an adverse event, such as hemorrhage, was confirmed by endoscopy. When no clear adverse events were present, eating was initiated on the second day following treatment. In all patients, proton pomp inhibitor was orally administered prior to the day on which the UW-EMR was performed.

(8) Endoscopy was performed one to three months postoperatively for follow-up observation, and the

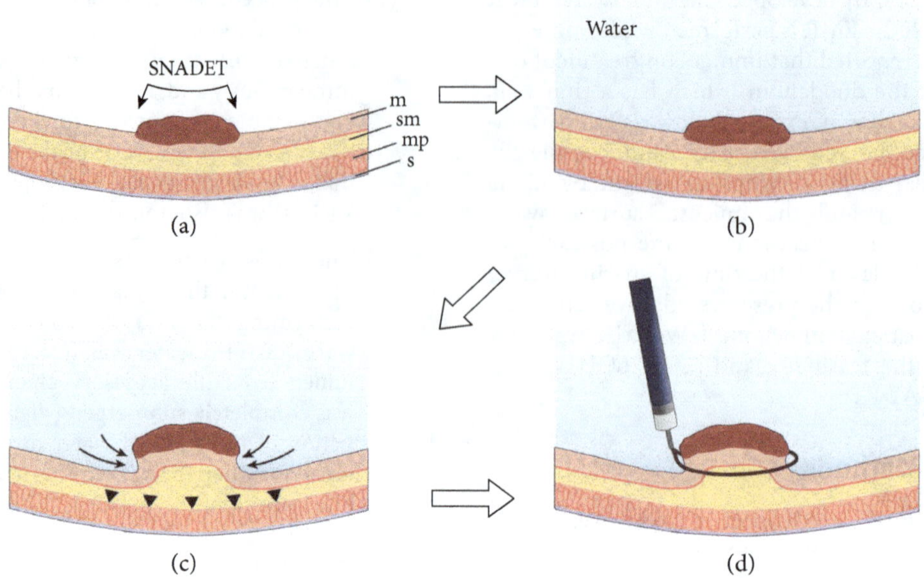

Figure 1: (a) The endoscope was inserted into the duodenum. m: mucosa, sm: submucosa, mp: muscularis propria, s: serosa. (b) After confirming the known tumor, slightly warm distilled water was injected into the duodenal lumen from the accessory channel, and the tumor was completely submerged. (c) The tumor was observed in underwater immersion and we observed until the lesion was slightly bulging from the mucosal surface (allow). During observation, the muscular layer was kept flat in a ring shape (allow head). (d) The snare was opened during underwater immersion and was subsequently pressed against the lesion site to confirm that the entire lesion entered the snare, and the lesion was strangulated. Resnaring was performed to confirm that the duodenal muscularis propria was not gripped, and the lesion was excised using an incision wave.

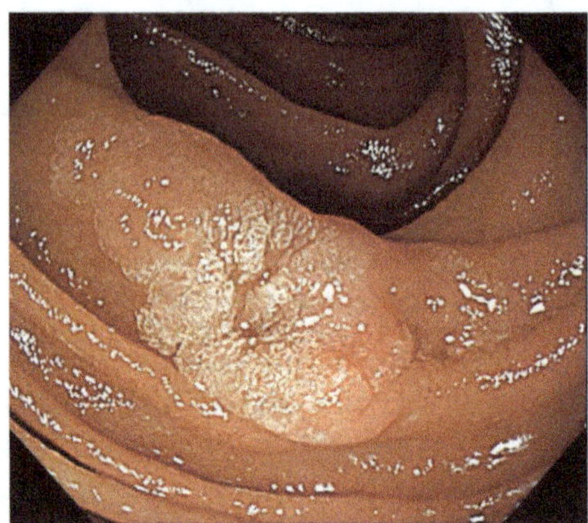

Figure 2: A slightly elevated lesion with a central irregular depression in the second part of duodenum was seen.

healing process of the wound site was evaluated. We also assessed the existence of any remnants.

2.4. Assessment of Adverse Events. We predominantly assessed bleeding and perforation as adverse events related to this procedure. In terms of time performing this assessment, adverse events were classified as either intraprocedural or postprocedural. A definition was created with reference to ESGE's Colorectal polypectomy and EMR guideline [7] as follows: (1) Intraprocedural bleeding/perforation is bleeding/perforation occurring during the procedure that persists for more than 60 s or requires endoscopic intervention. (2) Postprocedural bleeding/perforation is bleeding/perforation occurring after the procedure, up to 30 days post-UW-EMR, that results in an unplanned medical presentation, such as emergency department visit, hospitalization, or reintervention (repeat endoscopy, angiography, or surgery). In addition, the degree of the adverse event was defined as follows: (1) A mild event involves slight bleeding where hemostasis could be achieved using an endoscopic procedure without a blood transfusion. (2) A severe event involves all bleeding, except the above-mentioned bleeding, and all perforation. Furthermore, we also evaluated the type and degree of relevant adverse events aside from bleeding and perforation.

3. Results

3.1. Feasibility (Table 1). The sites of tumor occupation were as follows: duodenal bulb, one lesion (posterior wall, one lesion) and second part of duodenum, 15 lesions (anterior wall, two lesions; posterior wall, five lesions; left side wall, four lesions; right side wall, four lesions). Macroscopic findings indicated that 13 lesions were elevated and three were depressed.

The mean tumor diameter in the resected specimens was 10.5 mm (6–18 mm). Histological heteromorphism in the resected specimens revealed that seven patients had low-grade adenoma, seven had high-grade adenoma, and two had adenocarcinoma. The invasion depth of adenocarcinoma was mucosal carcinoma in all patients. Evaluation of the lateral stump of the tumor in the resected specimens revealed various results. One stump tested positive for high-grade

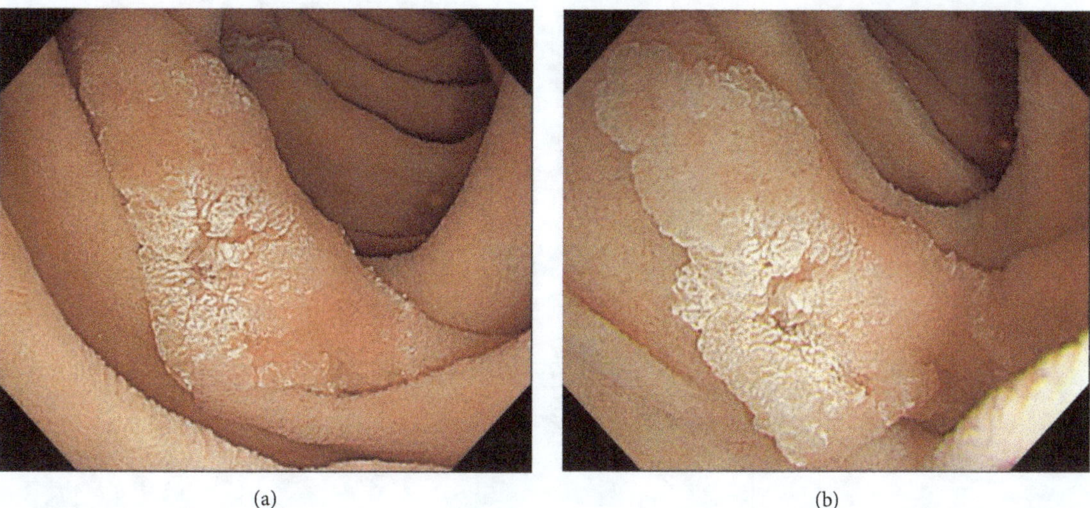

(a) (b)

FIGURE 3: (a) Slightly warm distilled water was injected into the duodenal lumen from the accessory channel, and the tumor was completely submerged. (b) The lesion was slightly bulging from the mucosal surface a few minutes after warm water injection, and the boundary between the tumor and the normal mucosal surface became morphologically clear.

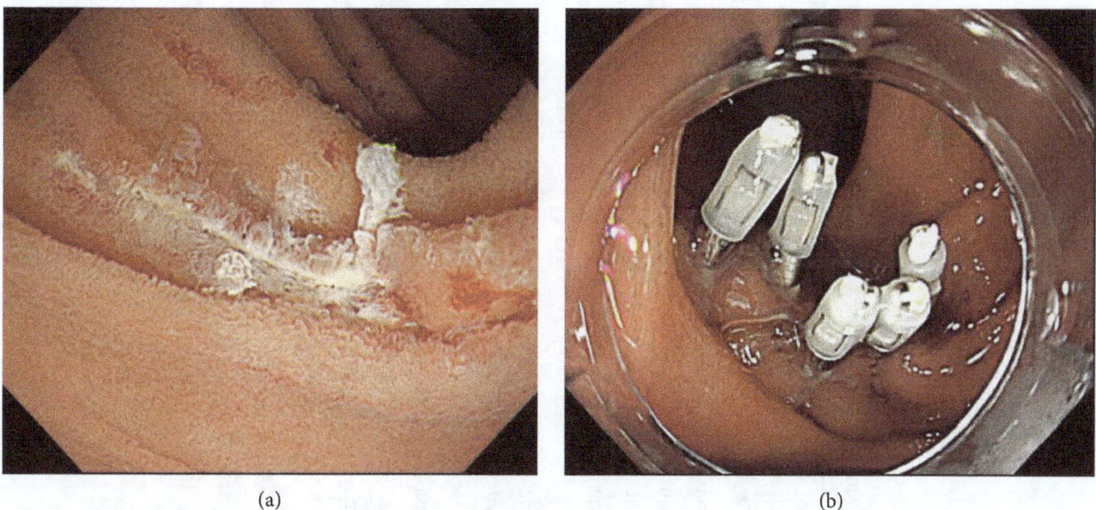

(a) (b)

FIGURE 4: (a) The lesion was resected using a snare under water. (b) After resection, it was endoscopically confirmed that there was no residual tumor, and then the resected surface was stitched using a hemoclip.

adenoma. In three lesions, the stump was diagnosed as negative for low-grade adenoma. However, evaluation of the other 12 lesions was difficult. En bloc resection was performed in 14 lesions (87.5%), but the remaining two lesions (12.5%) showed a remnant after initial the UW-EMR, and we performed additional resection on the same day. Fractional excision in two parts was performed for one lesion located on the left side wall of the second part of duodenum, and fractional excision in four parts was performed for one lesion located on the posterior wall of the second part of duodenum.

Endoscopic examination for follow-up observation was performed one to three months postoperatively (one patient received their endoscopic examination for follow-up observation one year postoperative because their postoperative diagnosis was low-grade adenoma). In two patients, small nodular lesions were observed in the UW-EMR scar. In case number 1 (second part of duodenum, posterior wall), a nodule was found in the scarred part when the endoscopy was performed for follow-up observation one month later, and adenocarcinoma was confirmed by biopsy in the same part (pathological diagnosis of resected specimen was adenocarcinoma). Fractional excision in four parts was performed in the present patient. However, in case number 12 (second part of duodenum, left side wall), en bloc resection was performed, but the results of the follow-up endoscopy performed six months after treatment revealed the presence of a white nodule in the scarred part, and a biopsy confirmed high-grade adenoma in the same part (pathological diagnosis of resected specimen revealed high-grade adenoma). In all cases, because the lesion was present in the scar after resection, additional endoscopic treatment was difficult and surgical resection was performed. In the 14 additional lesions, remnant recurrence during the mean observation period of 10.8 months (1–28 months) was not noted.

Table 1: Patient characteristics and therapeutic summary.

Case	Location	Macroscopic type	Size of snare	Biopsy diagnosis	Tumor size	Final diagnosis	Histological margin	En bloc or multiple resection	Recurrence (follow-up period)	Adverse event
1	2nd	Protuberance	20 mm	Group 4	13 mm	Aca	D/E	Multiple (4)	Recurrence (1 M)	(–)
2	2nd	Protuberance	27 mm	Adenoma	12 mm	LGA	D/E	En bloc	No (28 M)	(–)
3	2nd/2nd	Protuberance/protuberance	13 mm	Aca/undone	12 mm/6 mm	Aca/LGA	D/E/D/E	En bloc/En bloc	No (27 M)/No (27 M)	(–)/(–)
4	2nd	Protuberance	13 mm	Adenoma	11 mm	HGA	D/E	En bloc	OFD (10 M)	(–)
5	2nd	Protuberance	13 mm	Adenoma	9 mm	LGA	pHM0	En bloc	No (13 M)	(–)
6	2nd	Protuberance	13 mm	Group 4	8 mm	HGA	D/E	En bloc	No (12 M)	(–)
7	2nd	Protuberance	13 mm	Adenoma	10 mm	HGA	D/E	En bloc	No (12 M)	(–)
8	Bulb	Protuberance	13 mm	Hyperplastic	15 mm	LGA	D/E	En bloc	No (10 M)	Bleeding during UW-EMR
9	2nd	Protuberance	16 mm	Adenoma	15 mm	LGA	D/E	Multiple (2)	No (10 M)	Bleeding post-UW-EMR
10	2nd	Protuberance	13 mm	Adenoma	12 mm	HGA	D/E	En bloc	No (10 M)	(–)
11	2nd/2nd	Depress/depress	13 mm	Adenoma/HGA	7 mm/6 mm	LGA/HGA	pHM0/D/E	En bloc/En bloc	No (5 M)/No (5 M)	(–)/(–)
12	2nd	Protuberance	18 mm	Adenoma	8 mm	HGA	D/E	En bloc	Recurrence (1 M)	Bleeding during UW-EMR
13	2nd	Protuberance	13 mm	Adenoma	6 mm	HGA	pHM1	En bloc	No (1 M)	Bleeding during UW-EMR
14	2nd	Depress	13 mm	Adenoma	18 mm	LGA	pHM0	En bloc	No (1 M)	(–)

Aca: adenocarcinoma, LGA: low-grade adenoma, HGA: high-grade adenoma, D/E: difficulty of evaluation, OFD: other factors death.

4. Safety (Table 1)

With regard to adverse events, a minor intraprocedural event (minimal oozing of blood) was observed in three patients (case number 8, 12, and 13) and a minor postprocedural event (minimal oozing of the blood) in one (case number 9), but there were no serious adverse events, such as bleeding or perforation, that required blood transfusion. In the two patients who experienced an intraprocedural event, hemostasis was achieved by performing plication of the wound with a clip, and in the other patient, because minor oozing of blood was observed after wound plication, hypertonic saline-epinephrine solution was injected locally into the hemorrhage site to stop the bleeding. In one patient with postprocedural bleeding, minor oozing of blood from the wound was observed during the endoscopic observation performed the day following operative treatment, and hemostasis was achieved using APC cauterization.

5. Case Presentation

The patient was a 60-year-old woman (case number 3 on Table 1). There was one elevated lesion on both the left side wall and the right wall of the second part of duodenum (Figure 5), and because biopsy findings were suspected of adenocarcinoma, the patient visited our department for treatment. Along with small lesions for which biopsy was not performed, two lesions were collectively excised using UW-EMR (Figure 6). Four clips were used on the resected surface and one for plication. The postoperative course was favorable, and complications such as bleeding and perforation were not observed, even after resuming eating. She was discharged on postoperative day eight. Lesions in which adenocarcinoma was suspected during preoperative biopsy were revealed to be adenocarcinoma by the final pathological diagnosis of the resected specimens (Figures 7(a) and 7(b)), and the final pathological diagnosis of the other lesions was adenoma (Figures 7(c) and 7(d)). Follow-up endoscopic examination, which was performed one month after the UW-EMR, showed wound scarring in both lesions, and endoscopic findings suggesting recurrence were not observed (Figures 8(a) and 8(b)). Endoscopic examination subsequently performed at 6, 12, and 21 months after treatment revealed no recurrence (Figure 8(c)).

6. Discussion

ESD and EMR have been performed as endoscopic treatment of SNADET. In facilities with an experienced endoscopist, the risk of complications related to EMR is low and the procedure can be safely performed [8]. However, in the case of a lesion with a diameter of 20 mm or larger, there is a high possibility that fractional excision is performed in EMR, making it difficult to perform a pathological assessment after resection, and recurrence of the remnant after resection is a problem. In ESD, en bloc resection is possible for such large lesions, but because the duodenal muscularis propria is extremely thin, the intraoperative and delayed perforation rates are high [4]. Binmoeller et al. [5, 6] reported that by observing the tumor in underwater immersion in the UW-EMR, the deep muscular layer is kept flat in a ring shape, and the mucosa and submucosal layer of the tumor rise to the side of the intestinal lumen, filled with injected water so as to float from the muscular layer. Therefore, it is possible to grip the lesion with a snare without gripping the muscular layer. In addition, observation by insufflation revealed that the lesion part was extended and stretched along with the intestinal wall, and it is difficult to simply grip using the snare only. But, in the UW-EMR, the gastrointestinal wall of the lesion is in a relaxed state, so that gripping by snare becomes easier and a wider range of the lesion is available to be gripped, as compared to the use of a conventional EMR. In the present study, of the 14 patients (16 lesions) who underwent treatment, one lesion was present in the duodenal bulb and 15 lesions were present in the second part of the duodenum. Furthermore, these lesions were distributed in various parts of the second part of the duodenum. Of the target lesions in the present study, fractional excision had to be performed in two, but it was demonstrated that this method can be performed safely without causing serious complications up to the second part of the duodenum. Although clear guidelines for lesions indicated for treatment are needed in the future, this method may become a first-line therapy for SNADET.

Binmoeller et al. [5], who initially reported this method, regarded adenoma as the indication for UW-EMR. Therefore, even for laterally spreading duodenal adenoma with a large tumor diameter, treatment with fractional excision by this method was performed. By contrast, because we also regarded adenocarcinoma as an indication, considering the risk of remnant and pathological evaluation, lesions large enough to undergo en bloc resection (in principle, lesions less than 20 mm that can be gripped by snare) were indicated for treatment. Cases requiring planned fractional excision were excluded from the indication. As a result, when the tumor diameter was 20 mm or less, en bloc resection was possible in 87.5% of cases. However, en bloc resection could not be performed in two lesions (12.5%), and additional resection was performed. The sizes of these lesions were 15 mm and 13 mm, and even when compared to other lesions, their size allowed en bloc resection to be sufficiently performed. The two lesions in which fractional excision was performed were not particularly unique tumor sites in comparison with other lesions, but due to the curve of the duodenum and positional relation with the duodenal folds, it is possible that the identification of the area on the anal side was difficult, or alignment of the snare could not be sufficiently controlled. From this viewpoint, it appears necessary to attempt using a snare ring for under water immersion before treatment with this method. There are also various kinds of snares (e.g., round, oval, or semicircular shape; hard or soft material), and the selection of the device according to the size and lesion site is also important. It is the authors' opinion that, in any case, it is extremely important to establish a proper strategy before surgery.

In the patients in the present study in whom the procedure was performed, evaluation of the lateral stump was possible in only four lesions, and it was difficult to evaluate the

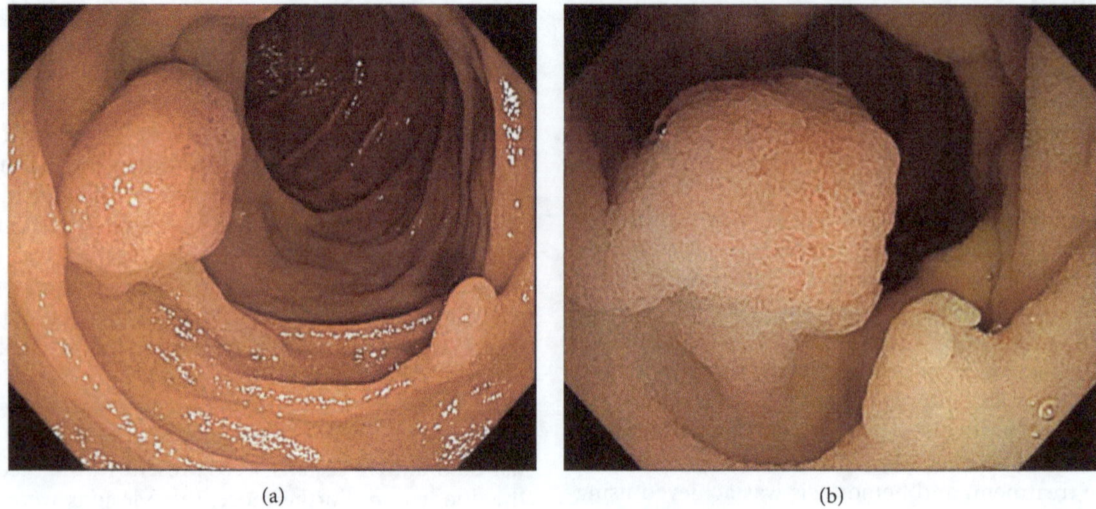

(a) (b)

FIGURE 5: (a) There was an elevated lesion on both the left side and the right wall of the second part of duodenum. (b) The boundary between the tumor and the normal mucosal surface became morphologically clear in underwater immersion.

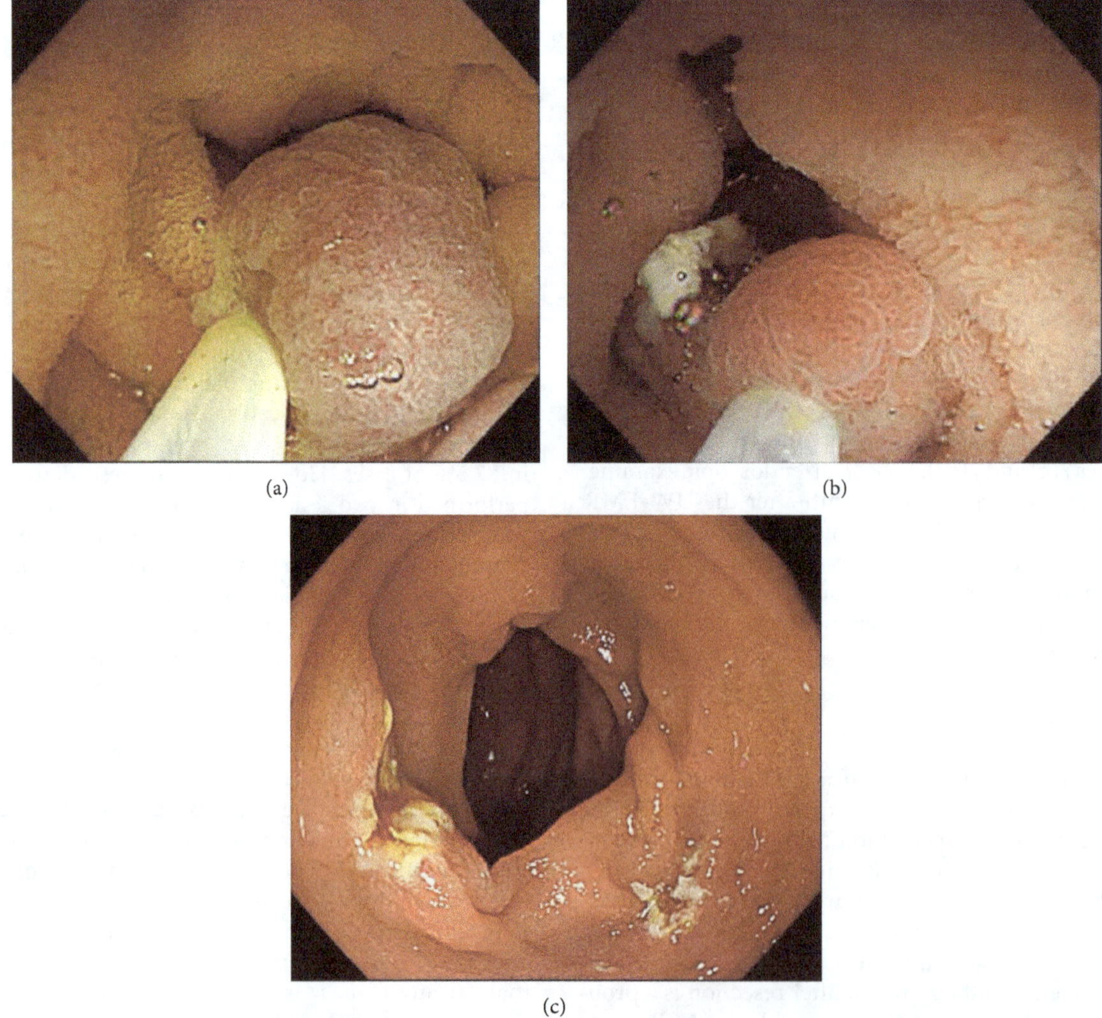

(a) (b)

(c)

FIGURE 6: (a, b) Two lesions were collectively excised using UW-EMR. (c) Minimal oozing of blood was seen after UW-EMR.

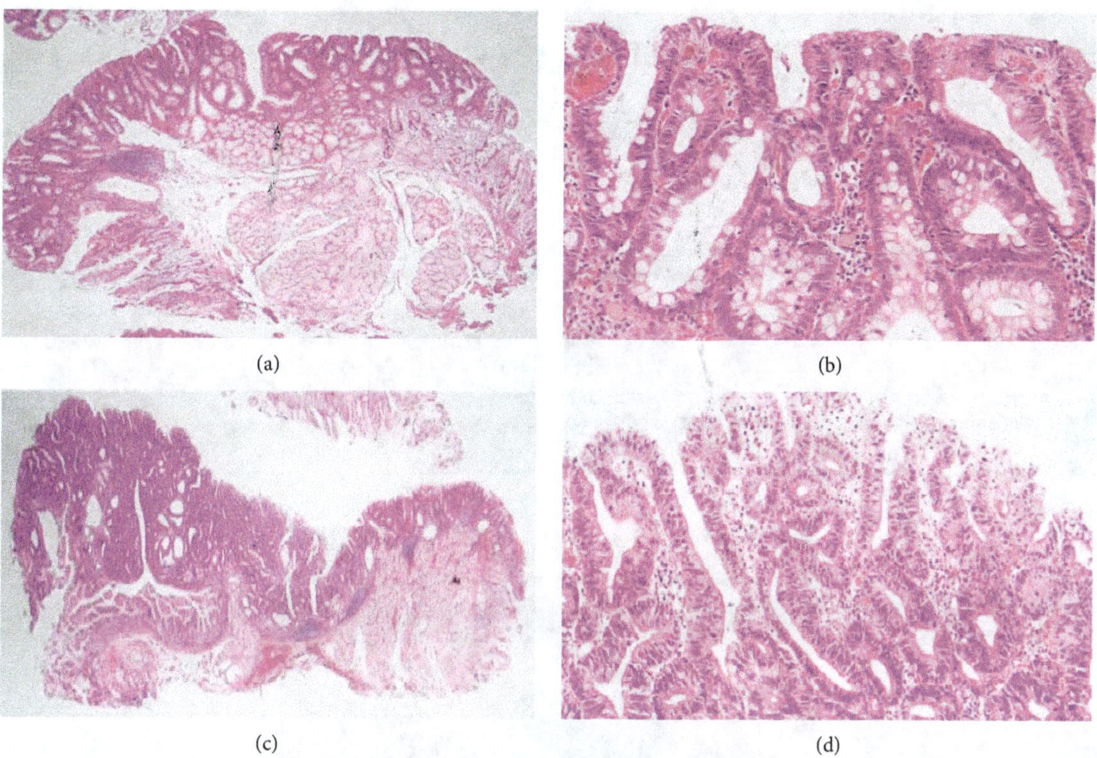

FIGURE 7: (a, b) Histopathological examination for larger lesion revealed that lesions in which adenocarcinoma was suspected during preoperative biopsy were revealed to be adenocarcinoma (HE staining, ×40 in (a), ×200 in (b)). (c, d) Histopathological examination for smaller lesion diagnosed as adenoma (HE staining, ×40 in (c), ×200 in (d)).

other 12 lesions. The reason for the difficulty in assessment in UW-EMRs appears to be related to the influence of thermal denaturation on the resected side surface by gripping the mucosal surface in an unexpanded state with the snare and performing the excision. Although it was endoscopically confirmed that there was no remnant at the time of the UW-EMR, careful follow-up observation, such as shortening of the observation period, may be necessary when the lateral stump in the resected specimen is difficult to evaluate. In fact, in the present study, we experienced recurrence in the remnant in two lesions (two patients). One lesion was adenocarcinoma for which fractional excision in four parts was performed. Because fractional excision seems to have a high risk of remnants, it is necessary to establish a solid strategy for collective resection for treatment, as previously mentioned. In cases where it is difficult to perform an en bloc resection, another treatment method should be considered without overly focusing on this method. However, in another lesion in which recurrence was noted, en bloc resection could be performed, but a nodule was confirmed in the scarred part of UW-EMR by endoscopy one month after treatment and a remnant was confirmed. Because this lesion was located in a site lateral to the superior duodenal angle where the duodenum had a large curve, observation of the anal side margin of the lesion could not be sufficiently performed, and snaring was performed in a state in which all lesions were not observed. When the entire image of the lesion is difficult to observe in one field of view, caution is needed with regard to the risk of the remaining remnants, and it is necessary to consider a treatment strategy without overly focusing on this method.

In the present study, 15 out of 16 lesions were preoperatively diagnosed by endoscopic biopsy, and the concordance rate of preoperative diagnosis and postoperative pathological diagnosis was 60% (9 out of 15 lesions). The problem of diagnostic accuracy of preoperative biopsy for SNADET has been previously indicated, and Goda et al. [9] and Kakushima et al. [10] reported a low proper diagnosis rate (68% and 74%, resp.). The appropriate diagnosis rate of preoperative diagnosis by endoscopy was higher (75% and 78%, resp.), which was due to recent improvements in endoscopic diagnostics and the development of diagnostic techniques using imaging enhancement, such as NBI and magnifying endoscopy. However, there is no established consensus regarding the criteria for endoscopic diagnosis of SNADET, and the fact that there are variations in diagnosis by surgeon and institution remains a problem. Of the types of SNADET, low-grade adenoma is also thought to be a lesion for which follow-up is possible [11], but at present, the proper diagnosis rate in endoscopic diagnosis and pathological diagnosis is low, and the possibility of malignancy cannot be denied, so it may be difficult to make the determination that follow-up is possible. Therefore, as the precision of preoperative diagnosis is low, endoscopic treatment may also be considered as a diagnostic treatment. In such a case, ESD, which is at a high risk of severe adverse event, cannot be used as a standard diagnostic treatment. However, in the present study, the safety of UW-EMR was strongly demonstrated, and from this viewpoint,

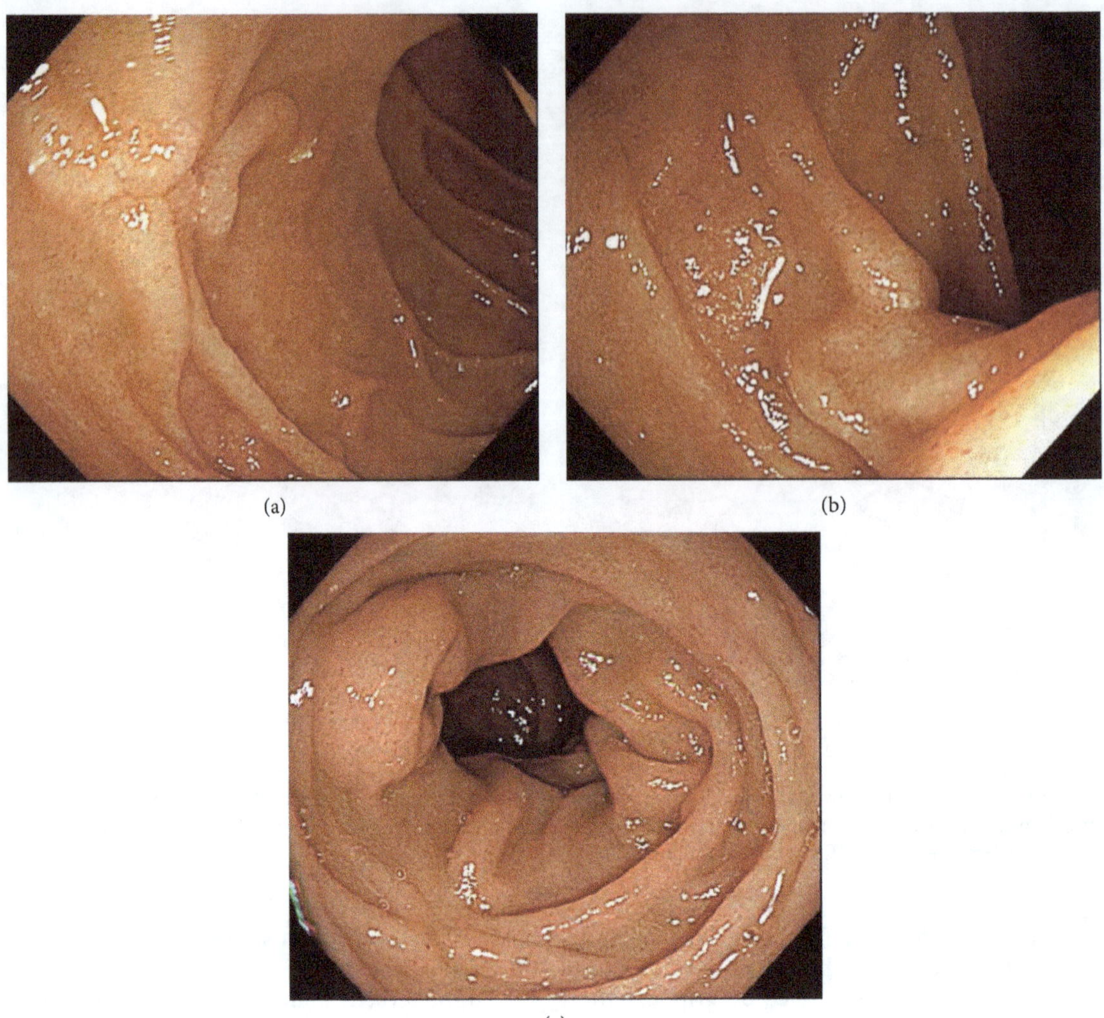

(a) (b) (c)

FIGURE 8: (a, b) Follow-up endoscopic examination, which was performed one month after the UW-EMR, showed wound scarring in both lesions without recurrence. (c) Endoscopic examination at 21 months after treatment showed no recurrence.

there is a possibility that it may become a standard treatment of SNADET. Endoscopic treatment for SNADET, including nonmalignant tumors especially such as adenoma, needs to be minimally invasive, and even with the ease of the procedure and the low risk of adverse events, UW-EMR may be a standard treatment for adenoma.

In conclusion, UW-EMR may be a feasible treatment method for SNADET, if its therapeutic indication is adequately considered. It is the authors' opinion that, especially in the case of adenoma with a tumor diameter less than 20 mm, it may be beneficial to actively consider the procedure. However, because the present study was both a retrospective and small case series study, to establish the utility, effectiveness, and safety of UW-EMR for treating SNADET in the future, it is necessary to conduct a prospective comparison study with ESD.

References

[1] D. Schottenfeld, J. L. Beebe-Dimmer, and F. D. Vigneau, "The epidemiology and pathogenesis of neoplasia in the small intestine," *Annals of Epidemiology*, vol. 19, no. 1, pp. 58–69, 2009.

[2] J. S. Chow, C. C. Chen, H. Ahsan, and A. I. Neugut, "A population-based study of the incidence of malignant small bowel tumors: SEER, 1973-1990," *International Journal of Epidemiology*, vol. 25, no. 4, pp. 722–728, 1996.

[3] J. R. Howe, L. H. Karnell, H. R. Menck, C. Scott-Conner, and The American College of Surgeons Commission on Cancer and the American Cancer Society, "Adenocarcinoma of the small bowel: review of the National Cancer Data Base, 1985-1995," *Cancer*, vol. 86, no. 12, pp. 2693–2706, 1999.

[4] S. Hoteya, N. Yahagi, T. Iizuka et al., "Endoscopic submucosal dissection for nonampullary large superficial adenocarcinoma/adenoma of the duodenum: feasibility and long-term outcomes," *Endoscopy International Open*, vol. 1, no. 1, pp. 2–7, 2013.

[5] K. F. Binmoeller, J. N. Shah, Y. M. Bhat, and S. D. Kane, ""Underwater" EMR of sporadic laterally spreading nonampullary duodenal adenomas (with video)," *Gastrointestinal Endoscopy*, vol. 78, no. 3, pp. 496–502.e1, 2013.

[6] K. F. Binmoeller, F. Weilert, J. Shah, Y. Bhat, and S. Kane, ""Underwater" EMR without submucosal injection for large sessile colorectal polyps (with video)," *Gastrointestinal Endoscopy*, vol. 75, no. 5, pp. 1086–1091, 2012.

[7] M. Ferlitsch, A. Moss, C. Hassan et al., "Colorectal polypectomy and endoscopic mucosal resection (EMR): European Society of Gastrointestinal Endoscopy (ESGE) clinical guideline," *Endoscopy*, vol. 49, no. 3, pp. 270–297, 2017.

[8] S. Nonaka, I. Oda, S. Abe et al., "Clinical outcomes of endoscopic resection for nonampullary duodenal tumor," *Progress of Digestive Endoscopy*, vol. 87, no. 1, pp. 53–57, 2015.

[9] K. Goda, D. Kikuchi, Y. Yamamoto et al., "Endoscopic diagnosis of superficial non-ampullary duodenal epithelial tumors in Japan: multicenter case series," *Digestive Endoscopy*, vol. 26, pp. 23–29, 2014.

[10] N. Kakushima, H. Kanemoto, K. Sasaki et al., "Endoscopic and biopsy diagnoses of superficial, nonampullary, duodenal adenocarcinomas," *World Journal of Gastroenterology*, vol. 21, no. 18, pp. 5560–5567, 2015.

[11] K. Okada, J. Fujisaki, A. Kasuga et al., "Sporadic nonampullary duodenal adenoma in the natural history of duodenal cancer: a study of follow-up surveillance," *The American Journal of Gastroenterology*, vol. 106, no. 2, pp. 357–364, 2011.

19

Efficacy and Safety of Endoscopic Intralesional Triamcinolone Injection for Benign Esophageal Strictures

Ya-Wu Zhang,[1,2,3] Feng-Xian Wei,[1,2,3] Xue-Ping Qi,[3] Zhao Liu,[4] Xiao-Dong Xu,[1,2,3] and You-Cheng Zhang[1,2,3]

[1]*Department of General Surgery, Lanzhou University Second Hospital, Lanzhou 730000, China*
[2]*Hepato-Biliary-Pancreatic Institute, Lanzhou University Second Hospital, Lanzhou 730000, China*
[3]*Lanzhou University Second Clinical Medical College, Lanzhou University, Lanzhou 730000, China*
[4]*The First Clinical Medical College of Lanzhou University, Lanzhou 730000, China*

Correspondence should be addressed to You-Cheng Zhang; zhangyouchengphd@163.com

Academic Editor: Aldona Dlugosz

Objectives. To evaluate the efficacy and safety of endoscopic intralesional triamcinolone injection (ITI) for benign esophageal strictures combined with endoscopic dilation (ED). *Methods.* Online databases including MEDLINE, EMBASE, the Cochrane Library, and Web of Science were comprehensively searched for prospective randomized control trials (RCTs) between 1966 and March 2018. A meta-analysis was conducted according to the methods recommended by the Cochrane Collaboration. *Results.* Six RCTs consisting of 176 patients were selected. Meta-analysis results showed that additional ITI had a significant advantage in terms of stricture rate and required ED sessions. Surgery-related and non-surgery-related strictures showed similar results. Additional ITI was not associated with significantly increased risk of complications. *Conclusions.* Our meta-analysis showed that additional ITI therapy was supposed to be effective and safe for benign esophageal strictures as it reduced the stricture rate and required ED sessions. However, more RCTs are necessary to support these findings.

1. Introduction

Surgical anastomosis, radiation therapy, Schatzki's rings, esophageal webs, corrosive injury, peptic injury, photodynamic therapy [1, 2], and endoscopic surgery can always induce benign esophageal strictures [3–5]. These injuries can induce edema, and finally lead to stricture formation through stimulating the proliferation of fibrotic tissue and/or accumulation of collagen [6]. Aside from resolving the severity of the stricture, the intended therapy also focused on the improvement of quality of life and avoidance of related complications, as well as the prevention of recurrences. Currently, endoscopic dilation (ED) is the first procedure adopted in clinical practice and is regarded as safe and effective, and the preferred initial treatment option irrespective of etiology [2, 7–9]. However, the procedure sometimes required frequent repetition due to a high risk of recurrence, and this severely influenced the patient's quality of life. Thus, a new therapeutic method is warranted to meet clinical demand.

In previous studies, oral administration and intralesional injection of corticosteroids have been used to soften scars and keloids with promising results, as it has pharmacological effects of inflammatory response inhibition and fibrotic tissue reduction [10, 11]. Some studies also investigated the efficacy of intralesional steroid injections for benign gastrointestinal strictures and proposed to augment the effect of ED [12–14]. Since the esophagus was a narrow tubular organ with a very high incidence and recurrence of stricture, local triamcinolone injection for esophageal strictures was supposed to reduce stricture recurrence by several studies [13, 14].

However, current studies about this issue were limited by small sample size or inconsistent data. We performed a meta-analysis including all prospective randomized controlled trials (RCTs) investigating the clinical efficacy and safety of intralesional triamcinolone injection (ITI) for benign esophageal strictures.

2. Methods

2.1. Inclusion Criteria. The following inclusion criteria were used to identify relevant studies: (1) Patients were individuals with benign esophageal strictures after surgery and/or corrosive injury. (2) Intervention was ITI in the treatment group, and comparison was saline injection (sham control) or no injection (blank control) in the control group. ED was performed conventionally mainly based on the demand of patients because of significant strictures (defined as failure of passing by an adult using a gastroscope of 8–9.8 mm diameter). (3) Outcome measures included stricture rate, ED sessions, dysphagia-free time, and treatment-related complications. Besides, clinical studies designed as RCTs were available without language limitation.

2.2. Search Strategy. Literature search was conducted in databases including MEDLINE (1966–Mar 2018), EMBASE (1978–Mar 2018), the Cochrane Library (1993–Mar 2018), and Web of Science (1985–Mar 2018). Search terms are as follows: (esophageal OR oesophagus OR esophagus) AND (stenoses OR stricture OR stenosis) AND (triamcinolone OR steroid OR corticosteroids injection). References of case reports, comparative studies, and reviews were also scanned to manually search relevant articles. Two reviewers independently reviewed the search results according to the inclusion criteria through screening the title and abstract. For potential studies, full-text papers were further evaluated independently for final inclusion. Disagreements between reviewers were resolved in consultation with a third reviewer (Zhang YC).

2.3. Data Extraction and Quality Assessment. Another two reviewers independently extracted the data including basic information, outcome measures, and methodological quality items. Any disagreements between the reviewers were resolved by discussion. Basic information included first author, publication year, sample size, average age of patients, intervention, comparison, dose of triamcinolone, diagnosis of patients, and follow-up periods. Outcomes included stricture rates, required dilation sessions, dysphagia-free time, and complications. Methodological quality items included randomization, allocation concealment, blinding, withdrawal and dropout, selective reporting result, and other biases. Quality assessment was performed independently by two reviewers according to the method and the tool of risk of bias recommended by the Cochrane Handbook [15].

2.4. Statistical Analysis. Review Manager (version 5.3, the Cochrane Collaboration, Copenhagen) was used to analyze data. For dichotomous outcomes, risk ratio (RR) with 95% confidence intervals (CI) was used. For continuous outcomes, standard mean difference (SMD) or mean difference (MD) were used. $P < 0.05$ was considered of statistical significance. The chi-square test was performed to assess the statistical heterogeneity across trials and I^2 value to assess the extent of inconsistency. When $I^2 > 50\%$, the random-effect model was used. If $I^2 \leqq 50\%$, the fixed-effect model was applied. Publication bias was explored using an inverted funnel plot.

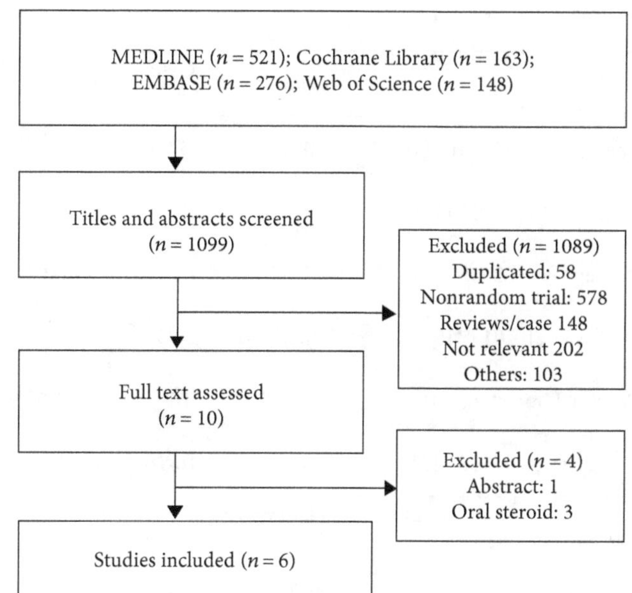

Figure 1: Flow chart of trial selection process.

3. Results

3.1. Literature Search Result and Study Characteristics. We identified 1099 citations from online databases and obtained 10 full texts of articles based on the titles, abstracts, and full-text evaluation. Finally, six studies enrolling 176 patients were included for quantitative analysis [16–21], as shown in Figure 1. Basic information of the included RCTs was listed in Table 1. The sample size ranged from 14 to 60 patients. Two trials adopted a sham control with saline injection [19, 21], and four trials adopted no injection. Five trials adopted bougie dilation, and only one trial adopted balloon dilation [18]. In the study of Ramage et al. [18], the patients received dilation 1-2 times in the past 18 months, which was reported comparable between the groups. The doses of intralesionally injected triamcinolone ranged at 20 mg, 32 mg, and 40 mg per patient, and one trial injected 5 mg of triamcinolone every 10 mm point around the stricture. The diagnosis included surgical injury in three trials, peptic and corrosive injury in two trials, and both surgical and corrosive injury in one trial. Quality assessment was shown in Figure 2, and the overall quality was moderate to high.

3.2. Stricture Rate. Five studies reported the stricture rate after steroid injection during follow-up [16–20]. Significant stricture was defined as failure of passing by an adult using a gastroscope of 8–9.8 mm diameter and the demand of a repeated dilation. Meta-analysis in a fixed-effect model showed that ITI significantly reduced the incidence of stricture compared with control, and stricture rates were 50% and 78% in the groups.

Subgroup analysis according to different stricture etiologies showed that the risks of surgery-related strictures and

Table 1: Characteristic of included randomized controlled trials.

Study	Country	Case (T/C, n)	Age (T/C, y)*	Intervention (T/C) T	Intervention (T/C) C	Dose	Diagnosis	Follow-up (months)
Takahashi et al. 2015 [16]	Brazil	7/7	39 (23–64)/ 46 (22–65)	ED + ITI	ED + saline injection	40 mg	Corrosive stenosis	12
Altintas et al. 2004 [17]	Turkey	10/11	49 (24–69)/ 45 (17–76)	ED + ITI	ED	32 mg	Corrosive, surgical, postradiotherapy	>6
Ramage et al. 2005 [18]	USA	15/15	66/67	ED + ITI	ED	20 mg	Corrosive esophageal stricture	>12
Hirdes et al. 2013 [19]	Netherlands	29/31	64 ± 9/62 ± 8	ED + ITI	ED + saline injection	20 mg	Anastomotic stricture	6
Pereira-Lima et al. 2015 [20]	Brazil	10/9	56 ± 8/52 ± 15	ED + ITI	ED	40 mg	Anastomotic stricture	6
Camargo et al. 2003 [21]	Japan	16/16	70 ± 10/71 ± 7	ED + ITI	ED	>30 mg	Endoscopic surgery stricture	>16

*Data were presented as mean ± standard deviation or median (range); T, treatment group; C, control group. ED, endoscopic dilation. ITI, intralesional triamcinolone injection.

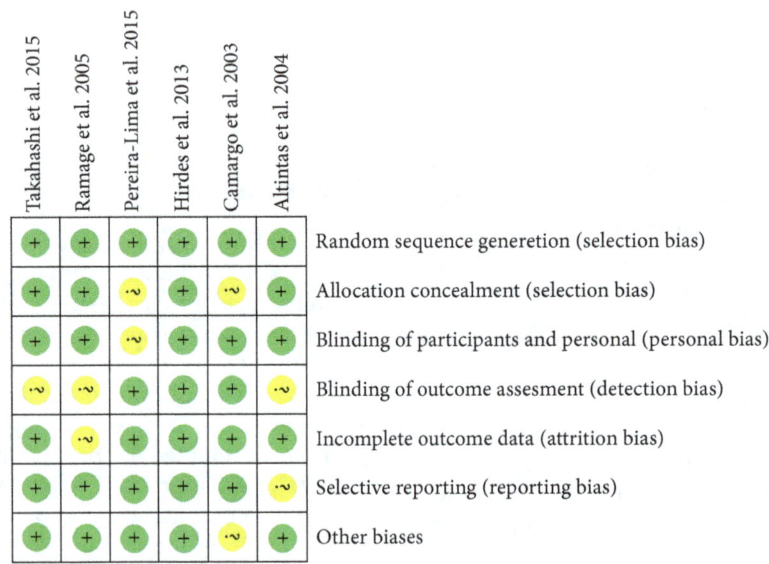

Figure 2: Summary of methodological quality of included studies.

non-surgery-related strictures were both reduced after ITI therapy, as shown in Figure 3.

3.3. Required ED Sessions. Four studies reported the number of required ED sessions during follow-up [16, 17, 19, 20]. Statistical heterogeneity was mild ($I^2 = 11\%$). Meta-analysis results showed that ITI significantly reduced the required ED sessions compared with the control.

Also, subgrouping according to different stricture etiologies showed that the number of required ED sessions was reduced after ITI therapy in the subgroup of surgery-related strictures. However, there was only one study including 21 patients in the subgroup of non-surgery-related strictures, and no significant difference was found, as shown in Figure 4.

3.4. Dysphagia-Free Time. Four studies reported the data of dysphagia-free time [16, 17, 19, 20]. There was a large heterogeneity across the trials ($I^2 = 88\%$), thus the random-effect model was used. No significant difference in dysphagia-free time was found between the groups.

After excluding the study causing the large heterogeneity [16], the I^2 value was reduced to 38% and fixed-effect model meta-analysis results of the remaining three studies showed that ITI significantly reduced the duration of dysphagia-free time compared with the control (Figure 5).

3.5. Complications. Injection-related complications were reported in two trials with a total of eight patients, and the others stated no related complications. Among them, two had perforations, one experienced bleeding, one had mucosal tearing, and four suffered from local infection. The adverse effects were similar between the patients treated with steroids and those without steroids. There was no statistically significant difference in the incidence of complications.

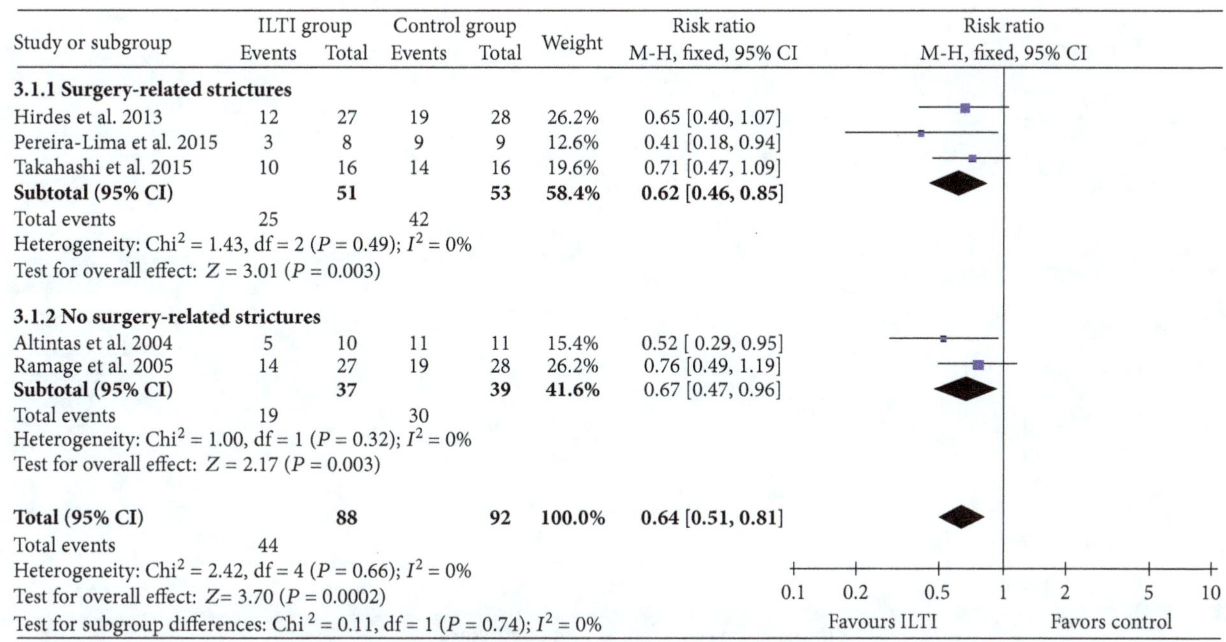

FIGURE 3: Forest plot of stricture rate between ITI and control.

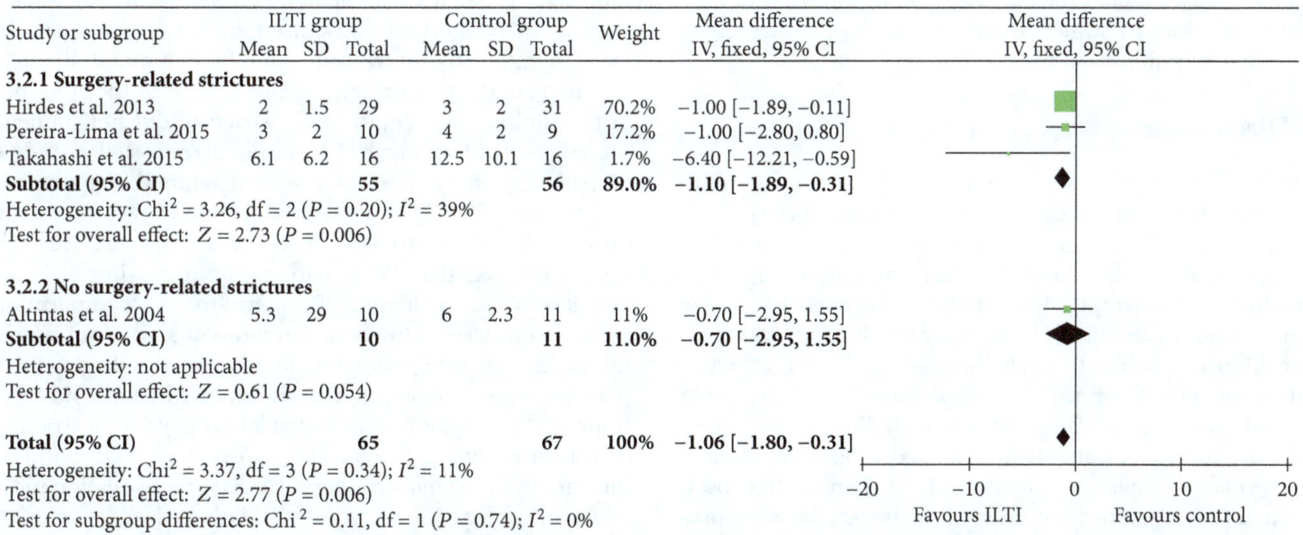

FIGURE 4: Forest plot of EBD sessions during follow-up between ITI and control.

Study or subgroup	ILTL group			Control group			Weight	Std. mean difference
	Mean	SD	Total	Mean	SD	Total		IV, random, 95% CI
Altintas et al. 2004	24	12.75	10	5.18	5.06	11	22.6%	1.90 [0.83, 2.97]
Hirdes et al. 2013	3.6	1.37	29	1.5	1.36	31	26.6%	1.59 [1.01, 2.18]
Pereira-Lima et al. 2015	12	2.74	15	10.1	1.28	14	25.2%	0.85 [0.09, 1.62]
Takahashi et al. 2015	3.5	4	16	6.1	5	16	25.7%	−0.56 [−1.27, 0.15]
Total (95% CI)			**70**			**72**	**100.0%**	**0.92 [−0.17, 2.01]**

Heterogeneity: $Tau^2 = 1.08$; $Chi^2 = 25.04$, df = 3 ($P < 0.0001$); $I^2 = 88\%$

Test for overall effect: $Z = 1.66$ ($P = 0.10$)

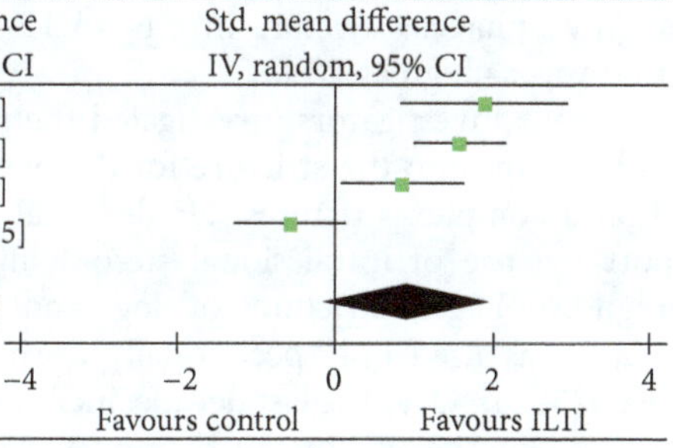

Std. mean difference IV, random, 95% CI: −4 −2 0 2 4; Favours control — Favours ILTI

FIGURE 5: Forest plot of dysphagia-free time between ITI and control.

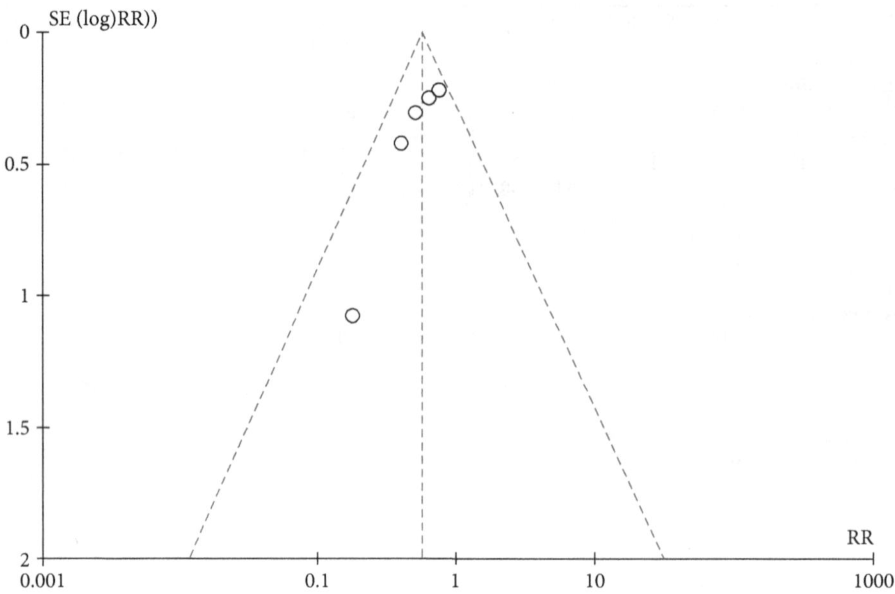

FIGURE 6: Inverted funnel plot of stricture rate.

3.6. Publication Bias. Due to the limited number of included studies, a publication bias test through an inverted funnel plot was only adopted for the outcome of the stricture rate. The shape was to some extent symmetrical, indicating a lower risk of publication bias (Figure 6).

4. Discussion

A benign esophageal stricture was diagnosed by clinical, radiological, and endoscopical features and biopsies [16, 22]. Therapeutic options for a benign stricture included ED, temporary stent placement, intralesional steroid injection, and incisional therapy. Among these methods, ED is the cornerstone treatment [1]. Esophageal dilation was performed using either through-the-scope balloons or wire-guided bougies. A defined esophageal diameter to be targeted by dilation is different from patients with different severities, but the majority of patients have considerable symptomatic improvement when a diameter of 15–18 mm has been reached [16–19]. However, most of the intractable strictures are often unsuccessful with a high incidence of recurrence, which then require repeated dilations [23, 24]. This would seriously influence the quality of life and also increase the risk of complication in these patients. As estimated by the current study, the recurrence rate of stricture in the control group of benign esophageal stricture in a 6- to 12-month follow-up period was as high as 78%.

Various investigators investigated the role of corticosteroid injection into the stricture for the prevention of recurrent and complex strictures. Holder et al. were the first to report the use of intralesional steroid injection (ISI) into benign esophageal strictures of dogs and children, and the therapy was used only occasionally during the 1970s and 1980s [25, 26]. Over the last decade, increasing interests were presented in the use of the therapy for refractory benign esophageal strictures [12, 13, 16, 18].

Some other large-scale comparative studies reported their primary results and findings as follows. Kochhar et al. reported 71 patients with benign esophageal stricture receiving ISI; all categories of stricture that required ED sessions were significantly decreased, while the luminal diameter was increased. Interestingly, it also indicated that the location, number, and length of the stricture did not influence the efficacy of treatment [13]. Lee et al. reported a study of 31 patients, where all of them were diagnosed by endoscopy and treated with ED and steroid injection in each of the four quadrants at the narrowest region of the stricture [12]. The results showed that ISI led to symptomatic improvement and less frequent dilation. Furthermore, no complications were encountered. However, Camargo et al. did not find an improvement in dilation frequency or dysphagia in 14 patients with corrosive strictures allocated to steroid injections [21]. A study that included 21 patients with strictures of various etiologies receiving preventive ED found an increase in dysphagia-free period and periodic dilation index, while no difference in required dilations [16]. So, for the difference across the studies, study design, kinds of etiology, and dose of steroid would be all potential factors that influenced the clinical outcomes.

The present meta-analysis of the high quality of RCTs only investigated the benign esophageal stricture of surgical and corrosive injuries, and the results showed that additional ITI was more helpful than ED alone for the management of the strictures, as it reduced the stricture rate and number of required ED sessions during follow-up. Subgroup analysis for etiology of surgery- or non-surgery-related strictures showed that ITI therapy seemed to achieve even better results for surgery-related strictures in all outcomes. Thus, it is supposed that when endoscopic ITI was applied with a conventional intention of ED, the outcomes of stricture control as well as patients' quality of life would be significantly improved. Regretfully, the meta-analysis indicated that the dysphagia-free time might not be prolonged, as the dysphagia-free time was determined by the time when a patient felt dysphagia and came to visit the surgeons. Meanwhile, dysphagia is a very subjective complaint, and the tolerance levels across patients may be very different. Thus, such negative results would be caused by the situations and by the insufficient test power of the relatively small sample size.

Obviously, there were no life-threatening or serious complications that occurred in patients undergoing quadrant injection. Additionally, our study did not find a significant difference in reported injection-related complications such as perforation, bleeding, mucosal laceration, and local infection. However, it was reported that ISI may increase the risk of candidal esophagitis [18]. Due to the rare incidence of complications, as well as our relatively small sample size, the current conclusion should be considered carefully, and high-risk patients need to be evaluated thoroughly in clinical practice.

The limitation of this meta-analysis included the small sample size of participants, which might be insufficient to achieve very strong results in aspects of dysphagia-free time and complications. There are also some differences in the included studies: (1) Even though both surgical and corrosive strictures were benign, without clear resolution of the mechanism they still might have possible differences in pathogenesis and pathophysiology, and this gave rise to different prognoses and heterogeneities, although subgroup analysis was performed with no significant statistical difference. (2) The detailed ITI procedure was not completely the same, and this might also influence the outcomes, although the interventions in each trial were comparable. (3) Both bougie dilation and balloon dilation were used to conduct the dilation, which may also partly influence the treatment efficacy, which could be difficult to avoid in the follow-up periods after more than six months.

5. Conclusions

Additional ITI therapy was supposed to be effective and safe for the management of benign esophageal strictures as it reduced the stricture rate and required ED sessions. However, the relatively small sample size of participants was included especially in the evaluation of safety, and larger-scale RCTs are still needed to support the findings.

Abbreviations

ITI: Intralesional triamcinolone injection
ISI: Intralesional steroid injection
ED: Endoscopic dilation
RCTs: Randomized control trials
SMD: Standard mean difference
MD: Mean difference.

Acknowledgments

The research is supported by the Cuiying Graduate Supervisor Applicant Training Program of Lanzhou University Second Hospital, the Natural Science Foundation of Gansu Province (no. 1606RJZA152) and Lanzhou University Second Hospital Research Grant no. YJZY2013-02.

References

[1] J. H. Kim, J. H. Shin, and H. Y. Song, "Benign strictures of the esophagus and gastric outlet: interventional management," *Korean Journal of Radiology*, vol. 11, no. 5, pp. 497–506, 2010.

[2] P. D. Siersema and L. R. H. de Wijkerslooth, "Dilation of refractory benign esophageal strictures," *Gastrointestinal Endoscopy*, vol. 70, no. 5, pp. 1000–1012, 2009.

[3] S. Hashimoto, M. Kobayashi, M. Takeuchi, Y. Sato, R. Narisawa, and Y. Aoyagi, "The efficacy of endoscopic triamcinolone injection for the prevention of esophageal stricture after endoscopic submucosal dissection," *Gastrointestinal Endoscopy*, vol. 74, no. 6, pp. 1389–1393, 2011.

[4] N. Hanaoka, R. Ishihara, Y. Takeuchi et al., "Intralesional steroid injection to prevent stricture after endoscopic submucosal dissection for esophageal cancer: a controlled prospective study," *Endoscopy*, vol. 44, no. 11, pp. 1007–1011, 2012.

[5] S. Kottewar, S. Siddique, R. M. Uhlich et al., "Sa1543 intra-lesional steroid injections in the treatment of benign recurrent esophageal strictures: a meta-analysis," *Gastrointestinal Endoscopy*, vol. 79, no. 5, article AB250, 2014.

[6] A. Repici, M. Conio, C. de Angelis et al., "Temporary placement of an expandable polyester silicone-covered stent for treatment of refractory benign esophageal strictures," *Gastrointestinal Endoscopy*, vol. 60, no. 4, pp. 513–519, 2004.

[7] P. D. Siersema, "Treatment options for esophageal strictures," *Nature Clinical Practice. Gastroenterology & Hepatology*, vol. 5, no. 3, pp. 142–152, 2008.

[8] J. C. Pereira-Lima, R. P. Ramires, I. Zamin, A. P. Cassal, C. A. Marroni, and A. A. Mattos, "Endoscopic dilation of benign esophageal strictures: report on 1043 procedures," *The American Journal of Gastroenterology*, vol. 94, no. 6, pp. 1497–1501, 1999.

[9] D. D. Ferguson, "Evaluation and management of benign esophageal strictures," *Diseases of the Esophagus*, vol. 18, no. 6, pp. 359–364, 2005.

[10] L. D. Ketchum, J. Smith, D. W. Robinson, and F. W. Masters, "The treatment of hypertrophic scar, keloid and scar contracture by triamcinolone acetonide," *Plastic and Reconstructive Surgery*, vol. 38, no. 3, pp. 209–218, 1966.

[11] B. H. Griffith, "The treatment of keloids with triamcinolone acetonide," *Plastic and Reconstructive Surgery*, vol. 38, no. 3, pp. 202–208, 1966.

[12] M. Lee, C. M. Kubik, C. D. Polhamus, C. E. Brady III, and S. C. Kadakia, "Preliminary experience with endoscopic intralesional steroid injection therapy for refractory upper gastrointestinal strictures," *Gastrointestinal Endoscopy*, vol. 41, no. 6, pp. 598–601, 1995.

[13] R. Kochhar and G. K. Makharia, "Usefulness of intralesional triamcinolone in treatment of benign esophageal strictures," *Gastrointestinal Endoscopy*, vol. 56, no. 6, pp. 829–834, 2002.

[14] A. Yeri, C. Christin, and O. Ravinder, "Efficacy of intralesional triamcinolone injections for benign refractory oesophageal strictures at Counties Manukau Health, New Zealand," *New Zealand Medical Journal*, vol. 128, no. 1416, pp. 44–50, 2015.

[15] J. P. T. Higgins and S. Green, *Cochrane Handbook for Systematic Reviews of Interventions Version 5.1.0 (Updated March 2011)*, The Cochrane Collaboration, 2011, http://www.cochrane-handbook.org.

[16] H. Takahashi, Y. Arimura, S. Okahara et al., "A randomized controlled trial of endoscopic steroid injection for prophylaxis of esophageal stenoses after extensive endoscopic submucosal dissection," *BMC Gastroenterology*, vol. 15, no. 1, p. 1, 2015.

[17] E. Altintas, S. Kacar, B. Tunc et al., "Intralesional steroid injection in benign esophageal strictures resistant to bougie dilation," *Journal of Gastroenterology and Hepatology*, vol. 19, no. 12, pp. 1388–1391, 2004.

[18] J. I. Ramage, A. Rumalla, T. H. Baron et al., "A prospective, randomized, double-blind, placebo-controlled trial of endoscopic steroid injection therapy for recalcitrant esophageal peptic strictures," *The American Journal of Gastroenterology*, vol. 100, no. 11, pp. 2419–2425, 2005.

[19] M. M. C. Hirdes, J. E. van Hooft, J. J. Koornstra et al., "Endoscopic corticosteroid injections do not reduce dysphagia after endoscopic dilation therapy in patients with benign esophagogastric anastomotic strictures," *Clinical Gastroenterology and Hepatology*, vol. 11, no. 7, pp. 795–801.e1, 2013.

[20] J. C. Pereira-Lima, M. Lemos Bonotto, G. D. Hahn et al., "A prospective randomized trial of intralesional triamcinolone injections after endoscopic dilation for complex esophagogastric anastomotic strictures," *Surgical Endoscopy*, vol. 29, no. 5, pp. 1156–1160, 2015.

[21] M. A. Camargo, L. R. Lopes, T. A. G. Grangeia, N. A. Andreollo, and N. A. Brandalise, "Use of corticosteroids after esophageal dilations on patients with corrosive stenosis: prospective, randomized and double-blind study," *Revista da Associação Médica Brasileira*, vol. 49, no. 3, pp. 286–292, 2003.

[22] A. Schoepfer, "Treatment of eosinophilic esophagitis by dilation," *Digestive Diseases*, vol. 32, no. 1-2, pp. 130–133, 2014.

[23] J. Alex Haller Jr., H. Gibbs Andrews, J. J. White, M. Akram Tamer, and W. W. Cleveland, "Pathophysiology and management of acute corrosive burns of the esophagus: results of treatment in 285 children," *Journal of Pediatric Surgery*, vol. 6, no. 5, pp. 578–584, 1971.

[24] J. A. O'neill, J. Betts, M. M. Ziegler, L. Schnaufer, H. C. Bishop, and J. M. Templeton, "Surgical management of reflux strictures of the esophagus in childhood," *Annals of Surgery*, vol. 196, no. 4, pp. 453–460, 1982.

[25] K. W. Ashcraft and T. M. Holder, "The experimental treatment of esophageal strictures by intralesional steroid injections," *The Journal of Thoracic and Cardiovascular Surgery*, vol. 58, pp. 685–691, 1969.

[26] T. M. Holder, K. W. Ashcraft, and L. Leape, "The treatment of patients with esophageal strictures by local steroid injections," *Journal of Pediatric Surgery*, vol. 4, no. 6, pp. 646–653, 1969.

20

Oral Health Impact Profile in Celiac Patients: Analysis of Recent Findings

Gabriele Cervino,[1] Luca Fiorillo,[1] Luigi Laino,[2] Alan Scott Herford,[3] Floriana Lauritano,[1] Giuseppe Lo Giudice,[1] Fausto Famà,[4] Rossella Santoro,[2] Giuseppe Troiano,[5] Gaetano Iannello,[1] and Marco Cicciù[1]

[1]*Department of Biomedical and Dental Sciences and Morphological and Functional Imaging, Messina University, 98100 Messina, Italy*
[2]*Multidisciplinary Department of Medical-Surgical and Odontostomatological Specialties, University of Campania "Luigi Vanvitelli", 80121 Naples, Italy*
[3]*Department of Maxillofacial Surgery, Loma Linda University, Loma Linda, CA 92354, USA*
[4]*Department of Human Pathology, University of Messina, 98100 Messina, Italy*
[5]*Departments of Clinical and Experimental Medicine, University of Foggia, 71121 Foggia, Italy*

Correspondence should be addressed to Marco Cicciù; mcicciu@unime.it

Academic Editor: Chiara Ricci

The increment of recording atypical oral manifestation in young patients often related to systematic disease is today a challenge for the therapists. Sometime, the presence of tooth enamel lesions correlated with soft tissue lesions is just a symptom or a trigger sign for a deeper and undetermined disease. Recently, high impact has been developed toward the influence of the diet as a controlled and modifiable factor in patients affected by celiac pathologies. The celiac disease (CD) is a chronic immune-mediated disorder triggered by the ingestion of gluten that appears in genetically predisposed patients. Gluten is a proline-rich and glutamine-rich protein present in wheat (gliadin), barley (hordein), and rye (secalin). The gluten-free diet (GFD) seems to better influence the oral health status of the CD patients. For this reason, the main objective of this revision was to analyze the international data highlighting the relationship between celiac patients and the oral health impact profile. A comprehensive review of the current literature was conducted according to the PRISMA guidelines by accessing the NCBI PubMed database. Authors conducted the search of articles in the English language published from 2008 to 2018. The first analysis with filters recorded 67 manuscripts accordingly with the selected keywords. Finally, a number of 16 appropriate published papers were comprehended in the review. The studies were different in terms of the structure, findings, outcomes, and diet quality evaluation, and for this reason, it was not possible to accomplish a meta-analysis of the recorded data. This manuscript offers some observational evidence to justify the advantages of gluten-free diets related to a better oral health status in the patients involved.

1. Introduction

Oral health is today considered one of the fundamental parameters related to the patient's general health and behavior. Oral health status allows individuals to run their daily activities (mastication, articulation, and socialization) without any pain, discomfort, and restriction. The patients' quality of life (QoL) is a caption currently applied in the medicine field to refer to social well-being and the effects of therapy on cancer patients. Specifically, in the dental practice, QoL, as it connected to the oral health, has only been recently employed [1–7].

The patients' general health condition is related to having no problems or diseases on all the anatomical structures, even involving the oral cavity functions or aesthetics. Today, great attention is focused on the prevention and maintenance of high standard of oral hygiene and control; however, some pathologies may be connected with systemic disease and not affect the oral cavity structures directly [3, 7–10].

Nowadays, even the current standard of performing diagnosis in oral lesions like teeth enamel defects or soft tissues and tongue lesions may be related to local affection or trauma; a deep knowledge of the patient anamnesis and clinical history is required in order to evaluate possible hidden causes strictly related to the diet or general health status. Therefore, it is well documented how many systemic diseases are somehow related to many oral manifestations and influence the individual quality of life [4, 9, 11–13].

Celiac disease (CD) is a long-term autoimmune disorder that affects the small intestine; this is caused by a constant intolerance to gluten proteins in genetically susceptible individuals. CD is caused by a reaction to gliadins and glutenins found in wheat. These protein-based factors may be responsible for a toxic event on the intestinal mucosa in genetically receptive subjects by triggering an immune-mediated reaction, related to the common villous atrophy and lymphocyte infiltrate in the small intestine mucosa recorded in CD. Common oral and dental manifestations of CD include mouth ulcers, in particular, recurrent aphthous ulcers, and dental enamel defects [13–16].

However, even if great important steps have been done in the field of quick diagnosis, CD is still not promptly diagnosed, because recently, the typical form of CD, characterized by modified absorption and gastrointestinal signs, is less recurrent compared with the atypical forms, often asymptomatic and involving extraintestinal clinical manifestations. A multidisciplinary evaluation and approach between clinicians, pediatricians, and gastroenterologists should be performed in order to underline all the extraintestinal possible manifestations of CD and to make an early diagnosis; recurrent aphthous ulcers, previously mentioned, could provide another clue to the possible presence of this disorder [17–20].

Numerous published papers underlined how specific oral signs and symptoms can be classified as risk factor signals for CD; however, only the internal specialist can perform the diagnosis, evaluate the presence of specific celiac antibodies, and demonstrate intestinal mucosa damages. However, the topic is still debated, and currently, the right frequency of these oral manifestations in potential celiac patients has not yet been classified and recorded [21–23].

However, it is widely recognized that, among these atypical signs of CD, there are certain oral manifestations which are surely interwoven to CD: tooth enamel lesions and defects, frequent aphthous stomatitis, delayed tooth eruption, multiple caries, angular cheilitis, atrophic glossitis, dry mouth, and burning tongue. For this reason, dentists and the first dental visits play a fundamental role in detecting symptoms related to CD and for the next medical treatments [23, 24].

About the treatments and the prevention of such oral manifestations, recently published investigations underlined how the gluten-free diet may favor an improvement of the general health condition of celiac and no celiac patients. Moreover, numerous epidemiological and clinical studies recorded a decrease of oral CD manifestations connected with the gluten-free diet of the involved patients [25–33].

The aim of the present revision is to examine the data of the last ten years' literature about oral manifestations of celiac disease and how gluten-free diet may definitely influence the conditions of the oral health patients.

2. Methods of Screening

2.1. Protocol Development and Online Information Recording. The inclusion parameters for the current research were collected in a protocol and then submitted in advance and documented in CRD York website PROSPERO, a global prospective catalogue of revision manuscripts. The criteria and the formal structure of the present revision can be searched online with the CRD id and code: application number: CRD 92075.

The documents collected in the present paper followed the Preferred Reporting Items for Systematic Review and Meta-analysis (PRISMA) statement accordingly [34, 35].

2.2. Outcome Query. The following question was sentenced and structured according to the (PICO) study design:

(i) How can the celiac disease influence the oral health status of the patients?

2.3. Searches. The PubMed-Medline resource database was applied through advanced researches. The keywords and search inquiries used during the primary stage were as follows: "oral health gluten-free diet." Additional manually selected articles were included regarding the eligibility criteria. Figure 1 represents the flow diagram of the selected studies according to PRISMA guidelines and following the criteria for the investigated paper choice. Web searching and researches by hand were then executed in the field of gastroenterology, dentistry, and medicine journals, finding different international journals. The search was restricted to English language manuscripts.

2.4. Data Recorded from the Selected Manuscripts. The Medical Subject Headings (MeSH) was used for finding the keywords used in the present revision. The selected keywords ("oral health"[MeSH Terms] OR ("oral"[All Fields] AND "health"[All Fields]) OR "oral health"[All Fields]) AND ("glutens"[MeSH Terms] OR "glutens"[All Fields] OR "gluten"[All Fields]) AND ("celiac"[MeSH Terms] OR "diet"[All Fields]) were written in the selected database.

2.5. Selections of the Papers. Three separate researchers, of three Italian universities (Messina, Foggia, and Naples Universities), singularly screened the full-text manuscripts for deciding inclusion and exclusion criteria. Reviewers compared decisions about criteria, parameters, and selected papers. During the step of reviewing the manuscripts, a complete independent two-fold revision was undertaken.

Reviewers compared their results and data. A fourth qualified chief reviewer (Loma Linda University) was then contacted when agreement could not be obtained at the first step of paper revisions.

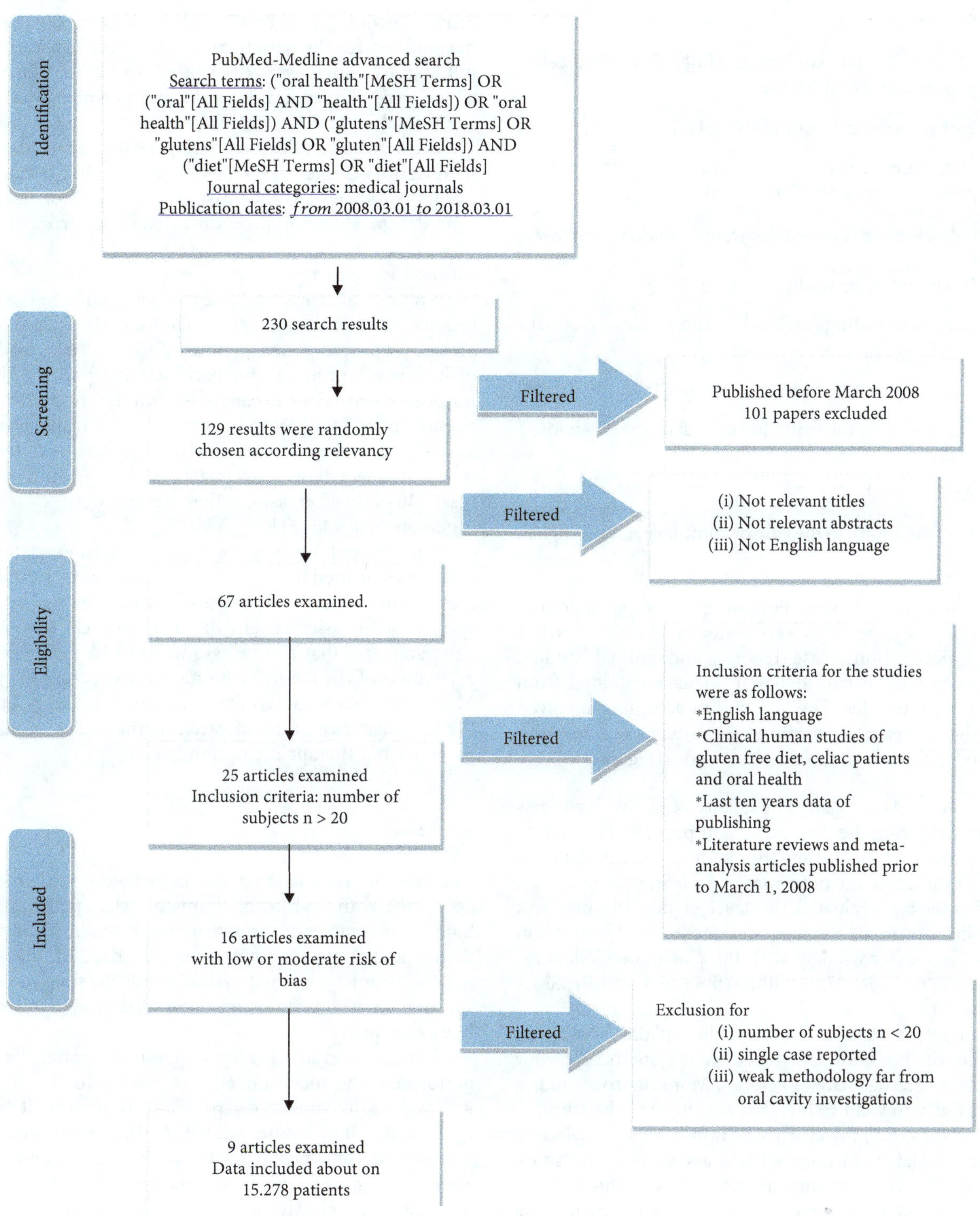

FIGURE 1: PRISMA flow chart diagram, including all the screening methodology, and revision progresses.

The papers recorded in the present revision highlighted clinical researches over celiac patients printed in the English style. Letters, editorials, case reports, animal studies and degrees, and PhD thesis were not included in the revision process.

2.6. Studies Involved in the Revision. The design of recording data involved all human prospective and retrospective clinical studies, split-mouth cohort studies, case–control papers, and case series manuscripts, published between March 2008 and March 2018, about gluten-free diet, oral disease, and celiac patients.

2.7. Exclusion and Inclusion Criteria. The applied inclusion criteria for the studies were as follows:

(i) English language

(ii) Clinical human studies of gluten-free diet, celiac patients, and oral health

(iii) Last ten year data of publishing

(iv) Literature reviews and meta-analysis articles published prior to March 1, 2008

The following types of articles were excluded as follows:

(i) In vivo/in vitro studies

(ii) Studies of testing medication and/or new treatment methodologies

(iii) Studies of cancer in locations other than mentioned

(iv) Studies not relevant to our selected diagnostic methods

(v) Animal studies

(vi) No availability to the title or summary not in English words

2.8. Data Recording Design. Following the initial literature screening, all the paper titles were evaluated in order to delete irrelevant publications, case reports, and animal studies. Then studies were excluded based on data obtained from reading the summaries. The last step of screening involved reading the full texts to determine each study's selection following the inclusion and exclusion criteria. (Figure 1).

2.9. Risk of Bias Assessment. The quality of all involved texts was assessed during the data extraction process. The quality appraisal involved evaluating the methodological elements that might influence the outcomes of each study.

Each reviewer evaluated the level of possible bias risk during the information taking out method. This revision work was made accordingly with the Cochrane Collaboration's double tool for determining risk of bias and PRISMA rules [34, 35].

Differences in risks of bias can help explain variation in the results of the studies included in a systematic review (i.e., explain heterogeneity of results). More rigorous studies are more likely to yield results that are closer to the truth.

Risk of bias (e.g., the absence of information or selective reports on variables of interest) was assessed on the study level. The risks were indicated as lack of precise information of interest related to the keywords selected. Finally, the researches selected for the revision were then recorded in modest, moderate, significant, and unclear risk.

3. Outcomes

3.1. Paper Recording and Possible Bias. The PRISMA flow diagram describes the revision steps for screening the papers and reaching the selected ones (Figure 1). The initial web and hand searches performed on PubMed-Medline and Oral Sciences Source produced a number of 230 findings. 101 references were not involved in the revision because they were printed before March 1, 2008. Then another 62 papers were not selected for the data because they were not available on full text. 67 papers were discovered on full-text form, 25 of which were merged in this work, and then after final screening, a total of 9 full-text papers.

During the last deep screening section, from the last 16 manuscripts, some researches were excluded because they were recorded as a unique case report ($n = 2$) or not significant design study or procedures were far from the topic ($n = 5$). So finally, 9 papers were recorded and screened in this revision paper.

No meta-analyses could be performed due to the heterogeneity between the studies (different study designs, control groups, and observation periods) Table 1. The possible risk of bias was considered for each selected papers. The final number of the selected papers was limited from 25 full-text papers to 9. The inclusion criteria were really restrictive, and for this reason also, the risk of bias was low. Ten types of research were evaluated as having minor risk of bias [36–44] whereas another seven were classified as moderate risk [45–51].

The present investigation of the data extracted from researches printed in English only could detect a publication bias. About possible bias, some of the selected papers did not specify the inclusion criteria of the patient selection. Another key parameter that can be assumed as bias is related to the evaluation of the clinical condition for selecting the patient. Moreover, data recorded from the eight studies pointed out the heterogeneity of the research methods, selections of the patients, and therapeutic options.

4. Results

The present systematic review discovered gluten-free diet is associated with oral health status of celiac patients. Due to high heterogeneity of the researches, it was not realizable to do meta-analysis for comparing the data of the selected papers. Due to poor material, it is not possible to establish specific oral health status related to diet or systemic diseases like celiac patients.

Moreover, even wide screening and research have been performed; the inclusion criteria related to the "oral cavity" was really inclusive, and for this reason, it was not possible to state some guidelines that may significantly increase the oral health status of the CD patients just by applying a gluten-free diet. Some papers with low risk of bias [36–44] clearly analyzed the correlation between gluten-free diet and oral health status of celiac patients. However, the data of those researches are not significant and finally suggested some recommendations and not guidelines. Specifically, because the disease involves the gastrointestinal area, the high part of the researches firstly investigated the microbiota related to the anatomical area far from the oral cavity area. Therefore, all the data extracted from the present revision clearly underlined how a diet associated with no gluten may favor high standard of oral health quality delaying gingival oral disease due to the alteration of the oral microbiota.

TABLE 1: CD and OH parameters recorded in the studies with low risk of bias (CD = celiac disease, PD = parodontal disease, OH = oral health, DDE = developmental defects of enamel, DED = dental enamel defects, and AGA = antigliadin antibodies).

References	Year	Author	Subjects (n)	Type of correlation	Result	Statistic
[36]	2018	Spinell et al.	6661	PD and CD	There is no significant correlation between PD and CD.	$P = 0.67$
[37]	2017	van Gils et al.	5522	CD and xerostomia; CD and OH	OHIP-14 and XI tests were performed.	$P < 0.001$ for both
[38]	2013	Rivera et al.	20	CD and enamel hypoplasia; CD and aphthous ulcers; CD and delayed eruption	Oral manifestations. In the long list of clinical signs and symptoms that have been found significantly associated with CD are oral manifestations such as dental enamel hypoplasia, aphthous ulcers, and delayed eruption of teeth.	Reported as significant values, insufficient extrapolated statistical data
[39]	2013	Shteyer et al.	90	CD and enamel defects; CD and aphthous stomatitis, DMFT	A high prevalence of enamel hypoplasia (66%) was found in children with CD. Plaque index was significantly lower in the celiac-treated group.	$P < 0.05$
[40]	2012	Mina et al.	25	CD and OH, enamel alteration	DMFT, enamel alterations, gingival index, and oral hygiene were evaluated in this study.	$P < 0.0001$
[41]	2010	Tsami et al.	35	CD and OH	The periodontal treatment need of children and adolescents with CD was high, most of them needed treatment for gingivitis (60.01%), and only a few subjects had a healthy periodontium (34.29%).	$P < 0.05$
[42]	2018	Souto-Souza et al.	2840	CD and OH; CD and enamel alterations	This meta-analysis indicated a high prevalence of DDE among celiac patients with a significant association of DDE with this population when compared to healthy people.	$P = 0.014$
[43]	2016	Sóñora et al.	21	CD and enamel defects	These results strongly suggest a pathological role for antibodies to gliadin in enamel defect dentition for both deciduous and permanent teeth.	Insufficient extrapolated statistical data
[44]	2012	Muñoz et al.	64	CD and enamel defects	This work describes structural similarities between gliadins and proline-rich enamel proteins and shows that potential cross-reactions of AGA could take place during amelogenesis in untreated patients. Further work is underway to study the biological effects of AGA on enamel formation to evaluate their putative role in the pathogenesis of DED in untreated CD.	$P = 0.045$

4.1. Oral Soft Tissue Manifestations. Oral soft tissue manifestations in CD-affected patients are reported in literature. Oral manifestations that interest gums such as aphthous ulcers or recurrent aphthosis are correlated to celiac disease-affected patients. These manifestations are more frequent in CD patients than in normal population [38, 39].

4.2. Dental Manifestations. Dental hard tissue manifestations in CD patients are various; we can find alterations on the enamel and teeth structure. Some studies report enamel hypoplasia, enamel defect or enamel and dental structure alterations [38–40, 42–44], this condition puts CD patients in condition of discomfort, lowering their general conditions of oral health and expelling them to other debilitating diseases.

4.3. Oral Health. Another series of oral manifestations is present in CD patients which does not affect soft tissue or the dental structure. Some studies evaluated the oral health of patients through self-administered tests like the OHIP-14 test (Oral Health Impact Profile 14) or XI test (Xerostomia inventory). Studies reported abnormalities in general oral health like DMFT index (Decayed, Missing, Filled Teeth); some other studies reported anomalies like delayed eruption and parodontal disease [36–42].

5. Discussion

The purpose of this review was to systematically overview published studies restricted to oral health and gluten-free diet in order to evaluate how a diet without gluten may influence the oral health status of celiac patients, following the brief report of the 16 papers classified with moderate and low risks of bias.

Spinell et al. [36] recently investigated whether celiac disease was associated with periodontitis or periodontal diseases among a population of US adult patients. In this large research, the National Health and Nutrition Examination Survey (NHANES) authors between 2009 and 2012 enrolled about 6661 subjects with full-mouth periodontal examination and serological testing for antitissue transglutaminase (tTg) and antiendomysial (EMA) antibodies. CD was defined as (i) self-reported physician diagnosis while on a gluten-free diet or (ii) tTg levels > 10.0 U/ml and positive EMA results. Positive serology without self-reported diagnosis was defined as undiagnosed CD (UdxCD). Authors concluded how CD is associated with modestly lower levels of mean periodontal disease but was not associated with periodontitis in a significant way. Larger studies are necessary to enhance precision and strengthen conclusions.

The oral health status and the xerostomia of celiac patients were investigated by van Gils et al. [37] in a study involving a population of about 740 patients with CD and 270 comparison participants. The Oral Health Impact Profile 14 (OHIP-14) and Xerostomia Inventory (XI) were screened and recorded. This study showed that oral health problems are more commonly experienced in adult patients with CD than in the comparison group. Collaboration between dentists and gastroenterologists is recommended to increase detection of undiagnosed CD.

De Angelis et al. [45] analyzed how the oral and intestinal bacteria metabolize dietary components, affecting human health by producing harmful or beneficial metabolites, which are involved in the incidence and progression of several intestinal-related and nonrelated diseases. Moreover, the authors stated how dietary regimens with fibers are the most effective to benefit the metabolism profile, and a profitable use of diet is fundamental in order to provide benefits to human health, both directly and indirectly, through the activity of the gut microbiota.

In a different revision paper, Cenit et al. [46] evaluated how in mature normal subjects, the GFD is connected with a low intake of complex polysaccharides caused shifts in the gut microbiota structure. Therefore, the authors concluded that microbiota imbalances have been recorded not only in untreated CD subjects but also in patients following a GFD. Moreover, typical bacterial strains isolated from subjects with active and nonactive CD have been shown to increase virulence features. These alterations may be significant for increasing CD pathogenesis by contributing to the disease onset.

Galipeau and Verdu [47] recorded significant findings in their review underlining and effective evidence between intestinal dysbiosis and CD; however, the main limit of the present investigation was related to the analysis of the manuscripts classified in the revision. It was determined evidence demonstrating causality is lacking. Therefore, it remains unclear whether general changes in microbial composition or the presence or absence of particular members of the microbiota play a direct role in CD pathogenesis, and so the diet is not fundamental in the CD developments.

Rivera et al. [38] in their research studied how CD continues to be an unsolved puzzle and a much-debated topic in the recent literature. Knowing the important health implications that CD can have, not only in an individual's health but also in the overall quality of life of these individuals and their families, is of vital importance. As clinicians, it is very important to be aware of the potential presentations, especially in terms of oral health, that CD can have and the consequences it can lead to in overall health status. When suspected, it is extremely important to refer the patient to a gastroenterologist for further evaluation, diagnosis, and, in the case of a positive work up, initiation of treatment with a GFD.

Shteyer et al. [39] made an interesting report studying the oral health status and quality in relation to GFD in children with CD. The results showed that newly diagnosed children with CD have more dental plaque and caries than the control groups, and children receiving GFD had lower dental plaque and better oral hygiene. These results should raise pediatric gastroenterologists' awareness toward oral health–related issues in children with CD. However, the data of the present investigation were not clear if the enamel defects were genetic or due to the low oral health conditions of the CD patients.

Mina et al. [40] in their study highlighted the main difference among CD children who did or did not comply with a gluten-free diet and control children are the presence of

Table 2: Selected papers in which there is a direct correlation between CD and oral health alterations or disease.

References	Author and year	Subjects (n)	Oral health status and symptoms
[36]	Spinell et al. 2018	6661	Periodontitis
[37]	van Gils et al. 2017	5522	Periodontitis and xerostomia
[38]	Rivera et al. 2013	/	Enamel hypoplasia; aphthous ulcers, delayed dental eruption
[39]	Shteyer et al. 2013	90	Enamel defects; aphthous stomatitis
[42]	Souto-Souza et al. 2018	2840	Enamel alterations
[43]	Sóñora et al. 2016	21	Enamel defects
[44]	Muñoz et al. 2012	64	Enamel defects

PMNs in the oral mucosa and protein salivary patterns; these findings could be considered as markers for CD, in conjunction with other signs and symptoms. The GFD seems to improve the oral health quality reducing the gingival inflammation.

Tsami et al. [41] inspected the factors that influence the oral hygiene and the periodontal treatment needs of children and adolescents with celiac disease (CD). It was found that the periodontal treatment need of children and adolescents with CD correlated with factors that related to the presence of a second medical condition and to the personal oral hygiene habits. CD seems to not have significant influence on the oral health status of the CD adolescents. Additionally, the oral hygiene level and periodontal status of children with CD do not have any specific characteristics, but they have similarities to the oral hygiene level and periodontal status of the children of the general population.

da Silva et al. [48] made a brief review of the literature about CD and analyzed a clinical case, and for this reason, this paper was not included in the final 9 papers. However, the management of the case was typical. A 39-year-old woman reported the presence of many symptoms. She also noted the appearance of symptomatic lesions in the mouth. These lesions had a mean duration of a month and occurred in any region of the oral mucosa, particularly on the tongue. Topical treatment was instituted for the oral lesions with immediate relief of the symptoms. The diagnosis of celiac disease was established by means of a medical clinical exam. A multidisciplinary approach and management with the involvement of a gastroenterologist and other health professionals, such as dentists, are important for diagnosing the disease and guiding the patient with celiac disease to achieve a good quality of life.

Francavilla et al. [49], thanks to advances in understanding the immunopathogenesis of CD, have proposed different kinds of treatment options alternative to the GFD. Some of these therapies try to decrease the immunogenicity of gluten-containing grains by modifying the grain itself or by applying oral enzymes to break down immunogenic peptides that usually remain intact during digestion.

Bascuñán et al. [50] evaluated how the only effective and safe treatment of celiac disease continues being the so-called gluten-free diet (GFD). Although GFD poses difficulties to patients in family, social, and working contexts, deteriorating his/her quality of life. The diet must be not only free of gluten but also healthy to avoid nutrient, vitamins, and mineral deficiencies or excess. Overweight/obesity frequency has increased. Authors concluded how nutritional education by a trained nutritionist is of great relevance to achieving long-term satisfactory health status and good compliance.

Theethira and Dennis [51] underlined how it is important to have regular follow-up visits and lab work to detect and treat nutritional deficiencies after initiation of the GFD. Indisputably, the GFD is the cornerstone of treatment for CD. Keeping these nutritional concerns in mind, a patient with CD can enjoy a healthy, well-rounded diet that improves and maximizes overall health and well-being.

Souto-Souza et al. [42] investigated the relationship between developmental defects of enamel and celiac disease. In their meta-analysis, it was observed how subjects with CD had a significantly higher prevalence of enamel defects matched with healthy people. The most important findings of this paper are that only developmental defects of enamel diagnosed using Aine's method were strictly related to CD. In a sensitivity analysis involving the deciduous, mixed, and permanent dentitions, only individuals with deciduous dentition were observed to have association with the disease. Then patients with enamel developmental defects should be screened for the possibility of having celiac disease.

Sóñora et al. [43], based on previously reported cross-reactivity of antibodies to gliadin with the enamel proteins, amelogenin and ameloblastin, investigated the ability of anti-gliadin IgG to recognize enamel organ structures. Strong staining of the enamel matrix and of the layer of ameloblasts was observed with serum samples from women with celiac disease. The results strongly advise a pathological position for antibodies to gliadin in enamel defect dentition for both deciduous and permanent teeth, considering that IgG can be transported through the placenta during fetal tooth development. Muñoz et al. [44] in their research classified the pathogenesis of enamel anomalies in permanent teeth of subjects affected by CD. The studies using ELISA and western blotting, for reactivity of sera from patients with CD against gliadin and peptides obtained from enamel, confirm that the antibodies against gliadin generated in patients with CD can react in vitro with an important enamel protein. The involvement of antigliadin serum in the pathogenesis of enamel defects in children with untreated CD can be hypothesized on the basis of these new results (Table 2).

Hypoplasia of the enamel, xerostomia, and oral gingival lesions are the most common symptoms reflected in the recorded manuscripts. The tooth enamel defects can be a clinical sign that can be useful for performing quick diagnosis of CD, but the defect can be managed only by dental conservative treatment, and a GFD cannot modify these clinical conditions. After all, xerostomia and oral ulcers and gingival lesions, other clinical signs of CD disease, can be topically treated by dental care, but in those case, a GFD diet seems to favor an increase of the oral health status of the CD patients.

6. Conclusions

Reading the selected papers, it is possible to screen about 15,000 CD patients. Even if this number is large, at the same time, it is not significative and representative, because the studies presented high heterogeneity criteria and methods for evaluations.

Authors' Contributions

GC is the author responsible for the paper writing. ASH is the chief reviewer for collecting data, and he is the native English speaker for the language proof and revision. LF, FF, and FL were responsible for collecting data and tables. GLG and GI were responsible for funding acquisition data. GT, RS, and LL were responsible for editing, original data, and text preparation. MC was responsible for the supervision.

References

[1] R. Nenna, C. Tiberti, L. Petrarca et al., "The celiac iceberg: characterization of the disease in primary schoolchildren," *Journal of Pediatric Gastroenterology and Nutrition*, vol. 56, no. 4, pp. 416–421, 2013.

[2] C. Catassi, I. M. Ratsch, E. Fabiani et al., "Coeliac disease in the year 2000: exploring the iceberg," *The Lancet*, vol. 343, no. 8891, pp. 200–203, 1994.

[3] P. Mariani, M. G. Viti, M. Montouri et al., "The gluten-free diet: a nutritional risk factor for adolescents with celiac disease?," *Journal of Pediatric Gastroenterology and Nutrition*, vol. 27, no. 5, pp. 519–523, 1998.

[4] K. Rostami, D. Aldulaimi, and M. Rostami-Nejad, "Gluten free diet is a cure not a poison!," *Gastroenterology and Hepatology from bed to bench*, vol. 8, no. 2, pp. 93-94, 2015.

[5] F. Germano, E. Bramanti, C. Arcuri, F. Cecchetti, and M. Cicciù, "Atomic force microscopy of bacteria from periodontal subgingival biofilm: Preliminary study results," *European Journal of Dentistry*, vol. 7, no. 2, pp. 152–158, 2013.

[6] S. Husby, S. Koletzko, I. R. Korponay-Szabó et al., "European Society for Pediatric Gastroenterology, Hepatology, and Nutrition guidelines for the diagnosis of coeliac disease," *Journal of Pediatric Gastroenterology and Nutrition*, vol. 54, no. 4, pp. 572-573, 2012.

[7] A. Fasano and C. Catassi, "Current approaches to diagnosis and treatment of celiac disease: an evolving spectrum," *Gastroenterology*, vol. 120, no. 3, pp. 636–651, 2001.

[8] P. H. Green and B. Jabri, "Coeliac disease," *Lancet*, vol. 362, no. 9381, pp. 383–391, 2003.

[9] W. J. Maloney, G. Raymond, D. Hershkowitz, and G. Rochlen, "Oral and dental manifestations of celiac disease," *The New York State Dental Journal*, vol. 80, no. 4, pp. 45–48, 2014.

[10] G. Campisi, C. di Liberto, A. Carroccio et al., "Coeliac disease: oral ulcer prevalence, assessment of risk and association with gluten-free diet in children," *Digestive and Liver Disease*, vol. 40, no. 2, pp. 104–107, 2008.

[11] P. Bucci, F. Carile, A. Sangianantoni, F. D'Angiò, A. Santarelli, and L. Lo Muzio, "Oral aphthous ulcers and dental enamel defects in children with coeliac disease," *Acta Paediatrica*, vol. 95, no. 2, pp. 203–207, 2006.

[12] L. Trotta, F. Biagi, P. I. Bianchi et al., "Dental enamel defects in adult coeliac disease: prevalence and correlation with symptoms and age at diagnosis," *European Journal of Internal Medicine*, vol. 24, no. 8, pp. 832–834, 2013.

[13] K. Cantekin, D. Arslan, and E. Delikan, "Presence and distribution of dental enamel defects, recurrent aphthous lesions and dental caries in children with celiac disease," *Pakistan Journal of Medical Sciences*, vol. 31, no. 3, pp. 606–609, 2015.

[14] M. A.-A. El-Hodhod, I. A. El-Agouza, H. Abdel-Al, N. S. Kabil, and K. A. E.-M. Bayomi, "Screening for celiac disease in children with dental enamel defects," *ISRN Pediatrics*, vol. 2012, Article ID 763783, 7 pages, 2012.

[15] M. Bossù, A. Bartoli, G. Orsini, E. Luppino, and A. Polimeni, "Enamel hypoplasia in coeliac children: a potential clinical marker of early diagnosis," *European Journal of Paediatric Dentistry*, vol. 8, no. 1, pp. 31–37, 2007.

[16] I. D. Hill, M. H. Dirks, G. S. Liptak et al., "Guideline for the diagnosis and treatment of celiac disease in children: recommendations of the North American Society for Pediatric Gastroenterology, Hepatology and Nutrition," *Journal of Pediatric Gastroenterology and Nutrition*, vol. 40, no. 1, pp. 1–19, 2005.

[17] U. Krupa-Kozak, L. Markiewicz, G. Lamparski, and J. Juśkiewicz, "Administration of inulin-supplemented gluten-free diet modified calcium absorption and caecal microbiota in rats in a calcium-dependent manner," *Nutrients*, vol. 9, no. 7, p. 702, 2017.

[18] K. Rostami, J. Bold, A. Parr, and M. Johnson, "Gluten-free diet indications, safety, quality, labels, and challenges," *Nutrients*, vol. 9, no. 8, p. 846, 2017.

[19] A. Avşar and A. G. Kalayci, "The presence and distribution of dental enamel defects and caries in children with celiac disease," *Turkish Journal of Pediatrics*, vol. 50, no. 1, pp. 45–50, 2008.

[20] E. O. Páez, P. J. Lafuente, P. B. García, J. M. Lozano, and J. C. L. Calvo, "Prevalence of dental enamel defects in celiac patients with deciduous dentition: a pilot study," *Oral Surgery, Oral Medicine, Oral Pathology, Oral Radiology, and Endodontology*, vol. 106, no. 1, pp. 74–78, 2008.

[21] L. Elli, V. Rossi, D. Conte et al., "Increased mercury levels in patients with celiac disease following a gluten-free regimen," *Gastroenterology Research and Practice*, vol. 2015, Article ID 953042, 6 pages, 2015.

[22] C. L. A. A. R. D. WIERINK, D. E. van DIERMEN, I. H. A. AARTMAN, and H. S. A. HEYMANS, "Dental enamel defects in children with coeliac disease," *International Journal of Paediatric Dentistry*, vol. 17, no. 3, pp. 163–168, 2007.

[23] S. Acar, A. A. Yetkiner, N. Ersin, O. Oncag, S. Aydogdu, and C. Arikan, "Oral findings and salivary parameters in children

with celiac disease: a preliminary study," *Medical Principles and Practice*, vol. 21, no. 2, pp. 129–133, 2012.

[24] N. Tian, L. Faller, D. A. Leffler et al., "Salivary gluten degradation and oral microbial profiles in healthy individuals and celiac disease patients," *Applied and Environmental Microbiology*, vol. 83, no. 6, article e03330, p. 16, 2017.

[25] A. Quagliariello, I. Aloisio, N. Bozzi Cionci et al., "Effect of bifidobacterium breve on the intestinal microbiota of coeliac children on a gluten free diet: a pilot study," *Nutrients*, vol. 8, no. 10, p. 660, 2016.

[26] M. C. Cenit, Y. Sanz, and P. Codoñer-Franch, "Influence of gut microbiota on neuropsychiatric disorders," *World Journal of Gastroenterology*, vol. 23, no. 30, pp. 5486–5498, 2017.

[27] L. Elli, L. Roncoroni, and M. T. Bardella, "Non-celiac gluten sensitivity: time for sifting the grain," *World Journal of Gastroenterology*, vol. 21, no. 27, pp. 8221–8226, 2015.

[28] L. Elli, F. Branchi, C. Tomba et al., "Diagnosis of gluten related disorders: celiac disease, wheat allergy and non-celiac gluten sensitivity," *World Journal of Gastroenterology*, vol. 21, no. 23, pp. 7110–7119, 2015.

[29] F. Penagini, D. Dilillo, F. Meneghin, C. Mameli, V. Fabiano, and G. Zuccotti, "Gluten-free diet in children: an approach to a nutritionally adequate and balanced diet," *Nutrients*, vol. 5, no. 11, pp. 4553–4565, 2013.

[30] V. M. P. Macho, A. S. Coelho, D. M. Veloso e Silva, and D. J. C. . Andrade, "Oral manifestations in pediatric patients with coeliac disease—a review article," *The Open Dentistry Journal*, vol. 11, no. 1, pp. 539–545, 2017.

[31] E. Bramanti, M. Cicciù, G. Matacena, S. Costa, and G. Magazzù, "Clinical evaluation of specific oral manifestations in pediatric patients with ascertained versus potential coeliac disease: a cross-sectional study," *Gastroenterology Research and Practice*, vol. 2014, Article ID 934159, 9 pages, 2014.

[32] M. Moreno, A. Rodríguez-Herrera, C. Sousa, and I. Comino, "Biomarkers to monitor gluten-free diet compliance in celiac patients," *Nutrients*, vol. 9, no. 1, p. 46, 2017.

[33] L. Elli, V. Discepolo, M. T. Bardella, and S. Guandalini, "Does gluten intake influence the development of celiac disease-associated complications?," *Journal of Clinical Gastroenterology*, vol. 48, no. 1, pp. 13–20, 2014.

[34] D. Moher, A. Liberati, J. Tetzlaff, D. G. Altman, and The PRISMA Group, "Preferred reporting items for systematic reviews and meta-analyses: the PRISMA statement," *PLoS Medicine*, vol. 6, no. 7, article e1000097, 2009.

[35] J. P. T. Higgins, D. G. Altman, P. C. Gotzsche et al., "The Cochrane Collaboration's tool for assessing risk of bias in randomised trials," *BMJ*, vol. 343, article d5928, 2011.

[36] T. Spinell, F. DeMayo, M. Cato et al., "The association between coeliac disease and periodontitis: results from NHANES 2009–2012," *Journal of Clinical Periodontology*, vol. 45, no. 3, pp. 303–310, 2018.

[37] T. van Gils, G. Bouma, H. J. Bontkes, C. J. J. Mulder, and H. S. Brand, "Self-reported oral health and xerostomia in adult patients with celiac disease versus a comparison group," *Oral Surgery, Oral Medicine, Oral Pathology, Oral Radiology*, vol. 124, no. 2, pp. 152–156, 2017.

[38] E. Rivera, A. Assiri, and S. Guandalini, "Celiac disease," *Oral Diseases*, vol. 19, no. 7, pp. 635–641, 2013.

[39] E. Shteyer, T. Berson, O. Lachmanovitz et al., "Oral health status and salivary properties in relation to gluten-free diet in children with celiac disease," *Journal of Pediatric Gastroenterology and Nutrition*, vol. 57, no. 1, pp. 49–52, 2013.

[40] S. Mina, C. Riga, A. I. Azcurra, and M. Brunotto, "Oral ecosystem alterations in celiac children: a follow-up study," *Archives of Oral Biology*, vol. 57, no. 2, pp. 154–160, 2012.

[41] A. Tsami, P. Petropoulou, J. Panayiotou, Z. Mantzavinos, and E. Roma-Giannikou, "Oral hygiene and periodontal treatment needs in children and adolescents with coeliac disease in Greece," *European Journal of Paediatric Dentistry*, vol. 11, no. 3, pp. 122–126, 2010.

[42] D. Souto-Souza, M. E. da Consolação Soares, V. S. Rezende, P. C. de Lacerda Dantas, E. L. Galvão, and S. G. M. Falci, "Association between developmental defects of enamel and celiac disease: a meta-analysis," *Archives of Oral Biology*, vol. 87, pp. 180–190, 2018.

[43] C. Sóñora, P. Arbildi, C. Rodríguez-Camejo, V. Beovide, A. Marco, and A. Hernández, "Enamel organ proteins as targets for antibodies in celiac disease: implications for oral health," *European Journal of Oral Sciences*, vol. 124, no. 1, pp. 11–16, 2016.

[44] F. Muñoz, N. Del Río, C. Sóñora, I. Tiscornia, A. Marco, and A. Hernández, "Enamel defects associated with coeliac disease: putative role of antibodies against gliadin in pathogenesis," *European Journal of Oral Sciences*, vol. 120, no. 2, pp. 104–112, 2012.

[45] M. De Angelis, G. Garruti, F. Minervini, L. Bonfrate, P. Portincasac, and M. Gobbetti, "The food-gut human axis: the effects of diet on gut microbiota and metabolome," *Current Medicinal Chemistry*, vol. 24, no. 999, p. 1, 2017.

[46] M. Cenit, M. Olivares, P. Codoñer-Franch, and Y. Sanz, "Intestinal microbiota and celiac disease: cause, consequence or co-evolution?," *Nutrients*, vol. 7, no. 8, pp. 6900–6923, 2015.

[47] H. J. Galipeau and E. F. Verdu, "Gut microbes and adverse food reactions: focus on gluten related disorders," *Gut Microbes*, vol. 5, no. 5, pp. 594–605, 2014.

[48] P. C. da Silva, V. de Almeida Pdel, M. A. Machado et al., "Oral manifestations of celiac disease. A case report and review of the literature," *Medicina Oral, Patología Oral y Cirugía Bucal*, vol. 13, no. 9, pp. E559–E562, 2008.

[49] R. Francavilla, F. Cristofori, M. Stella, G. Borrelli, G. Naspi, and S. Castellaneta, "Treatment of celiac disease: from gluten-free diet to novel therapies," *Minerva Pediatrica*, vol. 66, no. 5, pp. 501–516, 2014.

[50] K. A. Bascuñán, M. C. Vespa, and M. Araya, "Celiac disease: understanding the gluten-free diet," *European Journal of Nutrition*, vol. 56, no. 2, pp. 449–459, 2017.

[51] T. G. Theethira and M. Dennis, "Celiac disease and the gluten-free diet: consequences and recommendations for improvement," *Digestive Diseases*, vol. 33, no. 2, pp. 175–182, 2015.

21

Factors Associated with Recurrent Ulcers in Patients with Gastric Surgery after More Than 15 Years

Monica Pantea,[1] Anca Negovan,[1] Claudia Banescu,[2] Simona Bataga,[1] Radu Neagoe,[3] Simona Mocan,[4] and Mihaela Iancu[5]

[1]*Clinical Science-Internal Medicine, University of Medicine and Pharmacy, Gheorghe Marinescu 38, Tirgu Mureş, 540139 Mures, Romania*
[2]*Center for Advanced Medical and Pharmaceutical Research, University of Medicine and Pharmacy, Gheorghe Marinescu 38, Tirgu Mureş, 540139 Mures, Romania*
[3]*Surgical Science, University of Medicine and Pharmacy, Gheorghe Marinescu 38, Tirgu Mureş, 540139 Mures, Romania*
[4]*Pathological Department, Emergency County Hospital, Gheorghe Marinescu 50, Tirgu Mures, 540136 Mures, Romania*
[5]*Department of Medical Informatics and Biostatistics, University of Medicine and Pharmacy "Iuliu Haţieganu", Louis Pasteur St., No. 6, 400349 Cluj-Napoca, Romania*

Correspondence should be addressed to Anca Negovan; ancanegovan@yahoo.com

Academic Editor: Riccardo Casadei

Aim. We aimed to establish the independent predictive factors (from *Helicobacter pylori* infection, biliary reflux, histologic features of the gastric mucosa, drugs, comorbidities, and social habits) for gastric stump ulcer occurrence more than 15 years after surgery. *Methods.* 76 patients with previous gastric surgery were included: 21 patients with gastric ulcer (marginal ulcer or ulcer of the rest of the gastric remnant—study group) and 55 controls (nonulcer group). *Results. Helicobacter pylori* infection tended to be higher in the control group than in the ulcer group (14.5% vs. 4.8%, $p = 0.43$), without statistical significance. Alcohol consumption had a significant positive association with ulcer ($p = 0.008$), while smoking ($p = 0.064$), low-dose aspirin ($p = 0.063$), and biliary reflux ($p = 0.106$) had a tendency toward statistical signification for positive association. On univariate analysis, smoking ($p = 0.048$, OR = 3.15, 95% CI: 1.01–9.93) and low-dose aspirin consumption ($p = 0.067$, OR = 2.63, 95% CI: 0.95–7.68) were significantly associated with ulcer. According to the multivariable regression model, alcohol consumption (OR = 6.68, 95% CI: 1.29–41.14) and biliary reflux (OR = 6.12, 95% CI: 1.36–38.26) remained significantly associated with increased odds of stump ulcer. *Conclusion.* Biliary reflux and alcohol consumption, but not *Helicobacter pylori* infection or gastrotoxic drug, seem to be the most important predictors for ulcer recurrence in patients with gastric surgery for peptic ulcer after more than 15 years.

1. Introduction

Peptic ulcer disease (PUD) represents a common pathology in gastroenterology practice, affecting 4 million people each year worldwide, with complications reported in 10–20% [1, 2]. The annual incidence of PUD ranges between 0.10% and 0.19% with a significant decline in the last decades [3], due to several therapeutic improvements such as the use of proton pomp inhibitors (PPI) and eradication therapy for *Helicobacter pylori* (*H. pylori*). Improved medical therapy and advanced therapeutic endoscopic techniques steadily decreased the need to perform surgical treatment on PUD patients over the last 20 years [4].

The most frequent endoscopic lesions after gastric surgery are marginal ulcers (MU), which occur on the anastomotic area with a frequency range from 0.6% to 16% [5–8]. The etiology of MU is still unclear, even if several factors have been studied, such as the role of *H. pylori* infection, the importance of surgical anastomosis, and other associated risk factors (biliary reflux) [9–11].

Studies of risk factors influencing the occurrence of complications in gastric stump (ulcers, cancers) are of clinical interest, with the increasing number of gastric surgeries in obese patients or for early gastric cancer [12–14]. The known risk factors for gastric ulcer and bleeding (*H. pylori* infection, gastrotoxic medication) should be questioned in patients with gastric resection to identify predisposing factors that can be different from those in the normal stomach [15]. Therefore, information about the specific features of histologic and endoscopic lesions in the gastric remnant will help to identify the appropriate surveillance and treatment strategies.

Albeit there is no published data available regarding the prevalence of resected gastric patients, the increased incidence of gastric surgery in the past, especially due to the high prevalence of *H. pylori* in Eastern European countries [1], suggests a relatively high prevalence of patients with gastric stump after PUD surgery in our population, with no defined predisposing factors for recurrent ulcer. With more than 10–20 years having passed from their surgeries and many of them having chronic diseases and treatments, they represent a population with a high risk for ulcer and bleeding in the gastric remnant.

The aim of the present work is to establish the independent predictive factors like *H. pylori* infection, biliary reflux, histologic features of the gastric mucosa, gastrotoxic treatment (nonsteroidal anti-inflammatory drugs (NSAIDs), antiplatelet therapy), comorbidities, and social habits for gastric stump ulcer occurrence.

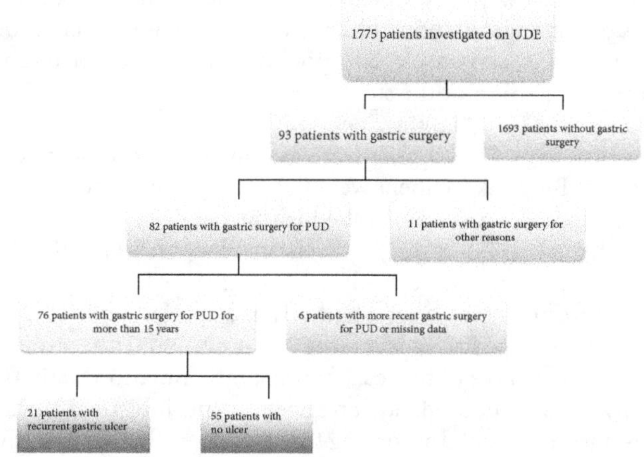

FIGURE 1: Flowchart of patient selection.

2. Materials and Methods

This is a cross-sectional study that investigates in the same time the possible predictive factors and disease occurrence. From a total of 1755 patients who underwent upper digestive endoscopy at the 3rd Medical Clinic in Tîrgu Mureş, Romania, between 2012 and 2015, 76 patients who presented with a history of gastric surgery for PUD of more than 15 years were prospectively recruited using an interview (Figure 1). No data regarding vagotomy was obtained due to the lack of medical records after more than 15 years.

Upper digestive endoscopy (UDE) was performed in all 76 patients with gastric surgery, and according to the presence of ulcers, they were divided into study (ulcer group) and control groups (nonulcer group). UDE was performed for digestive symptoms and anemia, for screening for bleeding risk before starting antithrombotic therapy or having major cardiovascular surgery, or for regular gastric stump complication (every 5 years). A written consent was obtained from every patient included in the study.

The ethical committee of the University of Medicine and Pharmacy of Tîrgu Mureş, Romania, approved this study.

2.1. Data Collection. Clinical and demographical data were collected from each patient. We registered the symptoms (heartburn, abdominal pain, vomiting, and nausea) or the presence of anemia in every patient. In order to investigate drug exposure, we used a structured interview and medical records. We recorded treatment with NSAIDs (ibuprofenum, diclofenacum, indometacinum, ketoprofenum, etc., as regular doses within two weeks prior to endoscopy) and antithrombotic therapy (low-dose aspirin (LDA) (75–125 mg/day) (available doses in Romania) and clopidogrelum (75 mg/day)), as well as anticoagulant therapy with acenocumarolum and low-weight molecular heparin (LWMH), at least 2 weeks before performing endoscopy. The reasons for antithrombotic therapies (clopidogrelum, LDA, and anticoagulants) were primary or secondary cardiovascular prevention for ischemic cardiac diseases or arrhythmias (with or without cardiac heart failure), cerebrovascular diseases, and peripheral arterial diseases. Regarding the medical therapy before surgery, none of the patients mentioned the treatment with PPI or *H. pylori* eradication therapy on interview. Some of them admitted having used other antiulcerogenic drugs (bismuth, magnesium or calcium carbonate, aluminum hydroxide, etc.). We used the medical records to check for medical prescriptions and to identify comorbidities (hypertension, ischemic and valvular heart disease, cerebrovascular disease, renal disease, liver disease, osteoarthritis, and diabetes mellitus). Patients with a decreased glomerular filtration rate (GFR) of less than 60 ml/min/1.73 m^2 were considered the chronic kidney disease group. Patients diagnosed on the basis of clinical and radiographic evidence as having a degenerative disorder of articular cartilage were included in the osteoarthritis group. We excluded patients with gastric surgery for other reasons (gastric cancer, bariatric surgery), patients with a gastric surgery within the last 15 years, or patients with lacking data. None of the recruited patients met the criteria to be evaluated for Zollinger-Ellison syndrome or gastrinoma. There were no available medical records or data regarding *H. pylori* infection before the surgery.

2.2. Endoscopy. A single examiner, blinded to drug exposure and symptoms, performed UDEs and carefully examined the gastric remnant and the efferent loop. A mucosa defect larger than 5 mm in diameter and extending into the deeper layers of the gastric wall was defined as ulcer, irrespective of the position in the gastric remnant or anastomotic area. At least 3 biopsies were taken from the gastric remnant, from the anastomosis and efferent side, and from the ulcers. Based on the endoscopic findings, we divided the patients into 2 groups: the study group (patients with ulcer) and the control group (patients without ulcer on UDE). The presence or absence of macroscopic bile pooling was noted on endoscopic intubation of the stomach.

2.3. Histology. The biopsies were examined for routine investigation. Biopsy specimens were fixed in 10% buffered formalin, routinely processed, embedded in paraffin, and stained with hematoxylin-eosin, PAS-Alcian blue, and Giemsa. *H. pylori* infection was considered negative if *H. pylori* was absent from all biopsy sites and positive if at least one histology test was positive, including the immunohistochemical study. The degree of mucosal chronic inflammation, activity, *H. pylori* infection, glandular atrophy, and intestinal metaplasia were classified according to the updated Sydney system, but the patients have been assigned according to the presence or absence of changes in the ulcer and nonulcer group. We also evaluated dysplasia according to the modified Vienna classification, but patients with dysplasia or neoplasia were excluded. Patients without important inflammation, but with prominent foveolar hyperplasia, fibromuscular replacement of the lamina propria, and congestion of superficial mucosal capillaries, were diagnosed with reactive gastropathy.

2.4. Statistical Analysis. The description of demographic and clinical characteristics was performed using absolute frequencies (number of cases) and relative frequencies (%). The bivariate analysis was realized using Fisher's exact test or chi-square tests. The crude odds ratio and associated 95% confidence interval (CI) were used to quantify the degree of association. An estimated significance level (p value) lower than 0.05 was considered statistically significant.

In order to establish the independent predictive factors for the occurrence of gastric stump ulcers, we used the binomial logistic regression as an appropriate statistical method. In the development of model prediction, we selected all variables with a p value smaller than 0.25 in the univariate regression analysis, along with all variables of known clinical importance. The presence of multicollinearity in the model was tested using variance inflation factors. The performance and consistency of the final model were assessed by McFadden's (R^2) coefficient, while the classification capacity was evaluated using receiver operating characteristic (ROC) curves and associated areas under the curve (AUC) as a measure. The values of AUC are comprised between 0.5 (no discrimination) and 1.0 (perfect classification), and according to the convention introduced by Hosmer and Lemeshow [16], values above 0.8 indicate an excellent discrimination ability for the model. The estimated AUC was accompanied by 95% associated confidence interval.

The level of statistical significance for all two-tailed tests was set to 0.05.

The advanced environment for statistical computing R (v.3.2.4, Vienna, Austria) was used for statistical analysis.

3. Results

3.1. Bivariate Analysis. The study was performed in 21 patients with gastric ulcer irrespective of localization (anastomotic area or the rest of the gastric remnant—study group) and 55 controls (nonulcer group). The distribution of demographical and clinical variables of interest (age, sex, smoking, alcohol consumption, *H. pylori* infection, drug consumption, biliary reflux, comorbidities, and symptomatology) is shown in Table 1.

Chi-square or Fisher's exact tests showed that alcohol consumption had a significant positive association with ulcer ($p = 0.008$), which indicated that patients who reported an alcohol consumption (≥10 units/week, 1 unit = 10 ml pure alcohol) were more likely to have a gastric ulcer than non-consumers. Regarding the habit of smoking ($p = 0.064$) and LDA consumption ($p = 0.063$), there was a tendency toward statistical signification for positive association.

Analyzing the frequency of histological findings in our groups, we found that the proportions of patients with reactive gastropathy were similar in ulcer and nonulcer groups (76.2% vs.70.9%, $p = 0.645$). Gastric atrophy and/or intestinal metaplasia were detected more frequently in patients with ulcer than in the control group, but the difference was not statistically significant (38.1% vs. 27.3%, $p = 0.358$).

In our study, 54 patients (71.05%) had Billroth I anastomosis and 19 patients (25%) had Billroth II anastomosis. The frequency of ulcer development was 90.5% in Billroth I anastomosis and 10.5% in Billroth II anastomosis.

3.2. Development of the Prediction Model. The univariable odds ratios, as a measure for the association between each studied predictor and gastric ulcer, are shown in Table 2.

From a total of 14 variables being considered potential predictors for gastric ulcer, 8 variables had $p < 0.25$ and were used for the first model selection. A preliminary main effects model was specified, and it was considered the final model, because we did not find other independent variables with $p \geq 0.25$ or significant interaction terms.

According to our multivariate regression analysis results (Table 3), the final multivariable ulcer gastric prediction model had the following as predictors: age, gender, smoking, NSAIDs, *H. pylori* infection, alcohol consumption, biliary reflux, chronic kidney diseases, respiratory diseases, and osteoarthritis. Each predictor had a variance inflation factor lower than 1.5, so there was no problem of multicollinearity.

There were two factors, alcohol consumption (OR = 6.68, 95% CI: 1.29–41.14) and the presence of biliary reflux (OR = 6.12, 95% CI: 1.36–38.26), that were significantly associated with increased odds of gastric stump ulcer. The presence of chronic kidney disease was also positively associated with gastric ulcer, with a tendency toward statistical significance ($p = 0.081$).

3.3. Model Performance. The model's McFadden's coefficient (R^2) was 0.390, and the model likelihood ratio test was significant (LR $\chi^2 = 24$, df = 9, $p = 0.0043$). The model also demonstrated an acceptable classification ability (AUC = 0.83, 95% CI: 0.73–0.93) (Figure 2) and a reasonable goodness-of-fit to data (Hosmer-Lemeshow test: $\chi^2 = 4.76$, df = 8, $p = 0.783$).

Table 1: The distribution of independent variables of interest in the studied groups.

Variables	Nonulcer group ($n = 55$) No. of cases (%)	Ulcer group ($n = 21$) No. of cases (%)	p value[a]
Gender			
Female	18 (32.7)	6 (28.6)	0.789
Male	37 (67.3)	15 (71.4)	
Age			
<60 years	15 (27.3)	7 (33.3)	0.778
≥60 years	40 (72.7)	14 (66.7)	
Smoking			
No	46 (83.6)	13 (61.9)	0.064
Yes[b]	9 (16.4)	8 (38.1)	
LDA[c]			
No	34 (61.8)	8 (38.1)	0.063
Yes	21 (38.2)	13 (61.9)	
Clopidrogrelum			
No	47 (85.5)	16 (76.2)	0.338
Yes	8 (14.5)	5 (23.8)	
NSAIDs[d]			
No	51 (92.7)	17 (81.0)	0.135
Yes	4 (7.3)	4 (19.0)	
Anticoagulants			
No	49 (89.1)	17 (81.0)	0.449
Yes	6 (10.9)	4 (19.0)	
H. pylori			
Negative	47 (85.5)	20 (95.2)	0.430
Positive	8 (14.5)	1 (4.8)	
Alcohol consumption[e]			
No	46 (83.6)	11 (52.4)	0.008
Yes	9 (16.4)	10 (47.6)	
Biliary reflux			
No	23 (41.8)	4 (19.0)	0.106
Yes	32 (58.2)	17 (81.0)	
Diabetes mellitus			
No	42 (76.4)	15 (71.4)	0.657
Yes	13 (23.6)	6 (28.6)	
Chronic kidney disease			
No	42 (76.4)	12 (57.1)	0.156
Yes	13 (23.6)	9 (42.9)	
Chronic liver disease			
No	33 (60.0)	10 (47.6)	0.439
Yes	22 (40.0)	11 (52.4)	
Respiratory disease			
No	44 (80.0)	13 (61.9)	0.139
Yes	11 (20.0)	8 (38.1)	
Osteoarthritis			
No	42 (76.4)	13 (61.9)	0.255
Yes	13 (23.6)	8 (38.1)	

Table 1: Continued.

Variables	Nonulcer group ($n = 55$) No. of cases (%)	Ulcer group ($n = 21$) No. of cases (%)	p value[a]
Symptoms[f]			
No	21 (38.2)	9 (42.9)	0.795
Yes	34 (61.8)	12 (57.1)	

[a]Obtained from chi-square or Fisher's exact test; [b]over 5 cigarettes/day including quitters during the past 5 years; [c]LDA = low-dose aspirin (75–125 mg/day); [d]NSAIDs: nonsteroidal anti-inflammatory drugs, regular daily doses; [e]more than 10 units/week, 1 unit = 10 ml pure alcohol; [f]symptoms = at least one symptom from upper abdominal pain, heartburn, and nausea/vomiting.

Table 2: Univariable odds ratio for considered independent variables of gastric ulcer.

Variables	p value[‡]	OR_{crude}	95% CI [lower limit, upper limit]
Independent variables			
Smoking[a]	0.048*	3.15	[1.01, 9.93]
LDA[b] (no)	0.067**	2.63	[0.95, 7.68]
Clopidrogrelum (no)	0.341	1.84	[0.49, 6.35]
NSAIDs[c] (no)	0.149***	3.00	[0.65, 13.99]
Anticoagulants (no)	0.353	1.92	[0.45, 7.57]
H. pylori (negative)	0.262	0.29	[0.02, 1.76]
Alcohol consumption[d]	0.007*	4.65	[1.54, 14.60]
Biliary reflux (absent)	0.071**	3.05	[0.98, 11.69]
Diabetes mellitus (absent)	0.657	1.29	[0.40, 3.93]
Chronic kidney disease (absent)	0.103***	2.42	[0.83, 7.09]
Chronic liver disease (absent)	0.332	1.65	[0.60, 4.61]
Respiratory disease (absent)	0.109***	2.46	[0.81, 7.45]
Osteoarthritis (absent)	0.211***	1.99	[0.66, 5.85]
Symptoms[e]	0.709	0.82	[0.30, 2.33]
Controls			
Gender (female)	0.728	1.22	[0.42, 3.88]
Age (<60 years)	0.603	0.75	[0.26, 2.30]

Note: the reference category for each variable was written in parenthesis. [‡]Estimated significance level obtained from Wald's test; $^{*}p < 0.05$, $^{**}p < 0.10$, $^{***}p < 0.25$. [a]<5 cigarettes/day, including quitters during the past 5 years; [b]LDA = low-dose aspirin (75–125 mg/day); [c]NSAIDs: nonsteroidal anti-inflammatory drugs, regular daily doses; [d]less than 10 units/week, 1 unit = 10 ml pure alcohol; [e]symptoms = the absence of any symptom from upper abdominal pain, heartburn, and nausea/vomiting; OR = odds ratio; CI = confidence interval.

4. Discussion

The potential complications after gastric resection are biliary reflux with consecutive gastropathy/gastritis, ulcers of the gastric remnant, nutritional disturbances, dumping syndrome, and "gastric stump cancers" [17–19]. Ulcers of the

TABLE 3: Multivariable odds ratio from the final logistic model of gastric ulcer.

Variables	OR_{adj}	95% CI [lower limit, upper limit]	p value‡
Independent variables			
NSAIDs (no)	4.76	[0.55, 43.65]	0.132
H. pylori (negative)	0.35	[0.02, 3.18]	0.387
Alcohol consumption (<10 U/week)	6.68	[1.29, 41.14]	0.013
Biliary reflux (absent)	6.12	[1.36, 38.26]	0.026
Chronic kidney disease (absent)	3.45	[0.84, 15.13]	0.081
Respiratory disease (absent)	1.79	[0.33, 9.43]	0.405
Osteoarthritis (absent)	2.69	[0.51, 14.73]	0.242
Controls			
Gender (female)	1.08	[0.22, 5.48]	0.911
Age (<60 years)	0.59	[0.14, 2.58]	0.425

Note: the reference category for each variable was written in parenthesis; OR_{adj} = adjusted OR; ‡estimated significance level obtained from Wald's test; NSAIDs: nonsteroidal anti-inflammatory drugs; CI = confidence interval.

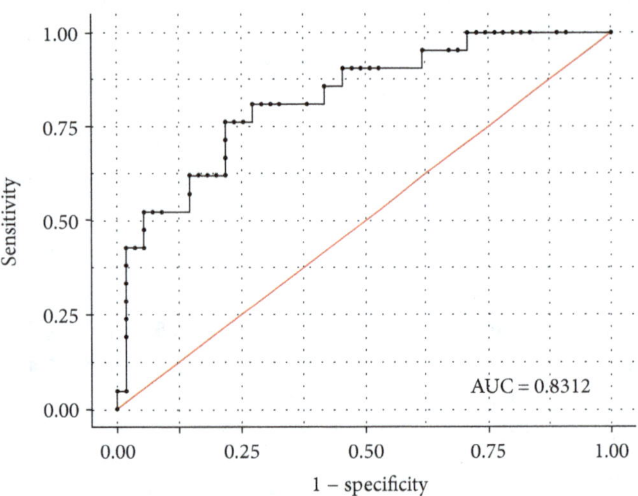

FIGURE 2: Discrimination ability of the logistic model (ROC curve). Note: the area under the curve demonstrated a good discrimination ability of the logistic model (good capacity of the logistic model to predict ulcer gastric presence correctly). The graph also showed sensitivity values versus 1 – specificity values for different cut-off classification probability values.

gastric stump are widely studied in the medical literature. In consecutively investigated patients, we noticed that the vast majority had been resected for ulcer more than 15 years before and some of them were in the "PPI era." We do not have a clear explanation, but it may be related to the "doctor's preference" for surgical therapy of ulcer-complicated episode instead of medical or endoscopic therapy in some Romanian hospitals, where medical therapeutic means were not fully available at that time. The most studied were MU, divided according to the time of discovery after surgery into early MU, occurring within 1 to 10 months after surgery [20, 21], and late MU, developing many years after gastrectomy [22]. The etiology of early MU seems to be linked to local tissue injury, the type of suture [22–24], local ischemia, and inflammatory reaction [22]. Nevertheless, the etiology of late MU ulcers is not very well known [12]. Our study questioned clinical and pathological predisposing factors for late recurrent gastric ulcers in patients with long-term gastric surgery for PUD, both in the anastomotic area (MU) and in the rest of the gastric remnant. Surprisingly, none of the known major risk factors for gastric ulcer (gastrotoxic drugs, *H. pylori* infection) remained predictors for recurrent ulcer in patients with previous gastric surgery for PUD in our work, except for alcohol consumption and biliary reflux.

We registered a frequency of ulcers of 27.6% among patients with gastric resection, similar to the data of Chung et al. who detected a prevalence of 27.1% [12]. The present observations suggest an increased frequency of recurrent ulcers in patients with more than 15 years after previous surgery investigated on UDE, as the reported PUD in the endoscopic population was 5.6% in an American study [25] and 12.5% in our endoscopic series (data not published). Despite the known predisposing factors discussed below, a possible individual predisposition or vulnerability of the gastric remnant, involving more subtle unknown environmental or genetic factors that unbalanced the protective and aggressive mechanisms of the gastric mucosa, can explain this observation [26, 27].

The relationship between the surgical reconstruction technique and ulcer formation is debatable according to the available published data. The majority of works suggest that patients with Billroth II anastomosis are more prone to developing endoscopic ulceration than patients with Billroth I, probably due to the increased bile reflux [12]. Another study found no significant difference between the two anastomosis models and ulcer occurrence [23]. Because the contingency table of Billroth I anastomosis, Billroth II anastomosis, and gastric ulcer contained observed frequencies lower than 5, we did not use the type of anastomosis as a factor in multivariate analysis, in order to avoid large standard errors of estimate.

Epidemiological and clinical research established that *H pylori* infection represents a major cause of peptic ulcers and gastric cancer on the normal stomach [2], but its role in developing gastric stump ulcer is still unclear [8, 9]. With a lower frequency (4.8%) in our ulcer group than in the non-ulcer group (14.5%), we found no statistically significant association between recurrent gastric ulcer and *H. pylori* infection in the gastric stump. The diminished role of *H. pylori* may be related to the low frequency of infection in the gastric stump. The spontaneous phenomenon of the germ clearance over the years seems to be a consequence of the antibacterial effect of the bile, the increase in gastric pH, or the replacement of normal mucosa with atrophic mucosa [28, 29].

Histological features in gastric mucosa samples (reactive gastropathy, active or inactive gastritis, and premalignant lesions) are not predictive for ulcer risk in resected patients. The most frequent histologic finding in resected patients was reactive gastropathy (72.4%), while inflammatory findings were rare (18.4%). The high frequency of gastric atrophy/intestinal metaplasia associated with a decreased acid secretion in the ulcer group and the low frequency of *H. pylori* infection and inflammation suggest the role of other factors instead of acid secretion or histological features in gastric stump ulcers. Even if *H. pylori*-related ulcer was the probable cause of the first complicated PUD in the majority of our patients, the long-term evolution of the disease, with the clearance of the germ, tends not to offer an efficient protection against recurrent ulcer.

The microenvironment is changing dramatically after gastric resection, especially due to biliary reflux, which becomes a permanent aggressor of the gastric layer, increasing the pH of the gastric content [28, 29]. The effect of chronic biliary reflux is the appearance of reflux gastritis, associated with histological changes. Even if the irritant effect of biliary reflux on the gastric mucosa is well known, its influence on developing gastric stump ulcer is not as well established as its role in gastric stump cancer [10, 29]. In our final regression model, biliary reflux remains a good predictor for ulcer, even if it is studied in the presence of other variables.

The use of NSAIDs and antithrombotic drugs is well known to increase the risk of gastric ulcer two- or threefold in the general population [1, 2]. It is believed that among patients with gastric resections, the use of the gastrotoxic medication has a similar effect. However, no controlled clinical studies on the consumption of NSAIDs and antiplatelet therapy have been conducted among patients with gastric resection for PUD, in order to determine the risk magnitude in this specific population. In our current research, the use of NSAIDs and LDA in the presence of other variables tended to influence the occurrence of ulcer in the gastric stump, possibly due to the complex interplay of aggressive mechanisms and other factors; their role did not reach statistical significance.

Although smoking or alcohol consumption are not the primary case of PUD, they have been reported as contributors to ulcer pathogenesis in some reports [30–33]. Several studies suggested that smoking and alcohol consumption might increase the risk of developing gastric ulcer among patients with the gastric stump, through different mechanisms. There was an influence of smoking on ulcer occurrence in our study, but not in the presence of other variables. Alcohol consumption (>10 units/week) remained a good predictor for ulcer recurrence in gastric-resected patients. Our observations support the different role of local aggressive factors in the gastric stump compared to the normal stomach, as alcohol consumption is not a major risk factor for gastric ulcer in the general population.

Symptoms were present in both the ulcer and nonulcer groups with comparable frequencies. Most of them can be explained by the presence of biliary reflux, common among patients with gastric resection [28], but the lack of specific premonitory symptoms for gastric stump severe lesions should be emphasized.

Concomitant diseases were not systematically investigated as predisposing factors for recurrent ulcers in patients with gastric surgery. Our previous work suggested the role of cerebrovascular diseases or congestive heart failure as independent risk factors for ulcer in nonresected aspirin consumers [33, 34]. Antithrombotic drug consumption was significantly associated with cardiovascular diseases, and on univariate analysis, antithrombotic drug consumption had the tendency toward statistical significance for ulcer occurrence, while cardiovascular diseases were not (using the chi-square test for the frequency of ischemic cardiac disease ($p = 0.690$) and for the frequency of heart failure ($p = 0.442$) in the studied groups). In the final regression model, we choose as an interest predictor drug consumption, but not cardiovascular diseases, in order to avoid the multicollinearity effect. Our findings suggest a possible influence of respiratory, articular, or renal chronic diseases on ulcer reoccurrence. When they were studied in the presence of other variables, only kidney diseases became a possible predictor for ulcer. Renal function impairment has been proved to increase the general risk for gastric ulcers and bleeding in several studies [34–36]. The possible described mechanisms are abnormal platelet function, mucosal integrity, or acid secretion in uremic patients that can promote local small bleeding and delay ulcer healing [35, 37], and these can also be available in the gastric remnant.

Despite its limitations—a study performed in an endoscopic population, with a relatively low number of cases, with no information on the vagotomy procedure or serological markers of decreased acid secretion—our study revealed the predictive role of the most known risk factors for ulcer development in the gastric stump. Because of the relatively small number of cases compared to the number of factors, the regression model must be retested in future studies in order to highlight the contribution of factors with a tendency toward statistical significance, to improve with another factors (such as the type of anastomosis) or to confirm known factors as *H. pylori* infection, reported to account for the majority of ulcers in our endoscopic population [38, 39].

To the best of our knowledge, there are no recently published reports regarding the interplay between clinical and histological factors in gastric stump ulcers, at more than 15 years after surgery. Our findings can offer a perspective on protective strategy development in gastric-resected patients irrespective of the cause and suggest that certain predisposing factors for gastric stump ulcer can be influenced.

5. Conclusions

Biliary reflux and alcohol consumption, but not *Helicobacter pylori* infection or gastrotoxic drug consumption, are the most important predictors for ulcer recurrence in patients with gastric surgery for peptic ulcer disease after more than 15 years.

Authors' Contributions

Monica Pantea and Anca Negovan contributed to this work.

References

[1] T. Milosavljević, M. Kostić-Milosavljević, M. Krstić, and A. Sokić-Milutinović, "Epidemiological trends in stomach-related diseases," *Digestive Diseases*, vol. 32, no. 3, pp. 213–216, 2014.

[2] H. Mitchell and P. Katelaris, "Epidemiology, clinical impacts and current clinical management of Helicobacter pylori infection," *The Medical Journal of Australia*, vol. 204, no. 10, pp. 376–380, 2016.

[3] W. J. den Hollander, C. Sostres, E. J. Kuipers, and A. Lanas, "*Helicobacter pylori* and nonmalignant diseases," *Helicobacter*, vol. 18, Supplement 1, pp. 24–27, 2013.

[4] C. W. Lee and G. A. Sarosi Jr., "Emergency ulcer surgery," *The Surgical Clinics of North America*, vol. 91, no. 5, pp. 1001–1013, 2011.

[5] M. M. Hutter, B. D. Schirmer, D. B. Jones et al., "First report from the American College of Surgeons Bariatric Surgery Center Network: laparoscopic sleeve gastrectomy has morbidity and effectiveness positioned between the band and the bypass," *Annals of Surgery*, vol. 254, no. 3, pp. 410–422, 2011.

[6] N. Runkel, M. Colombo-Benkmann, T. P. Hüttl, H. Tigges, O. Mann, and S. Sauerland, "Bariatric surgery," *Deutsches Ärzteblatt International*, vol. 108, no. 20, pp. 341–346, 2011.

[7] E. Passaro Jr, H. E. Gordon, and B. E. Stabile, "Marginal ulcer: a guide to management," *Surgical Clinics of North America*, vol. 56, no. 6, pp. 1435–1444, 1976.

[8] W. C. Chung, E. J. Jeon, K. M. Lee et al., "Incidence and clinical features of endoscopic ulcers developing after gastrectomy," *World Journal of Gastroenterology*, vol. 18, no. 25, pp. 3260–3266, 2012.

[9] Y. S. Lin, M. J. Chen, S. C. Shih, M. J. Bair, C. J. Fang, and H. Y. Wang, "Management of *Helicobacter pylori* infection after gastric surgery," *World Journal of Gastroenterology*, vol. 20, no. 18, pp. 5274–5282, 2014.

[10] W. C. Chung, E. J. Jeon, K. M. Lee et al., "Clinical outcomes of the marginal ulcer bleeding after gastrectomy: as compared to the peptic ulcer bleeding with non-operated stomach," *Gastroenterology Research and Practice*, vol. 2012, Article ID 624327, 6 pages, 2012.

[11] B. E. Schneider, L. Villegas, G. L. Blackburn, E. C. Mun, J. F. Critchlow, and D. B. Jones, "Laparoscopic gastric bypass surgery: outcomes," *Journal of Laparoendoscopic & Advanced Surgical Techniques Part A*, vol. 13, no. 4, pp. 247–255, 2003.

[12] K. Sun, S. Chen, J. Ye et al., "Endoscopic resection versus surgery for early gastric cancer: a systematic review and meta-analysis," *Digestive Endoscopy*, vol. 28, no. 5, pp. 513–525, 2016.

[13] W. Sun, X. Han, S. Wu, and C. Yang, "Endoscopic resection versus surgical resection for early gastric cancer: a systematic review and meta-analysis," *Medicine*, vol. 94, no. 43, article e1649, 2015.

[14] N. Puzziferri, T. B. Roshek III, H. G. Mayo, R. Gallagher, S. H. Belle, and E. H. Livingston, "Long-term follow-up after bariatric surgery: a systematic review," *JAMA*, vol. 312, no. 9, pp. 934–942, 2014.

[15] O. Jeong and Y. K. Park, "Clinicopathological features and surgical treatment of gastric cancer in South Korea: the results of 2009 nationwide survey on surgically treated gastric cancer patients," *Journal of Gastric Cancer*, vol. 11, no. 2, pp. 69–77, 2011.

[16] D. Hosmer and S. Lemeshow, *Applied Logistic Regression*, John Wiley & Sons, New York, 2000.

[17] V. N. Nikolopoulou, K. C. Thomopoulos, G. I. Theocharis, V. A. Arvaniti, and C. E. Vagianos, "Acute upper gastrointestinal bleeding in operated stomach: outcome of 105 cases," *World Journal of Gastroenterology*, vol. 11, no. 29, pp. 4570–4573, 2005.

[18] H. Hur, K. Y. Song, C. H. Park, and H. M. Jeon, "Follow-up strategy after curative resection of gastric cancer: a nationwide survey in Korea," *Annals of Surgical Oncology*, vol. 17, no. 1, pp. 54–64, 2010.

[19] H. Katai, "Function preserving surgery for gastric cancer," *International Journal of Clinical Oncology*, vol. 11, no. 5, pp. 357–366, 2006.

[20] J. Hedberg, H. Hedenström, S. Nilsson, M. Sundbom, and S. Gustavsson, "Role of gastric acid in stomal ulcer after gastric bypass," *Obesity Surgery*, vol. 15, no. 10, pp. 1375–1378, 2005.

[21] R. M. Dallal and L. A. Bailey, "Ulcer disease after gastric bypass surgery," *Surgery for Obesity and Related Diseases*, vol. 2, no. 4, pp. 455–459, 2006.

[22] A. Csendes, J. Torres, and A. M. Burgos, "Late marginal ulcers after gastric bypass for morbid obesity. Clinical and endoscopic findings and response to treatment," *Obesity Surgery*, vol. 21, no. 9, pp. 1319–1322, 2011.

[23] G. D. Pope, P. P. Goodney, K. W. Burchard et al., "Peptic ulcer/stricture after gastric bypass: a comparison of technique and acid suppression variables," *Obesity Surgery*, vol. 12, no. 1, pp. 30–33, 2002.

[24] J. C. Vasquez, D. Wayne Overby, and T. M. Farrell, "Fewer gastrojejunostomy strictures and marginal ulcers with absorbable suture," *Surgical Endoscopy*, vol. 23, no. 9, pp. 2011–2015, 2009.

[25] B. McJunkin, M. Sissoko, J. Levien, J. Upchurch, and A. Ahmed, "Dramatic decline in prevalence of Helicobacter pylori and peptic ulcer disease in an endoscopy-referral population," *The American Journal of Medicine*, vol. 124, no. 3, pp. 260–264, 2011.

[26] W. C. Chung, E. J. Jeon, D. B. Kim et al., "Clinical characteristics of *Helicobacter pylori*-negative drug-negative peptic ulcer bleeding," *World Journal of Gastroenterology*, vol. 21, no. 28, pp. 8636–8643, 2015.

[27] H. Yoon, S. G. Kim, H. C. Jung, and I. S. Song, "High recurrence rate of idiopathic peptic ulcers in long-term follow-up," *Gut and Liver*, vol. 7, no. 2, pp. 175–181, 2013.

[28] K. Fukuhara, H. Osugi, N. Takada et al., "Correlation between duodenogastric reflux and remnant gastritis after distal gastrectomy," *Hepato-Gastroenterology*, vol. 51, no. 58, pp. 1241–1244, 2004.

[29] H. Abe, K. Murakami, S. Satoh et al., "Influence of bile reflux and Helicobacter pylori infection on gastritis in the remnant gastric mucosa after distal gastrectomy," *Journal of Gastroenterology*, vol. 40, no. 6, pp. 563–569, 2005.

[30] S. Takeno, T. Hashimoto, K. Maki et al., "Gastric cancer arising from the remnant stomach after distal gastrectomy: a review," *World Journal of Gastroenterology*, vol. 20, no. 38, pp. 13734–13740, 2014.

[31] M. Yamada, F. L. Wong, S. Fujiwara, Y. Tatsukawa, and G. Suzuki, "Smoking and alcohol habits as risk factors for benign digestive diseases in a Japanese population: the radiation effects research foundation adult health study," *Digestion*, vol. 71, no. 4, pp. 231–237, 2005.

[32] P. Maity, K. Biswas, S. Roy, R. K. Banerjee, and U. Bandyopadhyay, "Smoking and the pathogenesis of gastroduodenal ulcer–recent mechanistic update," *Molecular and Cellular Biochemistry*, vol. 253, no. 1/2, pp. 329–338, 2003.

[33] A. Negovan, M. Iancu, V. Moldovan et al., "The contribution of clinical and pathological predisposing factors to severe gastro-duodenal lesions in patients with long-term low-dose aspirin and proton pump inhibitor therapy," *European Journal of Internal Medicine*, vol. 44, pp. 62–66, 2017.

[34] A. Negovan, M. Iancu, V. Moldovan et al., "Clinical risk factors for gastroduodenal ulcer in Romanian low-dose aspirin consumers," *Gastroenterology Research and Practice*, vol. 2016, Article ID 7230626, 8 pages, 2016.

[35] C. S. Bang, Y. S. Lee, Y. H. Lee et al., "Characteristics of nonvariceal upper gastrointestinal hemorrhage in patients with chronic kidney disease," *World Journal of Gastroenterology*, vol. 19, no. 43, pp. 7719–7725, 2013.

[36] J. C. Luo, H. B. Leu, K. W. Huang et al., "Incidence of bleeding from gastroduodenal ulcers in patients with end-stage renal disease receiving hemodialysis," *CMAJ*, vol. 183, no. 18, pp. E1345–E1351, 2011.

[37] J. Cheung, A. Yu, J. LaBossiere, Q. Zhu, and R. N. Fedorak, "Peptic ulcer bleeding outcomes adversely affected by end-stage renal disease," *Gastrointestinal Endoscopy*, vol. 71, no. 1, pp. 44–49, 2010.

[38] A. Negovan, M. Iancu, V. Moldovan, S. Mocan, and C. Banescu, "The interaction between GSTT1, GSTM1, and GSTP1 Ile105Val gene polymorphisms and environmental risk factors in premalignant gastric lesions risk," *BioMed Research International*, vol. 2017, Article ID 7365080, 9 pages, 2017.

[39] A. Negovan, M. Iancu, V. Moldovan et al., "Influence of MDR1 C3435T, CYP2C19*2 and CYP2C19*3 gene polymorphisms and clinical characteristics on the severity of gastric lesions: a case-control study," *Journal of Gastrointestinal and Liver Diseases*, vol. 25, no. 2, pp. 258–260, 2016.

22

Endosonographic Findings and the Natural Course of Chronic Gastric Anisakiasis: A Single-Center Experience

Eun Young Park,[1] Dong Hoon Baek,[1] Gwang Ha Kim,[1] Bong Eun Lee,[1] So-Jeong Lee,[2] and Do Youn Park[2]

[1]*Department of Internal Medicine, Pusan National University School of Medicine, and Biomedical Research Institute, Pusan National University Hospital, Busan, Republic of Korea*
[2]*Department of Pathology, Pusan National University School of Medicine, Busan, Republic of Korea*

Correspondence should be addressed to Gwang Ha Kim; doc0224@pusan.ac.kr

Academic Editor: Haruhiko Sugimura

Background. Chronic gastric anisakiasis is a rare, usually asymptomatic, and difficult to diagnose infection incidentally discovered during endoscopy, resembling a subepithelial tumor (SET). Because its endoscopic ultrasonography (EUS) findings are not established, it is occasionally misdiagnosed as gastrointestinal mesenchymal tumors and removed by endoscopic or surgical resection. We aimed to assess the characteristic EUS findings of chronic gastric anisakiasis and the clinical course during follow-up. *Methods.* The database of all patients who underwent EUS at Pusan National University Hospital (Busan, Korea) between January 2011 and December 2016 was retrospectively analyzed. A total of 28 SET cases with EUS features suggesting chronic gastric anisakiasis were included in the study. The EUS, histopathologic, and follow-up endoscopic features were analyzed. *Results.* On EUS, the lesions were mainly located in the submucosal and/or propria muscle layers. Twenty-seven lesions (27/28, 96%) showed hypoechoic echogenicity, and 22 lesions (22/28, 79%) were heterogeneous. Hyperechoic tubular structures suggesting denaturalized Anisakidae larvae were seen in 22 lesions (22/28, 79%). Endoscopic biopsies revealed significant eosinophil infiltration (≥30 per high-power field) in 12 lesions (12/21, 57%). During the median follow-up period of 9 months (range, 1–55 months), SETs decreased or subsided in 26 lesions (26/28, 93%) with no change in the size of the two lesions (2/28, 7%). *Conclusions.* Chronic gastric anisakiasis, although rare, should be included in the differential diagnoses for gastric SETs, especially in regions where raw fish is widely consumed. EUS findings suggesting chronic gastric anisakiasis are heterogeneously hypoechoic lesions with hyperechoic tubular structures, mainly in the submucosal and/or muscularis propria layers. Because chronic gastric anisakiasis decreases or subsides in most cases, follow-up endoscopy 6–12 months later is recommended.

1. Introduction

Anisakiasis is a parasitic disease caused by an accidental ingestion of the nematode larva of the Anisakidae family in uncooked saltwater fish. This disease is caused by eating infected raw, pickled, or salted fishes such as herring, mackerel, squid, salmon, bonito, tuna, and cuttlefish. The incidence of gastric anisakiasis in a population is directly related to the consumption of raw fish. Therefore, the infection is prevalent in regions where raw fish is widely consumed, especially in Far East Asia, including Korea.

Gastrointestinal anisakiasis was first reported in 1937 [1], and it most commonly occurs in the stomach with an incidence of 68–75% [2, 3]. Most cases are acute gastric anisakiasis causing cramping abdominal pain, nausea, and vomiting. The diagnosis of acute gastric anisakiasis is usually by endoscopic confirmation, which often reveals the presence of the Anisakidae larvae or mucosal changes such as edema, erosion, ulceration, and hemorrhage.

However, chronic gastric anisakiasis, a kind of parasitic eosinophilic granuloma, is a rare entity; it is usually asymptomatic and difficult to diagnose because the Anisakidae larva is absent, and it often appears as an incidental subepithelial tumor (SET) during endoscopy. Because its endoscopic ultrasonography (EUS) findings are not yet established, it is sometimes misdiagnosed as gastrointestinal mesenchymal

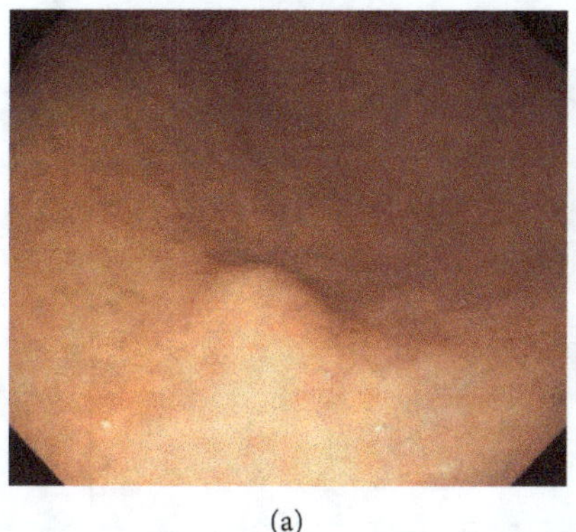
(a)

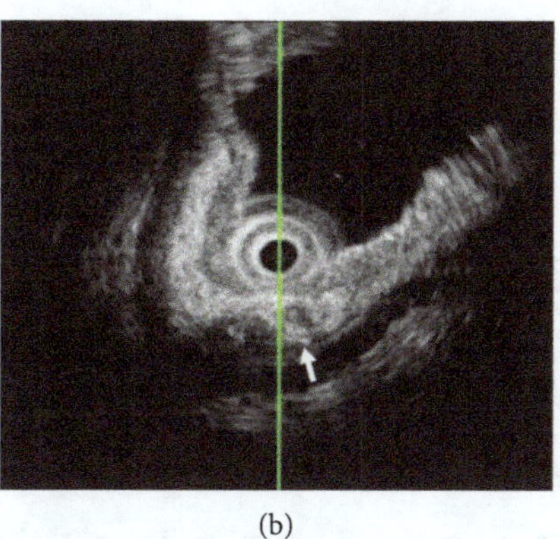
(b)

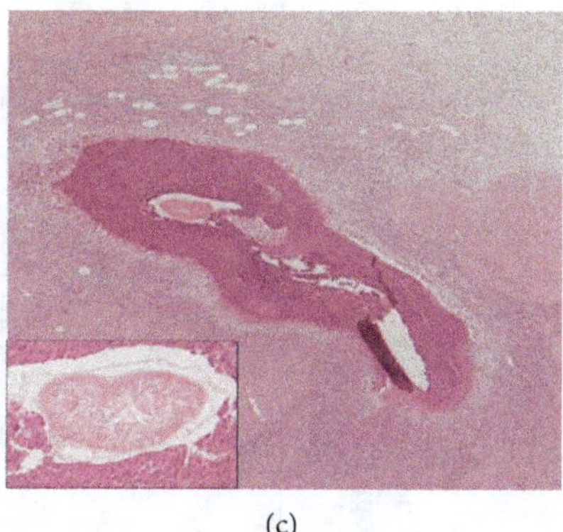
(c)

FIGURE 1: A case of chronic gastric anisakiasis histopathologically confirmed after surgical resection. (a) Endoscopy shows a subepithelial tumor-like lesion in the greater curvature of the gastric antrum. (b) On endoscopic ultrasonography, the lesion is a heterogeneously hypoechoic lesion in the submucosal layer. Hyperechoic tubular structures are seen inside the lesion (arrow). (c) Histopathological features of the resected specimen. Ill-defined granulomatous inflammation with marked eosinophil infiltration is seen in the submucosa (hematoxylin and eosin stain, ×40). Inside the granulomatous inflammation, the degenerated anisakiasis larva is observed (boxed area, hematoxylin and eosin stain, ×400).

tumors or heterotopic pancreas and it is removed by endoscopic or surgical resection [4, 5]. Recently, there have been few reports on the EUS findings of chronic gastric anisakiasis presenting as a SET and its natural course. Therefore, the aim of this study was to assess the characteristic EUS findings of chronic gastric anisakiasis and its clinical course during follow-up.

2. Methods

The database of all patients who underwent EUS at Pusan National University Hospital (Busan, Korea) between January 2011 and December 2016 was retrospectively analyzed. Based on our previous cases of histologically confirmed chronic gastric anisakiasis (Figure 1), we identified 38 SET cases with EUS features suggesting chronic gastric anisakiasis. Of these, 10 cases that did not undergo follow-up endoscopy were excluded. Ultimately, a total of 28 SET cases with EUS features were included in this study. The study protocol was reviewed and approved by the Institutional Review Board at Pusan National University Hospital (H-1801-017-063).

2.1. Endoscopic Ultrasonography. EUS was performed using a radial scanning ultrasound endoscope (GF-UM2000; Olympus, Tokyo, Japan) at 7.5 and 12 MHz or a 20 MHz catheter probe (UM3D-DP20-25R; Olympus). All examinations were performed under intravenous conscious sedation (using midazolam with or without propofol). Scanning of the tumor was performed after filling the stomach with 300–600 mL of deaerated water. At least five still images were obtained for each lesion during EUS, and these images were saved in our database.

The EUS images were reviewed by a single experienced endosonographer (G. H. Kim) who had previously performed more than 1000 examinations. The following EUS features were analyzed: (a) location, (b) gross shape using the Yamada classification [6], (c) presence of mucosal erosion on endoscopy, (d) maximal diameter, (e) pattern of tumor growth (intraluminal, mural, or extraluminal), (f) endosonographic layer of origin, (g) echogenicity (hypoechoic, isoechoic, or hyperechoic), (h) homogeneity (homogenous or heterogeneous), (i) distinctness of the borders (distinct or indistinct), and (j) presence of hyperechoic tubular structures indicating the presence of denaturalized Anisakidae larvae.

2.2. Histopathological Evaluation. Hematoxylin and eosin slides were reviewed for cases in which endoscopic biopsy was performed, and the histological features (eosinophil count per high-power field (HPF)) were recorded. Significant eosinophilic infiltration was defined as when the number of eosinophils was ≥30 per HPF [7].

2.3. Statistical Analyses. Variables were expressed as medians or range and simple proportions. Statistical significance was evaluated using χ^2 test or Fisher's exact test for categorical variables. A P value of <0.05 was considered statistically significant. The statistical analyses were conducted using IBM® SPSS® software, version 21.0 for Windows (IBM Corporation, Armonk, NY, USA).

3. Results

The 28 patients included 8 men and 20 women, age range from 25 to 76 years (median age: 53 years). Six patients presented with dyspepsia or epigastric pain. A SET was incidentally found during a routine health check-up in the other 22 patients who were asymptomatic. All patients except one had a history of marine raw fish intake within the previous 1 to 6 months.

Six lesions were located in the upper third of the stomach, 20 in the middle third, and one in the lower third (Table 1). Ten lesions (10/28, 35.7%) showed erosive change on the surface. As shown by the EUS, the lesions were mainly located in the third (submucosal) and/or fourth (propria muscle) layers and ranged from 3 mm to 25 mm in size (median size: 8 mm) (Table 2). A mural growth pattern was most commonly observed (23/28, 82%). Twenty-seven lesions (27/28, 96%) showed hypoechoic echogenicity, and

TABLE 1: Clinicopathologic and endosonographic features in 28 patients with chronic gastric anisakiasis.

Case	Sex	Age (years)	Location	Gross shape*	Erosion	Size (mm)	Growth pattern	EUS features				Hyperechoic tubular structures	Eosinophil no. on endoscopic biopsy†	Size on follow-up endoscopy	Follow-up period (months)
								Layer	Echogenicity	Homogeneity	Border				
1	M	27	Middle	I	–	7	Mural	3	Hypoechoic	Heterogeneous	Distinct	+	N-P	Decreased	1
2	M	41	Upper	I	–	3	Mural	3	Hypoechoic	Heterogeneous	Distinct	+	41	Subsided	26
3	M	43	Middle	I	+	9	Mural	3	Hypoechoic	Heterogeneous	Indistinct	+	37	Decreased	1
4	M	49	Middle	I	+	25	Intraluminal	2	Hypoechoic	Homogeneous	Indistinct	–	22	Subsided	32
5	M	51	Middle	I	–	17	Mural	3	Hypoechoic	Heterogeneous	Indistinct	+	64	Subsided	9
6	M	53	Middle	I	–	5	Mural	3	Hypoechoic	Homogeneous	Indistinct	–	5	Decreased	5
7	M	58	Middle	I	–	10	Mural	3	Hypoechoic	Heterogeneous	Distinct	+	45	Subsided	9
8	M	71	Middle	I	+	7	Mural	2, 3	Hypoechoic	Heterogeneous	Indistinct	+	18	Subsided	9
9	F	25	Upper	I	–	7	Mural	3	Hypoechoic	Heterogeneous	Indistinct	–	30	Same	22
10	F	42	Lower	I	–	11	Mural	2	Hypoechoic	Homogeneous	Distinct	–	107	Same	13
11	F	45	Middle	I	+	17	Mural	3, 4	Hypoechoic	Heterogeneous	Indistinct	+	500	Subsided	6
12	F	47	Middle	I	–	6	Mural	3	Hypoechoic	Homogeneous	Distinct	+	12	Subsided	14
13	F	49	Middle	I	–	7	Intraluminal	3, 4	Hypoechoic	Heterogeneous	Indistinct	+	N-P	Subsided	12
14	F	49	Middle	II	+	15	Mural	3, 4	Hyperechoic	Heterogeneous	Indistinct	+	56	Subsided	8
15	F	52	Middle	I	+	7	Mural	3	Hypoechoic	Heterogeneous	Indistinct	+	15	Subsided	18
16	F	52	Middle	I	+	6	Mural	3	Hypoechoic	Heterogeneous	Distinct	+	20	Decreased	1
17	F	53	Upper	I	–	9	Intraluminal	3	Hypoechoic	Heterogeneous	Distinct	+	N-P	Subsided	53
18	F	53	Middle	I	–	11	Mural	3	Hypoechoic	Heterogeneous	Indistinct	+	73	Subsided	7
19	F	55	Middle	I	–	16	Mural	3	Hypoechoic	Heterogeneous	Distinct	+	90	Decreased	3
20	F	57	Upper	I	+	8	Mural	2, 3	Hypoechoic	Homogeneous	Indistinct	–	370	Subsided	1
21	F	59	Upper	I	+	4	Mural	3, 4	Hypoechoic	Heterogeneous	Distinct	+	N-P	Decreased	55
22	F	59	Middle	I	–	6	Mural	3	Hypoechoic	Heterogeneous	Indistinct	+	N-P	Subsided	11
23	F	62	Upper	I	–	7	Mural	3	Hypoechoic	Heterogeneous	Distinct	+	N-P	Decreased	1
24	F	64	Middle	I	–	12	Mural	3	Hypoechoic	Heterogeneous	Distinct	–	N-P	Decreased	1
25	F	66	Middle	I	–	11	Mural	3, 4	Hypoechoic	Heterogeneous	Indistinct	+	5	Decreased	1
26	F	66	Middle	I	–	13	Mural	3, 4	Hypoechoic	Heterogeneous	Indistinct	+	25	Subsided	15
27	F	75	Middle	I	–	8	Intraluminal	2	Hypoechoic	Homogeneous	Indistinct	+	55	Decreased	1
28	F	76	Upper	I	+	8	Intraluminal	3	Hypoechoic	Heterogeneous	Indistinct	+	11	Subsided	19

*By Yamada classification [6]. †Per high-power field. N-P: not performed.

TABLE 2: Summary of endosonographic features of chronic anisakiasis.

EUS features	$N = 28$ (%)
Median size, mm (range)	8 (3–25)
Growth pattern	
Intraluminal	5 (18)
Mural	23 (82)
Layer	
Second layer	3 (11)
Second and third layers	2 (7)
Third layer	17 (61)
Third and fourth layers	6 (21)
Echogenicity	
Hypoechoic	27 (96)
Hyperechoic	1 (4)
Homogeneity	
Homogenous	6 (21)
Heterogeneous	22 (79)
Border	
Indistinct	17 (61)
Distinct	11 (39)
Hyperechoic tubular structure	
Present	22 (79)
Absent	6 (21)

22 lesions (22/28, 79%) were heterogeneous. The borders were indistinct in 17 lesions (17/28, 61%), and hyperechoic tubular structures were seen in 22 lesions (22/28, 79%). Endoscopic biopsies using the bite-on-bite technique were performed in 21 lesions, and the mean count of eosinophils per HPF was 76 (range, 5–500). Significant eosinophil infiltration (≥30 per HPF) was seen in 12 lesions (12/21, 57%). A representative case (case 11) is shown in Figure 2.

During the median follow-up period of 9 months (range, 1–55 months), SETs decreased or subsided in 26 lesions (26/28, 93%) and there was no change in the size of two lesions (2/28, 7%). Of the 26 lesions which decreased or subsided, 16 lesions subsided completely during the median follow-up period of 8 months (range, 5–39 months). Among those with the presence or absence of hyperechoic tubular structures, all 22 lesions (100%) with hyperechoic tubular structures decreased or subsided, and only 4 of the 6 lesions (67%) without hyperechoic tubular structures decreased or subsided ($P = 0.040$). Of the 12 lesions with significant eosinophil infiltration, 10 lesions (83%) decreased or subsided, and all 9 lesions (100%) without significant eosinophil infiltration decreased or subsided ($P = 0.486$).

4. Discussion

Chronic gastric anisakiasis results from the invasion of the mucosal or submucosal layer by Anisakidae larvae, causing abscesses or eosinophilic granulomas; it can appear as a form of SET [3]. In the present study, characteristic EUS findings of chronic gastric anisakiasis were heterogeneously hypoechoic lesions with hyperechoic tubular structures, occurring mainly in the submucosal and/or muscularis propria layer. Most SET lesions decreased or subsided on the follow-up endoscopy. To our knowledge, this study is the first report of the EUS features of chronic gastric anisakiasis presenting as a SET and its natural course.

Anisakiasis is a zoonotic disease caused by an infection with the larvae of the nematode Anisakis, which migrates into the human viscera. The adult Anisakis lives in the stomach of marine mammals such as whales and dolphins. Crustaceans are the first intermediary hosts. The second intermediary hosts include various species of fishes and cuttlefishes. Humans are only accidentally contaminated [1, 8]. During the previous last 30 years, the number of reported gastrointestinal anisakiasis in the world literature is up to 13,000 with most cases reported in Korea and Japan, where raw fish is widely consumed. Favored fishes of Korean, such as mackerels, cods, Alaska pollacks, scabbard fish, and squids, are reported to be heavily infected with *Anisakis simplex* [9]. As a result, almost all the patients in the present study (27 patients) had a history of marine raw fish ingestion.

The clinical symptoms of gastric anisakiasis are classified as acute or chronic infections [10]. Acute anisakiasis infection is due to the invasion of the gastric wall by the larvae. The most common symptoms of acute gastric anisakiasis are severe epigastric pain, anorexia, and vomiting within 12 hours of raw fish ingestion [3]. Using endoscopy, the larvae can be found in 50% of patients with acute gastric anisakiasis [11], and mucosal edema, erythema, erosion, or ulceration can also be seen [12, 13]. Although the infection regresses gradually, it is sometimes misdiagnosed as a gastric ulcer or gastric cancer [14, 15]. Chronic anisakiasis infection is often difficult to diagnose because its symptoms are mild and nonspecific and the larvae are denaturalized and absorbed in the submucosal layer [16]. The diagnosis is often made incidentally during an endoscopy or after the discovery of a mass in the abdomen [17]. In the present study, only 6 patients (21%) had nonspecific symptoms such as dyspepsia or epigastric pain; the remaining 21 patients (79%) were asymptomatic.

Histologic findings of chronic anisakiasis are classified into four types according to the duration of infection and degree of larval denaturalization [3, 18]. The first type is the phlegmon type where larvae are located in the submucosal layer with eosinophil, neutrophil, and histiocyte infiltrations. The second type is the chronic abscess type; larvae are denaturalized, and an abscess is formed by eosinophils and fibrin. The third type is the abscess-granulomatous type. This type develops 6 months after Anisakidae larvae infection and shows progressive granuloma and fibrosis. The fourth type is the granulomatous type where the abscess becomes a granuloma. Considering these histologic findings arising mainly from the submucosal layer, chronic gastric anisakiasis appears as a SET-like morphology on endoscopy as shown in the present study.

EUS findings of acute gastric anisakiasis are thickening of the gastric wall, mainly of the submucosal layer with low echoic change [19]. However, there have been few reports of chronic gastric anisakiasis appearing as a SET and its EUS findings [5]. According to the present study, EUS findings that

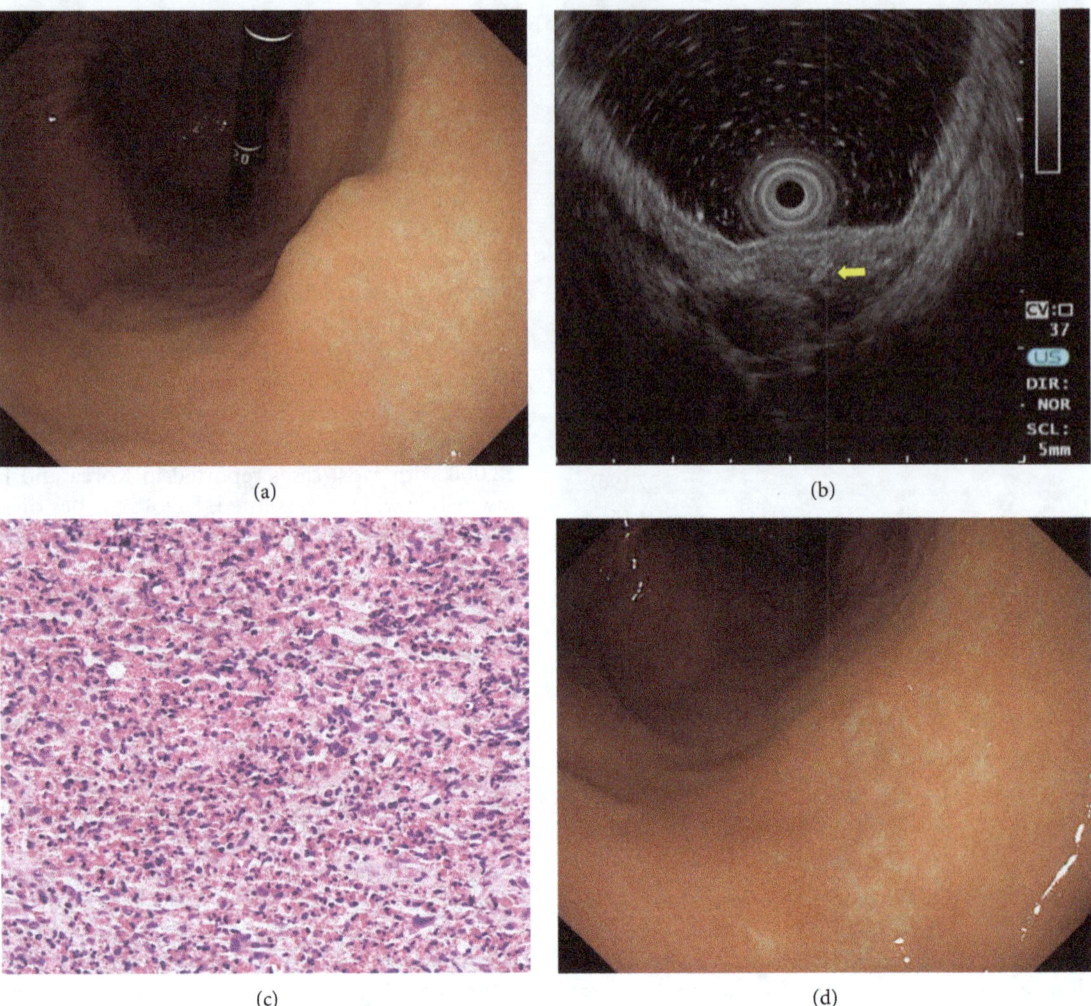

(a) (b) (c) (d)

Figure 2: A representative case of chronic gastric anisakiasis (case 11). (a) Initial endoscopy shows a subepithelial tumor-like lesion in the lesser curvature of the gastric midbody. (b) On endoscopic ultrasonography, the lesion is a heterogeneously hypoechoic lesion in the submucosal and muscularis propria layers. Hyperechoic tubular structures are seen inside the lesion (arrow). (c) Endoscopic biopsy reveals increased eosinophil infiltration (hematoxylin and eosin stain, ×400). (d) Follow-up endoscopy performed 6 months later shows that the lesion has subsided completely.

suggest chronic gastric anisakiasis are heterogeneously hypoechoic lesions with hyperechoic tubular structures, mainly in the submucosal and/or muscularis propria layer. These EUS findings are consistent with the aforementioned histologic findings of chronic anisakiasis: denaturalized larvae and abscess or granuloma formation in the submucosa. In particular, hyperechoic tubular structures are considered as indicative of the presence of a denaturalized larva. However, at a glance, these EUS findings are similar to those of gastric mesenchymal tumors, especially gastrointestinal stromal tumors [20, 21]. Therefore, some patients with chronic gastric anisakiasis undergo endoscopic or surgical resection to rule out the possibility of gastrointestinal stromal tumors [5, 22].

The role of endoscopic biopsy in chronic gastric anisakiasis is that endoscopic biopsy using the bite-on-bite technique enables us to obtain deep mucosal and submucosal tissues, which are the main pathologic sites of chronic anisakiasis. Thus, we could recognize the presence of eosinophils in all the lesions. However, eosinophils exist in the gastric mucosa of healthy persons or in some inflammatory conditions such as *Helicobacter pylori* gastritis and Crohn's disease. In a recent study involving the quantification of normal gastric eosinophil count, ≥30 eosinophils per HPF was suggested as the criteria of significantly increased eosinophils in gastric biopsies [7]. Based on these criteria, significant eosinophil infiltration was seen in 12 lesions (57%). The reason for this can be explained by the aforementioned histologic findings of chronic anisakiasis; as the time after the infection prolongs, the degree of eosinophil infiltration decreases.

Because chronic gastric anisakiasis is an inflammatory process, it is natural that the SET should decrease or subside. In addition, because the patients had a history of raw fish intake, characteristic EUS findings of chronic gastric anisakiasis, and significant eosinophil infiltration on biopsy, we decided to observe them rather than to perform endoscopic or surgical resection. As a result, most SETs (26/28, 93%) decreased or subsided; 16 lesions subsided completely during the median follow-up period of 8 months (range, 5–39 months). The median follow-up period for the 10 lesions, which decreased in size, was only 1 month (range, 1–55 months); in particular, the follow-up period for 9 lesions was less than 8 months. All lesions with hyperechoic tubular structures decreased or subsided. These results reveal that the lesions with hyperechoic tubular structures are in a relatively early state with the heavy inflammation of chronic anisakiasis compared to lesions without hyperechoic tubular structures.

This study had several limitations. First, there may have been potential selection or information biases resulting from the single-center retrospective nature of the study. Second, we did not confirm the Anisakidae larvae histopathologically. Immunologic methods using specific serum IgE antibody to *A. simplex* are reported to be helpful in the diagnosis of anisakiasis, but this antibody was detected in 25% of healthy controls and lacked specificity because of its cross-reactivity with other parasite antigens [23]. Furthermore, it is not generally available; thus, we could not utilize it in the present study. However, we experienced several cases of chronic gastric anisakiasis which was histopathologically confirmed by endoscopic or surgical resection, and then, we came to understand the EUS findings and corresponding histopathology of chronic anisakiasis. Finally, we did not perform endoscopic biopsies to evaluate the change in eosinophil counts on the follow-up endoscopy.

5. Conclusions

Although it is rare, chronic gastric anisakiasis should be included in the differential diagnoses for gastric SETs, especially in regions where raw fish is widely consumed. EUS findings suggesting chronic gastric anisakiasis include heterogeneously hypoechoic lesions with hyperechoic tubular structures, mainly in the submucosal and/or muscularis propria layers. In addition, endoscopic biopsy results showing significant eosinophil infiltration increase the possibility of chronic anisakiasis. Because chronic gastric anisakiasis decreases or subsides in most cases, follow-up endoscopy performed 6 to 12 months later is recommended.

Disclosure

This study was presented as a poster at the Korea Digestive Disease Week, Seoul, Republic of Korea, 23–25 November 2017. Eun Young Park and Dong Hoon Baek share co-first authorships.

Authors' Contributions

Gwang Ha Kim and Do Youn Park designed the research/study. Eun Young Park, Dong Hoon Baek, Gwang Ha Kim, and Bong Eun Lee collected the data. Eun Young Park, Dong Hoon Baek, and Gwang Ha Kim wrote the paper. Eun Young Park, Dong Hoon Baek, and So-Jeong Lee analyzed the data. Dong Hoon Baek and Gwang Ha Kim performed the study. Bong Eun Lee and So-Jeong Lee reviewed the data of the study population. All authors read and approved the final version of this manuscript.

Acknowledgments

This study was supported by a grant from the National R&D Program for Cancer Control, Ministry for Health, Welfare and Family Affairs, Republic of Korea (0920050) and by the Medical Research Center Program through the National Research Foundation Grant funded by the Korean Government (NRF-2015R1A5A2009656).

References

[1] P. H. Van Thiel, F. C. Kuipers, and R. T. Roskam, "A nematode parasitic to herring, causing acute abdominal syndromes in man," *Tropical and Geographical Medicine*, vol. 12, pp. 97–113, 1960.

[2] K. Ikeda, R. Kumashiro, and T. Kifune, "Nine cases of acute gastric anisakiasis," *Gastrointestinal Endoscopy*, vol. 35, no. 4, pp. 304–308, 1989.

[3] S. G. Kim, Y. J. Jo, Y. S. Park et al., "Four cases of gastric submucosal mass suspected as anisakiasis," *The Korean Journal of Parasitology*, vol. 44, no. 1, pp. 81–86, 2006.

[4] S. W. Park, Y. E. Joo, P. J. Jung et al., "Three cases of gastric anisakiasis mimicking submucosal tumor," *Korean Journal of Gastrointestinal Endoscopy*, vol. 32, no. 6, pp. 381–386, 2006.

[5] J. W. Choi, B. K. Park, Y. R. Kim et al., "Endoscopic ultrasonographic findings of two cases of parasitic eosinophilic granuloma in the stomach," *Korean Journal of Gastrointestinal Endoscopy*, vol. 30, pp. 267–272, 2005.

[6] T. Yamada and H. Ichikawa, "X-ray diagnosis of elevated lesions of the stomach," *Radiology*, vol. 110, no. 1, pp. 79–83, 1974.

[7] T. Lwin, S. D. Melton, and R. M. Genta, "Eosinophilic gastritis: histopathological characterization and quantification of the normal gastric eosinophil content," *Modern Pathology*, vol. 24, no. 4, pp. 556–563, 2011.

[8] H. Ishikura, K. Kikuchi, K. Nagasawa et al., "Anisakidae and anisakidosis," *Progress in Clinical Parasitology*, vol. 3, pp. 43–102, 1993.

[9] S. H. Choi, J. Kim, J. O. Jo et al., "*Anisakis simplex* larvae: infection status in marine fish and cephalopods purchased from the Cooperative Fish Market in Busan, Korea," *The Korean Journal of Parasitology*, vol. 49, no. 1, pp. 39–44, 2011.

[10] A. Alonso-Gómez, A. Moreno-Ancillo, M. C. López-Serrano et al., "*Anisakis simplex* only provokes allergic symptoms when the worm parasitises the gastrointestinal tract," *Parasitology Research*, vol. 93, no. 5, pp. 378–384, 2004.

[11] A. Repiso Ortega, M. Alcántara Torres, C. González de Frutos et al., "Gastrointestinal anisakiasis. Study of a series of 25 patients," *Gastroenterología y Hepatología*, vol. 26, no. 6, pp. 341–346, 2003.

[12] H. Ohtaki and R. Ohtaki, "Clinical manifestation of gastric anisakiasis," in *Gastric Anisakiasis in Japan: Epidemiology, Diagnosis, Treatment*, pp. 37–46, Springer, Tokyo, Japan, 1989.

[13] S. Kakizoe, H. Kakizoe, K. Kakizoe et al., "Endoscopic findings and clinical manifestation of gastric anisakiasis," *The American Journal of Gastroenterology*, vol. 90, no. 5, pp. 761–763, 1995.

[14] K. Hiramatsu, S. Kamiyamamoto, H. Ogino et al., "A case of acute gastric anisakiasis presenting with malignant tumor-like features: a large gastric vanishing tumor accompanied by local lymph node swelling," *Digestive Diseases and Sciences*, vol. 49, no. 6, pp. 965–969, 2004.

[15] D. B. Kang, W. C. Park, and J. K. Lee, "Chronic gastric anisakiasis provoking a bleeding gastric ulcer," *Annals of Surgical Treatment and Research*, vol. 86, no. 5, pp. 270–273, 2014.

[16] K. Fujisawa, T. Matsumoto, R. Yoshimura, S. Ayabe, and M. Tominaga, "Endoscopic finding of a large vanishing tumor," *Endoscopy*, vol. 33, no. 9, p. 820, 2001.

[17] M. Céspedes, A. Saez, I. Rodríguez, J. M. Pinto, and R. Rodríguez, "Chronic anisakiasis presenting as a mesenteric mass," *Abdominal Imaging*, vol. 25, no. 5, pp. 548–550, 2000.

[18] K. Kojima, T. Koyanagi, and K. Shiraki, "Pathological study of anisakiasis (parasitic abscess of the digestive tract)," *Nihon Rinsho*, vol. 24, no. 12, pp. 2314–2323, 1966.

[19] K. Sakai, A. Ohtani, H. Muta et al., "Endoscopic ultrasonography findings in acute gastric anisakiasis," *The American Journal of Gastroenterology*, vol. 87, no. 11, pp. 1618–1623, 1992.

[20] G. H. Kim, D. Y. Park, S. Kim et al., "Is it possible to differentiate gastric GISTs from gastric leiomyomas by EUS?," *World Journal of Gastroenterology*, vol. 15, no. 27, pp. 3376–3381, 2009.

[21] J. M. Yoon, G. H. Kim, D. Y. Park et al., "Endosonographic features of gastric schwannoma: a single center experience," *Clinical Endoscopy*, vol. 49, no. 6, pp. 548–554, 2016.

[22] J. H. Kang, E. J. Park, Y. B. Cho, Y. S. Kim, M. S. Lee, and C. S. Sim, "2 cases of submucosal tumors caused by gastric anisakiasis," *Korean Journal of Gastrointestinal Endoscopy*, vol. 19, no. 1, pp. 67–72, 1999.

[23] M. J. Perteguer, T. Chivato, A. Montoro, C. Cuellar, J. M. Mateos, and R. Laguna, "Specific and total IgE in patients with recurrent, acute urticaria caused by *Anisakis simplex*," *Annals of Tropical Medicine & Parasitology*, vol. 94, no. 3, pp. 259–268, 2000.

23

Predicting the Development of Gastric Neoplasms in a Healthcare Cohort by Combining *Helicobacter pylori* Antibodies and Serum Pepsinogen

Min-Sun Kwak, Goh Eun Chung, Su Jin Chung, Seung Joo Kang, Jong In Yang, and Joo Sung Kim

Department of Internal Medicine, Healthcare Research Institute, Healthcare System Gangnam Center, Seoul National University Hospital, Seoul, Republic of Korea

Correspondence should be addressed to Goh Eun Chung; gohwom@hanmail.net

Academic Editor: Maria P. Dore

Background. Helicobacter pylori (HP) and gastric atrophy are risk factors for gastric cancer. We evaluated whether the combination of serum HP antibody and pepsinogen (PG), which is indicative of gastric atrophy, could serve as a predictive marker for the development of gastric neoplasms in a Korean population. *Methods.* The subjects who had undergone health-screening examination with endoscopic follow-ups were classified into the following 4 groups according to serum PG status and *HP* antibody at baseline: group A (*HP* (−), normal PG), group B (*HP* (+), normal PG), group C (*HP* (+), atrophic PG), and group D (*HP* (−), atrophic PG). We compared the development of gastric neoplasms among the groups. *Results.* Of the 3297 subjects, 1239 (37.6%) were categorized as group A, 1484 (45.0%) as group B, 536 (16.3%) as group C, and 38 (1.2%) as group D. During the 5.6 years of mean follow-up period, the annual incidence of gastric neoplasms increased gradually by 0.06% in group A, 0.16% in group B, 0.38% in group C, and 0.49% in group D. A Cox proportional hazard model showed increased development of gastric neoplasms according to group (P for trend = 0.025). Compared to group A, the hazard ratio was 8.25 for group D (95% confidence interval 0.2–74.24), 5.35 for group C (1.68–17.05), and 2.65 for group B (0.86–8.14). *Conclusion.* The combination of serum PG and *HP* antibody is useful for predicting the development of gastric neoplasms, including cancer and adenoma, in a Korean population using endoscopic surveillance.

1. Introduction

Gastric cancer is one of the major causes of cancer-related death worldwide, and approximately 990,000 cases of gastric cancer are diagnosed annually [1]. In Eastern Asia, including Japan and South Korea, gastric cancer is the most prevalent cancer [2]. According to Correa's cascade, multiple processes, which are known as the gastritis–atrophy–metaplasia–dysplasia–cancer sequence, are responsible for the development of the intestinal type of gastric cancer, which is thought to represent a major route of stomach carcinogenesis in Eastern Asia [3, 4].

Helicobacter pylori (HP) infections and the associated chronic atrophic gastritis (CAG) are two well-known major risk factors for the development of gastric cancer [5, 6]. Previous studies have typically assessed gastric atrophy by measuring the pepsinogen (PG) levels in serum samples [7, 8]. Both PG I and II are produced by chief cells and mucous neck cells of the stomach, but PG II is also produced by pyloric gland cells [9, 10]. As gastric atrophy develops, chief cells are replaced by pyloric glands, leading to a decrease in the levels of PG I, while the levels of PG II remain relatively unaffected. Therefore, both low serum PG I and a low PG I/II ratio are recognized as serological markers of gastric atrophy [11].

In Japan, the ABCD prediction model, which combines the *HP* serology test and serum PG test, has been widely used to stratify the general population according to the risk of stomach cancer. This method is simple and less invasive than esophagogastroduodenoscopy. In the ABCD method,

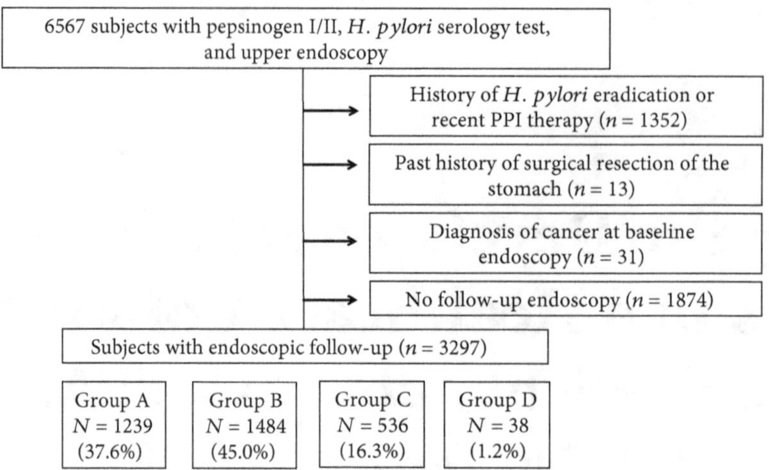

Figure 1: Flowchart of subjects in this study.

individuals are classified into four groups as follows: (1) immunoglobulin G (IgG) anti-*HP* antibody-negative and normal PG level (group A), (2) IgG anti-*HP* antibody-positive and normal PG level (group B), (3) IgG anti-*HP* antibody-positive and atrophic PG test (group C), and (4) IgG anti-*HP* antibody-negative and atrophic PG test (group D). A previous cross-sectional study revealed an increasing trend of gastric cancer in the order of group A to group D [8]. In Japan, a prospective study also demonstrated that the ABCD method predicts the development of gastric cancer [7]. In a recent meta-analysis, this four-risk group model, which combines the serum PG test and *HP* antibodies, was shown to categorize risk-stratified asymptomatic adults into the four risk groups of incident gastric cancer with moderate accuracy [6].

However, the ABCD method has several limitations. First, most studies were performed only in Japan [6], and there is a racial-ethnic difference in the occurrence of gastric cancer [12]. Second, the ABCD method was shown to be associated with gastric neoplasms, including not only gastric cancer but also gastric adenoma in cross-sectional analysis [13]. Because most premalignant gastric lesions can be treated with endoscopic treatment, evaluating the applicability of the ABCD method to predict not only gastric cancer but also gastric adenoma in a longitudinal study is important. Thus, this longitudinal cohort study aimed to evaluate whether or not the ABCD method, which combines serum PG and *HP* antibody tests, could predict the development of gastric cancer and gastric adenoma in a healthy Korean population using an annual or biennial endoscopic follow-up.

2. Methods

2.1. Study Population. In total, 6567 subjects who had undergone serum PG and *HP* IgG antibody testing and esophagogastroduodenoscopy on the same day during a health-screening examination at Seoul National University Hospital Gangnam Center between March 2008 and December 2009 were initially included. Overall, 1352 subjects with a prior history of *HP* eradication or recent proton-pump inhibitor therapy 1 month prior to enrollment and 13 subjects with a past history of gastric surgery were excluded. Thirty-one subjects who were diagnosed with gastric cancer at baseline and 1874 subjects without any follow-up endoscopy were also excluded (Figure 1). Subjects were encouraged to undergo an endoscopic examination annually to screen for the development of stomach cancer, and these follow-up data were analyzed in this study.

This study protocol conformed to the ethical guidelines of the 1975 Declaration of Helsinki and was approved by the Institutional Review Board of Seoul National University Hospital (1504-044-663). The need for informed consent was waived by the Institutional Review Board of Seoul National University Hospital because the researchers accessed only deidentified databases for analytical purposes.

2.2. Serum HP IgG Antibody Assay. Anti-*HP* antibody IgG (anti-*HP* Ab IgG) was measured using an enzyme-linked immunosorbent assay kit (Radim Diagnostics, Rome, Italy) and an automatic analyzer, Alisei® (Seac, Pomezia, Italy), which was previously validated in a nationwide Korean seroepidemiologic study [14, 15]. Anti-*HP* levels higher than 15 RU/mL were considered positive.

2.3. Serum PG Levels. Serum levels of PG I and II were measured using a latex-enhanced turbidimetric immunoassay (HBi Corp., Seoul, Korea, imported from Shima Laboratories, Tokyo, Japan), and the PG I-to-PG II ratios (PG I/II) were calculated. Serum PG status was defined as "atrophic" when both criteria of a serum PG I level $\leq$ 70 ng/mL and a PG I/II ratio $\leq$ 3.0 were simultaneously fulfilled, which is the most widely used definition [16]. All other cases were classified as "normal."

2.4. Classification of Subjects according to the ABCD Method. Subjects were classified into 4 groups according to the prediction by the ABCD method, which combined the serum PG status and *HP* antibody testing. According to the original ABC method, "atrophy" was defined as PGI $\leq$ 70 ng/mL and PG I/II $\leq$ 3 [7, 17]. Subjects were divided as follows: group

TABLE 1: Baseline characteristics of subjects according to the group.

	Total	Group A	Group B	Group C	Group D	P value
Number of subjects (%)	3297 (100%)	1239 (37.6%)	1484 (45.0%)	536 (16.3%)	38 (1.2%)	
H. pylori Ab		Negative	Positive	Positive	Negative	
Pepsinogen		Normal	Normal	Atrophic	Atrophic	
Age (years)[a]	51.3 ± 9.4	50.0 ± 9.6	51.0 ± 8.8	55.1 ± 9.4	53.3 ± 8.3	0.039
Male sex (%)	2326 (70.5%)	854 (68.9%)	1096 (73.9%)	353 (65.9%)	22 (57.9%)	<0.001
Pepsinogen I (ng/mL)[a]	57.8 ± 29.9	49.9 ± 25.5	71.0 ± 31.7	42.5 ± 16.3	19.3 ± 12.2	<0.001
Pepsinogen II (ng/mL)[a]	14.7 ± 9.1	8.9 ± 4.8	18.0 ± 10.0	19.3 ± 7.3	11.0 ± 4.9	0.013
Pepsinogen I/II ratio[a]	4.5 ± 1.8	5.8 ± 1.4	4.3 ± 1.3	2.2 ± 0.6	1.8 ± 0.9	<0.001
Follow-up duration (years)[a]	5.6 ± 2.0	5.6 ± 1.9	5.5 ± 2.0	5.5 ± 2.0	5.4 ± 2.0	0.404
Follow-up duration (months (median, range))	80 (12–104)	81 (12–103)	79 (12–104)	79 (12–104)	77 (22–102)	0.325

[a]Mean ± SD.

TABLE 2: Characteristics of incidental gastric cancer and adenoma during follow-up according to the group.

	Total	Group A (n = 1239)	Group B (n = 1484)	Group C (n = 536)	Group D (n = 38)
Incidence of gastric cancer	**15**	**1**	7	7	**0**
Intestinal type	12	0	6	6	0
Diffuse type	3	1	1	1	0
Incidence of gastric adenoma	**14**	**3**	**6**	**4**	**1**
Low-grade adenoma	10	2	4	3	1
High-grade adenoma	4	1	2	1	0
Annual incidence rate (%/year)	**0.16**	**0.06**	**0.16**	**0.38**	**0.49**

A (*HP* (−), normal PG status), group B (*HP* (+), normal PG status), group C (*HP* (+), atrophic PG status), and group D (*HP* (−), atrophic PG status).

2.5. Endoscopic Examination and Follow-Up. Fifteen experienced board-certified endoscopists performed esophagogastroduodenoscopy using GIF-H260 (Olympus, Tokyo, Japan), EG-405WR5, or EG-590WR (Fuji-non, Saitama, Japan). A follow-up endoscopy was recommended within 1 or 2 years. The endoscopists performed the endoscopic examination without knowledge of the serological data of the subjects. A gastric biopsy was performed when a lesion was suspected to be gastric cancer, and the biopsies were examined by expert gastrointestinal pathologists according to the World Health Organization (WHO) criteria [18]. Gastric adenoma was considered low-grade adenoma or high-grade adenoma according to the Vienna classification [19]. Gastric cancer was classified as a differentiated type (including well or moderately differentiated adenocarcinomas) and undifferentiated type (including poorly differentiated, signet-ring cell, and mucinous carcinomas) [20]. Gastric cancer was also classified according to Lauren's criteria as intestinal and diffuse types [21].

2.6. Statistical Analysis. The primary outcome in this study was the development of gastric cancer or adenoma. The data are expressed as the mean ± standard deviation or median (interquartile range) for continuous variables and frequency (%) for categorical variables. Analysis of variance (ANOVA) was used to analyze the continuous variables, and a Kruskal-Wallis test with Bonferroni's correction was used to analyze the categorical variables. The Kaplan-Meier method and Cox proportional hazard regression analysis were used to evaluate the development of gastric cancer or high-grade adenoma. All statistical analyses were conducted using SPSS 19 (SPSS Inc., Chicago, IL, USA). A two-tailed P value < 0.05 was considered statistically significant.

3. Results

3.1. Baseline Characteristics. In total, 3297 subjects were included in the analysis. Table 1 shows the baseline characteristics of the study subjects. The mean age was 51.3 years, and 70.5% of the subjects were male. Of the 3297 subjects, 1239 (37.6%) were categorized as group A, 1484 (45.0%) were categorized as group B, 536 (16.3%) were categorized as group C, and 38 (1.2%) were categorized as group D. The mean follow-up duration was 5.6 years.

3.2. Development of Gastric Neoplasms according to the HP Antibody and Serum PG Levels. Table 2 shows the development of gastric neoplasms during the follow-up period according to the groups. A total of 15 gastric cancers and 14 gastric adenomas developed among the 3297 subjects during the follow-up period. The mean age at diagnosis was 56.8 years, and 23 subjects (79.3%) were male. The annual

TABLE 3: Hazard ratio for the incidence of gastric adenoma and cancer by Cox regression analysis.

	Hazard ratio	95% confidence interval	*P* value
Group			
A	1		0.025[a]
B	2.65	0.86–8.14	0.088
C	5.35	1.68–17.05	0.005
D	8.25	0.92–74.24	0.060
Age	1.049	1.008–1.091	0.018
Male sex	1.716	0.692–4.254	0.244

[a]*P* for trend.

incidence rate of gastric neoplasms was 0.16%/year. Most gastric cancers were the intestinal type (12/15, 80%), and diffuse-type cancers developed in only 3 subjects (3/15, 20%). Regarding adenoma, 71.4% of the total cases developed low-grade adenoma. The annual incidence rate of gastric cancer or gastric adenoma also increased according to the ABCD group classification by 0.06% in group A, 0.16% in group B, 0.38% in group C, and 0.49% in group D.

The details regarding the incidental gastric neoplasms in the *HP*-negative subjects (group A) in this study are presented in Supplementary Table 1. One case exhibited a new *HP* infection during the follow-up period (1 year after enrollment) and developed high-grade adenoma 6 years later. The other female subjects had developed signet-ring cell carcinoma. Two cases with low-grade adenoma showed no evidence of pathological and serological *HP* infections during the follow-up period, and both cases were successfully treated with endoscopic mucosal resection.

3.3. Prediction of the Development of Gastric Neoplasms according to the ABCD Group. The Cox proportional hazard model (Table 3, Figure 2) showed an increased development of gastric neoplasms, including gastric cancer and adenoma, according to the group (*P* for trend = 0.025). Compared to group A, the hazard ratio was 8.25 for group D (95% confidence interval (CI) 0.2–74.24), 5.35 for group C (95% CI 1.68–17.05), and 2.65 for group B (0.86–8.14).

By considering only gastric cancer or high-grade adenoma, the Cox proportional hazard model (Table 4, Figure 3) showed an increased development of gastric cancer or high-grade adenoma according to the group (*P* for trend = 0.040). Compared to group A, the hazard ratio was 7.10 for groups C or D (95% confidence interval (CI) 1.48–34.01, *P* = 0.042) and 3.45 for group B (95% CI 0.74–16.01).

4. Discussion

This study showed an increased development of gastric neoplasms (including gastric adenoma and gastric cancer) in the order of group A (*HP* Ab (−)/atrophy (−) group) to group B (*HP* Ab (+)/atrophy (−) group), group C (*HP* Ab (+)/atrophy (+) group), and group D (*HP* Ab (−)/atrophy (+) group) during the follow-up period (mean of 5.6 years). To date, most studies evaluating the usefulness of the ABCD method have

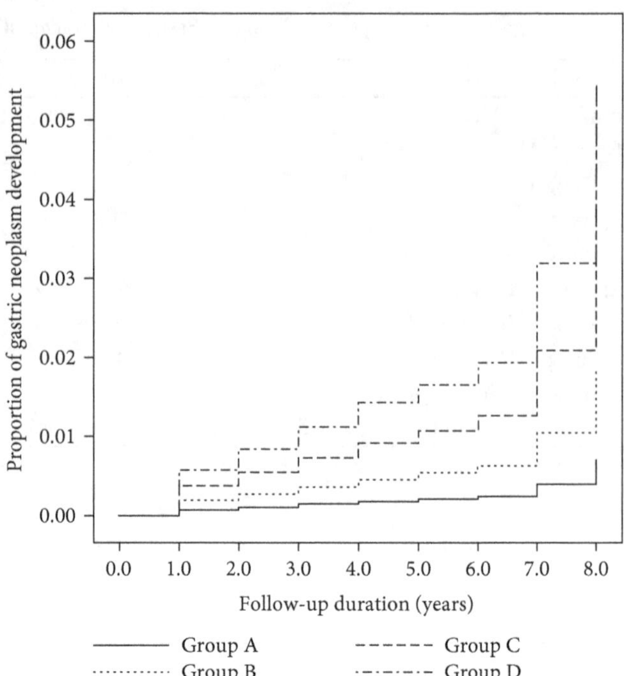

FIGURE 2: Incidence of gastric neoplasm according to the groups. This figure shows Cox regression analysis for the incidence of gastric cancer and gastric adenoma according to the groups (classified by *H. pylori* antibody status and pepsinogen status).

TABLE 4: Hazard ratio for the incidence of high-grade gastric adenoma and cancer by Cox regression analysis.

	Hazard ratio	95% confidence interval	*P* value
Group			
A	1		0.040[a]
B	3.45	0.74–16.01	0.114
C or D	7.10	1.48–34.01	0.014
Age	1.05	1.00-1.10	0.042
Male sex	2.45	0.71–8.53	0.158

[a]*P* for trend.

been performed in Japan, and this study confirmed the usefulness of the ABCD method in Korea, which is another area with a high prevalence of gastric cancer. Therefore, the ABCD method, which is noninvasive and conveniently combines the *HP* IgG antibody and serum PG levels, is useful for risk stratification of the development of gastric neoplasms in a Korean population.

Consistent with previous studies, compared to subjects in group A, the highest gastric neoplasm incidence was observed in group D, followed by group C and then group B with hazard ratios of 8.25, 5.35, and 2.65, respectively. Although there was a higher tendency of cancer development in group B than in group A, there was no statistically significant difference between these two groups (*P* = 0.088). Thus, the development of gastric cancer requires time in subjects with *HP* infections without atrophy because *HP*-induced

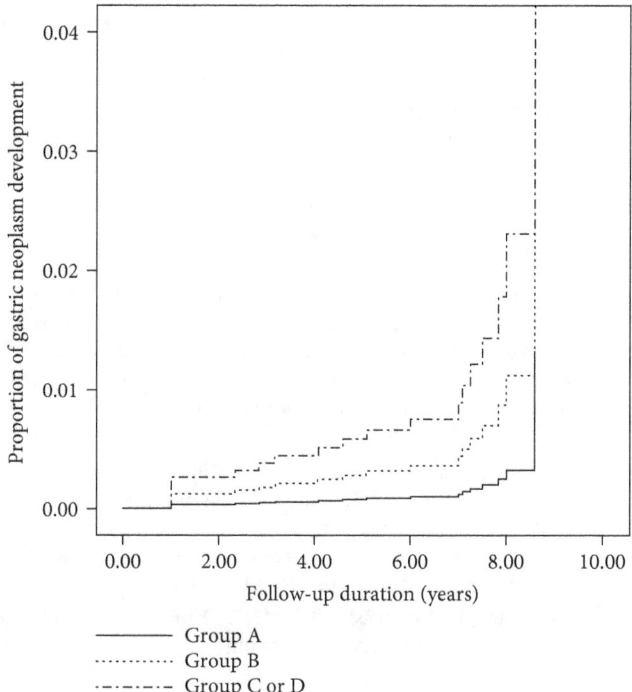

Figure 3: Incidence of gastric cancer and high-grade adenoma according to the groups. This figure shows Cox regression analysis for the incidence of gastric cancer and high-grade gastric adenoma according to the groups (classified by *H. pylori* antibody status and pepsinogen status).

gastric cancer usually develops through a gastritis-atrophy-metaplastic change. Previous studies with longer follow-up periods (more than 10 years) showed a significant difference in gastric cancer development between groups A and B [22], but studies with shorter follow-up periods showed a higher but not significant difference between group A and group B [7, 23].

In contrast to previous studies, the participants in group D did not develop gastric cancer or high-grade adenoma. In the present study, only 1 low-grade adenoma occurred in group D. However, this finding should not be considered evidence that the risk in group D is low in the Korean population because only a small number of subjects were categorized as group D ($n = 38$, 1.2%). In previous studies, the proportion of group D ranged from 0.7 to 6.3% [7, 22–24], and the proportion of group D was relatively low in this study. This finding might be related to a lower seroclearance of *HP* Ab in Korean subjects or an earlier development of stomach cancer in Korean subjects before the seroclearance of *HP* Ab. A previous meta-analysis similarly failed to show a significant difference between group C and group D [6]. A recent 20-year prospective study in Hisayama showed that the cumulative incidence of gastric cancer was significantly increased in groups B, C, and D. However, no significant difference was found between groups C and D, which is consistent with our results [22]. Thus, more large-scale long-term studies should be performed to draw a confirmative conclusion.

Although the incidence rate was extremely low, gastric cancer developed in group A. *HP*-negative gastric cancer is rare, is most likely to be a diffuse type, and lacks male dominancy [25]. Group A has been recently shown to include not only "true group A" but also subjects with endoscopic atrophy with a previous history of *HP* eradication and a spontaneous resolution of a previous *HP* infection [26–28]. More data should be collected to define *HP*-negative stomach cancer and identify the mechanism of cancer occurrence in these subjects.

This study has several strengths. First, this study was the first Korean large-scale longitudinal study with a follow-up period longer than 5 years. Most previous studies were performed in Japan. Because the occurrence of stomach cancer shows ethnic differences, validation in other populations might be helpful for the identification of the mechanism of gastric carcinogenesis. Second, the incidence of both gastric cancer and gastric adenoma was evaluated. Third, regular endoscopic surveillance was performed in this study, while most previous prospective studies evaluated the incidence of gastric cancer based on the double-contrast barium X-ray and PG test, followed by endoscopy. In this case, the incidence of cancer in groups C or D could be overestimated. Fourth, a previous history of *HP* eradication or PPI therapy could be thoroughly examined using a specific questionnaire.

This study also has several limitations. First, studies with longer follow-up duration should be conducted [29, 30]. Although the follow-up duration was more than 5 years in this study, a follow-up of these patients for more than 10–15 years may increase our understanding of the predictability of these serum markers. Second, although we excluded subjects who had a history of *HP* eradication at baseline, subjects who had eradication of *HP* during the follow-up period were not excluded. Third, subjects with new *HP* infections during the follow-up period were not excluded. Fourth, we showed baseline pepsinogen levels in this study, not the change of pepsinogen level during follow-up. Further study with follow-up pepsinogen levels might give more information about the change of functional status of the stomach according to the different risk subgroups. Fifth, we could not confirm whether the serum pepsinogen test reflects the severity of histological atrophy, because we did not perform routine biopsy for evaluation of gastric mucosa damage except for the presence of endoscopic abnormal lesions. However, correlation between serological evaluation by pepsinogen test and the severity of histological damage by operative link on gastritis assessment and operative link on gastritis/intestinal-metaplasia assessment staging system is well established [31].

In conclusion, this longitudinal cohort study showed that the ABCD method, which combines serum PG and *HP* antibody tests, is useful for predicting the development of gastric neoplasms, including cancer and adenoma, in a healthy Korean population using endoscopic surveillance.

Authors' Contributions

Min-Sun Kwak, Goh Eun Chung, and Su Jin Chung were responsible for research conception and design. Min-Sun Kwak, Goh Eun Chung, Su Jin Chung, Seung Joo Kang, Jong In Yang, and Joo Sung Kim were responsible for data acquisition. Min-Sun Kwak and Goh Eun Chung were responsible for data analysis and interpretation, statistical analysis, and drafting of the manuscript. Su Jin Chung, Seung Joo Kang, Jong In Yang, and Joo Sung Kim were responsible for critical revision of the manuscript. All authors were responsible for approval of the final manuscript.

References

[1] A. Jemal, F. Bray, M. M. Center, J. Ferlay, E. Ward, and D. Forman, "Global cancer statistics," *CA: a Cancer Journal for Clinicians*, vol. 61, no. 2, pp. 69–90, 2011.

[2] F. Bray, J. S. Ren, E. Masuyer, and J. Ferlay, "Global estimates of cancer prevalence for 27 sites in the adult population in 2008," *International Journal of Cancer*, vol. 132, no. 5, pp. 1133–1145, 2013.

[3] P. Correa, "Human gastric carcinogenesis: a multistep and multifactorial process—First American Cancer Society award lecture on cancer epidemiology and prevention," *Cancer Research*, vol. 52, no. 24, pp. 6735–6740, 1992.

[4] P. Correa and J. Houghton, "Carcinogenesis of *Helicobacter pylori*," *Gastroenterology*, vol. 133, no. 2, pp. 659–672, 2007.

[5] N. Uemura, S. Okamoto, S. Yamamoto et al., "*Helicobacter pylori* infection and the development of gastric cancer," *The New England Journal of Medicine*, vol. 345, no. 11, pp. 784–789, 2001.

[6] T. Terasawa, H. Nishida, K. Kato et al., "Prediction of gastric cancer development by serum pepsinogen test and *Helicobacter pylori* seropositivity in Eastern Asians: a systematic review and meta-analysis," *PLoS One*, vol. 9, no. 10, article e109783, 2014.

[7] H. Watabe, T. Mitsushima, Y. Yamaji et al., "Predicting the development of gastric cancer from combining *Helicobacter pylori* antibodies and serum pepsinogen status: a prospective endoscopic cohort study," *Gut*, vol. 54, no. 6, pp. 764–768, 2005.

[8] Y. Yamaji, T. Mitsushima, H. Ikuma et al., "Inverse background of *Helicobacter pylori* antibody and pepsinogen in reflux oesophagitis compared with gastric cancer: analysis of 5732 Japanese subjects," *Gut*, vol. 49, no. 3, pp. 335–340, 2001.

[9] I. M. Samloff and W. M. Liebman, "Cellular localization of the group II pepsinogens in human stomach and duodenum by immunofluorescence," *Gastroenterology*, vol. 65, no. 1, pp. 36–42, 1973.

[10] I. M. Samloff, "Cellular localization of group I pepsinogens in human gastric mucosa by immunofluorescence," *Gastroenterology*, vol. 61, no. 2, pp. 185–188, 1971.

[11] K. Miki, M. Ichinose, N. Kakei et al., "The clinical application of the serum pepsinogen I and II levels as a mass screening method for gastric cancer," *Advances in Experimental Medicine and Biology*, vol. 362, pp. 139–143, 1995.

[12] E. Lee, L. Liu, J. Zhang et al., "Stomach cancer disparity among Korean Americans by tumor characteristics: comparison with non-Hispanic whites, Japanese Americans, South Koreans, and Japanese," *Cancer Epidemiology, Biomarkers & Prevention*, vol. 26, no. 4, pp. 587–596, 2017.

[13] H. S. Choi, S. Y. Lee, J. H. Kim et al., "Combining the serum pepsinogen level and *Helicobacter pylori* antibody test for predicting the histology of gastric neoplasm," *Journal of Digestive Diseases*, vol. 15, no. 6, pp. 293–298, 2014.

[14] J. Y. Yim, N. Kim, S. H. Choi et al., "Seroprevalence of *Helicobacter pylori* in South Korea," *Helicobacter*, vol. 12, no. 4, pp. 333–340, 2007.

[15] S. J. Chung, S. H. Lim, J. Choi et al., "*Helicobacter pylori* serology inversely correlated with the risk and severity of reflux esophagitis in *Helicobacter pylori* endemic area: a matched case-control study of 5,616 health check-up Koreans," *Journal of Neurogastroenterology and Motility*, vol. 17, no. 3, pp. 267–273, 2011.

[16] M. Dinis-Ribeiro, G. Yamaki, K. Miki, A. Costa-Pereira, M. Matsukawa, and M. Kurihara, "Meta-analysis on the validity of pepsinogen test for gastric carcinoma, dysplasia or chronic atrophic gastritis screening," *Journal of Medical Screening*, vol. 11, no. 3, pp. 141–147, 2004.

[17] F. Kitahara, K. Kobayashi, T. Sato, Y. Kojima, T. Araki, and M. A. Fujino, "Accuracy of screening for gastric cancer using serum pepsinogen concentrations," *Gut*, vol. 44, no. 5, pp. 693–697, 1999.

[18] S. R. Hamilton and L. A. Aaltonene, "World Health Organization classification of tumours," in *Pathology and Genetics of Tumours of the Digestive System*, IARC Press, Lyon, 2000.

[19] R. J. Schlemper, R. H. Riddell, Y. Kato et al., "The Vienna classification of gastrointestinal epithelial neoplasia," *Gut*, vol. 47, no. 2, pp. 251–255, 2000.

[20] A. Japanese Gastric Cancer, "Japanese classification of gastric carcinoma—2nd English edition," *Gastric Cancer*, vol. 1, no. 1, pp. 10–24, 1998.

[21] B. Hu, N. El Hajj, S. Sittler, N. Lammert, R. Barnes, and A. Meloni-Ehrig, "Gastric cancer: classification, histology and application of molecular pathology," *Journal of Gastrointestinal Oncology*, vol. 3, no. 3, pp. 251–261, 2012.

[22] F. Ikeda, K. Shikata, J. Hata et al., "Combination of *helicobacter pylori* antibody and serum pepsinogen as a good predictive tool of gastric cancer incidence: 20-year prospective data from the Hisayama study," *Journal of Epidemiology*, vol. 26, no. 12, pp. 629–636, 2016.

[23] H. Ohata, S. Kitauchi, N. Yoshimura et al., "Progression of chronic atrophic gastritis associated with *Helicobacter pylori* infection increases risk of gastric cancer," *International Journal of Cancer*, vol. 109, no. 1, pp. 138–143, 2004.

[24] H. Charvat, S. Sasazuki, M. Inoue et al., "Prediction of the 10-year probability of gastric cancer occurrence in the Japanese population: the JPHC study cohort II," *International Journal of Cancer*, vol. 138, no. 2, pp. 320–331, 2016.

[25] T. Matsuo, M. Ito, S. Takata, S. Tanaka, M. Yoshihara, and K. Chayama, "Low prevalence of *Helicobacter pylori*-negative gastric cancer among Japanese," *Helicobacter*, vol. 16, no. 6, pp. 415–419, 2011.

[26] T. Boda, M. Ito, M. Yoshihara et al., "Advanced method for evaluation of gastric cancer risk by serum markers: determination of true low-risk subjects for gastric neoplasm," *Helicobacter*, vol. 19, no. 1, pp. 1–8, 2014.

[27] K. Miura, H. Okada, Y. Kouno et al., "Actual status of involvement of *Helicobacter pylori* infection that developed gastric

cancer from group a of ABC (D) stratification—study of early gastric cancer cases that underwent endoscopic submucosal dissection," *Digestion*, vol. 94, no. 1, pp. 17–23, 2016.

[28] K. Miki, "Gastric cancer screening by combined assay for serum anti-*Helicobacter pylori* IgG antibody and serum pepsinogen levels—"ABC method"," *Proceedings of the Japan Academy, Series B Physical and Biological Sciences*, vol. 87, no. 7, pp. 405–414, 2011.

[29] I. M. Modlin, M. Kidd, I. Latich, M. N. Zikusoka, and M. D. Shapiro, "Current status of gastrointestinal carcinoids," *Gastroenterology*, vol. 128, no. 6, pp. 1717–1751, 2005.

[30] T. Berge and F. Linell, "Carcinoid tumours. Frequency in a defined population during a 12-year period," *Acta Pathologica Microbiologica Scandinavica Section A Pathology*, vol. 84A, no. 4, pp. 322–330, 1976.

[31] X. Wang, B. Lu, L. Meng, Y. Fan, S. Zhang, and M. Li, "The correlation between histological gastritis staging- 'OLGA/OLGIM' and serum pepsinogen test in assessment of gastric atrophy/intestinal metaplasia in China," *Scandinavian Journal of Gastroenterology*, vol. 52, no. 8, pp. 822–827, 2017.

24

What Roles Do Probiotics Play in the Eradication of *Helicobacter pylori*? Current Knowledge and Ongoing Research

Han-Yi Song,[1] Long Zhou,[2] Dong-yan Liu,[3] Xin-Jie Yao,[1] and Yan Li[1]

[1]*Department of Gastroenterology, Shengjing Hospital of China Medical University, Shenyang, China*
[2]*Department of Orthopedics, Shengjing Hospital of China Medical University, Shenyang, China*
[3]*Medical Research Center, Shengjing Hospital of China Medical University, Shenyang, China*

Correspondence should be addressed to Yan Li; yanli0227@hotmail.com

Academic Editor: Chiara Ricci

With the rising global prevalence of antibiotic resistance, the eradication rate of *Helicobacter pylori* (HP) is continuing to decrease. Probiotics are beneficial to human health and may be an adjunct therapy to increase the eradication rate of HP, lower treatment-associated side effects, and reduce HP-associated gastric inflammation. However, inconsistent test results have prevented conclusions about the therapeutic prowess of probiotics for HP. The mechanisms of actions of probiotics include the production of substances that inhibit or kill HP or compete with HP for the adhesion site on gastric epithelial cells. Probiotics can also reduce the release of inflammatory factors by regulating the local immune response of the host. We searched the available literature for full-length articles focusing on the role of probiotics in HP management. This review presents the latest advances in this area.

1. Introduction

Helicobacter pylori (HP) is the main cause of chronic active gastritis, peptic ulcer, gastric mucosa-associated lymphoid tissue lymphoma, and gastric cancer. Dyspepsia, unexplained anemia, and idiopathic thrombocytopenic purpura are also closely related [1]. Approximately half of all humans harbor HP which is the most common cause of chronic gastritis worldwide. The 2015 Kyoto consensus suggested that HP gastritis is an infectious disease and those who test positive should receive treatment designed to eradicate the infection [2]. At present, no therapy regimen can guarantee 100% eradication of HP. The eradication rate is related to many factors, including therapeutic regimen, patient tolerance to adverse reactions, patient compliance, patient genetic polymorphism, smoking, diabetes, and other factors [3–5]. Among them, antibiotic resistance of HP is the main cause of the failure of HP eradication treatment [6]. The Maastricht V/Florence consensus suggested that in areas where clarithromycin resistance exceeds 15% or in areas with high clarithromycin and metronidazole resistance, a 10–14-day bismuth quadruple therapy is recommended as the first-line eradication regimen [7]. In North America, the average rates of resistance of HP to metronidazole, clarithromycin, and levofloxacin between 2009 and 2011 were 20%, 16%, and 31%, respectively, of isolates [8]. A recent study from China reported average metronidazole, clarithromycin, and levofloxacin resistance rates of HP of 63.8%, 28.9%, and 28%, respectively, of isolates [9]. Although increasing the dose and course of antibiotics can increase the eradication rate of HP, there can be consequences. Severe adverse reactions during antibiotic therapy can include diarrhea, constipation, bloating, nausea, abdominal pain, abdominal discomfort, dysbacteriosis of the intestinal flora, liver function damage, and fungal infection. The reported rate of adverse reactions during the eradication therapy ranges from 5 to 30%, with treatment discontinued in some cases. Furthermore, the increased prevalence of *Escherichia coli*-resistant strains, methicillin-resistant *Staphylococcus aureus*, and extended-spectrum beta-lactamase strains isolated from the intestine after HP eradication treatment has been described [10]. In addition, bismuth is neurotoxic, which restricts the use in children and the elderly. In patients, gastric mucosa is acquired by gastroendoscopy for the culture of HP to determine antibiotic susceptibility. The prudent selection of antibiotics according to the results of drug susceptibility testing can effectively increase the eradication rate of HP. However, the harsh HP growth conditions and long growth cycle do not guarantee the success of HP culture, which has hindered the widespread use of HP culture techniques [11]. Molecular biology techniques, such as polymerase chain reaction (PCR) and fluorescent labeling nucleic acid in situ hybridization (FISH), can be used to detect HP resistance sites in fresh or paraffin-embedded gastric mucosa tissues and feces, but only to clarithromycin and quinolones. Metronidazole resistance sites cannot be determined due to the complex drug resistance mechanisms that are involved [12].

These challenges have spurred exploration of new individualized approaches to treat HP infections. The many adjuvant HP eradication treatments that have emerged include an oral HP vaccine [13], Chinese herbal medicine [14], probiotics and periodontal scaling [15, 16], and gastric mucosal protective agents [17]. Among them, probiotics have received increasing attention in recent years because of their safety. A large number of clinical and basic studies have reported that some specific probiotics can boost the HP eradication rate and significantly reduce the adverse reactions during the eradication treatment, which facilitates improved patient compliance with the therapy [18–20]. These attributes should seemingly make probiotics a promising adjuvant treatment.

However, according to the 2016 Toronto consensus, there is insufficient evidence that the addition of probiotics can increase the HP eradication rates and reduce adverse reactions [21]. The 2017 ACG clinical guideline, which was based on evidence from a meta-analysis, reported that probiotics can indeed increase HP eradication rates and reduce the overall incidence of adverse reactions. However, the studies involved in the meta-analysis were mainly clinical trials conducted in China and were subject to a high risk of bias. Thus, currently, there is no conclusion about the best choice of probiotics as well as the dose and course of treatment [8]. The fifth Chinese HP consensus opinion pointed out that the conclusion that some probiotic strains can alleviate gastrointestinal side effects following HP eradication is widely accepted. Whether the addition of probiotics can increase the HP eradication rate requires confirmation in future well-designed studies. For now, the anti-HP mechanisms of probiotics remain unclear. In the context of the high global prevalence of antibiotic resistance, determination of the roles of probiotics in the eradication of HP is important, as is the feasibility of using bacteria to cure bacteria. Here, we have a review of the latest advances in the role of probiotics in the treatment of HP infections.

2. Definition and Classification of Probiotics

The Food and Agriculture Organization of the United Nations and the World Health Organization define probiotics as living microorganisms that are beneficial to life; can tolerate the effects of stomach acid, bile, and pancreatic juice; can colonize the host's gastrointestinal tract or reproductive system; induce host reactions; and balance the intestinal flora to improve health [22]. Currently, compound active probiotics composed of various kinds of microorganisms are widely used globally, mainly for the treatment of diarrhea caused by dysbacteriosis of the intestine and to regulate the body's immune functions.

In 2013, the International Probiotics and Prebiotics Science Association classified probiotics as follows: (1) bacteria in the genus *Lactobacillus*, including *Lactobacillus acidophilus*, *Clostridium butyricum*, *L. reuteri*, *L. bulgaricus*, *L. casei*, *L. paracasei L. rhamnosus*, *L. salivarius*, and *L. plantarum*; (2) bacteria in the genus *Bifidobacterium*, including *Bifidobacterium infantis*, *B. adolescentis*, *B. animalis*, *B. longum*, *B. breve*, and ovary double *Bacteroides*; (3) Gram-positive cocci, such as *Streptococcus thermophilus*, *S. faecalis*, and *Lactococcus*; and (4) yeast, such as *Saccharomyces boulardii*. At present, commercially available probiotic products include probiotic amended yogurt, encapsulated live bacteria, bacteria powder, oral liquids, and various preparations of single strains.

3. Theoretical Basis of Microecological Therapy

Human skin and gastrointestinal, respiratory, and urogenital tracts harbor huge numbers of colonized microbes, which are important in regulating the immune function of the human body to resist the colonization of pathogens [23]. These microorganisms include beneficial bacteria, conditional pathogens, and pathogenic bacteria, which have evolved to a normal state of microecological balance in the human body. The gastric environment is particularly harsh and difficult for microbiota to colonize. The common wisdom for a long time was that the stomach was sterile for approximately 80% of microbes are not cultivable. With the development of high-throughput sequencing technology, this view has been debunked. HP is not the only inhabitant of the gastric mucosa anymore; a non-HP microbial community has been recognized and is called gastric microbiota [24]. HP may be influenced in their pathogenicity by the community they live in [25]. The gastric microbiota belong mainly to the Proteobacteria, Firmicutes, Actinobacteria, and Fusobacterium phyla, the majority of which were Streptococcus and Staphylococcus [26]. HP infection can affect the balance of gastric microbiota, and microbial interactions are a major factor in regulating the indigenous microbiota. Reports showed that the gastric microbiota of HP-negative subjects has a higher diversity than that of HP-positive patients [27].

Adhesion and virulence factors of HP contribute to pathogenicity. Colonization of the stomach by HP affects the distribution and quantity of the original gastric bacteria and upsets the microecological balance, resulting in disease. For example, there are fewer lactobacilli in the HP-infected stomach compared to the stomach not infected with HP [23]. HP leads to a microecological imbalance principally because of its production of an antibacterial peptide called cecropin. This peptide can cause other bacteria to undergo "autogenic autolysis" [28]. The lack of competition from these bacteria allows HP to multiply unimpeded. A series of virulence factors are able to stimulate the gastric epithelial cells, resulting in apoptosis and inflammation. In the context of the global prevalence of antibiotic resistance, increasing the dose of antibiotics or prolonging the course of antibiotics to increase the eradication rate of HP is not an ideal method, because it can promote the further development of antibiotic resistance.

Microecological therapy has brought new ideas to the treatment of HP. Remodeling the microecological balance in the stomach can reduce HP colonization. Concerning an animal model of HP infection, sterile, immunodeficient, or knockout animals are the easiest to establish. The use of ordinary mice is hampered by the difficulty to establish a chronic HP infection. An analysis of the components of the gastric microbiota in sterile and normal mice revealed that the number of bacteria in the stomach of normal mice reached was up to 10×8 colony forming units (CFU)/g, with Lactobacillus dominating [29]. In an animal experiment conducted in China, normal mice received HP suspensions for 7 days. The resulting HP infection rate was 30%. If the mice were first fed with a mixture of gentamicin and azithromycin for 3 days to eliminate the original microbiota of the stomach, the 7-day administration of HP produced a 100% HP infection rate. After the gastric microbiota balance was remodeled by feeding the Lactobacillus and Bifidobacterium suspension for 7 days, the HP infection rate was reduced to 30% and HP colonization decreased significantly. Some experiments confirm that some components of the gastric microbiota have been shown to exert antibacterial properties and could drive HP conversing from a spiral to a coccoidal form [30, 31]. The findings support the speculation that the immune system and normal gastric microbiota can effectively antagonize the colonization of HP, while disruption of the gastric microbiota balance increases the susceptibility to HP infection. The data provide a theoretical basis for the clinical use of probiotics to increase the HP eradication rate.

4. Effect of Probiotics on HP Eradication

Many meta-analyses and clinical trials have confirmed that probiotic supplementation can increase the eradication rate of HP and reduce adverse reactions during eradication. It can be concluded from literature analysis that not all probiotics have antagonistic effects on HP and different probiotics have specific effects. The antagonistic effect of mixed strains of probiotics on HP was greater than that of a single strain. Probiotics alone cannot completely eliminate HP but can reduce the amount of HP load in the stomach, reduce the delta value of UBT, and alleviate gastric mucosal inflammation. More details on the role of probiotics on the HP eradication rate can be seen in Tables 1–4.

Some clinical trials proved that probiotics can reduce the DOB values of UBT, despite a complete eradication of HP not being obtained [32–34]. Whether DOB values quantitatively reflect the density of gastric HP is a controversial question. DOB value is affected by many factors, such as the density of HP colonization, urease activity, and gastric emptying. Different probiotics can reduce the DOB value by inhibiting urease activity [35] or decreasing the attachment of HP to the gastric mucosa, suppressing the HP density [36].

5. Action Mechanism of Probiotics

5.1. Production of Substances That Inhibit or Kill HP. The antagonistic mechanism of probiotics to HP is unclear. Probiotic microorganisms can produce a variety of substances that inhibit HP and induce the secretion of antibodies by the host. A partial list of the antibacterial compounds includes bacteriocins, lactic acid, acetic acid, and hydrogen peroxide (H_2O_2). Different probiotic strains produce different antibacterial substances. *Strep. lactis* can produce nisin. This positively charged molecule can combine with cell membranes by electrostatic and hydrophobic interactions followed by membrane insertion to form a permeable channel that preludes cell autolysis and death [56]. *Bacillus subtilis* produces the antibiotic amicoumacin A and similar isocoumarins, and *L. roche* produces a variety of reoterms that all inhibit the growth and activity of HP. One of the characteristics of HP is the secretion of urease, which breaks down urea in the stomach to produce ammonia and which neutralizes gastric acid to protect the bacteria from gastric acid damage. Most lactobacilli produce lactic acid, which can inhibit the activity of urease. Lactic acid is deleterious to HP. The morphological alteration that occurs is independent of pH [57]. Fujimura et al. cocultured an HP standard strain and *L. gasseri* OLL2716 on agar for 24 h. Electron microscopy examination revealed a spherical shape of HP. The bacteria had also lost their growth ability [58]. Another characteristic of HP is catalase activity. Probiotics can produce H_2O_2. Catalase action results in the production of many oxygen radicals, which are antibacterial due to their interference with HP enzyme activity. Live probiotics antagonize HP, but bacterial viability may not be a prerequisite for the deleterious activity. Heat-inactivated *L. johnsonii* No. 1088 (HK-LJ88) can kill HP *in vitro* and, when cocultured with HP for 24 h, can lead to altered HP morphology and lysis. Orally administered HK-LJ88 can reduce HP colonization in the mouse stomach. The anti-HP effect of HK-LJ88 does not involve coagglutination of the bacteria. Rather, some surface molecules of HK-LJ88 are not inactivated by the heat [59]. In another study on the coculture of HP with *L. acidophilus* CRL 639 for 24 hours, the latter appeared to be lysed and the released protein compounds deformed or killed HP [60].

5.2. Effect on HP Colonization in the Stomach. The colonization of HP in the gastric epithelium is a prerequisite for the disease. HP has multiple flagella at one end, which provide the mechanical for a bacterium to penetrate the thick layer of the mucus and colonize the surface of gastric epithelial cells rather than being excreted with the peristalsis of the stomach. The HP surface contains adhesions, such as neutrophil activator protein, fibrillar N-acetylneuraminyl lactose-binding hemagglutinin (NLBH), Bab A, Lewis antigen, heat shock protein, Alp A, and Alp B. The gastric epithelial cells contain mucin receptors, mucopolysaccharide receptors, Lewis blood group substances, glycolipid receptors, and other corresponding receptors. The binding of the HP adhesins to the receptors mediates the colonization of HP in the gastric mucosa. Identifying the ability of probiotic bacteria to colonize the gastric mucosa is the first step in

TABLE 1: Summary of meta-analysis of the effect of probiotics on the eradication rate of HP.

Author	Trials	Probiotic	Result
Jian et al. [37]	8 RCT (n = 1372)	Lactobacilli + triple therapy	Pooled eradication rate Probiotic: 82.26% (95% CI = 78.01–86.51%) No probiotic: 76.97% (95% CI = 73.11–80.83%) OR = 1.78 (95% CI = 1.21–2.62)
Sachdeva and Nagpal [38]	10 RCT (n = 963)	Multistrain (fermented milk) + triple or quadruple therapy	Eradication rates were improved by approximately 5–15% OR = 1.91 (95% CI: 1.38–2.67)
Dang et al.[39]	33 RCT (n = 4459), 9 RCT for children, 24 RCT for adults	Probiotics + triple therapy or sequential therapy or quadruple therapy	The pooled eradication rate in probiotic supplementation groups was significantly higher than that in controls (RR = 1.122, 95% CI = 1.086–1.159)
Szajewska et al.[40]	9 RCT (adult, n = 1708) 2 RCT (children, n = 330)	Saccharomyces boulardii + triple therapy	Eradication rate (adult) Probiotic: 80.0% (95% CI = 77–82) No probiotic: 71.0% (95% CI = 68–74) RR = 1.11, 95% CI = 1.06–1.17 Eradication rate (children) Probiotic: 87.5% No probiotic:77.2% RR = 1.13, 95% CI = 1.03–1.25
Zhang et al. [41]	45 RCT (n = 6997)	Probiotics + standard therapy	Eradication rate Probiotic: 82.31% No probiotics: 72.08% (RR: 1.11; 95% CI: 1.08–1.15) Side effects (RR = 0.59; 95% CI = 0.48–0.71) Probiotic: 21.44% No probiotic: 36.27%
Wen et al. [42]	17 RCT in Asian pediatric patients (n = 1932)	Multistrain probiotics + 14-day triple therapy	Bifidobacterium infantis + Clostridium butyricum was most beneficial for eradication rates (RR: 1.16, 95% CI: 1.07–1.26)
Losurdo et al. [43]	7 RCT (n = 517)	Probiotic strain alone	The mean weighted eradication rate was 14% (95% CI = 2%–25%) Lactobacilli: 16% (95% CI: 1%–31%) Saccharomyces boulardii: 12% (95% CI: 0%–29%) Multistrain: 14% (95% CI: 0%–43%)

screening probiotics that can antagonize HP adhesion and colonization. Such probiotics can compete with HP for the adhesion site of gastric epithelial cells to reduce the colonization of HP in the stomach. Mukai et al. found that *L. reuteri* affects the colonization of HP by the secretion of sialic acid gangliosides and thiolates that inhibit HP's glycolipid linkage with gastric epithelial cells, as well as competing with HP for the adhesion of asialo-ganglio-N-tetraosylceramide and sulfatide [61]. *In vitro* experiments confirmed that Lactobacillus can downregulate the expression of HP adhesin sabA and reduce the adhesion of HP to gastric mucosa [62]. Others demonstrated that the growth of Lactobacillus and HP in the stomach is antagonistic to each other. If Lactobacilli exist in the stomach, the amount of HP will be reduced [63]. HP infection does not necessarily lead to disease, which is related to the virulence and quantity of HP. Peptic ulcers do not develop when the HP density of the gastric antrum is $<10^5$ CFU/g [64]. The foregoing support the view that, while the oral administration of probiotics may well not completely eliminate HP, adhesion of HP can be reduced and gastric mucosal inflammation can be lessened. For children and elderly people who do not have digestive symptoms, oral administration of probiotics to reduce HP colonization is superior to traditional treatment.

5.3. Inhibition of Inflammation after HP Infection. HP infection leads to gastric mucosal inflammation. This can begin a pathway, which is termed the Correa cascade, from chronic gastritis to atrophic gastritis to intestinal metaplasia to atypical hyperplasia, culminating in gastric cancer. This is the most common pattern of evolution after gastric mucosal infection with HP. Urease, cytotoxin-associated gene A (CagA), vacuolating cytotoxin A (VacA), and neutrophil-activating protein (NAP) are common virulence factors of HP. As its name implies, NAP activates neutrophils. It also promotes the production of reactive oxygen species in neutrophils and mediates the adhesion of gastric epithelial cells to neutrophils, resulting the activation of gastric inflammation cascade reaction after HP infection. Interleukin- (IL-) 8 is the earliest discovered cytokine associated with HP gastritis. It is a chemotactic compound that can activate neutrophils, induce the degeneration and necrosis of gastric

TABLE 2: Summary of clinical trials using a single strain of probiotics with antibiotics.

Author	Study size	Probiotic	Study type	Result
Zhao et al. [44]	240	Saccharomyces boulardii	A prospective, randomized, controlled study	Eradication rate Probiotic: 85.0% No probiotic: 75.8% Adverse reaction decreases
Dore et al. [45]	45	Lactobacillus reuteri (DSM 17938)	A case report series	Eradication rate: 93.3%
Cekin et al. [18]	159	Bifidobacterium animalis subsp. lactis B94	Randomized, placebo-controlled study	Eradication rate Probiotic: 86.8% No probiotics: 70.8% Adverse reaction decreases
Zhu et al. [46]	240	Saccharomyces boulardii	Randomized clinical trial	Saccharomyces boulardii reduced the overall side effect rate, and there was no difference observed in efficacy on the eradication rate
Chen et al. [47]	105	Clostridium butyricum	Open-label, randomized clinical trial	No significant difference in eradication rates was observed. Supplementation of probiotics led to improvement of gastrointestinal symptoms

TABLE 3: Summary of clinical trials using mixtures of probiotics in association with triple therapy.

Author	Study size	Probiotics	Study type	Result
Du et al. [48]	228	L. acidophilus + S. faecalis + B. subtilis	Randomized Prospective Open	Eradication rate Probiotic: 79.5% No probiotics: 60.8% Adverse reaction decreases
Wang and Huang [49]	100	L. acidophilus + B. bifidum	Randomized Prospective Open	Probiotic: 83.7% No probiotics: 64.4%
Tongtawee et al. [50]	200	Lactobacillus delbrueckii + Streptococcus thermophillus	Double-blind Placebo-controlled Randomized	Probiotic: 90.8% No probiotics: 84.3%
Haghdoost et al. [51]	176	Lactobacillus + Bifidobacterium	Randomized Placebo-controlled study	Probiotic: 78.4% No probiotics: 64.8%

mucosa cells, and also stimulate mucosal monocytes and dendritic cells to produce tumor necrosis factor, IL-1, and IL-6. The dendritic cell activity produces an inflammatory cascade. These responses are insufficient to clear HP infection but cause chronic inflammation [65]. Virulence and inflammatory factors are now being used to prepare HP-associated vaccines. Animal studies have demonstrated the considerable (80%) effectiveness of oral vaccines based on NAP [66]. Some probiotic strains can also reduce the release of inflammatory factors by regulating the local immune response of the host and relieving the inflammatory response of the gastric mucosa. An *in vitro* study confirmed that HP-induced secretion of IL-8 in gastric epithelial cells can be reduced by *L. salivarius* [67]. Another study showed that the exopolysaccharide of *Strep. thermophilus* CRL1190 reduces the colonization of HP to AGS cells and also relieves the inflammatory response of AGS cells caused by HP [68]. The mechanism by which probiotics regulate mucosal immune responses is unclear. *L. reuteri* can inhibit the activation of nuclear factor-kappa B (NF-κB) and downstream factors by blocking the release of the tumor necrosis factor from macrophages. *L. acidophilus* can inhibit the expression of Smad7, inactivate the transduction of the NF-κB pathway, and weaken the HP-induced gastric mucosal inflammatory response [69]. *L. plantarum* and *L. acidophilus* applied prior to HP infection reduce the degree of gastritis. Phosphorylation of Janus kinase 2 and the expression of the cytostatic factor suppressors of cytokine signaling- (SOCS-) 2 and 3 are increased in the JAK-STAT pathway. SOCS-2 and SOCS-3 can inhibit a variety of signal transduction pathways, which reduces the release of inflammatory factors [70]. Probiotics can reduce the release of IL-8, interferon gamma, and other inflammatory factors by inhibiting the Toll-like receptor 4-NF-κB signaling pathway [71]. *L. salivarius* UCC118 and UCC119 can reduce the secretion of IL-8 by the gastric mucosa after HP infection. This effect has

TABLE 4: Summary of clinical trials using probiotics in the absence of antibiotics.

Author	Study size	Probiotic	Study type	Result
Sakamoto et al. [33]	31	Lactobacillus gasseri OLL2716	A randomized, controlled clinical trial	Value of UBT decreases. Examination of antral biopsies showed two- to 100-fold decreases in the numbers of HP, but in no case were bacteria eliminated completely.
Cruchet et al. [34]	326	Lactobacillus johnsonii La1	A double-blind, randomized, controlled clinical trial	A significant difference (DOB2–DOB1) was detected (−7.64 per thousand; 95% CI: −14.23 to −1.03)
Linsalata et al. [52]	22	Lactobacillus brevis	A randomized, double-blind, placebo-controlled study	Reduction in the UBT delta values
Imase et al. [36]	179	L. reuteri	A randomized, double-blind, crossover study	Administration of L. reuteri tablets significantly decreased UBT in HP-positive subjects
Rosania et al. [53]	80	A mixture of 8 different probiotics	Double-blind, placebo-controlled, randomized	Eradication rate Probiotic: 32.5% Placebo: 0%
Francavilla et al. [54]	100	L. reuteri DSM 17938 + L. reuteri ATCC PTA 6475	Double-blind, placebo-controlled, randomized	Probiotic: a decrease in the 13C-UBT value by 13% Placebo: a 4% increase
Holz et al. [55]	128 subjects, 47 twin pairs, and 34 singletons	L. reuteri DSM 17648	Placebo-controlled pilot study	Had unique properties as it specifically aggregates with planktonic HP in the stomach. It can significantly reduce the HP load after a 14-day oral treatment

nothing to do with the life or death of *L. salivarius*, but the probiotic body must be complete. *L. salivarius* UCC118 and UCC119 can destroy the type IV secretion system encoded by the cagPAI of the HP toxin-related gene and block the entry of the effector molecule cagA into host epithelial cells [72]. A probiotic mixture of *Enterococcus faecalis*, *B. longum*, and *L. acidophilus* reportedly tolerated the acidic environment in the stomach and survived for 8 hours. These three probiotics could not reduce the colonization of HP in the stomach but could reduce the release of inflammatory factors such as tumor necrosis factor-alpha, IL-1β, IL-10, IL-6, granulocyte colony-stimulating factor, and macrophage inflammatory protein 2 by inhibiting the NF-κB and mitogen-activated protein kinase signal transduction pathways [73]. Arginine is a substrate for the synthesis of nitric oxide, one of the strongest mediators of inflammation. The arginine deiminase activity following L. brevis administration causes arginine deficiency and prevents polyamine generation from proliferating cells [52].

6. Conclusion

With the deepening of the research on the intestinal microflora, microecological therapy is attracting increasing attention. Probiotics can help improve the eradication rate of HP and reduce the adverse reactions. However, not all probiotics but only some specific probiotic strains have such effects. Here are several research hurdles still to be surmounted. First, the gut microflora of humans is affected by various factors, such as the environment, diet, genetics, and lifestyle, and it is difficult to directly study the effects of probiotics on the human body. Second, due to the synergistic or antagonistic effect between bacteria, it is difficult to generalize the effects of certain probiotic strains in the different probiotic combinations. Third, due to the specificity of the strains and the inconsistent results of the research, the results to date can be questioned.

The results to date consistently support the prowess of probiotics in alleviating adverse reactions in the eradication of HP. However, questions remain. Can probiotics increase the eradication rate of HP? If so, what is the mechanism? Which probiotic strain has the best anti-HP effect? What is the best dose and the timing of medication (i.e., before or after eradication)? Is there a difference in efficacy between single strains and mixed strains? Are there side effects of supplemental exogenous probiotics? The answers await future basic and clinical studies.

Authors' Contributions

Han-Yi Song did the literature search, the design, and the writing. Long Zhou did the analysis and interpretation. Dong-yan Liu did the critical reviews. Xin-Jie Yao did the data collection and processing. Yan Li did the concept and supervision.

References

[1] P. Malfertheiner, F. Megraud, C. A. O'Morain et al., "Management of *Helicobacter pylori* infection–the Maastricht IV/Florence consensus report," *Gut*, vol. 61, no. 5, pp. 646–664, 2012.

[2] K. Sugano, J. Tack, E. J. Kuipers et al., "Kyoto global consensus report on *Helicobacter pylori* gastritis," *Gut*, vol. 64, no. 9, pp. 1353–1367, 2015.

[3] Y. A. Lin, H. Wang, Z. J. Gu et al., "Effect of CYP2C19 gene polymorphisms on proton pump inhibitor, amoxicillin, and levofloxacin triple therapy for eradication of *Helicobacter pylori*," *Medical Science Monitor*, vol. 23, pp. 2701–2707, 2017.

[4] D. Itskoviz, D. Boltin, H. Leibovitzh et al., "Smoking increases the likelihood of *Helicobacter pylori* treatment failure," *Digestive and Liver Disease*, vol. 49, no. 7, pp. 764–768, 2017.

[5] C. Horikawa, S. Kodama, K. Fujihara et al., "High risk of failing eradication of *Helicobacter pylori* in patients with diabetes: a meta-analysis," *Diabetes Research and Clinical Practice*, vol. 106, no. 1, pp. 81–87, 2014.

[6] D. Y. Graham, Y.–. C. Lee, and M.–. S. Wu, "Rational *Helicobacter pylori* therapy: evidence-based medicine rather than medicine-based evidence," *Clinical Gastroenterology and Hepatology*, vol. 12, no. 2, pp. 177–186.e3, 2014.

[7] P. Malfertheiner, F. Megraud, C. A. O'Morain et al., "Management of *Helicobacter pylori* infection-the Maastricht V/Florence Consensus Report," *Gut*, vol. 66, no. 1, pp. 6–30, 2016.

[8] W. D. Chey, G. I. Leontiadis, C. W. Howden, and S. F. Moss, "ACG clinical guideline: treatment of *Helicobacter pylori* infection," *The American Journal of Gastroenterology*, vol. 112, no. 2, pp. 212–239, 2017.

[9] Y. Hu, Y. Zhu, and N. H. Lu, "Primary antibiotic resistance of *Helicobacter pylori* in China," *Digestive Diseases and Sciences*, vol. 62, no. 5, pp. 1146–1154, 2017.

[10] I. Adamsson, C. Edlund, and C. E. Nord, "Impact of treatment of *Helicobacter pylori* on the normal gastrointestinal microflora," *Clinical Microbiology and Infection*, vol. 6, no. 4, pp. 175–177, 2000.

[11] N. Arslan, O. Yilmaz, and E. Demiray-Gurbuz, "Importance of antimicrobial susceptibility testing for the management of eradication in *Helicobacter pylori* infection," *World Journal of Gastroenterology*, vol. 23, no. 16, pp. 2854–2869, 2017.

[12] T. Nishizawa and H. Suzuki, "Mechanisms of *Helicobacter pylori* antibiotic resistance and molecular testing," *Frontiers in Molecular Biosciences*, vol. 1, no. 19, 2014.

[13] A. T. B. Abadi, "Vaccine against *Helicobacter pylori*: inevitable approach," *World Journal of Gastroenterology*, vol. 22, no. 11, pp. 3150–3157, 2016.

[14] F. Ma, Y. Chen, J. Li et al., "Screening test for anti-*Helicobacter pylori* activity of traditional Chinese herbal medicines," *World Journal of Gastroenterology*, vol. 16, no. 44, pp. 5629–5634, 2010.

[15] H. Y. Song and Y. Li, "Can eradication rate of gastric *Helicobacter pylori* be improved by killing oral *Helicobacter pylori*?," *World Journal of Gastroenterology*, vol. 19, no. 39, pp. 6645–6650, 2013.

[16] J. K. C. Yee, "Are the view of *Helicobacter pylori* colonized in the oral cavity an illusion?," *Experimental & Molecular Medicine*, vol. 49, no. 11, article e397, 2017.

[17] Y. Wang, B. Wang, Z. F. Lv et al., "Efficacy and safety of ecabet sodium as an adjuvant therapy for *Helicobacter pylori* eradication: a systematic review and meta-analysis," *Helicobacter*, vol. 19, no. 5, pp. 372–381, 2014.

[18] A. H. Cekin, Y. Sahinturk, F. Akbay Harmandar, S. Uyar, B. Oguz Yolcular, and Y. Cekin, "Use of probiotics as an adjuvant to sequential *H. pylori* eradication therapy: impact on eradication rates, treatment resistance, treatment-related side effects, and patient compliance," *The Turkish Journal of Gastroenterology*, vol. 28, no. 1, pp. 3–11, 2017.

[19] T. Kafshdooz, A. Akbarzadeh, A. Majdi Seghinsara, M. Pourhassan, H. T. Nasrabadi, and M. Milani, "Role of probiotics in managing of *Helicobacter pylori* infection: a review," *Drug Research*, vol. 67, no. 2, pp. 88–93, 2017.

[20] L. V. McFarland, Y. Huang, L. Wang, and P. Malfertheiner, "Systematic review and meta-analysis: multi-strain probiotics as adjunct therapy for *Helicobacter pylori* eradication and prevention of adverse events," *United European Gastroenterology Journal*, vol. 4, no. 4, pp. 546–561, 2016.

[21] C. A. Fallone, N. Chiba, S. V. van Zanten et al., "The Toronto consensus for the treatment of *Helicobacter pylori* infection in adults," *Gastroenterology*, vol. 151, no. 1, pp. 51–69.e14, 2016.

[22] C. Hill, F. Guarner, G. Reid et al., "Expert consensus document. The International Scientific Association for Probiotics and Prebiotics consensus statement on the scope and appropriate use of the term probiotic," *Nature Reviews Gastroenterology & Hepatology*, vol. 11, no. 8, pp. 506–514, 2014.

[23] R. L. Brown and T. B. Clarke, "The regulation of host defences to infection by the microbiota," *Immunology*, vol. 150, no. 1, pp. 1–6, 2017.

[24] G. Ianiro, J. Molina-Infante, and A. Gasbarrini, "Gastric microbiota," *Helicobacter*, vol. 20, pp. 68–71, 2015.

[25] V. Pereira, P. Abraham, S. Nallapeta, and A. Shetty, "Gastric bacterial flora in patients harbouring *Helicobacter pylori* with or without chronic dyspepsia: analysis with matrix-assisted laser desorption ionization time-of-flight mass spectroscopy," *BMC Gastroenterology*, vol. 18, no. 1, p. 20, 2018.

[26] I. Yang, S. Nell, and S. Suerbaum, "Survival in hostile territory: the microbiota of the stomach," *FEMS Microbiology Reviews*, vol. 37, no. 5, pp. 736–761, 2013.

[27] A. F. Andersson, M. Lindberg, H. Jakobsson, F. Bäckhed, P. Nyrén, and L. Engstrand, "Comparative analysis of human gut microbiota by barcoded pyrosequencing," *PLoS One*, vol. 3, no. 7, article e2836, 2008.

[28] J. Bylund, T. Christophe, F. Boulay, T. Nystrom, A. Karlsson, and C. Dahlgren, "Proinflammatory activity of a cecropin-like antibacterial peptide from *Helicobacter pylori*," *Antimicrobial Agents and Chemotherapy*, vol. 45, no. 6, pp. 1700–1704, 2001.

[29] M. Karita, Q. Li, D. Cantero, and K. Okita, "Establishment of a small animal model for human *Helicobacter pylori* infection using germ-free mouse," *The American Journal of Gastroenterology*, vol. 89, no. 2, pp. 208–213, 1994.

[30] C. Zaman, T. Osaki, T. Hanawa, H. Yonezawa, S. Kurata, and S. Kamiya, "Analysis of the microbial ecology between *Helicobacter pylori* and the gastric microbiota of Mongolian gerbils," *Journal of Medical Microbiology*, vol. 63, pp. 129–137, 2014.

[31] Y. Khosravi, Y. Dieye, M. F. Loke, K. L. Goh, and J. Vadivelu, "*Streptococcus mitis* induces conversion of *Helicobacter pylori* to coccoid cells during co-culture in vitro," *PLoS One*, vol. 9, no. 11, article e112214, 2014.

[32] P. Michetti, G. Dorta, P. H. Wiesel et al., "Effect of whey-based culture supernatant of *Lactobacillus acidophilus (johnsonii)* La1 on *Helicobacter pylori* infection in humans," *Digestion*, vol. 60, no. 3, pp. 203–209, 1999.

[33] I. Sakamoto, M. Igarashi, K. Kimura, A. Takagi, T. Miwa, and Y. Koga, "Suppressive effect of *Lactobacillus gasseri* OLL 2716 (LG21) on *Helicobacter pylori* infection in humans," *The Journal of Antimicrobial Chemotherapy*, vol. 47, no. 5, pp. 709-710, 2001.

[34] S. Cruchet, M. C. Obregon, G. Salazar, E. Diaz, and M. Gotteland, "Effect of the ingestion of a dietary product containing *Lactobacillus johnsonii* La1 on *Helicobacter pylori* colonization in children," *Nutrition*, vol. 19, no. 9, pp. 716–721, 2003.

[35] M. J. Salas-Jara, E. A. Sanhueza, A. Retamal-Díaz, C. González, H. Urrutia, and A. García, "Probiotic *Lactobacillus fermentum* UCO-979C biofilm formation on AGS and Caco-2 cells and *Helicobacter pylori* inhibition," *Biofouling*, vol. 32, no. 10, pp. 1245–1257, 2016.

[36] K. Imase, A. Tanaka, K. Tokunaga, H. Sugano, H. Ishida, and S. Takahashi, "*Lactobacillus reuteri* tablets suppress *Helicobacter pylori* infection–a double-blind randomised placebo-controlled cross-over clinical study," *Journal of the Japanese Association for Infectious Diseases*, vol. 81, no. 4, pp. 387–393, 2007.

[37] J. Zou, J. Dong, and X. Yu, "Meta-analysis: *Lactobacillus* containing quadruple therapy versus standard triple first-line therapy for *Helicobacter pylori* eradication," *Helicobacter*, vol. 14, no. 5, pp. 97–107, 2009.

[38] A. Sachdeva and J. Nagpal, "Effect of fermented milk-based probiotic preparations on *Helicobacter pylori* eradication: a systematic review and meta-analysis of randomized-controlled trials," *European Journal of Gastroenterology & Hepatology*, vol. 21, no. 1, pp. 45–53, 2009.

[39] Y. Dang, J. D. Reinhardt, X. Zhou, and G. Zhang, "The effect of probiotics supplementation on *Helicobacter pylori* eradication rates and side effects during eradication therapy: a meta-analysis," *PLoS One*, vol. 9, no. 11, article e111030, 2014.

[40] H. Szajewska, A. Horvath, and M. Kolodziej, "Systematic review with meta-analysis: *Saccharomyces boulardii* supplementation and eradication of *Helicobacter pylori* infection," *Alimentary Pharmacology & Therapeutics*, vol. 41, no. 12, pp. 1237–1245, 2015.

[41] M. M. Zhang, W. Qian, Y. Y. Qin, J. He, and Y. H. Zhou, "Probiotics in *Helicobacter pylori* eradication therapy: a systematic review and meta-analysis," *World Journal of Gastroenterology*, vol. 21, no. 14, pp. 4345–4357, 2015.

[42] J. Wen, P. Peng, P. Chen et al., "Probiotics in 14-day triple therapy for Asian pediatric patients with *Helicobacter pylori* infection: a network meta-analysis," *Oncotarget*, vol. 8, no. 56, pp. 96409–96418, 2017.

[43] G. Losurdo, R. Cubisino, M. Barone et al., "Probiotic monotherapy and *Helicobacter pylori* eradication: a systematic review with pooled-data analysis," *World Journal of Gastroenterology*, vol. 24, no. 1, pp. 139–149, 2018.

[44] H. M. Zhao, H. J. Ou-Yang, B. P. Duan et al., "Clinical effect of triple therapy combined with *Saccharomyces boulardii* in the treatment of *Helicobacter pylori* infection in children," *Chinese Journal of Contemporary Pediatrics*, vol. 16, no. 3, pp. 230–233, 2014.

[45] M. P. Dore, S. Soro, C. Rocchi, M. F. Loria, S. Bibbò, and G. M. Pes, "Inclusion of *Lactobacillus reuteri* in the treatment of *Helicobacter pylori* in Sardinian patients: a case report series," *Medicine*, vol. 95, no. 15, article e3411, 2016.

[46] X. Y. Zhu, J. Du, J. Wu, L. W. Zhao, X. Meng, and G. F. Liu, "Influence of *Saccharomyces boulardii* sachets combined with bismuth quadruple therapy for initial *Helicobacter pylori* eradication," *Zhonghua Yi Xue Za Zhi*, vol. 97, no. 30, pp. 2353–2356, 2017.

[47] L. Chen, W. Xu, A. Lee et al., "The impact of *Helicobacter pylori* infection, eradication therapy and probiotic supplementation on gut microenvironment homeostasis: an open-label, randomized clinical trial," *eBioMedicine*, vol. 35, pp. 87–96, 2018.

[48] Y.-Q. Du, T. Su, J.-G. Fan et al., "Adjuvant probiotics improve the eradication effect of triple therapy for *Helicobacter pylori* infection," *World Journal of Gastroenterology*, vol. 18, no. 43, pp. 6302–6307, 2012.

[49] Y. H. Wang and Y. Huang, "Effect of *Lactobacillus acidophilus* and *Bifidobacterium bifidum* supplementation to standard triple therapy on *Helicobacter pylori* eradication and dynamic changes in intestinal flora," *World Journal of Microbiology and Biotechnology*, vol. 30, no. 3, pp. 847–853, 2014.

[50] T. Tongtawee, C. Dechsukhum, W. Leeanansaksiri et al., "Effect of pretreatment with *Lactobacillus delbrueckii* and *Streptococcus thermophillus* on tailored triple therapy for *Helicobacter pylori* eradication: a prospective randomized controlled clinical trial," *Asian Pacific Journal of Cancer Prevention*, vol. 16, no. 12, pp. 4885–4890, 2015.

[51] M. Haghdoost, S. Taghizadeh, M. Montazer, P. Poorshahverdi, A. Ramouz, and S. Fakour, "Double strain probiotic effect on *Helicobacter pylori* infection treatment: a double-blinded randomized controlled trial," *Caspian Journal of Internal Medicine*, vol. 8, no. 3, pp. 165–171, 2017.

[52] M. Linsalata, F. Russo, P. Berloco et al., "The influence of lactobacillus brevis on ornithine decarboxylase activity and polyamine profiles in *Helicobacter pylori*-infected gastric mucosa," *Helicobacter*, vol. 9, no. 2, pp. 165–172, 2004.

[53] R. Rosania, M. Filomena Minenna, F. Giorgio et al., "Probiotic multistrain treatment may eradicate *Helicobacter pylori* from the stomach of dyspeptics: a placebo-controlled pilot study," *Inflammation & Allergy Drug Targets*, vol. 11, no. 3, pp. 244–249, 2012.

[54] R. Francavilla, L. Polimeno, A. Demichina et al., "*Lactobacillus reuteri* strain combination in *Helicobacter pylori* infection: a randomized, double-blind, placebo-controlled study," *Journal of Clinical Gastroenterology*, vol. 48, no. 5, pp. 407–413, 2014.

[55] C. Holz, A. Busjahn, H. Mehling et al., "Significant reduction in *Helicobacter pylori* load in humans with non-viable *Lactobacillus reuteri* DSM17648: a pilot study," *Probiotics and Antimicrobial Proteins*, vol. 7, no. 2, pp. 91–100, 2015.

[56] E. H. Lee, I. Khan, and D. H. Oh, "Evaluation of the efficacy of nisin-loaded chitosan nanoparticles against foodborne pathogens in orange juice," *Journal of Food Science and Technology*, vol. 55, no. 3, pp. 1127–1133, 2018.

[57] P. S. Hsieh, Y. C. Tsai, Y. C. Chen, S. F. Teh, C. M. Ou, and V. A. E. King, "Eradication of *Helicobacter pylori* infection by the probiotic strains *Lactobacillus johnsonii* MH-68 and *L. salivarius* ssp. *salicinius* AP-32," *Helicobacter*, vol. 17, no. 6, pp. 466–477, 2012.

[58] S. Fujimura, A. Watanabe, K. Kimura, and M. Kaji, "Probiotic mechanism of *Lactobacillus gasseri* OLL2716 strain against *Helicobacter pylori*," *Journal of Clinical Microbiology*, vol. 50, no. 3, pp. 1134–1136, 2012.

[59] Y. Aiba, H. Ishikawa, M. Tokunaga, and Y. Komatsu, "Anti-*Helicobacter pylori* activity of non-living, heat-killed form of lactobacilli including *Lactobacillus johnsonii* no.1088," *FEMS Microbiology Letters*, vol. 364, no. 11, 2017.

[60] G. L. Lorca, T. Wadström, G. Font de Valdez, and Å. Ljungh, "*Lactobacillus acidophilus* autolysins inhibit *Helicobacter pylori* in vitro," *Current Microbiology*, vol. 42, no. 1, pp. 39–44, 2001.

[61] T. Mukai, T. Asasaka, E. Sato, K. Mori, M. Matsumoto, and H. Ohori, "Inhibition of binding of *Helicobacter pylori* to the glycolipid receptors by probiotic *Lactobacillus reuteri*," *FEMS Immunology and Medical Microbiology*, vol. 32, no. 2, pp. 105–110, 2002.

[62] N. de Klerk, L. Maudsdotter, H. Gebreegziabher et al., "Lactobacilli reduce *Helicobacter pylori* attachment to host gastric epithelial cells by inhibiting adhesion gene expression," *Infection and Immunity*, vol. 84, no. 5, pp. 1526–1535, 2016.

[63] A. García, K. Sáez, C. Delgado, and C. L. González, "Low co-existence rates of *Lactobacillus* spp. and *Helicobacter pylori* detected in gastric biopsies from patients with gastrointestinal symptoms," *Revista Española de Enfermedades Digestivas*, vol. 104, no. 9, pp. 473–478, 2012.

[64] S. Khulusi, M. A. Mendall, P. Patel, J. Levy, S. Badve, and T. C. Northfield, "*Helicobacter pylori* infection density and gastric inflammation in duodenal ulcer and non-ulcer subjects," *Gut*, vol. 37, no. 3, pp. 319–324, 1995.

[65] H. W. Fu, "*Helicobacter pylori* neutrophil-activating protein: from molecular pathogenesis to clinical applications," *World Journal of Gastroenterology*, vol. 20, no. 18, pp. 5294–5301, 2014.

[66] B. Satin, G. del Giudice, V. Della Bianca et al., "The neutrophil-activating protein (HP-NAP) of *Helicobacter pylori* is a protective antigen and a major virulence factor," *The Journal of Experimental Medicine*, vol. 191, no. 9, pp. 1467–1476, 2000.

[67] A. M. Kabir, Y. Aiba, A. Takagi, S. Kamiya, T. Miwa, and Y. Koga, "Prevention of *Helicobacter pylori* infection by Lactobacilli in a gnotobiotic murine model," *Gut*, vol. 41, no. 1, pp. 49–55, 1997.

[68] G. Marcial, J. Villena, G. Faller, A. Hensel, and G. F. de Valdéz, "Exopolysaccharide-producing *Streptococcus thermophilus* CRL1190 reduces the inflammatory response caused by *Helicobacter pylori*," *Beneficial Microbes*, vol. 8, no. 3, pp. 451–461, 2017.

[69] Y.-J. Yang, C. C. Chuang, H. B. Yang, C. C. Lu, and B. S. Sheu, "*Lactobacillus acidophilus* ameliorates *H. pylori*-induced gastric inflammation by inactivating the Smad7 and NFκB pathways," *BMC Microbiology*, vol. 12, no. 1, p. 38, 2012.

[70] J. S. Lee, N. S. Paek, O. S. Kwon, and K. B. Hahm, "Anti-inflammatory actions of probiotics through activating suppressor of cytokine signaling (SOCS) expression and signaling in *Helicobacter pylori* infection: a novel mechanism," *Journal of Gastroenterology and Hepatology*, vol. 25, no. 1, pp. 194–202, 2010.

[71] C. Zhou, F. Z. Ma, X. J. Deng, H. Yuan, and H. S. Ma, "Lactobacilli inhibit interleukin-8 production induced by *Helicobacter pylori* lipopolysaccharide-activated Toll-like receptor 4," *World Journal of Gastroenterology*, vol. 14, no. 32, pp. 5090–5095, 2008.

[72] K. A. Ryan, A. M. O'Hara, J. P. van Pijkeren, F. P. Douillard, and P. W. O'Toole, "*Lactobacillus salivarius* modulates cytokine induction and virulence factor gene expression in *Helicobacter pylori*," *Journal of Medical Microbiology*, vol. 58, no. 8, pp. 996–1005, 2009.

[73] H. J. Yu, W. Liu, Z. Chang et al., "Probiotic BIFICO cocktail ameliorates *Helicobacter pylori* induced gastritis," *World Journal of Gastroenterology*, vol. 21, no. 21, pp. 6561–6571, 2015.

Staffing at Ambulatory Endoscopy Centers in the United States: Practice, Trends, and Rationale

Deepak Agrawal[1] and **Rajeev Jain**[2]

[1]Department of Medicine, Division of Digestive and Liver Diseases, University Texas Southwestern Medical Center, Dallas, TX, USA
[2]Texas Digestive Disease Consultants, Dallas, TX, USA

Correspondence should be addressed to Deepak Agrawal; dagrawal4321@gmail.com

Academic Editor: Paolo Gionchetti

Background. Endoscopy nurse (RN) has a pivotal role in administration and monitoring of moderate sedation during endoscopic procedures. When sedation for the procedure is administered and monitored by an anesthesia specialist, the role of an RN is less clear. The guidelines on this issue by nursing and gastroenterology societies are contradictory. *Methods.* Survey study of endoscopy lab managers and directors at outpatient endoscopy units in Texas. The questions related to staffing patterns for outpatient endoscopies and responsibilities of different personnel assisting with endoscopies. *Results.* Responses were received from 65 endoscopy units (response rate 38%). 63/65 (97%) performed at least a few cases with an anesthesia specialist. Of these, 49/63 (78%) involved only an endoscopy technician, without an additional RN in the room. At 12/49 (25%) units, the RN performed tasks of an endoscopy technician. At 14/63 (22%), an additional RN was present during endoscopic procedures and performed tasks not directly related to patient care. *Conclusions.* Many ambulatory endoscopy units do not have an RN present at all times when sedation is administered by an anesthesia specialist. An RN, when present, did not perform tasks commensurate with the education and training. This has implications about optimal utilization of nurses and cost of performing endoscopies.

1. Introduction

Endoscopies at the ambulatory surgical centers (ASCs) are well-established models of care offering convenience, efficiency, and economy for low-risk endoscopies. For ASCs to be successful, it is important to keep quality and patient satisfaction high and costs low. Optimal staffing of the endoscopy units is, therefore, essential. The endoscopy team usually consists of a registered nurse (RN) who administers moderate sedation and an endoscopy technician who assists with technical procedural-related activities such as taking biopsies and removing polyps. The person performing the tasks of a technician may be another RN or a trained unlicensed person. In the last few years, more and more endoscopists prefer sedation with propofol, which is faster and shorter acting [1]. Propofol sedation qualifies as deep sedation since spontaneous breathing can be affected and per regulations in the United States can be administered only by an anesthesia specialist. This raises questions about the role of an RN during endoscopic procedures since their main responsibility of administering sedation is now taken over by an anesthesia specialist. Endoscopy units outside United States have different staffing models but have the same concerns about costs and efficiency of health care.

The American Society of Gastrointestinal Endoscopy (ASGE) guidelines state that when an anesthesia specialist is responsible for sedation [2], an additional RN is not needed while the Society of Gastroenterology Nurses and Associates (SGNA) recommends the presence of an RN to assist the endoscopy team [3]. These contradictory statements are not supported by any references or data. The practice patterns, thus, have emerged based on opinions, perceptions, needs, and wants. With increasing health care costs and decreasing reimbursements for procedures, optimal resource utilization has become an important issue [4]. Furthermore, there is a significant shortage of RNs in the United States and optimal utilization of their knowledge and expertise is important.

We conducted a survey of ambulatory surgical centers (ASCs) and endoscopy units in Texas, United States, to determine the practice patterns regarding type of sedation (moderate vs. deep), staffing of endoscopy units, and the role of RNs during procedure when sedation is administered by an anesthesia specialist.

2. Methods

A questionnaire was constructed after open-ended interviewing of gastroenterologists and nurses from two institutions. The responses were reviewed by additional gastroenterologists and nurse managers from three different institutions, not included in the study, for linguistic, internal, and external validation of the questionnaire. An online version of the survey was created using https://www.surveymonkey.com/. The questions asked included type of endoscopy unit (ambulatory versus hospital based); number of endoscopic procedures performed per month; type of procedures; percentage of patients with different American Society of Anesthesiologists (ASA) classification; method of sedation; and personnel present in the endoscopy room during procedure and their responsibilities during procedure.

The names of ambulatory surgical centers performing endoscopies were obtained from the Texas Department of State Health Services [5]. An email with hyperlink to the survey was sent to the managers or directors of the endoscopy units. If no response was received after one week, the endoscopy units were contacted with a phone call to make sure they had received the survey. If email addresses were unavailable, the survey was faxed to the endoscopy unit. All data were obtained anonymously. This research was granted exemption by the Institutional Review Board of the University of Texas Southwestern Medical Center.

Data were summarized using descriptive statistics. Response rates were calculated as number of surveys with responses divided by number of surveys distributed. All the data supporting the results are shown in the paper and can be applicable from the corresponding author.

3. Results

The surveys were distributed to 172 endoscopy units and responses received from 65 (response rate 38%). Details of the ASCs are shown in Table 1.

Table 1: Characteristics of endoscopy units surveyed.

	Range	Mean
Number of procedure rooms	2–5	3.4
Number of procedures performed in a month	220–1350	796
Percent of procedures that are		
Upper endoscopies	20–50%	32%
Colonoscopies	50–90%	68%
Others	0–3%	<1%
ASA classification of patients		
ASA 1	20–35%	24%
ASA 2	25–60%	41%
ASA 3	15–45%	35%
ASA 4	0-1%	<1%
Percent of procedures in an endoscopy unit with an anesthesia specialist	0%–100%	72%

3.1. Use of an Anesthesia Specialist. Overall, 63/65 (97%) of endoscopy units performed cases with an anesthesia specialist. Of these, 30 (46%) endoscopy units performed 100% of their procedures and 15 (23%) performed 75–99% of their procedures with deep sedation administered by an anesthesia specialist. Two endoscopy units performed their cases only with moderate sedation and did not use an anesthesia specialist.

3.2. Use of RNs. Of the endoscopy units that performed their cases with an anesthesia specialist, 49/63 (78%) involved only an endoscopy technician, without an additional RN in the room. At 12/49 (25%) endoscopy units, the RN performed tasks of an endoscopy technician. The other endoscopy units had a "floating nurse" who was available, if needed.

At 14/63 (22%), an additional RN was present during endoscopic procedures and performed tasks not directly related to patient care. The responsibilities of RNs included at least one of the following: performing a time out before the procedure, documenting endoscopic accessories used, and documenting/labeling pathology samples. At some units, RNs had additional responsibilities. For example, at 7/26 (27%) endoscopy units, the RNs helped with consents before the procedures. At 2/26 (8%) endoscopy units, the RNs completed the preliminary endoscopy report or discharge instructions after discussions with the endoscopist.

Twenty-six endoscopy units had at least one RN present during endoscopy, when sedation was administered by an anesthesia specialist (12 endoscopy units had 1 RN and 14 units had 2 RNs). The reasons given by endoscopy units for having an RN along with anesthesia specialists included regulatory requirement to have an RN in the room (18/26, 69%), complete documentation requirements (17/26, 65%), improved patient safety (4/26, 15%), and need for an RN for submucosal injections (3/26, 12%). At the 37 endoscopy units without an RN, submucosal injections were mainly performed by the technician assisting with the procedures except at 7 (19%) units where a floating RN was called, as needed. At two endoscopy units, the technician was allowed to assist with submucosal injection of saline and dye but not diluted epinephrine.

4. Discussion

ASCs avoid urgent circumstances and high-risk patients and are especially well suited for care-process standardization. Reducing variation and standardizing workflows that allow staff to work at their level of training and scope of practice is necessary to provide high quality, cost-effective care. Conflicting statements from professional societies or ambiguous statements from credentialing and regulatory bodies can create confusion about standards of practice. We highlight such an issue in our study, which although focused on endoscopy is applicable to other procedures at ASCs.

What should be the appropriate staffing during endoscopy when endoscopy sedation is provided by an anesthesia specialist? What should be the role of an RN in this situation? The American Society of Gastrointestinal Endoscopy states, "When endoscopy is with an anesthesia specialist, one endoscopy staff member is required to assist the endoscopist with the technical portion of the procedure. This person may be an unlicensed active personnel (UAP), licensed practical nurse (LPN) or an RN. The presence of an RN is not mandatory in this setting" [2, 6]. The Society of Gastroenterology Nurses and Associates in their minimum RN staffing position statement states, "When an anesthesia specialist is providing the sedation, the RN will remain in the procedure room to assist the healthcare team" [3]. The contradictory position statements are confusing for physicians, nurses, management of endoscopy units, and accreditation organizations and introduce variation in standards of care and resource utilization.

The issue highlighted in our study, while focused on endoscopy, has a more generalized appeal for other procedures at ASCs. Conflicting statements from professional societies or ambiguous statements from credentialing and regulatory bodies are not uncommon. Our survey is the first study, to our knowledge, to determine how ASCs choose to staff their endoscopy units and the rationale for their approach. Our results show that, when an anesthesia specialist administers sedation, less than one fourth of the ambulatory endoscopy units have an RN present during the procedure. Most of them instead have a "floating" nurse who is available to help as needed. Notably, the change in staffing model of not having an RN in the room appears to be a recent trend. ASGE survey from 2013 had reported that in ambulatory endoscopy units, an RN was present in the room along with anesthesiology provider 62% of the time [7]. We speculate that this may be in response to decreasing reimbursements and emphasis on optimizing resource utilization [8].

The responsibilities of an RN, when present in the room along with an anesthesia specialist, mainly included performing a surgical time out, documenting endoscopic accessories used (for billing purposes), and/or helping with pathology samples—none of which require a person to have nursing knowledge or expertise. When an RN was not present, these tasks were completed by the endoscopy technician and/or anesthesia specialist. The increasing documentation requirements and paperwork sometimes necessitates an additional person in the room, other than a technician. Some endoscopy units used the floating RN or another technician for these tasks.

One of the arguments of having an RN in the room along with the anesthesia specialist is increased patient safety. The premise of such an argument would be that deep sedation by an anesthesiologist has more complications compared to moderate sedation by an RN and that an extra RN is needed helpful to respond to these complications. There is no data to support these premises. Before the current regulation that administration of propofol can only be performed by an anesthesia specialist, RNs administered propofol under the endoscopist's supervision. This was referred to as nurse-administered propofol sedation (NAPS), the safety of which has been well established in many prospective and retrospective studies [9, 10]. Notably, in these studies, no additional RN was present.

Another reason why endoscopy units need RNs during the procedure is the belief that regulations require that submucosal injection of saline, epinephrine, and dyes into the gastrointestinal wall can only be performed by a nurse and not an unlicensed personnel (UAP) or a technician. The regulations on what licensed and unlicensed personnel are permitted to do during a procedure are determined by the state but the directives are often not stated clearly. The Joint Commission, the Accreditation Association for Ambulatory Health Care, and Centers for Medicare and Medicaid Services do not define the specific qualifications or number of staff required [11–13]. Rather, they generalize that the staff be adequate in number with appropriate training and supervision. In the state of Texas, a surgical technician can inject submucosal normal saline or dye as long as the technician is deemed competent to do so and performs tasks under continuous and direct physician supervision [14]. In our survey, many respondents believed that having an RN in the room along with an anesthesia specialist was per state or federal regulations and accreditation guidelines. Few respondents commented that they thought the use of an RN in addition to the anesthesia specialist was standard of care. Our survey shows that the majority of the endoscopy units in Texas do not have an additional RN in the room along with anesthesia provider and thus would be considered a standard of care [15].

The question if an RN should be present at all times during the procedure is important and especially relevant in present health care scenario where there is severe shortage of RNs and endoscopy units are under pressure to provide more cost-efficient care to the patients. A recent report by American Association of Colleges of Nursing estimates the nursing shortage to be 260,000 by year 2025 [16]. In our survey, few respondents specifically commented on having difficulty hiring RNs. Declining reimbursements, bundled payments, and reference pricing have now made it imperative to reevaluate the costs of endoscopic procedures [4, 8, 17, 18]. An ASGE survey of endoscopy units in the US reported that clinical full-time equivalents (FTEs) in one endoscopic procedure have increased from 4.1 in 2008 to 4.7 in 2011—a 15% increase while the reimbursements have decreased. Clinical labor represents more than 40% of the total endoscopy unit cost [7]. More importantly, patients now bear the burden of increased costs due to high deductible plans or copays.

When an anesthesia specialist administers sedation, RNs present in the room did not perform tasks commensurate with their training and experience. Endoscopy nurses are a valuable resource and their knowledge and expertise can be utilized in more important ways. For example, the endoscopy nurses can be helpful in tracking quality indicators of endoscopy. The endoscopy nurse can also help improve communication about endoscopic procedures with the patients. In a recent study, patients at a safety-net hospital, who gave informed consent for an endoscopy after an educational class given by nurses, reported being better informed about the procedure compared to patients who were consented in the gastroenterology clinic [19].

Our study has limitations. First, the study was conducted in the United States and may not be applicable to endoscopy units in other countries, which have different regulatory requirements. Second, our study population was restricted to ambulatory endoscopy units, which affects generalizability of the results to endoscopy units within a hospital. This was intentional to ensure homogeneity of patient population across different endoscopy units. For example, the patients were mostly ASA I and II and less likely to include complex indications. Second, we surveyed only endoscopy units in the state of Texas. We did so to avoid regional variations in policies and regulations regarding scope of practice for surgical technicians, LPNs, and RNs. Fourth limitation is the possibility of information bias. Response bias could have occurred if endoscopy units that do not use an RN in the endoscopy unit were more likely to respond. However, we believe that our data is more representative of the current trends than nonresponse bias. A 2012 survey of endoscopy practices conducted by ASGE showed that nationwide 66% endoscopy units use propofol for sedation which is very similar to our data. Even, if there is some response bias, our survey shows the feasibility and safety of procedure with an anesthesia specialist without an RN in the room. Finally, our survey does not address the issue of safety of endoscopic procedure with different staffing models.

In conclusion, our study highlights different endoscopy staffing models and how different endoscopy units are adapting to the changes in health care—increasing demand for the more expensive deep sedation, decreasing reimbursements and nursing shortage. Interests and safety of the patients come first and endoscopy units should ensure that the staff assisting with the procedures are well trained. Most ambulatory endoscopy units now do not have an RN present at all times when sedation is administered by an anesthesia specialist. This staffing model meets the regulatory requirements in the US, is not associated with any adverse outcome, and may allow more appropriate utilization of endoscopy nurses.

Additional Points

Biostatistics Statement. Simple descriptive statistics was used.

Ethical Approval

This study was granted exemption by the Institutional Review Board of the University of Texas Southwestern Medical Center.

References

[1] H. Liu, D. A. Waxman, R. Main, and S. Mattke, "Utilization of anesthesia services during outpatient endoscopies and colonoscopies and associated spending in 2003-2009," *Journal of the American Medical Association*, vol. 307, no. 11, pp. 1178–1184, 2012.

[2] ASGE Standards of Practice Committee, R. Jain, S. O. Ikenberry et al., "Minimum staffing requirements for the performance of GI endoscopy," *Gastrointestinal Endoscopy*, vol. 72, no. 3, pp. 469-470, 2010.

[3] Society of Gastroenterology Nurses and Associates, *Minimum Registered Nurse Staffing for Patient Care in the Gastrointestinal Endoscopy Unit*, 2010.

[4] S. D. Dorn and C. J. Vesy, "Medicare's revaluation of gastrointestinal endoscopic procedures: implications for academic and community-based practices," *Clinical Gastroenterology and Hepatology*, vol. 14, no. 7, pp. 924–928.e1, 2016.

[5] Texas Department of State Health Services, *Ambulatory Surgical Centers*, 2017.

[6] ASGE Ensuring Safety in the Gastrointestinal Endoscopy Unit Task Force, A. H. Calderwood, F. J. Chapman et al., "Guidelines for safety in the gastrointestinal endoscopy unit," *Gastrointestinal Endoscopy*, vol. 79, no. 3, pp. 363–372, 2014.

[7] American Society of Gastrointestinal Endoscopy-Endoscopic Operations Survey, *2012 Data Book and Analysis*.

[8] American Gastroenterology Association, *CMS Cuts Reimbursements to Colonoscopy*.

[9] D. K. Rex, V. P. Deenadayalu, E. Eid et al., "Endoscopist-directed administration of propofol: a worldwide safety experience," *Gastroenterology*, vol. 137, no. 4, pp. 1229–1237, 2009.

[10] J. J. Vargo, L. B. Cohen, D. K. Rex et al., "Position statement: nonanesthesiologist administration of propofol for GI endoscopy," *Gastroenterology*, vol. 137, no. 6, pp. 2161–2167, 2009.

[11] Joint Commission on Accreditation of Healthcare Organizations, *Standards for Ambulatory Care*, Joint Commission Resources, Oakbrook Terrace, IL, USA, 2009.

[12] Accreditation Association for Ambulatory Health Care, *Accreditation Handbook for Ambulatory Health Care 2009*, Skokie, IL, USA, 2009.

[13] *Ambulatory Surgical Centers - State Operations Manual*, Centers for Medicare and Medicaid Serives, 2015, https://www.cms.gov/Regulations-and-Guidance/Guidance/Manuals/downloads/som107ap_l_ambulatory.pdf.

[14] Association of Surgical Technologists, *Texas Surgical Assistant Scope of Practice Laws*.

[15] P. Moffett and G. Moore, "The standard of care: legal history and definitions: the bad and good news," *Western Journal of Emergency Medicine*, vol. 12, no. 1, pp. 109–112, 2011.

[16] American Association of College of Nursing, *Nursing Shortage*, American Association of College of Nursing, 2017, http://www.aacnnursing.org/Portals/42/News/Factsheets/Nursing-Shortage-Factsheet-2017.pdf.

[17] J. V. Brill, R. Jain, P. S. Margolis et al., "A bundled payment framework for colonoscopy performed for colorectal cancer screening or surveillance," *Gastroenterology*, vol. 146, no. 3, pp. 849–853.e9, 2014.

[18] J. C. Robinson and K. MacPherson, "Payers test reference pricing and centers of excellence to steer patients to low-price and high-quality providers," *Health Affairs*, vol. 31, no. 9, pp. 2028–2036, 2012.

[19] D. Siao, J. L. Sewell, and L. W. Day, "Assessment of delivery methods used in the informed consent process at a safety-net hospital," *Gastrointestinal Endoscopy*, vol. 80, no. 1, pp. 61–68, 2014.

26

Only Surgical Treatment to Be Considered for Adhesive Small Bowel Obstruction: A New Paradigm

Nicolas Tabchouri,[1] David Dussart,[1] Urs Giger-Pabst,[2] Nicolas Michot,[1] Frederic Marques,[1] Meriem Khalfallah,[1] Petru Bucur,[1] Louise Barbier,[1] Aurore Kraemer-Bucur,[1] Mihane Nayeri,[1] Julien Thiery,[1] Celine Bourbao-Tournois,[1] Pascal Bourlier,[1] Ephrem Salamé,[1] and Mehdi Ouaïssi[1]

[1]*Department of Digestive, Oncological, Endocrine, Hepato-Biliary and Pancreatic Surgery, and Liver Transplantation, Trousseau Hospital, University Hospital of Tours, France*
[2]*Department of General Surgery & Therapy Center for Peritoneal Carcinomatosis, St. Mary's Hospital, University Hospital of the Ruhr-University Bochum, Herne, Germany*

Correspondence should be addressed to Mehdi Ouaïssi; m.ouaissi@chu-tours.fr

Academic Editor: Roberto Caronna

Background. Adhesive small bowel obstruction (SBO) represents a heavy burden in healthcare systems worldwide and is associated with significant morbidity and mortality. Although conservative treatment alone can lead to SBO resolution in most cases, its optimal duration is still a matter of debate. The aim of this study was to analyze different SBO evolution patterns in order to further determine when to switch to surgical treatment. *Study Design.* All patients who were admitted for adhesive SBO between 2011 and 2016 were reviewed. Patients who had immediate surgery (IS), a successful medical treatment (SMT), and a failed medical treatment (FMT) were compared in terms of overall morbidity, mortality, and SBO recurrence. *Results.* Overall 154 patients were identified, including 23 (14.9%) in IS, 27 (17.5%) in FMT, and 104 (67.6%) in SMT groups. In terms of comorbidities, patients were similar in all groups. Overall morbidity rates were highest in IS and FMT groups (30% and 33%, respectively, vs. 4% in the SMT group, $p < 0.001$) whereas mortality rate was highest in the FMT group (22% vs. 0% and 0% in IS and SMT groups, respectively, $p < 0.001$). SBO recurrence rate was highest in the SMT group (22% vs. 4% and 7% in IS and FMT groups, respectively, $p = 0.042$). *Conclusion.* FMT seems to be associated with similar overall morbidity compared with IS but with increased postoperative mortality. Patient frailty seems to be worsened by prolonged inefficient medical treatment.

1. Introduction

Peritoneal adhesions are the underlying cause of 32% of acute intestinal obstructions and of 65%–75% of small bowel obstructions (SBO) and represent a major unresolved public health issue and burden [1]. In patients with abdominal pain, SBO is a common cause that accounts for 4% of all emergency department admissions and 20% of emergency surgical procedures [2]. Mortality rates of patients surgically treated for SBO remain surprisingly high (5–10%) [1, 3–5].

Conservative SBO treatment was acknowledged by published reports and clinical practice when patients did not present any sign of strangulation, peritonitis, or severe intestinal impairment and when computed tomography (CT scan) revealed no small bowel feces sign, free intraperitoneal fluid, or mesenteric edema [6]. However, no consensus has been reached regarding conservative treatment duration or when to switch to operative treatment in case of failure. Despite two large cohort studies demonstrating that mortality rates were increased in SBO patients undergoing surgery with a 24-hour delay [5, 7], the 2013 World Society of Emergency Surgery recommendations state that surgical treatment should be considered in the absence of SBO resolution after a 72-hour nonoperative management duration [6].

These conflicting results are due to the usually heterogeneous nature of patients' inclusion. Very few data were reported in the literature about short- or long-term outcome of patients which have had a failure of medical treatment of SBO. The present study aimed at determining results of different surgical managements of SBO in the same surgical team with homogeneous management with a focus on the specificity of the group of patients which have a failure of their medical treatment.

2. Methods

2.1. Study Population and Data Collection. From January 2011 to May 2016, all consecutive patients treated for adhesive SBO at the University Hospital of Tours were identified and retrospectively included. During the study period, the first admission for SBO was defined as the index date. Other causes for SBO including malignancy, volvulus, postoperative ileus (within 1 month), inflammatory bowel disease, large bowel obstruction, hernia, radiation-related obstruction, and Meckel's diverticulum were excluded [8–11]. At initial admission, CT scan and blood work were performed for all patients.

2.2. SBO Management. SBO surgical treatment upon admission (immediate surgery (IS)) was decided based on clinical evaluation (spontaneous and/or provoked abdominal pain, abdominal guarding, hemodynamic choc, signs of strangulation, peritonitis, and fever) and imaging severity signs (such as free intraperitoneal fluid, mesenteric edema, lack of small bowel feces sign, bowel strangulation, devascularized bowel, necrosis, and perforation) [6]. When severity signs were absent, patients were treated medically (with intravenous hydration, fasting, nasogastric tube drainage, and analgesics) and were clinically and biologically reevaluated every 6 hours. Failed medical treatment (FMT) was diagnosed if severity signs appeared or if SBO resolution was not reached and led to secondary surgical treatment (the decision to switch to surgical treatment was left at each physician's discretion). Patients treated medically and who died before undergoing surgery were accounted for as FMT patients. Each patient was admitted and reevaluated by the same senior surgeon. Patients were therefore divided into three groups: immediate surgery (IS), failed medical treatment (FMT), and successful medical treatment (SMT). These groups, which represented three different SBO profiles and evolution patterns, were then compared.

2.3. Study Variables. The following baseline demographic and clinical characteristics were collected: age, gender, BMI, comorbidities, previous surgical procedures, American Society of Anesthesiologist (ASA) score and Charlson comorbidity index (CCI) [12, 13]. Clinical, biological (including C-reactive protein (CRP), electrolyte fluid analysis, and white blood cell (WBC) count), and CT scan evaluation and results upon admission were collected, as well as clinical and biological results at each reevaluation. Medical treatment duration was noted in all FMT patients. The following intraoperative and postoperative variables were also collected: operative duration, adhesion type (single band or extensive intra-abdominal adhesions), small bowel injury occurrence, and whether or not resection was required. We also recorded whether or not surgical treatment was performed during the night (between 6:30 pm and 6:30 am).

2.4. Postoperative Outcomes. Postoperative morbidity and mortality were assessed at 30 days following surgery using Clavien-Dindo classification. Severe postoperative complications were defined as Clavien-Dindo > 2 [14]. Anastomotic leakage, intra-abdominal abscess, and postoperative collections were searched for if patient presented with signs of sepsis, using CT scan. Other postoperative complications were also collected such as hemorrhage, anastomosis stenosis, and other infectious and cardiorespiratory complications. Therapeutic management of postoperative complications was also recorded. Postoperative bowel recovery was determined by flatus, passage of stool, and oral intake recovery. In the SMT group, median time to flatus and oral intake recovery was collected. Total in-hospital stay and readmission rates were collected. Readmissions due to SBO recurrence as well as subsequent therapeutic management were specifically recorded. Patients who were not readmitted were contacted by phone in order to assess any SBO recurrence symptoms. Follow-up was updated to May 2016. Further analyses were performed in the FMT group according to medical treatment duration (<48 h and >48 h).

2.5. Statistical Analysis. Baseline characteristics of the studied population and intraoperative and postoperative outcomes were analyzed. Categorical variables were compared using the chi-squared test or Fischer's exact test when appropriate. Bonferroni's correction was also used whenever appropriate. Continuous variables were compared using Student's *t*-test or the Mann-Whitney *U* test whenever appropriate. Categorical variables were expressed as numbers (percentages) and continuous variables as means (±standard deviation (SD) or range). All statistical analyses were performed using IBM SPSS Statistics version 20 (IBM SPSS Inc., Chicago, IL, USA), and statistical significance was accepted at the 0.05 level.

3. Results

3.1. Baseline Characteristics (Table 1). Overall, 154 patients presenting with adhesive SBO were included in the study period. Median age was 74 (16–104) years and there were 85 men (55.2%). All patients had a previous abdominal surgery by open procedure. Immediate surgery (IS group) was required in 23 (14.9%) patients, and failed medical treatment was observed in 27 (17.5%) patients (FMT group). In 104 (67.6%) patients, medical treatment was sufficient and led to SBO resolution (SMT group). In terms of comorbidities, atrial fibrillation was significantly more frequent in the SMT group (IS, 4.3%; FMT, 7.4%; and SMT, 18.3%; $p = 0.001$) and chronic obstructive pulmonary disease was significantly more frequent in IS (IS, 13%, FMT: 0%, and SMT: 2.9%; $p = 0.038$). Charlson comorbidity index was not significantly different between the three groups. In terms of

TABLE 1: Demographic characteristics and initial SBO clinical, radiological, and biological presentations.

	IS ($n = 23$)	FMT ($n = 27$)	SMT ($n = 104$)	Total ($n = 154$)	P
Demographic characteristics					
Age (years)	69 (25–97)	70 (22–104)	76 (16–99)	74 (16–104)	0.115
Gender (M/F)	9/14	12/15	65/39	85/69	0.052
BMI (kg/m^2)	23.5 (16.9–81)	20.3 (16.5–30.9)	23.1 (14.8–40.1)	23.8 (14.8–40.1)	**0.004**
ASA score, n (%)					
1–2	19 (82.6)	19 (70.4)	83 (79.8)	121 (78.6)	
3–4	4 (17.4)	8 (29.6)	21 (20.2)	33 (21.4)	0.497
Previous SBO, n (%)	14 (60.9)	4 (14.8)	41 (39.4)	59 (38.4)	**0.004**
Comorbidity, n (%)					
Diabetes mellitus, n (%)	0	2 (7.4)	17 (16.4)	19 (12.3)	0.068
Renal failure, n (%)	1 (4.3)	2 (7.4)	13 (12.5)	20 (12.9)	0.437
Peripheral arterial disease, n (%)	4 (17.3)	3 (11.1)	19 (18.3)	26 (16.9)	0.788
Coronary disease, n (%)	2 (8.7)	2 (7.4)	15 (14.4)	19 (12.3)	0.520
Atrial fibrillation, n (%)	1 (4.3)	2 (7.4)	34 (32.7)	37 (24.1)	**0.001**
Previous stroke, n (%)	2 (8.7)	2 (7.4)	7 (6.7)	11 (7.1)	0.113
Elevated blood pressure, n (%)	12 (52.2)	6 (22.2)	45 (43.3)	63 (40.9)	0.069
COPD, n (%)	3 (13.0)	0	3 (2.9)	6 (3.9)	**0.038**
Performance status, n (%)					
(i) 0	6 (26.1)	8 (29.6)	23 (22.1)	37 (24.1)	
(ii) 1	8 (34.8)	9 (33.3)	46 (44.3)	63 (40.9)	
(iii) 2	8 (34.8)	5 (18.5)	23 (22.1)	36 (23.4)	0.542
(iv) 3	1 (4.3)	3 (11.1)	10 (9.6)	14 (9.1)	
(v) 4	0	2 (7.4)	2 (1.9)	4 (2.6)	
Charlson comorbidity index, n (%)					
(i) 0	13 (56.5)	13 (48.1)	41 (39.4)	67 (43.5)	
(ii) 1–2	9 (39.1)	9 (33.3)	37 (35.6)	55 (35.7)	0.243
(iii) 3–4	1 (4.3)	3 (11.1)	23 (22.1)	27 (17.5)	
(iv) ≥5	0	2 (7.4)	3 (2.8)	5 (3.2)	
Clinical presentation					
Spontaneous abdominal pain, n (%)	22 (95.6)	11 (40.1)	56 (53.9)	89 (57.8)	**<0.001**
Provoked abdominal pain, n (%)	22 (95.6)	25 (92.6)	73 (70.2)	120 (77.9)	**0.004**
Radiological presentation					
Free peritoneal fluid, n (%)	13 (56.5)	8 (29.6)	13 (12.5)	34 (22.1)	**<0.001**
Feces sign, n (%)	19 (82.6)	3 (11.1)	20 (19.2)	42 (27.3)	**<0.001**
Devascularized bowel, n (%)	19 (82.6)	1 (3.7)	2 (1.9)	22 (14.3)	**<0.001**
Biological presentation					
WBC count (G/L)	13.5 (8.3–18.9)	10.2 (5.3–15.6)	10.8 (4.9–17.1)	11.1 (6.2–17.5)	**0.042**
CRP (mg/L)	32	39.8	26.7	29.8	0.304

SBO: small bowel obstruction; IS: immediate surgery; FMT: failed medical treatment; SMT: successful medical treatment; BMI: body mass index; ASA: American Society of Anesthesiologists; COPD: chronic obstructive pulmonary disease; WBC: white blood cells; CRP: C-reactive protein. Continuous variables are presented as mean (range).

clinical presentation, spontaneous and provoked abdominal pain was significantly more frequent in the IS group compared to the FMT and SMT groups (95% vs. 40% and 54%, $p < 0.001$ and 96% vs. 93% and 70%, $p = 0.004$, respectively). IS patients presented with significantly more intraperitoneal fluid, feces sign, and devascularized bowel compared with FMT and SMT patients ($p < 0.001$). In terms of biological evaluation, WBC count was significantly increased in the IS group ($p = 0.040$).

3.2. Surgical Treatment. In the FMT group, the decision to switch to surgical treatment was taken because of persistence or worsening of abdominal pain ($n = 7$, 26%), lack of SBO resolution after a 48-hour period of time ($n = 17$, 63%), and SBO recurrence after feeding reintroduction during the same in-hospital stay ($n = 3$, 11%). In the FMT group, 2 (7.4%) patients died before reaching the operative room. Surgical treatment consisted of open procedures in all cases. Extensive adhesiolysis and small bowel resection were required in 40%

TABLE 2: Outcome according to different SBO therapeutic managements.

	IS ($n = 23$)	FMT ($n = 27$)	SMT ($n = 104$)	Total ($n = 154$)	P
Single band adhesion, *n* (%)	13 (56.5)	17 (63.0)	—	30 (60.0)	0.774
Extensive adhesions, *n* (%)	10 (43.5)	10 (37.0)	—	20 (40.0)	0.640
Associated bowel resection, *n* (%)	5 (21.7)	4 (14.8)	—	9 (18.0)	0.715
Night shift surgery, *n* (%)	17 (73.9)	13 (48.1)	—	30 (60.0)	1.000
Operative time (min)	120 (70–180)	117 (70–160)	—	120 (70–172)	0.871
Short-term outcome					
Overall complications, *n* (%)	7 (30.4)	9 (33.3)	4 (3.8)	31 (20.1)	**<0.001**
Grade I–II, *n* (%)	5 (21.7)	2 (7.4)	3 (2.9)	10 (6.5)	**0.004**
Grade III–IV, *n* (%)	2 (8.7)	1 (3.7)	1 (0.9)	4 (3.8)	**0.010**
Reoperation, *n* (%)	0	1 (3.7)	0	1 (0.65)	—
Mortality, *n* (%)	0	6 (22.2)	0	6 (3.9)	**<0.001**
Anastomotic leak, *n* (%)	1 (4.3)	3 (11.1)	0	4 (2.6)	**0.005**
Peritonitis, *n* (%)	0	2 (7.4)	0	2 (1.3)	**0.009**
Intra-abdominal collection, *n* (%)	1 (4.3)	1 (3.7)	0	2 (1.3)	0.119
Superficial abscess, *n* (%)	1 (4.3)	1 (3.7)	0	2 (1.3)	0.119
Cardiac failure, *n* (%)	0	0	0	0	1.000
Pulmonary complication, *n* (%)	0	2 (7.4)	0	2 (1.3)	**0.009**
Urinary infection, *n* (%)	4 (17.4)	4 (14.8)	1 (0.9)	9 (5.8)	**0.001**
Long-term outcome					
Follow-up (months)	47 (2–147)	34 (2–57)	34 (2–179)	34.7 (2–179)	0.648
SBO recurrence, *n* (%)	1 (4.3)	2 (7.4)	23 (22.1)	26 (16.9)	**0.042**
Stoma requirement, *n* (%)	1 (4.3)	2 (7.4)	0	3 (1.9)	**0.031**
Anastomotic stenosis, *n* (%)	1 (4.3)	0	0	1 (0.6)	0.057

SBO: small bowel obstruction; IS: immediate surgery; FMT: failed medical treatment; SMT: successful medical treatment. Continuous variables are presented as mean (range).

and 18% of all patients who underwent surgical SBO treatment (IS and FMT groups, $n = 50$). Most surgical procedures (IS and FMT groups) were performed during the night ($n = 30$, 60%). In the FMT group, mean medical treatment duration was 4 ± 2 days; in FMT, 33% ($n = 9$) and 67% ($n = 18$) of patients were treated ≤48 h and >48 h, respectively.

3.3. Postoperative Morbidity and Mortality. Overall morbidity and mortality rates are presented in Table 2. There was no intraoperative death. Six patients (6.7%) died postoperatively from pancreatitis ($n = 1$), cardiorespiratory complication ($n = 3$), and peritonitis ($n = 2$). Overall postoperative morbidity rate was 12.9% ($n = 20$) and was significantly different between the 3 groups. Ten (6.5%) patients presented with grade I–II postoperative complications according to Clavien-Dindo classification and 10 (6.5%) with grade III–IV complications. In the IS group, one (4.3%) patient presented with an anastomotic leak, one (4.3%) with an intra-abdominal abscess, 4 (17.3%) with a urinary infection, and one (4.4%) with an incisional abscess. Mortality rate was null.

In the FMT group, mortality rate was 22.2% ($n = 6$): one (3.7%) patient died of pancreatitis, 2 (7.4%) before undergoing surgery, one (3.7%) due to cardiorespiratory complication (requiring critical care), and 2 (7.4%) due to anastomotic leak occurrence (redo surgery was not performed in both latter patients due to very advanced age: 95 and 104 years old). In the SMT group, one (0.9%) patient needed intensive care for hemodynamic instability. Two (1.8%) patients presented with a catheter-related skin infection and one (0.9%) with a urinary infection.

The FMT group was further analyzed according to conservative treatment duration (failure less than 48 hours following medical treatment introduction (FMT < 48 h, $n = 9$) and failure more than 48 hours following introduction (FMT > 48 h, $n = 18$)). Observed mortality rates were 33% ($n = 3$) in FMT < 48 h vs. 16.6% ($n = 3$) in FMT > 48 h, $p = 0.367$.

3.4. SBO Recurrence. SBO recurrence was observed in 27 (16.9%) patients. In the SMT group, 23 (22.1%) patients presented with SBO recurrence vs. one (4.3%) and 2 (7.4%) in the IS and FMT groups, respectively ($p = 0.042$). SBO recurrence surgical treatment was required in 4 (3.8%) SMT patients vs. $n = 2$ (7.4%) and $n = 1$ (4.3%) patients in the FMT and IS groups, respectively. Median follow-up duration in the entire population was 34 months (2–179) and was not significantly different between the three groups. Median time to SBO recurrence was 38 months (1–172) Table 2.

4. Discussion

If adhesive SBO medical treatment is widely accepted as a potential therapeutic option, the exact duration before deciding to switch to a surgical treatment in case of failure has yet to be determined. In clinical practice, SBO management is based on physical examination (mainly pain severity), CT scan results, patient comorbidity, and surgeon's clinical experience. The World Society of Emergency Surgery has published recommendations regarding SBO management in 2013, stating that surgical treatment should be proposed whenever medical treatment failed to achieve SBO resolution 72 hours following introduction [6]. But, most physicians prefer a conservative management in SBO patients presenting with important comorbidities, believing this will decrease mortality rates compared with surgical treatment. Indeed, surgeons do not seem to strictly abide by these recommendations and medical treatment duration can go up to 9 days according to some [3, 15]. The present study sought to analyze different adhesive SBO profiles and their respective outcomes in order to further improve therapeutic management.

In this series, IS patients presented with significantly more grade III–IV postoperative complications compared with FMT patients (9% vs. 4%, $p = 0.010$), but mortality rates were highest in FMT patients (0% vs. 22%, $p = 0.042$). Although age and comorbidities were not different between the groups, the occurrence of grade III–IV postoperative complications seemed to lead to impaired survival in patients who previously underwent medical treatment (FMT) compared with those who immediately underwent surgery (IS). A prolonged medical treatment might therefore be responsible of increasing patient frailty and decreasing their resistance in case of postoperative complications' occurrence.

Common arguments against early surgical treatment when confronted with adhesive SBO include worsened outcome compared with successful medical treatment and an increased SBO recurrence rate [7, 16]. Current analysis was not in accordance with these arguments, showing that grade III–IV–V postoperative complications were higher in initially medically treated patients, and SBO recurrence rate was highest in the SMT group. Indeed, although most published studies have reported increased postoperative complications in operatively managed SBO patients compared with medically managed patients, one possible explanation may be that surgically treated FMT patients should be taken into account differently than IS patients [9]. Because of profile difference between IS and FMT patients, we chose to separately analyze their outcomes. When comparing IS and SMT patients, the present results are in accordance with other published reports. Compared with IS patients, SMT patients presented with less severe postoperative complications but postoperative mortality was similar [7, 16]. Whereas regardless of medical treatment duration, FMT patients presented with worse outcomes (morbidity and mortality) compared with IS patients. Weaknesses of the study include its retrospective design and its relatively low number of cases (compared with other published reports) [7, 9]. However, strengths include the fact that patients were divided into 3 groups (IS, FMT, and SMT) unlike most authors who analyzed results according to 2 groups (medical and surgical treatment). Indeed, separating patients into 3 groups has led to identify patients with considerably impaired outcome (FMT).

The present results revealed a lower recurrence rate in SBO patients who were surgically treated (IS + FMT, $n = 3$, 6%) compared with SMT patients ($n = 23$, 22.1%, $p = 0.042$). This is in accordance with other published series. The alleged "paradox" arising from "surgical treatment induced adhesions" should no longer be considered a valid argument in choosing therapeutic management [1].

5. Conclusions

FMT seems to be associated with similar overall morbidity compared with IS but with increased postoperative mortality and recurrence rates of SBO. Patient frailty seems to be worsened by prolonged inefficient medical treatment. This study showed that SBO should be treated earlier by surgery in order to decrease mortality rates and recurrences of SBO.

Authors' Contributions

Nicolas Tabchouri and David Dussart contributed equally.

References

[1] M. Ouaïssi, S. Gaujoux, N. Veyrie et al., "Post-operative adhesions after digestive surgery: their incidence and prevention: review of the literature," *Journal of Visceral Surgery*, vol. 149, no. 2, pp. e104–e114, 2012.

[2] F. Catena, S. Di Saverio, F. Coccolini et al., "Adhesive small bowel adhesions obstruction: evolutions in diagnosis, management and prevention?," *World Journal of Gastrointestinal Surgery*, vol. 8, no. 3, pp. 222–231, 2016.

[3] J. E. Keenan, R. S. Turley, C. C. McCoy, J. Migaly, M. L. Shapiro, and J. E. Scarborough, "Trials of nonoperative management exceeding 3 days are associated with increased morbidity in patients undergoing surgery for uncomplicated adhesive small bowel obstruction," *Journal of Trauma and Acute Care Surgery*, vol. 76, no. 6, pp. 1367–1372, 2014.

[4] C. T. Aquina, A. Z. Becerra, C. P. Probst et al., "Patients with adhesive small bowel obstruction should be primarily managed by a surgical team," *Annals of Surgery*, vol. 264, no. 3, pp. 437–447, 2016.

[5] A. N. Kothari, J. L. Liles, C. J. Holmes et al., ""Right place at the right time" impacts outcomes for acute intestinal obstruction," *Surgery*, vol. 158, no. 4, pp. 1116–1127, 2015.

[6] S. Di Saverio, F. Coccolini, M. Galati et al., "Bologna guidelines for diagnosis and management of adhesive small bowel obstruction (ASBO): 2013 update of the evidence-based guidelines from the world society of emergency surgery ASBO working group," *World Journal of Emergency Surgery*, vol. 8, no. 1, p. 42, 2013.

[7] P. G. Teixeira, E. Karamanos, P. Talving, K. Inaba, L. Lam, and D. Demetriades, "Early operation is associated with a survival benefit for patients with adhesive bowel obstruction," *Annals of Surgery*, vol. 258, no. 3, pp. 459–465, 2013.

[8] S. Hajibandeh, S. Hajibandeh, N. Panda et al., "Operative versus non-operative management of adhesive small bowel obstruction: a systematic review and meta-analysis," *International Journal of Surgery*, vol. 45, pp. 58–66, 2017.

[9] J.-J. Duron, S. T. du Montcel, A. Berger et al., "Prevalence and risk factors of mortality and morbidity after operation for adhesive postoperative small bowel obstruction," *American Journal of Surgery*, vol. 195, no. 6, pp. 726–734, 2008.

[10] S. B. S. Sajja and M. Schein, "Early postoperative small bowel obstruction," *British Journal of Surgery*, vol. 91, no. 6, pp. 683–691, 2004.

[11] G. Miller, J. Boman, I. Shrier, and P. H. Gordon, "Readmission for small-bowel obstruction in the early postoperative period: etiology and outcome," *Canadian Journal of Surgery*, vol. 45, no. 4, pp. 255–258, 2002.

[12] W. D. Owens, J. A. Felts, and E. L. Spitznagel Jr., "ASA physical status classifications: a study of consistency of ratings," *Anesthesiology*, vol. 49, no. 4, pp. 239–243, 1978.

[13] M. E. Charlson, P. Pompei, K. L. Ales, and C. R. MacKenzie, "A new method of classifying prognostic comorbidity in longitudinal studies: development and validation," *Journal of Chronic Diseases*, vol. 40, no. 5, pp. 373–383, 1987.

[14] D. Dindo, N. Demartines, and P.-A. Clavien, "Classification of surgical complications: a new proposal with evaluation in a cohort of 6336 patients and results of a survey," *Annals of Surgery*, vol. 240, no. 2, pp. 205–213, 2004.

[15] M. J. Lee, A. E. Sayers, T. R. Wilson et al., "Current management of small bowel obstruction in the UK: results from the National Audit of Small Bowel Obstruction clinical practice survey," *Colorectal Disease*, vol. 20, no. 7, pp. 623–630, 2018.

[16] B. T. Fevang, D. Jensen, K. Svanes, and A. Viste, "Early operation or conservative management of patients with small bowel obstruction?," *The European Journal of Surgery*, vol. 168, no. 8, pp. 475–481, 2002.

Current Management of Pancreatic Neuroendocrine Tumors: From Demolitive Surgery to Observation

Ilenia Bartolini,[1] Lapo Bencini,[2] Matteo Risaliti,[1] Maria Novella Ringressi,[1] Luca Moraldi,[2] and Antonio Taddei[1]

[1]*Department of Surgery and Translational Medicine, AOU Careggi, University of Florence, Largo Brambilla 3, 50134 Florence, Italy*
[2]*Department of Oncology, AOU Careggi, Largo Brambilla 3, 50134 Florence, Italy*

Correspondence should be addressed to Ilenia Bartolini; ilenia.bartolini@gmail.com

Academic Editor: Alessandro Zerbi

Incidental diagnosis of pancreatic neuroendocrine tumors (PanNETs) greatly increased in the last years. In particular, more frequent diagnosis of small PanNETs leads to many challenging clinical decisions. These tumors are mostly indolent, although a percentage (up to 39%) may reveal an aggressive behaviour despite the small size. Therefore, there is still no unanimity about the best management of tumor smaller than 2 cm. The risks of under/overtreatment should be carefully evaluated with the patient and balanced with the potential morbidities related to surgery. The importance of the Ki-67 index as a prognostic factor is still debated as well. Whenever technically feasible, parenchyma-sparing surgeries lead to the best chance of organ preservation. Lymphadenectomy seems to be another important prognostic issue and, according to recent findings, should be performed in noninsulinoma patients. In the case of enucleation of the lesion, a lymph nodal sampling should always be considered. The relatively recent introduction of minimally invasive techniques (robotic) is a valuable option to deal with these tumors. The current management of PanNETs is analysed throughout the many available published guidelines and evidences with the aim of helping clinicians in the difficult decision-making process.

1. Introduction

In the last decades, the incidental diagnosis of neoplasms has been greatly increased due to the widespread use of advanced imaging techniques. Indeed, the diagnosis of pancreatic neuroendocrine tumors (PanNETs) has increased fourfold to sevenfold [1]. Furthermore, the size of these lesions at diagnosis has considerably decreased [2, 3], and the detection of tumors < 2 cm ranges from 26% to 61% [4, 5].

Pancreatic neuroendocrine tumors comprised less than 5% of all pancreatic tumors and 7% of all NETs [6, 7] being the second most common pancreatic neoplasm, with an overall incidence of approximately 5 : 1,000,000 new cases/year and an estimated prevalence of 1 : 100,000 people [7, 8]. Actually, they probably represent up to 10% of pancreatic tumors [9]. Moreover, their prevalence at autopsy ranges from 0.8% to 10% [10].

The great majority of PanNETs are sporadic (noninherited), while 10–30% of the patients develop a PanNETs within a genetic syndrome. The most frequent syndrome is multiple endocrine neoplasia (MEN) type 1 [11] while other rare genetic conditions are MEN4, Von Hippel-Lindau disease, neurofibromatosis 1 (von Recklinghausen's syndrome), and tuberous sclerosis [11–13].

Up to 90% of PanNETs are classified as nonfunctional (NF-PanNETs). This group includes also patients presenting with high hormone levels without symptoms. However, a considerable part of these patients (up to 60%) have a metastatic disease at diagnosis, while 21% present a locally advanced disease [10, 14]. Those patients who have nonspecific symptoms complain for abdominal pain, weight loss, or mass effect related to the pancreatic tumor or to the distant spread [13].

Functional PanNETs (F-PanNETs) comprehend insulinomas (35–40% of F-PanNETs) manifesting with the classical Whipple's triad (fasting hypoglycemia, symptoms of hypoglycemia, and immediate relief of symptoms after the administration of glucose) [12], gastrinomas (16–30%) with the Zollinger-Ellison syndrome (multiple peptic ulcers, esophageal reflux, and diarrhea), glucagonomas (<10%) with the "4D syndrome" (dermatitis, diabetes, deep vein thrombosis, and depression), and VIPomas (<10%) related to the Verner-Morrison syndrome (watery diarrhea, achlorhydria, and hypokalemia). The remaining 5% are somatostatinomas, related to combined symptoms such as diabetes, diarrhea, steatorrhea, anemia, and weight loss [11, 15].

From a curative perspective, all patients presenting with F-PanNETs should be evaluated for surgery in the absence of serious concomitant illnesses, despite the tumor dimension. The surgical approach, whenever possible, is the best recognized option to cure the syndromes and to increase the oncologic outcome after optimal medical control of the symptoms [13, 15, 16]. Similarly, bigger NF-PanNETs in fit-for-surgery patients are good candidates for resection. Conversely, there is still an ongoing debate between surgical resection versus observation in the presence of small NF-PanNETs (≤2 cm).

The aim of this paper is to focus on the management of sporadic PanNETs as highlighted by different guidelines and previously published papers.

2. Diagnosis and Prognosis of PanNETs

Diagnosis of PanNETs is widely increasing, mostly as incidental, due to the more and more frequent use of high resolution imaging examinations associated with a greater awareness of these pathologies [13, 17]. According to the paper written by Kuo and Salem [1] based on the American Surveillance, Epidemiology and End Results (SEER), the diagnosis of PanNETs smaller than 2 cm has risen from 12% in 1988 to 20% in 2009. A more recent paper on the same database that included 64,971 patients with a NET from 1973 to 2012 showed a global increase in the diagnosis of NETs of sixfold. Nevertheless, within patients with a known tumor grade (70%), 51% had a G1 NET and 16% had a G2 NET. G1 NETs showed the major increase in incidence. Within the patients with a known stage, 52% had a localized disease at diagnosis. This trend was seen across all sites and pancreas as well [17].

The traditional laboratory workup in NF-PanNETs [13] comprehends chromogranin A (CgA), with a sensitivity of 72–100% and a specificity of 50–80%, and neuron-specific enolase (NSE) (sensitivity of 30–40% and a specificity of up to 100%). Their combined evaluation adds strength to their single diagnostic power [18]. However, the routine use of CgA is still questioned for its limited importance in the presence of small lesions. Other tests, such as transcript multianalyte assays, appear as promising and more sensitive and efficient when compared to the single CgA analysis [19, 20]. The appropriate hormone evaluation is to be included if a functional tumor is suspected.

Radiologic imaging comprehends CT (computed tomography) scan or magnetic resonance imaging (MRI), endoscopic ultrasound (EUS) with a fine-needle biopsy [21], and somatostatin receptor-based imaging to localize/stage the neoplasm [13, 16, 22].

Larghi and colleagues [23] performed a prospective study evaluating feasibility and yield of the 19-gauge needle biopsy under EUS guidance. Despite the small sample (30 patients, 10 operated), they found a rate of 83.3% of concordance between preoperative and postoperative Ki-67 indexes.

Mitotic count and Ki-67 expression were the important items to be taken into account in the 2010 WHO classification. Grades 1 and 2 were considered as differentiated tumors (90%, Ki-67< 20%), while Grade 3 were classified as neuroendocrine carcinomas (NEC) [24]. However, more recent evidences [25, 26] demonstrated heterogeneous biology within the G3 subgroup, in which few well-differentiated tumors with Ki-67 > 20% showed a mild prognosis. The updated 2017 WHO classification [27] properly classified these tumors as well-differentiated G3-NETs rather than poorly differentiated G3-NEC [28, 29]. The use of immunohistochemical markers may help in differentiating these two subgroups. This distinction has a therapeutic and prognostic value in such tumors, although their rarity leads to the need of further studies to completely validate this new classification. Moreover, the 2017 WHO classification established the threshold of the Ki-67 index at 3% between G1 and G2 NETs [27]. Furthermore, since the Ki-67 index seems to be not sufficient to classify these tumors, the inclusion of some other genetic mutation analyses is expected in the upcoming classifications [25].

Nevertheless, some different Ki-67 index cut-offs between G1 and G2 have also been proposed (3–10%) [30, 31], and different classification systems have been suggested and revised over the years.

According to a robust comparative study including more than 1000 patients, the American Joint Committee on Cancer (AJCC, 7th edition), the World Health Organization (WHO) 2010, and the European Neuroendocrine Tumor Society (ENETS) classification systems all resulted to be independent prognostic factors for survival, although the ENETS TNM seemed to be the most accurate if compared to the others [32]. On the other hand, Strosberg and coworkers [33] reported the validity of the AJCC system in a study involving 425 patients, reporting a 5-year OS rate of 92%, 84%, 81%, and 57% in case of stages 1 to 4, respectively.

Luo et al. [34, 35] proposed a modified ENETS TNM system using the ENETS TNM definition associated with the AJCC staging definition. Subsequently, their data was validated according to the North American SEER registry, within multicentric series including thousands of patients. However, the AJCC released the 8th edition with the new TNM staging system identical to the ENETS TNM [29].

Several other independent prognostic factors have been recently recognized:

(i) The presence of calcification at preoperative imaging seems to be related to tumor grade and metastatic lymph node numbers.

(ii) Distant metastases and their progression time are survival predictors, independent from the Ki-67 index [36].

(iii) Lymph node involvement and lymph node ratio are both related to the tumor recurrence after surgery.

(iv) The absence of symptoms in NF-PanNETs seems related with a better prognosis, independent from the tumor stage [13].

(v) Peritumoral vascular invasion is recently known as an independent prognostic factor [36].

(vi) Older age, with different cut-off (55–75 years), is related with a higher mortality rate [37, 38].

The median and the 5-year overall survival (OS) for patients affected by NF-PanNETs are 38 months and 43%, respectively [39]. The tumor spread is another important prognostic factor, with the median OS falling from 124, 70, and 23 months for patients with localized disease, regional tumor involvement, and metastatic disease, respectively [39].

Interestingly, less than 10% of pancreatic insulinomas are frankly malignant. However, the diameter > 2 cm and Ki-67 > 2% are both predictors of liver metastasis, with the median survival of less than 2 years in this evidence [15]. Furthermore, up to 40% of the patients with gastrinomas develop liver metastasis, representing the most important prognostic factor (10-year OS of 10–20% for metastatic disease and 90–100% for without metastasis) [15].

3. Surgery versus Observation of NF-PanNETs

Specific criteria to definitively and unequivocally predict the behaviour of PanNETs have not been found yet. Consequently, the heterogeneous and often unpredictable behaviour of PanNETs leads to a difficult management of these patients.

The most used criteria are size or change in size during the years, morphological aspect, grade, and Ki-67 expression [12, 40]. In brief, the risk of overtreatment (unnecessary pancreatic resection for an indolent neoplasm) should be carefully balanced with the risk of undertreatment (missing the opportunity to cure a mild to more aggressive disease).

Unfortunately, pancreatic surgery still has significant mortality, ranging from 1% to 10% [41], and morbidity, including perioperative and long-term complications (i.e., diabetes, pancreatic exocrine impairment), of up to 50–60%, even in high volume centers [40, 42–46].

Some authors suggested a nonoperative management through a "wait-and-see" policy of "small" NF-PanNETs [2, 36, 47, 48]. The prolonged careful observation of these lesions could avoid pancreatic surgery and its related frequent complications, because most of the small NF-PanNETs are indolent despite a chance of 10% of nodal involvement [47]. Nevertheless, patients with growing tumors during the follow-up may receive subsequent surgery without changes in OS and disease-free survival (DFS) rates [47].

Sadot and colleagues [2] published a matched case-control study of patients with PanNETs smaller than 3 cm who were observed (104 patients) and compared to those who underwent upfront resection (77 patients). Twenty-five per cent of the patients in the observation group underwent subsequent tumor resection after a median interval of 30 months. No patients died for the neoplasm after a median follow-up of 44 months in either group. Interestingly, the authors did not found any difference in OS between the two groups, although the incidence of "salvage surgery" was higher than those reported by other authors. This difference may be related with the chosen bigger cut-off of 3 cm. Nevertheless, in 65% of the cases, indication to surgery was given according to patients' (38%) or physicians' (27%) preferences. They concluded that observation for stable, small, incidentally discovered PanNETs could be reasonable, in selected patients [2].

According to the updated ENET guidelines [13], some patients with NF-PanNETs ≤2 cm could be safely managed conservatively. Additional criteria for the nonoperative approach should be the presence of G1-low G2 tumor, pancreatic head localization, and no signs of malignancy at imaging. In patients with G2 NF-PanNETs of 2 cm, surgery should be recommended. Similarly, patients with tumor bigger than 2 cm should be evaluated for surgery routinely. The presence of concomitant illnesses and patients' age or wishes should be also considered. However, in the case of surveillance, EUS and MRI should be mandatory to be repeated every 6 months (12 months if no changes are discovered). If an increase of 0.5 cm (or more) in the size of the lesion occurs, patients should be reevaluated for surgery [13].

The comparison between observation and upfront surgery in a small case series (35 patients) reported by Rosenberg et al. [49] showed the absence of significant progression in the observed tumors smaller than 2 cm. Unfortunately, the reported median follow-up was only 27.8 months when dealing with mild aggressive tumors. Interestingly, the same authors found no strict relation between Ki-67 index and aggressive behaviour, although many patients had an unknown tumor grade (73% and 5% for observation and resected groups, resp.). However, other authors did not recommend the routine evaluation of Ki-67 in small PanNETs due to its limited value in case of the tumor biopsy [47]. Similarly, the results of a French multicenter study involving 80 patients reported how the tumor size was an independent predictor of malignancy, while the Ki-67 index was not. Again, 18% of the patients had no Ki-67 index evaluation. Furthermore, the authors found that a size cut-off of 1.7 cm had a very high sensitivity and specificity to predict a malignant behaviour (92% and 75%, resp.) [50].

Zhang et al. [51] in a case series of 249 patients (193 resected and 56 observed) reported a significant OS benefit for the resected group. However, the surgical approach became significant predictor of OS for tumors > 1.5 cm only. Analogue size cut-off values were reported in other papers [52].

Conversely, the American National Comprehensive Cancer Network (NCCN) guidelines [16] recommend surgery in every NF-PanNET bigger than 1 cm, and they stated that observation can be considered in incidentally discovered, low-grade NF-PanNETs smaller than 1 cm. Additional factors for conservative management include the surgical risk, the tumor site, and the patient comorbidities, especially

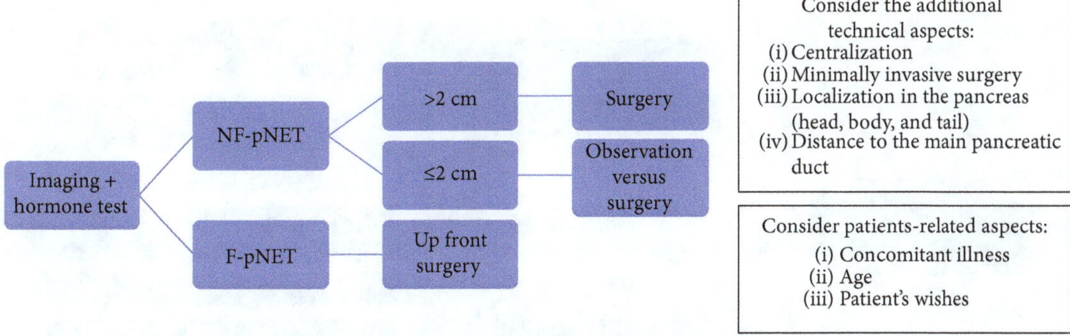

FIGURE 1: Summary and proposal of a management flow chart in PanNETs.

when dealing with small asymptomatic tumor [16]. Probably, the more aggressive surgical approach of the Cancer Network professionals could be justified by the target which obtains the best chance of tumor survival for this kind of malignancies.

Similarly, the Canadian National Expert Group suggested a surgical approach for every healthy patients with resectable disease. Surveillance may be considered only in NF-PanNETs smaller than 2 cm, with a low Ki-67 index measured on EUS-FNA samples and no signs of tumor local or distant spread [53].

The rationale for a more aggressive approach (routine surgery) is that some small (<2 cm) high-grade tumors have a frankly malignant behaviour (9% to 39%) [1, 37, 54–58]. Nevertheless, a proper histological examination of the tumor (including mitotic and Ki-67 indexes) is possible only on the resected specimen. Therefore, some authors believe that an upfront surgical treatment, whenever possible (patients fit for surgery), is the best chance of cure, despite the size of the tumor, providing the longer survival [54, 59].

Kuo and Salem [1] reported a population-level analysis of PanNETs <2 cm using the SEER database. They found the presence of some extrapancreatic tumor spread, nodal involvement, or distal metastasis in 17.9%, 27.3%, and 9.1% of the cohort, respectively. The tumor grade (unknown in 47.9%) and patient race were the most significant predictor of DFS. However, the DFS at 5, 10, and 15 years was 89.7%, 80%, and 70.6, respectively.

Gratian and colleagues [54] reported a large population study using the National Cancer Data Base including 1854 patients with NF-PanNETs ≤ 2 cm diagnosed between 1998 and 2011. Tumors ≤ 0.5 cm in their maximum size presented at diagnosis with nodal or distant metastases in 33% and 11% of cases, respectively. Nevertheless, tumor size was positively associated with distant tumor spread. The five-year OS was 27.6% for the observation group versus 83.0%, 72.3%, and 86% ($p < 0.01$) for distal pancreatectomies (DP), pancreaticoduodenectomies (PD), and total pancreatectomies (TP), respectively.

In a recently published review and meta-analysis, Sallinen et al. [41] criticized the low quality of the previously published studies. In this issue, the authors focused the attention on the lack of important data in most of the published articles, including unacceptable low rates of confirmed diagnosis of PanNETs (46% in the studies about sporadic PanNETs). Therefore, definitive conclusions might actually not be drawn. Moreover, the criteria applied in the wait-and-see policy of control arms might include patients' and surgeons' wishes. Nevertheless, the tumor growth was seen in 22% of the patients with sporadic PanNETs (pooled estimate) while none developed metastasis during follow-up period [41]. In the same review, the surgery rate during the follow-up ranged from 3 to 25% with 43% of the patients operated for their or surgeons' preferences rather than for objective parameters. The authors also analysed the huge differences between the results of case series and the studies based on oncological databases. The lack of data regarding tumor-related history and the influence of external factors such as insurance status and the presence of many selection biases led to an underreporting of patients with less aggressive neoplasms. Nevertheless, most of such type databases reported a malignant potential even in small tumors (>0.5 cm) [1, 56, 59, 60]. Lastly, the authors concluded that the brand-new acquisitions on Pan-NETs could lead to a more restrictive indication to surgery [41]. Similar considerations were reported by others [61].

A proposal of an algorithm is outlined in Figure 1.

4. Resective Surgery

4.1. Lesion Localization. The preoperative exact localization of the lesion within the pancreatic gland is of crucial importance. According to recent papers, PET (positron emission tomography)/CT with ^{68}Ga-labeled somatostatin analogues should be the examination of choice for both staging and localization in noninsulinoma PanNETs and has replaced the suboptimal octreoscan, with a sensitivity and a specificity of 86–100% and 79–100%, respectively [13]. Conversely, sensitivity of PET/CT with ^{68}Ga-labeled somatostatin analogues is reported to be around 25% in case of insulinomas [13], reflecting up to 10% of these tumors having a negative preoperative imaging workup. For these patients, selective intra-arterial injection of calcium with hepatic venous insulin gradients has been advocated, although more recent, noninvasive methods of localization have been developed for insulinomas [22]. Several new cellular targets and tracers such as enxendin-4 or ^{18}F-FDOPA (6-[18F]-L-fluoro-L-3,4-dihydroxyphenylalanina) have been employed [22].

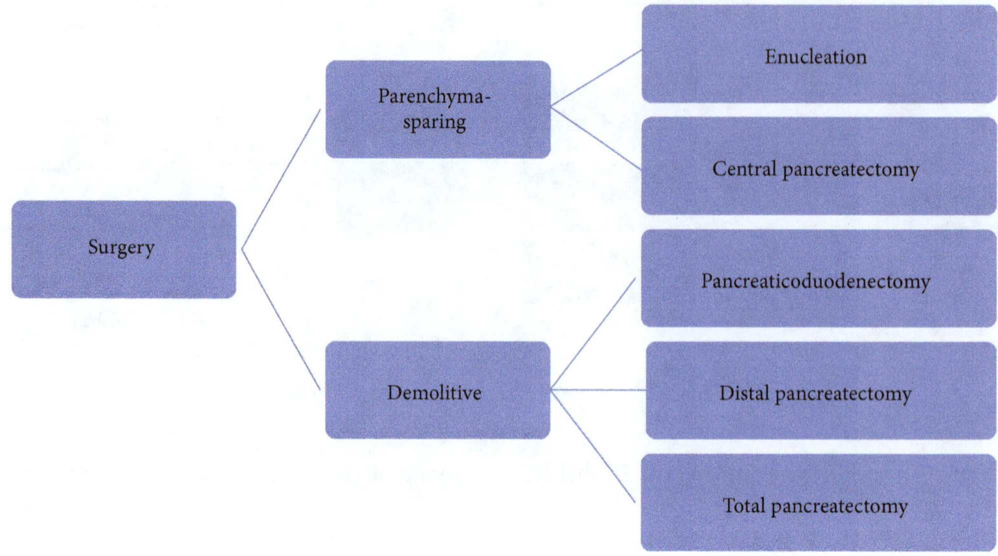

FIGURE 2: Summary of all surgical options available to deal with PanNETs. A tailored, single-patient, focused approach remains the best option.

Benign insulinomas usually express glucagon-like peptide-1 receptors (GLP-1R), and imaging with different radiolabelled-exendin-4 compounds (i.e., ^{68}Ga-NOTA-exendin-4) is recommended, with a sensitivity up to 90%. In case of high suspicion of well-differentiated metastatic insulinoma, somatostatin receptor imaging (i.e., ^{68}Ga-DOTA-octreotate (^{68}Ga-DOTATATE) PET/CT) is also advisable to complete the staging and to assess the feasibility of medical treatment, with a sensitivity of up to 80%. Similarly, ^{18}F-FDOPA after premedication with carbidopa may be used, although its role is still controversial [22]. Conversely, FDG-PET (2-[^{18}F]fluoro-2-deoxy-D-glucose) is used in the presence of high-grade metastatic insulinomas. Moreover, the shift from GLP-1R to SSTR to FDG avidity is described as a "triple-flop" phenomenon, reflecting a progression from benignity to malignity [22].

The sensitivity of intraoperative ultrasound (IOUS) in the detection of small p-NETs is similar to that of EUS, but if combined with direct palpation, its sensitivity rises to 97% [62].

4.2. Parenchymal-Sparing Operations versus Demolitive Operations. There are many different surgical options to deal with PanNETs, ranging from simple enucleation (EN) to a total pancreatectomy [14] (Figure 2).

Obviously, demolitive operations may lead to an unnecessary removal of a huge amount of healthy pancreatic parenchyma and lead to life-threatening postoperative complications, including death.

A rationale strategy for small low-grade malignant tumors could be to remove the tumor only, conserving as much glandular tissue as possible and avoiding lesions of the main pancreatic duct [57, 63–65].

Obviously, the oncological results, including both OS and disease-free survival (DFS), should be equivalent between EN and demolitive surgery, with a proper and detailed surveillance program. Most of the case series and review articles comparing EN and standard surgery reported no differences in the OS and local and distant recurrence rates [66–70]. Some authors reported suboptimal results after EN in terms of increased recurrences in more aggressive tumors located in the head of the pancreas [64]. To achieve these excellent oncologic results, a careful patient selection is required to reserve major pancreatic resection to the more aggressive, large-sized tumors with nodal involvement [63, 67, 71, 72]. The maintenance of the pancreatic endocrine and exocrine functions is the major long-term benefit related to limited surgery (i.e., enucleations) compared to major pancreatic resections (pancreaticoduodenectomy, PD; distal pancreatectomy, DP; and total pancreatectomy, TP) [63, 66, 68, 69, 73–75].

Despite their apparent scarce invasiveness, the major drawback of EN is the high complication rate, mostly related to postoperative pancreatic fistulas (POPFs) [72, 76]. Fortunately, most of them are classified as low grade [63] according to the guidelines of the International Study Group for Pancreatic Fistula (ISGPF) [77] and amenable to be managed conservatively, at the price of prolonged hospital stay and increased costs [72].

The incidence of POPFs is globally reported to be superior after EN with respect to major pancreatic resections, especially if the lesion lied in the head (18%–50% versus 12%) [64, 66–69, 72, 74, 78]. There are many possible explanations to this high rate of POPFs. Firstly, these lesions are often associated with a nondilated pancreatic duct within a soft and friable pancreas. Secondly, the lack of specialization and centralization in high volume hospitals is proven to be related to worst perioperative outcomes. Finally, the localization of the p-NET in the head is a risk factor for POPF after EN, due to the presence of a bigger pancreatic duct.

Interestingly, another concern is represented by tumors arising from the pancreatic head, in which some surgeons could be tempted to push on the technical limits of EN, in order to avoid the challenging PD.

Zhang and coworkers [75] in their case series of 119 patients receiving enucleation (91% for PanNETs) reported that NYHA (New York Heart Association) class II or III and operative time longer than 180 min were both independent risk factors for POPF development.

Compared with major resection, perioperative outcomes of EN were at least equal if not superior, except for a higher rate of POPF. Moreover, minimally invasive EN had a significative shorter operation time and a shorter length of hospital stay if compared to open enucleation [70]. Furthermore, minimally invasive ENs have better results compared to other parenchyma-preserving procedures such as central pancreatectomy, pancreatic head resection, dorsal pancreatectomy, and middle-preserving pancreatectomy [12, 14, 42, 63, 66–69, 71, 73].

Despite the theoretical previous mentioned indications for EN, tumors should also be at least 2-3 mm far from the main pancreatic duct in order to avoid direct injuries and the development of a POPF [63, 70, 75, 76, 79–81]. Preoperative MRCP associated with IOUS and, eventually, intraoperative frozen section examination are all powerful tools to assure the exact location and to confirm the low aggressivity of the lesions [72, 74, 75, 80].

When considering the group of F-PanNET only, EN is considered safe for insulinomas, while gastrinomas were usually candidates to a major pancreatic resection with formal lymphadenectomy due the higher risk of lymph node metastasis (60–90%) and locoregional involvement [16]. Enucleation plus lymphadenectomy, could be considered acceptable only for small exophytic gastrinomas of the pancreatic head, if other preoperative signs of malignancies were excluded [13, 16, 82].

Some authors suggested that EN is a feasible approach in selected (≤2 cm, G1, superficial) NF-PanNETs [53, 65, 75, 83]. Conversely, this approach could lead to a questionable oncological outcome. Indeed, the tumor size seems to be directly related to the probability of lymph node metastasis. Interestingly, NF-PanNETs smaller than 2 cm have a low (7%–26%) but measurable risk of lymph node metastases. In summary, the updated NCCN guidelines and others indicate the cut-off value of 2 cm in diameter to perform pancreatic EN [16, 39]. Significant tumor growth in the previous 3–6 months is another parameter that contraindicates an EN outside specific cases [82].

An impressive meta-analysis collecting 1148 patients (38% of EN and 62% of major resections; minimally invasive technique employed in 25.5% and 22.4%, resp.) with p-NETs or other cystic neoplasms, found that duration of surgery, length of hospital stay, and organ impairment favored EN. Nevertheless, the POPF's rate was significantly higher in the EN group, although morbidity and mortality did not differ [42].

Zhou et al. [70] performed a systematic review including 1316 pancreatic EN for benign or low-grade malignant pancreatic tumors (65.6% of PanNETs) with an overall morbidity of 50.3%, POPF representing the most frequent complication (38.1%). Reoperations were 3.7%; mortality and recurrence were 0.3% and 2.3%, respectively. Endocrine and exocrine insufficiencies were observed in only 2.4% and 1.1% of the patients, respectively. Interestingly, in the studies in which EN was compared to demolitive surgery, an equivalent DFS between the two approaches was found.

4.3. Lymphadenectomy. The importance of a formal regional lymphadenectomy is still under debate for PanNETs. Franko et al. [84] published a large population study using the SEER database including 2158 patients with PanNETs diagnosed between 1973 and 2004. Tumor size and nodal status were not found to be predictors of OS. These results are consistent with other earlier papers [38, 54, 85], although it could be related to inadequate lymph node sampling.

More recently, some authors suggested a routinary nodal sampling in PanNETs in order to reduce the possibility of tumor understaging rather than to prolong survival itself [83]. Interestingly, the NCCN guidelines focus on the importance of a correct lymphadenectomy, underlining the possibility of nodal metastasis even in the presence of small (1-2 cm) tumors [16]. Conversely, Yoo and colleagues [86] found that routinary lymphadenectomy may be considered as an overtreatment and not necessary in NET G1.

Other papers reported that node involvement and lymph node ratio are both related to the tumor recurrence after surgery [58, 87–90]. Therefore, a formal lymphadenectomy should be considered in all noninsulinoma F-PanNETs [13], since insulinomas do not require a formal lymphadenectomy for their benignity (up to 90% of the patients) [13]. Nevertheless, Sharpe and colleagues [59] found that lymph nodal positivity (29% of patients who underwent surgery) was associated with a higher mortality rates. In the presence of a suspected gastrinoma, formal regional lymphadenectomy may improve survival reducing the persistence or the spread of the disease [15, 88].

In the presence of NF-PanNETs, tumor size seems to relate with the chance of nodal involvement and, consequently, the need of clearance [16, 39, 91]. Interestingly, an extended lymphadenectomy (beyond or far from the pancreas) was not demonstrated to be of great help, even in the presence of more advanced tumors [92].

4.4. Extensive Surgery and Systemic Therapy. The role of splenectomy is another debated issue, although most of the authors agree that it should be avoided if splenic vessels are not involved in the neoplastic tissue [93].

In the presence of advanced or metastatic F-PanNETs, palliative surgery may be indicated to relieve symptoms. To achieve this, the removal of at least 90% of tumor load is advocated. Unresectable liver metastasis could be managed by palliative treatments, including transarterial chemoembolization (TACE), radiofrequency ablation (RFA), or cryoablation [15].

NF-PanNETs with vascular involvement could have a prognostic benefit after demolitive resection in selected patients (up to 62% of 10-year OS rate) with a low morbidity rate [85, 94] if performed in high volume centers.

Distant metastases (mostly in the liver) are detected at the time of first diagnosis in about 30% of the patients and in up to 70% in referral centers due to patient preselection toward more complex situations [16, 95].

In case of liver metastasization, surgery may be indicated in well-differentiated G1-G2 PanNETs [95] and when the primary and metastatic tumors are judged as resectable in one- or two-stage surgery. Accurate evaluation of the volume of the future liver remnant should be performed preoperatively, and the surgical plan should be confirmed with the intraoperative ultrasound evaluation [95]. Of course, a simultaneous PD and a major hepatectomy should be avoided to limit perioperative life-threatening complications.

In the case of a planned two-stage surgery, hepatectomy should be performed as the first step, in order to reduce the risk of perihepatic sepsis [13, 16]. Nevertheless, the presence of suspected additional metastatic sites should be excluded before planning any surgical resection, and the presence of concomitant important comorbidities should be taken into consideration [95]. This very aggressive management (in selected patients) leads to an OS of up to 60–80% with morbidity and mortality rate of 30% and 0–5%, respectively [65, 95, 96]. Surgical debulking with palliative intent may also be considered in very selected patients suffering from NF-PanNETs [16].

Pancreatic G3 NEC are usually indicated for medical treatment (mostly based on cisplatin and etoposide) because of high rate of distant metastasis. Systemic therapy is also indicated in nonresectable disease [95]. Patient's characteristics such as the presence of symptoms, comorbidities, and general conditions together with tumor characteristics (histology, stage, and radiotracer uptake) are the parameters to consider in a multidisciplinary team to make a correct choice of medical treatment.

There are three main different groups of medical therapies available: somatostatin analogues (octreotide, lanreotide), molecularly targeted treatment (everolimus, sunitinib), and chemotherapy with cytostatic/cytotoxic drugs (5-fluorouracil (5-FU), capecitabine, dacarbazine, oxaliplatin, streptozotocin, and temozolomide). Although chemotherapy is pushed afterwards more tolerable and manageable in G1-2 PanNETs, in the case of symptomatic, high burden or G2 rapidly-progressing NETs or NEC, it is still the preferred choice as first-line therapy as the only effective therapy.

There are different commonly used regimens (i.e., temozolomide alone or combined with capecitabine or different combination of 5-FU, doxorubicin, and streptozotocin), although there is not a wide consensus on the best protocol. Most of them are under experimentation in ongoing trials [16].

In the next future, conventional chemotherapy might be tailored on each patient according to the tumor biology, including molecular and genetic patterns.

A recently recognized form of treatment is the peptide receptor radionuclide therapy with labelled somatostatin analogues. Main indications are advanced, inoperable G1 or G2 tumors. Patients with G3 tumors expressing somatostatin receptor may receive this treatment in the presence of the progression of disease or in case of a failure of previous therapies [15, 97].

5. Minimally Invasive Surgical Techniques

The well-known advantages of laparoscopy include decrease in postoperative pain, lesser blood loss, lower depression of the immune system leading to faster recovery, and definitively, earlier start of adjuvant therapies if required. Nevertheless, due to its intrinsic complexity, the widespread adoption of such techniques in pancreatic surgery was slower if compared to other subspecialities [98–100].

The robotic technology could overcome some of the technical limitations of pure laparoscopy. The EndoWrist system (instruments articulated with 7 degrees of freedom), motion scaling and tremor filtration, stable and high-definition 3D vision, and ergonomic surgeon position are the main advantages. Some other tools are particularly powerful in pancreatic surgery. An ultrasound flexible integrated probe can be moved by the console surgeon and seen together with operative field in a picture-in-picture mode. The adoption of the near-infrared technology and the fluorescence guidance (Firefly® Technology) is a promising tool for tumor localization, although further evidence is needed to confirm its routinary employment for PanNETs. Intraoperative US together with the fluorescence guidance are both crucial for the localization of the lesions and to define their relation with the surrounding healthy tissue or structures.

All these features partially overcome the absence of a tactile feedback [80]. Further, the last generation of da Vinci Xi® robot (Intuitive Surgical, Sunnyvale, California) has several additional technical advantages as compared to the older systems. However, the major drawbacks and limitations of robotic system are the long operative time and the increased costs. The theoretical reduction of hospital stay and the prompter return to daily activities could balance the economic perspective [12, 51].

Indications for the adoption of the minimally invasive surgery do not obviously differ from those for open or laparoscopic surgery, although may lead to a widening of surgical indications in patients suffering for comorbidities at greater risk of postoperative complications. Moreover, more aggressive PanNETs could be managed safely through a minimally invasive approach, achieving the same oncological results [101].

From a comparative perspective, robotic surgery resulted to be safe, feasible, and at least equal to laparoscopy in pancreatic surgery, resulting in low morbidity and short hospital stay [46, 102–104]. Interestingly, duration of robotic EN is shorter than open EN in most of the published studies [68, 70, 81, 105].

Parenchyma-sparing operations could also be associated with the use of a minimally invasive technique to achieve the less clinical impact for the patients. Conversely, some limited case series reported robotic multivisceral resections for metastatic Pan-NET [106].

Unfortunately, there are very few statistically powered studies comparing open, laparoscopic, and robotic techniques in the area of PanNETs. Most of the experiences are reported in wider case series, often merged with different pancreatic tumors (i.e., cystic lesions) [55, 103, 104]. Moreover, many studies comparing minimally invasive techniques had a mixture of pure laparoscopy and robotics limiting the power of any specific comparison [74, 78, 81, 103, 105, 107]. A robust agreement among surgeons tends to recommend the laparoscopic technique to resect insulinomas [98, 108].

Zhang and colleagues [93] presented their initial experience comparing 43 and 31 patients undergoing robotic or laparoscopic DP for PanNETs. They found a significantly higher rate of spleen preservation (79.1 versus 48.4%, $p = 0.006$), lower risk of excessive blood loss, and greater number of lymph node harvested in the robotic group. All the other perioperative outcomes were comparable.

6. Follow-Up

The classical follow-up of patients with PanNETs should include clinical examination, appropriate biochemical markers, and imaging techniques such as CT scan and MRI. Somatostatin receptor-based imaging or PET scan should not be routinary used for surveillance [16].

The scheduling of the exams should be modified according to the tumor grade and stage and tailored in each patient after a multidisciplinary round [39]. Patients with a final histopathological confirmation of localized Pan-NET G1 with R0 surgery could avoid longer follow-up. All the other patients should receive tests once or twice a year for 10 years [16]. Patients with NEC should be reassessed every 3–6 months with advanced imaging.

Unfortunately, most of the patients with an advanced Pan-NET will experience some tumor progression. NCCN guidelines reported a global disease recurrence ranging from 21 to 42% [16]. The Ki-67 index is related to tumor spread, with an increasing risk of progression of 2% for each Ki-67 unit [109].

7. Conclusions

The incremental incidental diagnosis of small- to medium-size PanNETs has been leading to many challenging clinical decisions. There is still no unanimity about the optimal management of tumor smaller than 2 cm. Most of these tumors have a good prognosis, although the single behaviour is not always predictable. Specific prognostic criteria are still under examination.

The importance of the Ki-67 index as a prognostic factor to drive any decision-making process is still under debate. The tumor size (with different cut-off values) and the location within the pancreatic gland (head, body, and tail) together with the patient age and wishes and the presence of concomitant illnesses are all parameters to be considered for management. The possibility of under/overtreatment is often possible, leading to any delay in the correct management or to the development of life-threatening complications.

The brand-new available publications and guidelines have, however, made the decision algorithm increasingly easier to understand.

Whenever technically adequate and feasible, the parenchyma-sparing pancreatic resections should be preferred especially in young patients. Pancreatic enucleation is the procedure of choice to avoid perioperative morbidities and to preserve organ function in the long term (endocrine and exocrine). Lymphadenectomy or, at least, lymph nodal sampling seems to be important prognostic factor and should be considered routinely.

Despite its relatively new introduction, most of the pancreatic surgery could be achieved through a minimally invasive approach minimizing postoperative impairment but in the hands of experienced surgeons. The robotic platform is a valuable option in order to overcome the intrinsic limits of traditional laparoscopy.

The role of hospital centralization, the multidisciplinary approach, and the surgeon-related volume of activity are also of crucial impact for the final outcomes.

References

[1] E. J. Kuo and R. R. Salem, "Population-level analysis of pancreatic neuroendocrine tumors 2 cm or less in size," *Annals of Surgical Oncology*, vol. 20, no. 9, pp. 2815–2821, 2013.

[2] E. Sadot, D. L. Reidy-Lagunes, L. H. Tang et al., "Observation versus resection for small asymptomatic pancreatic neuroendocrine tumors: a matched case-control study," *Annals of Surgical Oncology*, vol. 23, no. 4, pp. 1361–1370, 2016.

[3] O. M. Sandvik, K. Søreide, E. Gudlaugsson, J. T. Kvaløy, and J. A. Søreide, "Epidemiology and classification of gastroenteropancreatic neuroendocrine neoplasms using current coding criteria," *British Journal of Surgery*, vol. 103, no. 3, pp. 226–232, 2016.

[4] A. Cheema, J. Weber, and J. R. Strosberg, "Incidental detection of pancreatic neuroendocrine tumors: an analysis of incidence and outcomes," *Annals of Surgical Oncology*, vol. 19, no. 9, pp. 2932–2936, 2012.

[5] R. Bettini, S. Partelli, L. Boninsegna et al., "Tumor size correlates with malignancy in nonfunctioning pancreatic endocrine tumor," *Surgery*, vol. 150, no. 1, pp. 75–82, 2011.

[6] K. Oberg, U. Knigge, D. Kwekkeboom, A. Perren, and on behalf of the ESMO Guidelines Working Group, "Neuroendocrine gastro-entero-pancreatic tumors: ESMO Clinical Practice Guidelines for diagnosis, treatment and follow-up," *Annals of Oncology*, vol. 23, Supplement_7, pp. vii124–vii130, 2012.

[7] B. Lawrence, B. I. Gustafsson, A. Chan, B. Svejda, M. Kidd, and I. M. Modlin, "The epidemiology of gastroenteropancreatic neuroendocrine tumors," *Endocrinology and Metabolism Clinics of North America*, vol. 40, no. 1, pp. 1–18, 2011.

[8] J. C. Yao, M. Hassan, A. Phan et al., "One hundred years after "carcinoid": epidemiology of and prognostic factors for neuroendocrine tumors in 35,825 cases in the United States," *Journal of Clinical Oncology*, vol. 26, no. 18, pp. 3063–3072, 2008.

[9] M. Fraenkel, M. K. Kim, A. Faggiano, and G. D. Valk, "Epidemiology of gastroenteropancreatic neuroendocrine tumours," *Best Practice & Research Clinical Gastroenterology*, vol. 26, no. 6, pp. 691–703, 2012.

[10] T. R. Halfdanarson, K. G. Rabe, J. Rubin, and G. M. Petersen, "Pancreatic neuroendocrine tumors (PNETs): incidence, prognosis and recent trend toward improved survival," *Annals of Oncology*, vol. 19, no. 10, pp. 1727–1733, 2008.

[11] R. F. de Wilde, B. H. Edil, R. H. Hruban, and A. Maitra, "Well-differentiated pancreatic neuroendocrine tumors: from genetics to therapy," *Nature Reviews Gastroenterology & Hepatology*, vol. 9, no. 4, pp. 199–208, 2012.

[12] J. B. Liu and M. S. Baker, "Surgical management of pancreatic neuroendocrine tumors," *Surgical Clinics of North America*, vol. 96, no. 6, pp. 1447–1468, 2016.

[13] M. Falconi, B. Eriksson, G. Kaltsas et al., "ENETS consensus guidelines update for the management of patients with functional pancreatic neuroendocrine tumors and non-functional pancreatic neuroendocrine tumors," *Neuroendocrinology*, vol. 103, no. 2, pp. 153–171, 2016.

[14] L. R. McKenna and B. H. Edil, "Update on pancreatic neuroendocrine tumors," *Gland Surgery*, vol. 3, no. 4, pp. 258–275, 2014.

[15] R. T. Jensen, G. Cadiot, M. L. Brandi et al., "ENETS Consensus Guidelines for the management of patients with digestive neuroendocrine neoplasms: functional pancreatic endocrine tumor syndromes," *Neuroendocrinology*, vol. 95, no. 2, pp. 98–119, 2012.

[16] National Comprehensive Cancer Network, "Neuroendocrine and adrenal tumor (version 2.2018)," https://www.nccn.org/professionals/physician_gls/pdf/neuroendocrine.pdf.

[17] A. Dasari, C. Shen, D. Halperin et al., "Trends in the incidence, prevalence, and survival outcomes in patients with neuroendocrine tumors in the United States," *JAMA Oncology*, vol. 3, no. 10, pp. 1335–1342, 2017.

[18] Y. Lv, X. Han, C. Zhang et al., "Combined test of serum CgA and NSE improved the power of prognosis prediction of NF-pNETs," *Endocrine Connections*, vol. 7, no. 1, pp. 169–178, 2018.

[19] M. Kidd, L. Bodei, and I. M. Modlin, "Chromogranin A: any relevance in neuroendocrine tumors?," *Current Opinion in Endocrinology, Diabetes, and Obesity*, vol. 23, no. 1, pp. 28–37, 2016.

[20] I. M. Modlin, I. Drozdov, D. Alaimo et al., "A multianalyte PCR blood test outperforms single analyte ELISAs (chromogranin A, pancreastatin, neurokinin A) for neuroendocrine tumor detection," *Endocrine-Related Cancer*, vol. 21, no. 4, pp. 615–628, 2014.

[21] B. Weynand, I. Borbath, V. Bernard et al., "Pancreatic neuroendocrine tumour grading on endoscopic ultrasound-guided fine needle aspiration: high reproducibility and interobserver agreement of the Ki-67 labelling index," *Cytopathology*, vol. 25, no. 6, pp. 389–395, 2014.

[22] D. A. Pattison and R. J. Hicks, "Molecular imaging in the investigation of hypoglycaemic syndromes and their management," *Endocrine-Related Cancer*, vol. 24, no. 6, pp. R203–R221, 2017.

[23] A. Larghi, G. Capurso, A. Carnuccio et al., "Ki-67 grading of nonfunctioning pancreatic neuroendocrine tumors on histologic samples obtained by EUS-guided fine-needle tissue acquisition: a prospective study," *Gastrointestinal Endoscopy*, vol. 76, no. 3, pp. 570–577, 2012.

[24] D. S. Klimstra, R. Armold, C. Capella et al., "Neuroendocrine neoplasms of the pancreas," in *WHO Classification of Tumours of the Digestive System*, F. T. Bosman, F. Carneiro, R. H. Hruban, and N. D. Theise, Eds., pp. 322–326, IARC Press, Lyon, 2010.

[25] X. Han, X. Xu, H. Ma et al., "Clinical relevance of different WHO grade 3 pancreatic neuroendocrine neoplasms based on morphology," *Endocrine Connections*, vol. 7, no. 2, pp. 355–363, 2018.

[26] M. Milione, P. Maisonneuve, F. Spada et al., "The clinicopathologic heterogeneity of grade 3 gastroenteropancreatic neuroendocrine neoplasms: morphological differentiation and proliferation identify different prognostic categories," *Neuroendocrinology*, vol. 104, no. 1, pp. 85–93, 2017.

[27] R. V. Lloyd, R. Y. Osamura, G. Klöppel, and J. Rosai, *WHO Classification of Tumours of Endocrine Organs*, IARC Press, Lyon, 2017.

[28] O. Basturk, Z. Yang, L. H. Tang et al., "The high-grade (WHO G3) pancreatic neuroendocrine tumor category is morphologically and biologically heterogenous and includes both well differentiated and poorly differentiated neoplasms," *The American Journal of Surgical Pathology*, vol. 39, no. 5, pp. 683–690, 2015.

[29] E. K. Bergsland, E. A. Woltering, G. Rindi et al., "Neuroendocrine tumors of the pancreas. American Joint Committee on Cancer 2017," in *AJCC Cancer Staging Manual*, M. B. Amin, S. Edge, F. Greene, D. R. Byrd, R. K. Brookland, M. K. Washington, J. E. Gershenwald, C. C. Compton, K. R. Hess, D. C. Sullivan, J. M. Jessup, J. D. Brierley, L. E. Gaspar, R. L. Schilsky, C. M. Balch, D. P. Winchester, E. A. Asare, M. Madera, D. M. Gress, and L. R. Meyer, Eds., pp. 407–419, Springer, 2017.

[30] K. Lowe, A. Khithani, E. Liu et al., "Ki-67 labeling: a more sensitive indicator of malignant phenotype than mitotic count or tumor size?," *Journal of Surgical Oncology*, vol. 106, no. 6, pp. 724–727, 2012.

[31] N. A. Hamilton, T. C. Liu, A. Cavatiao et al., "Ki-67 predicts disease recurrence and poor prognosis in pancreatic neuroendocrine neoplasms," *Surgery*, vol. 152, no. 1, pp. 107–113, 2012.

[32] G. Rindi, M. Falconi, C. Klersy et al., "TNM staging of neoplasms of the endocrine pancreas: results from a large international cohort study," *Journal of the National Cancer Institute*, vol. 104, no. 10, pp. 764–777, 2012.

[33] J. R. Strosberg, A. Cheema, J. Weber, G. Han, D. Coppola, and L. K. Kvols, "Prognostic validity of a novel American Joint Committee on Cancer Staging Classification for pancreatic neuroendocrine tumors," *Journal of Clinical Oncology*, vol. 29, no. 22, pp. 3044–3049, 2011.

[34] G. Luo, A. Javed, J. R. Strosberg et al., "Modified staging classification for pancreatic neuroendocrine tumors on the basis of the American Joint Committee on Cancer and European Neuroendocrine Tumor Society Systems," *Journal of Clinical Oncology*, vol. 35, no. 3, pp. 274–280, 2017.

[35] G. Luo, K. Jin, H. Cheng et al., "Revised nodal stage for pancreatic neuroendocrine tumors," *Pancreatology*, vol. 17, no. 4, pp. 599–604, 2017.

[36] L. Landoni, G. Marchegiani, T. Pollini et al., "The evolution of surgical strategies for pancreatic neuroendocrine tumors (Pan-NENs): time-trend and outcome analysis from 587 consecutive resections at a high-volume institution," *Annals of Surgery*, 2017.

[37] J. Cherenfant, S. J. Stocker, M. K. Gage et al., "Predicting aggressive behavior in nonfunctioning pancreatic neuroendocrine tumors," *Surgery*, vol. 154, no. 4, pp. 785–793, 2013.

[38] K. Y. Bilimoria, M. S. Talamonti, J. S. Tomlinson et al., "Prognostic score predicting survival after resection of pancreatic

neuroendocrine tumors: analysis of 3851 patients," *Annals of Surgery*, vol. 247, no. 3, pp. 490–500, 2008.

[39] M. Falconi, D. K. Bartsch, B. Eriksson et al., "ENETS Consensus Guidelines for the management of patients with digestive neuroendocrine neoplasms of the digestive system: well-differentiated pancreatic non-functioning tumors," *Neuroendocrinology*, vol. 95, no. 2, pp. 120–134, 2012.

[40] J. Chabot, "Editorial: pancreatic neuroendocrine tumors: primum non nocere," *Surgery*, vol. 159, no. 1, pp. 348-349, 2016.

[41] V. Sallinen, T. Y. S. le Large, S. Galeev et al., "Surveillance strategy for small asymptomatic non-functional pancreatic neuroendocrine tumors – a systematic review and meta-analysis," *HPB: The Official Journal of the International Hepato Pancreato Biliary Association*, vol. 19, no. 4, pp. 310–320, 2017.

[42] F. J. Hüttner, J. Koessler-Ebs, T. Hackert, A. Ulrich, M. W. Büchler, and M. K. Diener, "Meta-analysis of surgical outcome after enucleation *versus* standard resection for pancreatic neoplasms," *British Journal of Surgery*, vol. 102, no. 9, pp. 1026–1036, 2015.

[43] G. Balzano, A. Zerbi, G. Capretti, S. Rocchetti, V. Capitanio, and V. di Carlo, "Effect of hospital volume on outcome of pancreaticoduodenectomy in Italy," *British Journal of Surgery*, vol. 95, no. 3, pp. 357–362, 2008.

[44] G. A. Gooiker, V. E. P. P. Lemmens, M. G. Besselink et al., "Impact of centralization of pancreatic cancer surgery on resection rates and survival," *British Journal of Surgery*, vol. 101, no. 8, pp. 1000–1005, 2014.

[45] T. Hata, F. Motoi, M. Ishida et al., "Effect of hospital volume on surgical outcomes after pancreaticoduodenectomy: a systematic review and meta-analysis," *Annals of Surgery*, vol. 263, no. 4, pp. 664–672, 2016.

[46] L. Bencini, M. Annecchiarico, M. Farsi et al., "Minimally invasive surgical approach to pancreatic malignancies," *World Journal of Gastrointestinal Oncology*, vol. 7, no. 12, pp. 411–421, 2015.

[47] S. Gaujoux, S. Partelli, F. Maire et al., "Observational study of natural history of small sporadic nonfunctioning pancreatic neuroendocrine tumors," *The Journal of Clinical Endocrinology and Metabolism*, vol. 98, no. 12, pp. 4784–4789, 2013.

[48] L. C. Lee, C. S. Grant, D. R. Salomao et al., "Small, nonfunctioning, asymptomatic pancreatic neuroendocrine tumors (PNETs): role for nonoperative management," *Surgery*, vol. 152, no. 6, pp. 965–974, 2012.

[49] A. M. Rosenberg, P. Friedmann, J. del Rivero, S. K. Libutti, and A. M. Laird, "Resection versus expectant management of small incidentally discovered nonfunctional pancreatic neuroendocrine tumors," *Surgery*, vol. 159, no. 1, pp. 302–310, 2016.

[50] N. Regenet, N. Carrere, G. Boulanger et al., "Is the 2-cm size cutoff relevant for small nonfunctioning pancreatic neuroendocrine tumors: a French multicenter study," *Surgery*, vol. 159, no. 3, pp. 901–907, 2016.

[51] I. Y. Zhang, J. Zhao, C. Fernandez-del Castillo et al., "Operative versus nonoperative management of nonfunctioning pancreatic neuroendocrine tumors," *Journal of Gastrointestinal Surgery*, vol. 20, no. 2, pp. 277–283, 2016.

[52] Y. Kishi, K. Shimada, S. Nara, M. Esaki, N. Hiraoka, and T. Kosuge, "Basing treatment strategy for non-functional pancreatic neuroendocrine tumors on tumor size," *Annals of Surgical Oncology*, vol. 21, no. 9, pp. 2882–2888, 2014.

[53] S. Singh, C. Dey, H. Kennecke et al., "Consensus recommendations for the diagnosis and management of pancreatic neuroendocrine tumors: guidelines from a Canadian National Expert Group," *Annals of Surgical Oncology*, vol. 22, no. 8, pp. 2685–2699, 2015.

[54] L. Gratian, J. Pura, M. Dinan, S. Roman, S. Reed, and J. A. Sosa, "Impact of extent of surgery on survival in patients with small nonfunctional pancreatic neuroendocrine tumors in the United States," *Annals of Surgical Oncology*, vol. 21, no. 11, pp. 3515–3521, 2014.

[55] M. Lombardi, N. de Lio, N. Funel et al., "Prognostic factors for pancreatic neuroendocrine neoplasms (pNET) and the risk of small non-functioning pNET," *Journal of Endocrinological Investigation*, vol. 38, no. 6, pp. 605–613, 2015.

[56] A. B. Haynes, V. Deshpande, T. Ingkakul et al., "Implications of incidentally discovered, nonfunctioning pancreatic endocrine tumors: short-term and long-term patient outcomes," *Archives of Surgery*, vol. 146, no. 5, pp. 534–538, 2011.

[57] P. Finkelstein, R. Sharma, O. Picado et al., "Pancreatic neuroendocrine tumors (panNETs): analysis of overall survival of nonsurgical management versus surgical resection," *Journal of Gastrointestinal Surgery*, vol. 21, no. 5, pp. 855–866, 2017.

[58] C. Ricci, R. Casadei, G. Taffurelli et al., "The role of lymph node ratio in recurrence after curative surgery for pancreatic endocrine tumours," *Pancreatology*, vol. 13, no. 6, pp. 589–593, 2013.

[59] S. M. Sharpe, H. in, D. J. Winchester, M. S. Talamonti, and M. S. Baker, "Surgical resection provides an overall survival benefit for patients with small pancreatic neuroendocrine tumors," *Journal of Gastrointestinal Surgery*, vol. 19, no. 1, pp. 117–123, 2015.

[60] G. Kloppel, "Classification and pathology of gastroenteropancreatic neuroendocrine neoplasms," *Endocrine-Related Cancer*, vol. 18, Supplement 1, pp. S1–16, 2011.

[61] S. Partelli, R. Cirocchi, S. Crippa et al., "Systematic review of active surveillance versus surgical management of asymptomatic small non-functioning pancreatic neuroendocrine neoplasms," *The British Journal of Surgery*, vol. 104, no. 1, pp. 34–41, 2017.

[62] S. Weinstein, T. Morgan, L. Poder et al., "Value of intraoperative sonography in pancreatic surgery," *Journal of Ultrasound in Medicine*, vol. 34, no. 7, pp. 1307–1318, 2015.

[63] H. G. Beger, M. Siech, B. Poch, B. Mayer, and M. H. Schoenberg, "Limited surgery for benign tumours of the pancreas: a systematic review," *World Journal of Surgery*, vol. 39, no. 6, pp. 1557–1566, 2015.

[64] A. P. J. Jilesen, C. H. J. van Eijck, O. R. C. Busch, T. M. van Gulik, D. J. Gouma, and E. J. M. N. van Dijkum, "Postoperative outcomes of enucleation and standard resections in patients with a pancreatic neuroendocrine tumor," *World Journal of Surgery*, vol. 40, no. 3, pp. 715–728, 2016.

[65] F. M. Watzka, C. Laumen, C. Fottner et al., "Resection strategies for neuroendocrine pancreatic neoplasms," *Langenbeck's Archives of Surgery*, vol. 398, no. 3, pp. 431–440, 2013.

[66] S. C. Pitt, H. A. Pitt, M. S. Baker et al., "Small pancreatic and periampullary neuroendocrine tumors: resect or enucleate?," *Journal of Gastrointestinal Surgery*, vol. 13, no. 9, pp. 1692–1698, 2009.

[67] R. Casadei, C. Ricci, D. Rega et al., "Pancreatic endocrine tumors less than 4 cm in diameter: resect or enucleate?

A single-center experience," *Pancreas*, vol. 39, no. 6, pp. 825–828, 2010.

[68] C. E. Cauley, H. A. Pitt, K. M. Ziegler et al., "Pancreatic enucleation: improved outcomes compared to resection," *Journal of Gastrointestinal Surgery*, vol. 16, no. 7, pp. 1347–1353, 2012.

[69] T. Hackert, U. Hinz, S. Fritz et al., "Enucleation in pancreatic surgery: indications, technique, and outcome compared to standard pancreatic resections," *Langenbeck's Archives of Surgery*, vol. 396, no. 8, pp. 1197–1203, 2011.

[70] Y. Zhou, M. Zhao, L. Wu, F. Ye, and X. Si, "Short- and long-term outcomes after enucleation of pancreatic tumors: an evidence-based assessment," *Pancreatology*, vol. 16, no. 6, pp. 1092–1098, 2016.

[71] V. Sallinen, C. Haglund, and H. Seppänen, "Outcomes of resected nonfunctional pancreatic neuroendocrine tumors: do size and symptoms matter?," *Surgery*, vol. 158, no. 6, pp. 1556–1563, 2015.

[72] F. Faitot, S. Gaujoux, L. Barbier et al., "Reappraisal of pancreatic enucleations: a single-center experience of 126 procedures," *Surgery*, vol. 158, no. 1, pp. 201–210, 2015.

[73] C. Sperti, V. Beltrame, A. C. Milanetto, M. Moro, and S. Pedrazzoli, "Parenchyma-sparing pancreatectomies for benign or border-line tumors of the pancreas," *World Journal of Gastrointestinal Oncology*, vol. 2, no. 6, pp. 272–281, 2010.

[74] S. Crippa, L. Boninsegna, S. Partelli, and M. Falconi, "Parenchyma-sparing resections for pancreatic neoplasms," *Journal of Hepato-Biliary-Pancreatic Sciences*, vol. 17, no. 6, pp. 782–787, 2010.

[75] T. Zhang, J. Xu, T. Wang, Q. Liao, M. Dai, and Y. Zhao, "Enucleation of pancreatic lesions: indications, outcomes, and risk factors for clinical pancreatic fistula," *Journal of Gastrointestinal Surgery*, vol. 17, no. 12, pp. 2099–2104, 2013.

[76] K. Heeger, M. Falconi, S. Partelli et al., "Increased rate of clinically relevant pancreatic fistula after deep enucleation of small pancreatic tumors," *Langenbeck's Archives of Surgery*, vol. 399, no. 3, pp. 315–321, 2014.

[77] C. Bassi, G. Marchegiani, C. Dervenis et al., "The 2016 update of the International Study Group (ISGPS) definition and grading of postoperative pancreatic fistula: 11 years after," *Surgery*, vol. 161, no. 3, pp. 584–591, 2017.

[78] K. B. Song, S. C. Kim, D. W. Hwang et al., "Enucleation for benign or low-grade malignant lesions of the pancreas: single-center experience with 65 consecutive patients," *Surgery*, vol. 158, no. 5, pp. 1203–1210, 2015.

[79] C. Brient, N. Regenet, L. Sulpice et al., "Risk factors for postoperative pancreatic fistulization subsequent to enucleation," *Journal of Gastrointestinal Surgery*, vol. 16, no. 10, pp. 1883–1887, 2012.

[80] K. S. Choi, J. C. Chung, and H. C. Kim, "Feasibility and outcomes of laparoscopic enucleation for pancreatic neoplasms," *Annals of Surgical Treatment and Research*, vol. 87, no. 6, pp. 285–289, 2014.

[81] J. B. Jin, K. Qin, H. Li et al., "Robotic enucleation for benign or borderline tumours of the pancreas: a retrospective analysis and comparison from a high-volume centre in Asia," *World Journal of Surgery*, vol. 40, no. 12, pp. 3009–3020, 2016.

[82] A. S. Ore, C. E. Barrows, M. Solis-Velasco, J. Shaker, and A. J. Moser, "Robotic enucleation of benign pancreatic tumors," *Journal of Visualized Surgery*, vol. 3, p. 151, 2017.

[83] M. Falconi, A. Zerbi, S. Crippa et al., "Parenchyma-preserving resections for small nonfunctioning pancreatic endocrine tumors," *Annals of Surgical Oncology*, vol. 17, no. 6, pp. 1621–1627, 2010.

[84] J. Franko, W. Feng, L. Yip, E. Genovese, and A. J. Moser, "Non-functional neuroendocrine carcinoma of the pancreas: incidence, tumor biology, and outcomes in 2,158 patients," *Journal of Gastrointestinal Surgery*, vol. 14, no. 3, pp. 541–548, 2010.

[85] D. J. Birnbaum, O. Turrini, L. Vigano et al., "Surgical management of advanced pancreatic neuroendocrine tumors: short-term and long-term results from an international multi-institutional study," *Annals of Surgical Oncology*, vol. 22, no. 3, pp. 1000–1007, 2015.

[86] Y. J. Yoo, S. J. Yang, H. K. Hwang, C. M. Kang, H. Kim, and W. J. Lee, "Overestimated oncologic significance of lymph node metastasis in G1 nonfunctioning neuroendocrine tumor in the left side of the pancreas," *Medicine*, vol. 94, no. 36, article e1404, 2015.

[87] G. Lamberti, C. Ceccarelli, N. Brighi et al., "Determination of mammalian target of rapamycin hyperactivation as prognostic factor in well-differentiated neuroendocrine tumors," *Gastroenterology Research and Practice*, vol. 2017, Article ID 7872519, 9 pages, 2017.

[88] G. W. Krampitz, J. A. Norton, G. A. Poultsides, B. C. Visser, L. Sun, and R. T. Jensen, "Lymph nodes and survival in pancreatic neuroendocrine tumors," *Archives of Surgery*, vol. 147, no. 9, pp. 820–827, 2012.

[89] X. Zhang, L. Lu, Y. Shang et al., "The number of positive lymph node is a better predictor of survival than the lymph node metastasis status for pancreatic neuroendocrine neoplasms: a retrospective cohort study," *International Journal of Surgery*, vol. 48, pp. 142–148, 2017.

[90] S. Partelli, S. Gaujoux, L. Boninsegna et al., "Pattern and clinical predictors of lymph node involvement in nonfunctioning pancreatic neuroendocrine tumors (NF-PanNETs)," *JAMA Surgery*, vol. 148, no. 10, pp. 932–939, 2013.

[91] Y. M. Hashim, K. M. Trinkaus, D. C. Linehan et al., "Regional lymphadenectomy is indicated in the surgical treatment of pancreatic neuroendocrine tumors (PNETs)," *Annals of Surgery*, vol. 259, no. 2, pp. 197–203, 2014.

[92] C. Conrad, O. C. Kutlu, A. Dasari et al., "Prognostic value of lymph node status and extent of lymphadenectomy in pancreatic neuroendocrine tumors confined to and extending beyond the pancreas," *Journal of Gastrointestinal Surgery*, vol. 20, no. 12, pp. 1966–1974, 2016.

[93] J. Zhang, J. Jin, S. Chen et al., "Minimally invasive distal pancreatectomy for PNETs: laparoscopic or robotic approach?," *Oncotarget*, vol. 8, no. 20, pp. 33872–33883, 2017.

[94] S. P. Haugvik, K. J. Labori, A. Waage, P. D. Line, Ø. Mathisen, and I. P. Gladhaug, "Pancreatic surgery with vascular reconstruction in patients with locally advanced pancreatic neuroendocrine tumors," *Journal of Gastrointestinal Surgery*, vol. 17, no. 7, pp. 1224–1232, 2013.

[95] M. Pavel, E. Baudin, A. Couvelard et al., "ENETS Consensus Guidelines for the management of patients with liver and other distant metastases from neuroendocrine neoplasms of foregut, midgut, hindgut, and unknown primary," *Neuroendocrinology*, vol. 95, no. 2, pp. 157–176, 2012.

[96] X. M. Keutgen, N. Nilubol, J. Glanville et al., "Resection of primary tumor site is associated with prolonged survival in

metastatic nonfunctioning pancreatic neuroendocrine tumors," *Surgery*, vol. 159, no. 1, pp. 311–319, 2016.

[97] M. H. Kulke, L. B. Anthony, D. L. Bushnell et al., "NANETS treatment guidelines: well-differentiated neuroendocrine tumors of the stomach and pancreas," *Pancreas*, vol. 39, no. 6, pp. 735–752, 2010.

[98] A. Al-Kurd, K. Chapchay, S. Grozinsky-Glasberg, and H. Mazeh, "Laparoscopic resection of pancreatic neuroendocrine tumors," *World Journal of Gastroenterology*, vol. 20, no. 17, pp. 4908–4916, 2014.

[99] P. Drymousis, D. A. Raptis, D. Spalding et al., "Laparoscopic versus open pancreas resection for pancreatic neuroendocrine tumours: a systematic review and meta-analysis," *HPB: The Official Journal of the International Hepato Pancreato Biliary Association*, vol. 16, no. 5, pp. 397–406, 2014.

[100] S. P. Haugvik, I. P. Marangos, B. I. Røsok et al., "Long-term outcome of laparoscopic surgery for pancreatic neuroendocrine tumors," *World Journal of Surgery*, vol. 37, no. 3, pp. 582–590, 2013.

[101] G. G. Fernandez Ranvier, D. Shouhed, and W. B. Inabnet III, "Minimally invasive techniques for resection of pancreatic neuroendocrine tumors," *Surgical Oncology Clinics of North America*, vol. 25, no. 1, pp. 195–215, 2016.

[102] L. Milone, D. Daskalaki, X. Wang, and P. C. Giulianotti, "State of the art of robotic pancreatic surgery," *World Journal of Surgery*, vol. 37, no. 12, pp. 2761–2770, 2013.

[103] A. H. Zureikat, A. J. Moser, B. A. Boone, D. L. Bartlett, M. Zenati, and H. J. Zeh III, "250 robotic pancreatic resections: safety and feasibility," *Annals of Surgery*, vol. 258, no. 4, pp. 554–562, 2013.

[104] U. Boggi, N. Napoli, F. Costa et al., "Robotic-assisted pancreatic resections," *World Journal of Surgery*, vol. 40, no. 10, pp. 2497–2506, 2016.

[105] Y. Shi, C. Peng, B. Shen et al., "Pancreatic enucleation using the da Vinci robotic surgical system: a report of 26 cases," *The International Journal of Medical Robotics and Computer Assisted Surgery*, vol. 12, no. 4, pp. 751–757, 2016.

[106] M. L. Calin, A. Sadiq, G. Arevalo et al., "The first case report of robotic multivisceral resection for synchronous liver metastasis from pancreatic neuroendocrine tumor: a case report and literature review," *Journal of Laparoendoscopic & Advanced Surgical Techniques*, vol. 26, no. 10, pp. 816–824, 2016.

[107] F. Tian, X. F. Hong, W. M. Wu et al., "Propensity score-matched analysis of robotic versus open surgical enucleation for small pancreatic neuroendocrine tumours," *British Journal of Surgery*, vol. 103, no. 10, pp. 1358–1364, 2016.

[108] A. P. Su, N. W. Ke, Y. Zhang et al., "Is laparoscopic approach for pancreatic insulinomas safe? Results of a systematic review and meta-analysis," *Journal of Surgical Research*, vol. 186, no. 1, pp. 126–134, 2014.

[109] F. Panzuto, L. Boninsegna, N. Fazio et al., "Metastatic and locally advanced pancreatic endocrine carcinomas: analysis of factors associated with disease progression," *Journal of Clinical Oncology*, vol. 29, no. 17, pp. 2372–2377, 2011.

Permissions

All chapters in this book were first published in GRP, by Hindawi Publishing Corporation; hereby published with permission under the Creative Commons Attribution License or equivalent. Every chapter published in this book has been scrutinized by our experts. Their significance has been extensively debated. The topics covered herein carry significant findings which will fuel the growth of the discipline. They may even be implemented as practical applications or may be referred to as a beginning point for another development.

The contributors of this book come from diverse backgrounds, making this book a truly international effort. This book will bring forth new frontiers with its revolutionizing research information and detailed analysis of the nascent developments around the world.

We would like to thank all the contributing authors for lending their expertise to make the book truly unique. They have played a crucial role in the development of this book. Without their invaluable contributions this book wouldn't have been possible. They have made vital efforts to compile up to date information on the varied aspects of this subject to make this book a valuable addition to the collection of many professionals and students.

This book was conceptualized with the vision of imparting up-to-date information and advanced data in this field. To ensure the same, a matchless editorial board was set up. Every individual on the board went through rigorous rounds of assessment to prove their worth. After which they invested a large part of their time researching and compiling the most relevant data for our readers.

The editorial board has been involved in producing this book since its inception. They have spent rigorous hours researching and exploring the diverse topics which have resulted in the successful publishing of this book. They have passed on their knowledge of decades through this book. To expedite this challenging task, the publisher supported the team at every step. A small team of assistant editors was also appointed to further simplify the editing procedure and attain best results for the readers.

Apart from the editorial board, the designing team has also invested a significant amount of their time in understanding the subject and creating the most relevant covers. They scrutinized every image to scout for the most suitable representation of the subject and create an appropriate cover for the book.

The publishing team has been an ardent support to the editorial, designing and production team. Their endless efforts to recruit the best for this project, has resulted in the accomplishment of this book. They are a veteran in the field of academics and their pool of knowledge is as vast as their experience in printing. Their expertise and guidance has proved useful at every step. Their uncompromising quality standards have made this book an exceptional effort. Their encouragement from time to time has been an inspiration for everyone.

The publisher and the editorial board hope that this book will prove to be a valuable piece of knowledge for researchers, students, practitioners and scholars across the globe.

List of Contributors

Hui Yang, Ling Li, Rong-Ping Zhang and Xu Liu
Biomedical Engineering Center, Kunming Medical University, Kunming 650500, China

Yi Lu and Zhong-Kun Ren
Neurosurgery, The 1st Affiliated Hospital of Kunming Medical University, Kunming 650032, China

Xiao-Feng Zeng
School of Forensic Medicine, Kunming Medical University, Kunming 650500, China

Dario Raimondo
Gastroenterology and Endoscopy Unit, Fondazione Istituto G. Giglio, Contrada Pietra Pollastra Pisciotto, 90015 Cefalù, Italy

Domenico Albano
Department of Radiology, DIBIMED, University of Palermo, Via del Vespro 127, 90127 Palermo, Italy

Valentina Guarnotta
Section of Cardio-Respiratory and Endocrine-Metabolic Diseases, Biomedical Department of Internal and Specialist Medicine (DIBIMIS), University of Palermo, Piazza delle Cliniche 2, 90127 Palermo, Italy

Melania Blasco
Internal Medicine Unit, Fondazione Istituto G. Giglio, Contrada Pietra Pollastra Pisciotto, 90015 Cefalù, Italy

Sergio Testai
Radiology Unit, Fondazione Istituto G. Giglio, Contrada Pietra Pollastra Pisciotto, 90015 Cefalù, Italy

Marcello Giuseppe Spampinato
Surgery Unit, Fondazione Istituto G. Giglio, Contrada Pietra Pollastra Pisciotto, 90015 Cefalù, Italy

Mario Trompetto
Department of Colorectal Surgery, Clinic S. Rita, Vercelli, Italy

Pierlorenzo Pallante
Institute of Experimental Endocrinology and Oncology (IEOS), National Research Council (CNR), Via S. Pansini 5, Naples, Italy

Raffaella Capasso
Department of Medicine and Health Sciences, University of Molise, Via Francesco de Sanctis 1, 86100 Campobasso, Italy

Alfonso De Stefano
Department of Abdominal Oncology, Division of Abdominal Medical Oncology, Istituto Nazionale per lo Studio e la Cura dei Tumori, "Fondazione G. Pascale, " IRCCS, Naples, Italy

Isacco Maretto
1st Surgical Clinic, Department of Surgical, Oncological, and Gastroenterological Sciences, University of Padua, Padua, Italy

Florian Kurtz, Florian Struller, Philipp Horvath and Alfred Königsrainer
Dept. of General Surgery, Karls-Eberhard University Tübingen, Germany

Marc A. Reymond
Dept. of General Surgery, Karls-Eberhard University Tübingen, Germany
National Center for Pleura and Peritoneum, Comprehensive Cancer Center South-Western Germany, Tübingen, Stuttgart, Germany

Wiebke Solass and Hans Bösmüller
Institute of Pathology, Karls-Eberhard University Tübingen, Germany

Yongming Wang and Xiaoyu Li
Ministry of Education Key Laboratory of Child Development and Disorders, Children's Hospital, Chongqing Medical University, Chongqing, China
Department of Neonatology, Children's Hospital, Chongqing Medical University, Chongqing, China

Chunbao Guo
Ministry of Education Key Laboratory of Child Development and Disorders, Children's Hospital, Chongqing Medical University, Chongqing, China
Department of Pediatric General Surgery and Liver Transplantation, Children's Hospital, Chongqing Medical University, Chongqing, China

Wenhui Mo, Jingjing Li, Kan Chen, Yujing Xia, Sainan Li, Xiya Lu, Wenwen Wang and Chuanyong Guo
Department of Gastroenterology, Shanghai Tenth People's Hospital, Tongji University School of Medicine, Shanghai 200072, China

Chengfen Wang
Putuo District People's Hospital, Tongji University School of Medicine, Shanghai 200060, China

Ling Xu
Department of Gastroenterology, Shanghai Tongren Hospital, Shanghai Jiaotong University School of Medicine, Shanghai 200336, China

Mujian Teng
Department of Hepatobiliary Surgery, Qianfoshan Hospital Affiliated to Shandong University, Jinan, China

Weiwei Zhang
Department of Hepatobiliary Surgery, Qianfoshan Hospital Affiliated to Shandong University, Jinan, China
Department of General Surgery, Shanghai Public Health Clinical Center, Fudan University, Shanghai, China

Baochi Liu, Qiling Liu, Xin Liu, Yanhui Si and Lei Li
Department of General Surgery, Shanghai Public Health Clinical Center, Fudan University, Shanghai, China

Daniela Pugliese, Luisa Guidi and Alessandro Armuzzi
IBD Unit, Presidio Columbus Fondazione Policlinico Universitario A. Gemelli IRCCS Università Cattolica, Rome 00168, Italy

Annalisa Aratari, Stefano Festa and Claudio Papi
IBD Unit, S. Filippo Neri Hospital, Rome 00135, Italy

Pietro Manuel Ferraro
Nephrology, Presidio Columbus Fondazione Policlinico Universitario A. Gemelli IRCCS Università Cattolica, Rome 00168, Italy

Rita Monterubbianesi and Maria Lia Scribano
IBD Unit, San Camillo Forlanini Hospital, Rome 00152, Italy

Yuting Qian, Tingting Bai, Juanjuan Li, Yi Zang, Tong Li, Mingping Xie, Qi Wang, Lifu Wang and Ruizhe Shen
Department of Gastroenterology, Ruijin Hospital Affiliated to Shanghai Jiaotong University School of Medicine, 197 Second Ruijin Road, Shanghai 200025, China

Ilenia Bartolini, Maria Novella Ringressi, Filippo Melli, Matteo Risaliti, Giacomo Batignani, Paolo Bechi and Antonio Taddei
Department of Surgery and Translational Medicine, University of Florence, AOU Careggi, Largo Brambilla 3, 50134 Florence, Italy

Marco Brugia and Enrico Mini
Department of Experimental and Clinical Medicine, AOU Careggi, Largo Brambilla 3, 50134 Florence, Italy

Luca Boni
Clinical Trials Coordinating Center of Istituto Toscano Tumori, AOU Careggi, Largo Brambilla 3, 50134 Florence, Italy

Wan-fu Lin, Yu-ren Zhang, Huan Wang, He-tong Zhao, Bin-bin Cheng and Chang-quan Ling
Department of Traditional Chinese Medicine, Changhai Hospital, Second Military Medical University, Shanghai 200433, China

Mao-feng Zhong
Graduate School of Shanghai University of Traditional Chinese Medicine, Shanghai 201203, China

Priscilla S. P. Oliveira and Daniela O. Magro
Department of Surgery, Medical Sciences School, Campinas State University, Campinas 13083-887, Brazil

Michel G. Camargo, Carlos A. R. Martinez and Claudio S. R. Coy
Department of Surgery, Medical Sciences School, Campinas State University, Campinas 13083-887, Brazil
Diagnostic Center of Diseases of the Digestive System-Gastrocentro, Medical Sciences School, Campinas State University,Campinas 13083-878, Brazil

Rita B. Carvalho
Diagnostic Center of Diseases of the Digestive System-Gastrocentro, Medical Sciences School, Campinas State University,Campinas 13083-878, Brazil

Ken Ito, Naoki Okano, Seiichi Hara, Kensuke Takuma, Kensuke Yoshimoto,Susumu Iwasaki, Yui Kishimoto and Yoshinori Igarashi
Division of Gastroenterology and Hepatology, Toho University Omori Medical Center, Tokyo, Japan

Hyeong Su Kim and Jung Han Kim
Division of Hemato-Oncology, Department of Internal Medicine, Kangnam Sacred-Heart Hospital, Hallym UniversityMedical Center, Hallym University College of Medicine, Seoul, Republic of Korea

Bum Jun Kim
Division of Hemato-Oncology, Department of Internal Medicine, Kangnam Sacred-Heart Hospital, Hallym UniversityMedical Center, Hallym University College of Medicine, Seoul, Republic of Korea
Department of Internal Medicine, National Army Capital Hospital, The Armed Forces Medical Command, Sungnam,Gyeonggi-do, Republic of Korea

Hyun Joo Jang
Division of Gastroenterology, Department of Internal Medicine, Dongtan Sacred-Heart Hospital, Hallym University Medical Center, Hallym University College of Medicine, Hwasung, Gyeonggi-do, Republic of Korea

Mladen Pavlovic
Department of Surgery, Faculty of Medical Sciences, University of Kragujevac, Serbia

Nevena Gajovic, Gordana Radosavljevic, Jelena Pantic, Nebojsa Arsenijevic and Ivan Jovanovic
Center for Molecular Medicine and Stem Cell Research, Faculty of Medical Sciences, University of Kragujevac, Serbia

Milena Jurisevic
Department of Pharmacy, Faculty of Medical Sciences, University of Kragujevac, Serbia

Slobodanka Mitrovic
Department of Pathology, Faculty of Medical Sciences, University of Kragujevac, Serbia

Cicilia Marcella and Rui Hua Shi
Department of Gastroenterology, Southeast University Affiliated Zhongda Hospital, Nanjing 210009, China

Shakeel Sarwar
Department of Orthopedics, Southeast University Affiliated Zhongda Hospital, Nanjing 210009, China

Laszlo Markasz and Helene Engstrand Lilja
Department of Women's and Children's Health, Uppsala University, Uppsala, Sweden

Alkwin Wanders
Department of Biomedical Sciences, Umeå University, Umeå, Sweden

Laszlo Szekely
Department of Laboratory Medicine, Division of Pathology, Karolinska Institute, Stockholm, Sweden

Goro Shibukawa, Atsushi Irisawa, Ai Sato, Yoko Abe, Akane Yamabe, Noriyuki Arakawa, Yusuke Takasaki, Takumi Maki, Yoshitsugu Yoshida, Ryo Igarashi, Shogo Yamamoto and Tsunehiko Ikeda
Department of Gastroenterology, Aizu Medical Center, Fukushima Medical University, Aizuwakamatsu, Japan

Hiroshi Hojo
Department of Pathology, Aizu Medical Center, Fukushima Medical University, Aizuwakamatsu, Japan

Ya-Wu Zhang, Feng-Xian Wei, Xiao-Dong Xu and You-Cheng Zhang
Department of General Surgery, Lanzhou University Second Hospital, Lanzhou 730000, China
Hepato-Biliary-Pancreatic Institute, Lanzhou University Second Hospital, Lanzhou 730000, China
Lanzhou University Second Clinical Medical College, Lanzhou University, Lanzhou 730000, China

Xue-Ping Qi
Lanzhou University Second Clinical Medical College, Lanzhou University, Lanzhou 730000, China

Zhao Liu
The First Clinical Medical College of Lanzhou University, Lanzhou 730000, China

Gabriele Cervino, Luca Fiorillo, Floriana Lauritano, Giuseppe Lo Giudice, Gaetano Iannello and Marco Cicciù
Department of Biomedical and Dental Sciences and Morphological and Functional Imaging, Messina University,98100 Messina, Italy

Luigi Laino and Rossella Santoro
Multidisciplinary Department of Medical-Surgical and Odontostomatological Specialties, University of Campania "Luigi Vanvitelli",80121 Naples, Italy

Alan Scott Herford
Department of Maxillofacial Surgery, Loma Linda University, Loma Linda, CA 92354, USA

Fausto Famà
Department of Human Pathology, University of Messina, 98100 Messina, Italy

Giuseppe Troiano
Departments of Clinical and Experimental Medicine, University of Foggia, 71121 Foggia, Italy

Monica Pantea, Anca Negovan and Simona Bataga
Clinical Science-Internal Medicine, University of Medicine and Pharmacy, Gheorghe Marinescu 38, Tirgu Mureş, 540139 Mures, Romania

Claudia Banescu
Center for Advanced Medical and Pharmaceutical Research, University of Medicine and Pharmacy, Gheorghe Marinescu 38,Tirgu Mureş, 540139 Mureş, Romania

Radu Neagoe
Surgical Science, University of Medicine and Pharmacy, Gheorghe Marinescu 38, Tirgu Mureş, 540139 Mures, Romania

Simona Mocan
Pathological Department, Emergency County Hospital, Gheorghe Marinescu 50, Tirgu Mures, 540136 Mures, Romania

Mihaela Iancu
Department of Medical Informatics and Biostatistics, University of Medicine and Pharmacy "Iuliu Haţieganu", Louis Pasteur St.,No. 6, 400349 Cluj-Napoca, Romania

Eun Young Park, Dong Hoon Baek, Gwang Ha Kim and Bong Eun Lee
Department of Internal Medicine, Pusan National University School of Medicine, and Biomedical Research Institute,Pusan National University Hospital, Busan, Republic of Korea

So-Jeong Lee and Do Youn Park
Department of Pathology, Pusan National University School of Medicine, Busan, Republic of Korea

Min-Sun Kwak, Goh Eun Chung, Su Jin Chung, Seung Joo Kang, Jong In Yang and Joo Sung Kim
Department of Internal Medicine, Healthcare Research Institute, Healthcare System Gangnam Center, Seoul National University Hospital, Seoul, Republic of Korea

Han-Yi Song, Xin-Jie Yao and Yan Li
Department of Gastroenterology, Shengjing Hospital of China Medical University, Shenyang, China

Long Zhou
Department of Orthopedics, Shengjing Hospital of China Medical University, Shenyang, China

Dong-yan Liu
Medical Research Center, Shengjing Hospital of China Medical University, Shenyang, China

Deepak Agrawal
Department of Medicine, Division of Digestive and Liver Diseases, University Texas Southwestern Medical Center, Dallas, TX, USA

Rajeev Jain
Texas Digestive Disease Consultants, Dallas, TX, USA

Nicolas Tabchouri, David Dussart, Nicolas Michot, Frederic Marques, Meriem Khalfallah, Petru Bucur, Louise Barbier, Aurore Kraemer-Bucur,Mihane Nayeri, Julien Thiery, Celine Bourbao-Tournois, Pascal Bourlier, Ephrem Salamé and Mehdi Ouaïssi
Department of Digestive, Oncological, Endocrine, Hepato-Biliary and Pancreatic Surgery, and Liver Transplantation,Trousseau Hospital, University Hospital of Tours, France

Urs Giger-Pabst
Department of General Surgery and Therapy Center for Peritoneal Carcinomatosis, St. Mary's Hospital, University Hospital of the Ruhr-University Bochum, Herne, Germany

Ilenia Bartolini, Matteo Risaliti, Maria Novella Ringressi and Antonio Taddei
Department of Surgery and Translational Medicine, AOU Careggi, University of Florence, Largo Brambilla 3, 50134 Florence, Italy

Lapo Bencini and Luca Moraldi
Department of Oncology, AOU Careggi, Largo Brambilla 3, 50134 Florence, Italy

Index

www.ingramcontent.com/pod-product-compliance
Lightning Source LLC
Chambersburg PA
CBHW080410190526
45161CB00003B/195

9781632418906